Handbook of Laboratory Animal Science

Volume I

Selection and Handling of Animals in Biomedical Research

Edited by
Per Svendsen and Jann Hau

CRC Press

Boca Raton   Ann Arbor   London   Tokyo

Library of Congress Cataloging-in-Publication Data

Handbook of laboratory animal science / edited by Per Svendsen, Jann
  Hau.
       p. cm.
     Includes bibliographical references and indexes.
     Contents: v. 1. Selection and handling of animals in biomedical
research — v. 2. Animal models.
      ISBN 0-8493-4378-X (v. 1). — ISBN 0-8493-4390-9 (v. 2)
      1. Laboratory animals. 2. Animal experimentation. 3. Animal
models in research. I. Svendsen, Per. II. Hau, Jann.
QL55.H36 1994
599′.00724—dc20
          93-39121
          CIP

PREFACE

Research involving laboratory animals is an important factor in the advancement of the medical, veterinary, agricultural, and biological sciences. All drugs prescribed for humans or animals have been developed and tested in laboratory animals; new surgical techniques and materials are developed and tested in laboratory animals before they are accepted for humans or domestic animals; and our knowledge in physiology, microbiology, and pathology is based on experiments with laboratory animals.

In 1959 W. M. S. Russel and R. L. Burch formulated the principles of humane experimental technique. The experimenter should aim at reducing the number of animals used, replace experiments on live animals with alternative methods, and refine the techniques to reduce discomfort to the animals. Reduction, replacement, and refinement have since become the cornerstones of laboratory animal science.

In 1975 the first regular university course in laboratory animal science in Denmark was offered at Odense University Medical School, and a textbook was published in Danish. Courses are now given at both undergraduate and post-graduate levels at most Scandinavian universities. With the advancement of laboratory animal science, the original textbook has become insufficient and the demand for a revision obvious. Rather than rewriting the book ourselves, we decided to ask a group of scientists, mainly from the Scandinavian countries, to contribute to a completely new textbook.

In many countries, a specific course in laboratory animal science is now required for scientists who wish to perform experiments on animals. It is our hope that this textbook can be useful also outside the Scandinavian countries.

The editors wish to thank all the authors for their contributions and for their valuable assistance as reviewers. The laborious task of revising and correcting the language was performed by Bodil Svendsen. We wish to thank her for this valuable contribution.

Per Svendsen
Biomedical Laboratory
Odense University
Odense, Denmark

Jann Hau
Laboratory Animal Science and Welfare
The Royal Veterinary College
London, United Kingdom

THE EDITORS

Per Svendsen is Associate Professor in Laboratory Animal Science and Head of the Biomedical Laboratory of the Medical Faculty, University of Odense, Denmark.

Dr. Svendsen graduated in veterinary medicine from The Royal Veterinary and Agricultural University, Copenhagen, Denmark in 1963. Following research fellowships at the Department of Physiology, New York State Veterinary College at Cornell University, where he completed a Masters degree in physiology and surgery, and at the Department of Surgery at the Royal Veterinary and Agricultural University in Copenhagen, he earned his doctorate in ruminant pathophysiology.

In 1970 he joined the Department of Physiology at the University of Nairobi in Kenya, where he taught physiology to veterinary and agriculture students. In 1974 he joined the newly established medical faculty at the University of Odense in Denmark, where he established the Biomedical Laboratory and the centralized laboratory animal facility. From 1987 to 1989, Dr. Svendsen taught surgery at the Faculty of Veterinary Science at Sokoine University of Agriculture in Morogoro, Tanzania.

Dr. Svendsen has published more than 100 scientific papers and chapters in textbooks. He has published textbooks in animal physiology and ethology and, together with Dr. Hau, he published *Forsøgsdyr og dyreforsøg*, a Danish textbook in laboratory animal science.

Dr. Svendsen's current research interests include digestive physiology, mainly concerning pancreatic and hepatic secretions, and fetal physiology.

Jann Hau, Dr. med., is Professor in Laboratory Animal Science and Welfare at The Royal Veterinary College, University of London, UK.

Dr. Hau is a biologist who specialized in laboratory animal science and did his doctorate at The Medical Faculty, University of Odense, Denmark. Following research fellowships at Odense University he joined the Department of Pathology, The Royal Veterinary and Agricultural University (RVAU) in Copenhagen as Associate Professor and Head of the Laboratory Animal Science Unit in 1983. He was later Head of the Department of Pathology and Dean of the Faculty of Animal Husbandry and Veterinary Science at the RVAU.

In 1991 he joined the Royal Veterinary College in London as Professor in the newly established London University Chair in Laboratory Animal Science and Welfare.

Dr. Hau is responsible for the undergraduate and postgraduate teaching in laboratory animal science and welfare which includes a 1-year Master of Science course specialized in Laboratory Animal Science.

Dr. Hau has organized several international meetings on laboratory animal science. He is the editor-in-chief of Scandinavian Journal of Laboratory Animal Science and editor for the laboratory animals section in the journal Animal Welfare. He is a member of a number of laboratory animal science societies including LASA, ScandLAS, and AALAS.

Dr. Hau has published more than 200 scientific papers and chapters in books and, together with Dr. Svendsen, he wrote the first Danish textbook on laboratory animals and animal experiments published in 1981, 1985, and 1989.

Dr. Hau's current research interests include development of laboratory animal models for studies of biological mechanisms in reproductive physiology, and development of methods to assess long-term stress and welfare state in animals. These studies include ethology as well as studies of physiological and immunological changes associated with changes in the welfare of the animal. Dr. Hau has also concentrated on research projects that are focused on ways to replace, reduce, and refine the use of animals in antibody production.

CONTRIBUTORS

Andre Chwalibog
Division of Animal Nutrition
Department of Animal Science and Animal
  Health
The Royal Veterinary and Agricultural
  University
Frederiksberg, Denmark

Melvin B. Dennis, Jr.
Department of Comparative Medicine
University of Washington
Seattle, Washington

Ann Detmer
AgroLab
Scandinavia AB
Kristianstad, Sweden

Karin Erb
Fertility Clinic
Odense University Hospital
Odense, Denmark

Stian Erichsen
National Institute of Public Health
Oslo, Norway

Ricardo Ernesto Feinstein
Department of Pathology
The National Veterinary Institute
Uppsala, Sweden

Richard T. Fosse
Laboratory Animal Veterinary Services
University of Bergen
Bergen, Norway

Frederik Dagnæs-Hansen
Bomholtgaard, Ltd.
Ry, Denmark

Axel Kornerup Hansen
Laboratory Animal Department
Panum Institute
University of Copenhagen
Copenhagen, Denmark

Jann Hau
Laboratory Animal Science and Welfare
Royal Veterinary College
London, England

Annelise Hem
Laboratory Animal Department
The Norwegian Cancer Research Institute
The Norwegian Radium Hospital
Oslo, Norway

Jens Juul Holst
Department of Medical Physiology
The Panum Institute
University of Copenhagen
Copenhagen, Denmark

Steinar Hunskaar
Division for General Practice
Department of Public Health and Primary
  Health Care
University of Bergen
Bergen, Norway

Krister Iwarsson
Laboratory Animal Unit
Karolinska Institute
Stockholm, Sweden

Otto Kugelberg
Unit for Laboratory Animal Science and
  Service
Swedish Medical Research Council
Stockholm, Sweden

Lennart Lindberg
Animal Resources
National Veterinary Institute
Uppsala, Sweden

Bodil Lissau
Gea, Ltd.
Frederiksberg, Denmark

Karl Johan Öbrink
Department of Physiology and Medical
  Biophysics
Biomedical Center
Uppsala University
Uppsala, Sweden

H.P. Olesen
Institute for Experimental Research in Surgery
University of Copenhagen
Copenhagen, Denmark

Kai H. O. Pelkonen
Deparment of Physiology
Univrsity of Kuopio
Kuopio, Finland

Claes Rehbinder
Department of Pathology
The National Veterinary Institute
Uppsala, Sweden

Peter Sandøe
Department of Education, Philosophy, and
  Rhetoric
University of Copenhagen
Copenhagen, Denmark

Adrian J. Smith
Laboratory Animal Unit
Norwegian College of Veterinary Medicine
Oslo, Norway

Dag R. Sørensen
Laboratory Animal Unit
The National Hospital
Oslo, Norway

Daniel A. Steinbrüchel
Department of Thoracic and Cardiovascular
  Surgery
Aarhus University Hospital
Aarhus, Denmark

Per Svendsen
Biomedical Laboratory
Odense University
Odense, Denmark

Gerald L. Van Hoosier, Jr.
Department of Comparative Medicine
University of Washington
Seattle, Washington

Aage Vølund
Novo Research Institute
Bagsværd, Denmark

Tage Waller
Laboratory Animal Unit
Karolinska Institute
Stockholm, Sweden

Lars Wass
Unit for Laboratory Animal Science and Service
Swedish Medical Research Council
Stockholm, Sweden

TABLE OF CONTENTS

Chapter 1

Animal Research and Ethics

Peter Sandøe

CONTENTS

INTRODUCTION

Most scientists involved in biomedical research nowadays recognize that the use of animals in research poses an ethical problem. On the one hand most of the animals used are sentient beings who may suffer because of the experiments. Research, on the other hand, may help to solve major human problems; for example, it may help scientists to find ways of alleviating, curing, or preventing major human diseases.

Many scientists do, however, seem to have doubts about how to deal with ethical problems. And therefore they seek advice from outside their own circle. They may call in a politician or they may, as the editors of this volume have done, ask a philosopher for a contribution. But what can a philosopher do to solve an ethical problem?

Before answering this question it may be useful to distinguish between the following two forms of ethics (the terms are inspired by Riesman[1]):

- *Radar Ethics* — Moral constraints are thought of as something coming from "the outside" to which the person in question has to adjust.
- *Gyroscope Ethics* — Moral constraints are self-imposed, on the basis of the person's own moral reflections.

Some scientists seem to think that all they need is radar ethics. Science helps society to gain important knowledge; and so, many scientists find that it is up to society to decide which ethical limits there should be concerning the ways in which the knowledge may be obtained, e.g., whether and to which extent laboratory animals may be used in painful experiments.

If this was the attitude of the readers of this book, this chapter should have been written by a politician rather than a philosopher. A good politician who is aware of the feelings of the electorate will be able, much better than the philosopher, to say what is expected of scientists working with animals, and what kind of legal restrictions in the use of laboratory animals may be anticipated in the future.

There are, however, good reasons why scientists ought not to think that all they need is radar ethics. Let me just briefly mention three such reasons:

- The scientist has a personal moral responsibility for what he does and cannot just leave it to society to decide what is right and wrong.
- Generally scientists prefer self-discipline to very stringent and elaborate rules concerning what they may and may not do. But self-discipline presupposes that the scientist himself is able to decide how far it is ethically defensible to go.
- To ensure a rational public discussion concerning ethics and the use of animals in research those who know how and why animals are used ought to contribute to the discussion. But scientists can only contribute if they are willing to engage in moral reflections.

0-8493-4378-X/94/$0.00+$.50
© 1994 by CRC Press Inc.

I doubt that anyone will want to dispute these reasons. My experience is, however, that many scientists are still suspicious of the idea of engaging in moral reflections. The root of this suspicion may be expressed in the following manner: "Moral reflections are subjective and emotional, whereas the scientist is supposed to be objective and emotionally unbiased." Of course, there is *a sense* in which moral reflections are subjective and emotional. Unlike science they are not concerned with finding facts about a mind-independent reality. Rather, their aim is to find out what our attitudes should be, if we think rationally and impartially about the matters at issue. But if we try as hard as we can to think rationally and impartially about our attitudes to animal experimentation, our attitudes will be as objective and emotionally unbiased as they can be — and much more so than they usually are. Even a scientist should not ask for more.

The task of the philosopher then is to work out various ways in which to think rationally and impartially about the fundamental moral question at issue: to what extent can we morally justify the use of animals in biomedical research?

THE BASIC ISSUE

Much of the public discussion concerning the use of animals in biomedical research does not center around basic ethical principles. Rather it is about whether or not animal experiments give us new and reliable results, whether there are cheaper and better alternatives, and whether, even if animal experiments are needed, the same results could be achieved by means of a smaller number of experiments and/or by treating the animals in a way that causes less suffering.

To engage in this discussion, important as it may be, is to sidestep the basic moral issue; i.e., I assume that any decent person would agree that if we could be reasonably sure to achieve the same results at the same or even at a lower cost by cutting down the use of animals in painful or lethal experiments we should, of course, do so.

Where the interesting and controversial moral issue begins is when we have experiments which satisfy the following three conditions:

- We have all reason to believe that the experiments may give us some new and useful results. Results may be useful in many ways, but let me here assume that they serve to prevent, alleviate, or cure serious human diseases.
- It is not possible to carry through the experiments without causing serious harm to the involved animals.
- We have no reason to believe that the same results could be achieved by alternative methods, by experiments involving a smaller number of animals, or by experiments causing less harm to the animals.

To have an easy way of referring to biomedical experiments satisfying these three conditions, let me call them *harmful but vital*. I am sure that not all harmful animal experiments conducted within biomedical research are vital. But I am in no doubt that a substantial number of them are. Examples from experimental surgery, neuroscience, and toxicology spring to my mind. And I am sure that many of the chapters in these volumes will confirm my views about the usefulness of animal experimentation. Let me here just say a little about the concept of harm. One may distinguish between three different kinds of harm,[2] (1) suffering, (2) deprivation, and (3) death.

By *deprivation* I mean the prevention of behavior and activities which are pleasant or otherwise desirable; for example, for animals of most species, lack of exercise and opportunities for exploration may be considered a deprivation.

It is interesting that suffering and death are normally rated quite differently according to whether they befall a human being or an animal. According to the common view death is much worse for a human being than most kinds of suffering, whereas with animals it is the other way round. The reason for this may be that we put less weight on human suffering than we do on animal suffering, or it may be that we find the death of a human being much worse than the death of an animal. There is no doubt that the latter explanation is the right one. Actually, we also tend to put less weight on animal suffering than we do on human suffering, but at least we view them as comparable entities.

Some people even seem to think that the killing of an animal poses no ethical problem as long as it is done "humanely" — that is, in such a way that the animal does not experience any pain, anxiety, or the like. Therefore, allegedly, there is no reason to worry about the number of animals used in experiments as long as the animals do not suffer and are humanely killed at the end of the experiment.

Most people, however, do worry about the number of animals killed for the sake of research. With some kinds of animals people feel badly about any killing except when the animal is old or sick. This is particularly the case with apes. Thus, research foundations in the U.S. have set up various retirement arrangements for their chimpanzee research subjects, enabling the animals to live out their lives in suitable conditions.

The reason why people worry particularly about the killing of apes is probably that these animals are more "human-like" than any other animals. Since we take human life to be of immense ethical importance, we allegedly ought to extend this importance to cover also the apes. However, it may be doubted whether this will solve the ethical problems relating to the killing of animals. Rather it seems that this will just move the problem. The next step would be to explain what the morally relevant difference is between killing an ape and killing a dog or a rat. This, I am sure, is no easy task.

The common views on the killing of humans and animals, as I have tried to indicate, clearly need critical discussion. But it will lead me too far astray to pursue the discussion here. Good discussions may be found elsewhere.[3,4]

Most people in our society will, I think, deplore the fact that some vital experiments are harmful, but if the experiments really are vital they will consider them to be morally justified. They will say that the harm inflicted on the animals is a necessary evil, which is morally outweighed by the benefit achieved.

Strictly speaking, however, in many cases it is not true that the *only* way to achieve the relevant results is by means of harmful experiments on animals. Often it might also be possible to achieve the same results by means of experiments on *humans*. And since the results are mostly to be used in *human* medicine, the experiments would in most cases be more relevant and more reliable if they were conducted on humans.

To make the discussion more realistic, let me give an example of an actual experiment conducted on human beings — an experiment which appears to have been both harmful and vital. The example is an odontological experiment conducted in Sweden between 1947 and 1951. The main aim of the experiment was to establish a correlation between the development of caries and the intake of different sorts of food containing carbohydrates. The experiment was conducted on patients from Vipeholms Sjukhus, a hospital for the mentally deficient. The mental deficiency of the subjects of the experiment varied from an almost complete lack of intelligent life to only a minor deficiency.[5]

The subjects were divided into groups, which were all given the same basic diet and (apart from a control group) in addition were fed different kinds of drinks or food containing carbohydrate. The groups were given these drinks and foods at different times, either during meals or between meals. The experiment yielded a number of highly interesting and significant results; for example, that the incidence of caries will only increase if sweets are eaten between meals, and that sweets which "stick" to the teeth cause more caries than sweet substances that do not.

The Swedish government supported the experiments financially and the results formed the basis of a very efficient information campaign. There is no doubt that the experiments had a serious purpose, were conducted in accordance with common scientific standards, and resulted in some obvious benefits in the form of increased dental health in the Swedish population.

Of course, these benefits were paid for by harm inflicted on the research subjects. Some of them developed more caries than they would otherwise have done, and the sweet diets must have given rise to other sorts of inconvenience.

Is an experiment of this kind ethically justified? Most people would probably give a negative answer to this question. Also, according to official ethical guidelines, this experiment would be rejected. Thus, the Declaration of Helsinki[6] says:

> Every biomedical research project involving human subjects should be preceded by careful assessment of predictable risks in comparison with foreseeable benefits to the subjects or to others. Concern for the interests of the subject must always prevail over the interests of science and society.

Clearly, in the Swedish experiments the interests of the patients from Vipeholms Sjukhus did not prevail over the interests of science and society.

Another problem about these experiments is the lack of informed consent of the subjects involved. According to the Declaration of Helsinki, the doctor should "obtain the subject's freely-given informed consent, preferably in writing. ... Where physical or mental incapacity makes it impossible to obtain informed consent ... permission from the responsible relative replaces that of the subject in accordance with national legislation".

Even if permission could be granted by the responsible relatives, it may be claimed that it is unethical to conduct the experiment on mentally handicapped persons. Thus, according to a Danish Commission appointed by the Minister for Health, "research should not be conducted on ... mentally handicapped persons, which could likewise be conducted on legally competent persons".[7] This claim may be backed up by two considerations. The first is that informed consent is a condition which is so important that it should only be dispensed with if there is no other way to carry out the relevant experiments. The other is that if it is not possible to find competent persons who are willing to participate in an experiment, then the experiment is probably against the interests of those participating.

It seems that there are several reasons that will serve to convince most people that the Swedish experiment and other similar harmful experiments involving human subjects are not ethically justified.

This leaves me with the following two propositions:

- It is morally justified to use animals in harmful experiments as long as these experiments are vital.
- It is *never* morally justified to use human beings in harmful experiments, even when the experiments are vital and the harm is only slight.

To be able to maintain both propositions without having double moral standards one must be able to state a relevant difference between humans and other animals; i.e., one must explain what it is about humans that gives their interests a moral significance that we are not willing to ascribe to the animals. This I take to be the basic ethical issue in discussions about the use of animals in research.

IS THERE A RELEVANT DIFFERENCE?

In the history of philosophy there have been a number of attempts to establish a difference between humans and animals on the basis of which it may be claimed that man has ethical priority. Nearly all the attempts consist in pointing to an intellectual or mental ability which distinguishes man from animals. It could be that man is rational, that he is intelligent, or that he possesses a free will.

Let me as an example assume that the relevant difference is that man is more intelligent than other animals. It is surely correct that nearly all humans are more intelligent than all other animals. But there are exceptions. For example, the most deficient of the patients used in the above-mentioned Swedish experiments are described by the director of the hospital in the following way:

> In members of the lowest group, both the urge to move around and the ability to interact with the surroundings have never exceeded a minimum. Individuals within this group are reflex-beings who barely have psychological reactions. They lack the instinct of self-preservation and the urge to move around. They lack the ability consciously to influence their surroundings and live absolutely dependent on the environment without the care of which they would soon succumb.

(Translated from Petersson.[8])

I think that one would be hard put to claim that the rodents, dogs, cats, and monkeys normally used in experiments are less intelligent than these humans. And if one insists that intelligence is the decisive moral dividing line, I cannot see how one can resist the conclusion that morally speaking it would be more right to use mentally deficient humans in experiments than to use laboratory animals.

Without doing so here I shall maintain that a similar line of argument may be carried through for all the other attempts to use a difference in mental ability as a reason for saying that harmful experiments, if vital, may be conducted on animals but never on humans.

Reflecting on the possibility of using mentally deficient humans in experiments which cause suffering may, by the way, serve to cast doubt on the whole idea of seeing mental ability as the morally relevant difference. Why should lack of intelligence make suffering less bad? In some cases it seems to be the other way round. For example, you can tell an intelligent person that something painful is only going to last for some time, and this may help him to bear with it. Whereas with a young child, a mentally deficient human, or an animal this is not possible, and fear may therefore be added to pain.

At this stage of the argument some will react by saying that humans are humans and animals are animals — and that this is the essential, morally relevant difference. But if we allow this to count as a relevant difference, we shall also have to allow as relevant other differences which most of us see as completely irrelevant. Take the racist — would we accept it as a serious candidate for a morally relevant difference between white people and black people if he said that whites are whites and blacks are blacks?

Or what about the sexist who says that men are men and women are women — and that therefore men should have more rights than women?

To use mere membership of a certain species as a reason for saying that it is morally justified to use some animals (e.g., rodents) but not others (e.g., humans) in harmful experiments is a kind of unwarranted discrimination, "speciesism", which in principle is not different from other kinds of arbitrary discrimination such as racism and sexism.[9]

Talking about speciesism, I cannot but mention the widespread ranking of research animals, according to which, for example, mice and rats are considered to be "lower animals" than, for example, dogs and cats, and therefore as far as possible should replace these "higher" animals. However, there seems to be no intrinsic difference between the animals mentioned which can serve as a morally relevant reason for discriminating among them. I think that scientists have a duty to help fight this absurd kind of discrimination.

I have now discussed two ways of justifying the claim that humans have moral priority and that harmful experiments may sometimes be conducted on animals but never on humans. One is by means of a difference in intellectual or other mental abilities and the other by means of a mere difference in species. And I have argued that neither of these will do the job.

If one wishes to justify the view that humans have moral priority, it must be by means of some other kind of difference between humans and animals. I think that there is at least one other such justification which is worth discussing. This justification takes as its starting point the idea that humans need to cooperate. An essential precondition of our wealthy and comfortable life is that we can share the work. This allows us, among other things, to enjoy the advantages of specialization and large-scale operations. Also, it is necessary for our welfare that each of us can feel safe and trust that agreements will be kept. Morality may be seen as a means of securing these things.

Accordingly, the essence of morality is egoism. When I have to show consideration for other people, it is really for my own sake. By respecting the rules of morality I am contributing to the maintenance of a society which is essential to my welfare. And if I try to free-wheel I will be punished by loneliness, poverty — and maybe even confinement.

On the basis of this view of morality there appears a relevant difference between humans and animals. I am dependent on the respect and cooperation of other people. And if I treat my fellow humans badly, they will also treat me badly, whereas the animal community will not strike back if, for example, I use some of its members in painful experiments. From an egoistic point of view I only need to treat the animals well enough for them to be fit for the experiments.

This justification for giving humans moral priority over animals fits well into parts of the morality prevalent in our society and logically it is also nice and coherent. The only problem about it is that it presupposes a kind of egoism that most of us find difficult to maintain with a clear conscience.

Animals are not the only beings that we do not owe moral consideration, according to this view. It is also the case with all the humans whose cooperation and respect we can do without. Thus, according to this view, we do not owe any moral consideration to future generations. And we need only care about weak individuals to the extent that this serves as a kind of insurance of decent treatment — should we ourselves be placed in the same situation. Therefore we may also be able to justify experiments on humans like those conducted at Vipeholms Sjukhus.

However, if one feels that other people have a right to consideration, whether or not this serves one's own personal interests, then one cannot use the outlined view as a defense of harmful animal experiments. But since I cannot prove that other people have such a right to consideration, I will leave the view as an option.

If the arguments presented here are sound, one seems to be stuck with the following three options concerning the justification of harmful animal experiments:

- *The Egoist Option* — Harmful animal experiments are justified because they will not harm myself. Consequently, it may also be possible to justify harmful experiments on humans — that is, if these experiments are compatible with my own egoistic interests.[10]
- *The Perfectionist Option* — Harmful animal experiments are justified because animals are less intelligent or lack some other mental capacity found in normal humans. Consequently, harmful experiments on mentally deficient humans may also be justified.[11,12]
- *The Egalitarian Option* — To harm an animal is, morally speaking, on a par with harming a human. It may be possible to justify harmful animal experiments by reference to their beneficial consequences, but then harmful experiments on normal human beings may also be justified.[13]

Thus, the moral reflections presented here leave open more than one option. However, it is important to notice that even though there is not one option which is *the* right or *the* true one, at least one possibility has been ruled out. There is no option which allows you to say *both* that sometimes harmful animal experiments are morally justified, and that harmful experiments on humans never are.

At this point some of my readers may feel tempted to say that maybe it was not such a brilliant idea to engage in moral reflections after all. Perhaps one should simply stick to radar ethics. In that case, all that is necessary to defend the two propositions, is the observation that most people in our society actually think that harmful animal experiments are sometimes morally justified, while harmful experiments on humans never are. I do, however, hope that the intellectual honesty of my readers will tell them that this is much too easy a way out of the problem. Either one must try to argue that an important option has been overlooked (attempts are still being made[14]) or one must choose one of the three options outlined.

Personally, I think that the egalitarian option is by far the most attractive of the three, and I shall therefore end with a few brief remarks about what follows from the view that, morally speaking, suffering and other kinds of harm are equally bad whether they befall a human or an animal.

THE EGALITARIAN OPTION

If one accepts the egalitarian option, a great deal of moral reflection is still needed to find out to what extent harmful experiments may be justified. Among other things we need to find out to what extent harmful experiments on human beings may be justified.

Some people will say that however great the benefit, we are never allowed to harm an innocent human being as a means of achieving it. A human being may only be experimented on if the experiment is thought to benefit or at least not to harm the subject and if the subject gives his informed consent. Animals are not able to give their consent, and it therefore follows from the egalitarian option that we are never justified in using animals in harmful experiments.[15]

Few of us are willing to accept the ethical principle underlying such a view. Most of us, for example, think that war may be morally justified, even though it will inevitably cause harm to innocent people. So it appears that most of us think that sometimes we may be justified in doing things of which the foreseeable consequence is that innocent people will be harmed, as long as the beneficial consequences are great enough. By analogy, harmful experiments on animals may be justified if they really are a necessary means to a great benefit, for example finding the cure for a serious disease.

However, according to the egalitarian option, if the same benefits can be achieved in a way that causes less harm by using humans instead of animals, humans should be used.[16] I am aware that this last conclusion comes up against a massive psychological barrier in most people. We just cannot bring ourselves to think that, for example, the suffering of a human is morally on a par with the suffering of an animal. We are naturally biased in favor of humans. However, this bias should not be taken to imply that there is anything wrong with the egalitarian conclusion. Rather it should be seen as an unfortunate psychological limitation on our side.

An analogy may make this view appear more credible than it initially seems: while I am writing this, people are starving to death in Africa. Most people in my part of the world could, without any great personal sacrifice, save the lives of several people. Nonetheless few, if any, of us make the small necessary changes in spending and lifestyle necessary to save these people. Should we on the basis of this behavior conclude that the life of an African, morally speaking, is not worth some trivial changes in our lifestyle? No, we should of course conclude that we have an unfortunate bias in favor of our own trivial desires. In my view the right way to handle such psychological limitations is by admitting their existence and then trying to organize things in a way that enables us to limit their influence as much as possible. And the best way to do this may be to set ourselves some relatively limited goals which we may be able to live up to psychologically.

LIMITED EGALITARIAN GOALS

Roughly speaking there seem to be two ways to pursue the egalitarian option. One is by limiting the demand for animal experiments, the other is by improving the conditions for animals used in experiments. I shall end the chapter by saying a little about each of these two strategies.

LIMITING THE DEMAND FOR ANIMAL EXPERIMENTS

A large number, if not the majority, of animal experiments are required by national or international authorities. Pharmaceuticals, food, and other products must often be tested for toxicity and carcinogenicity, among other things, before they can be marketed. The demand for such animal experiments can be limited without any risk to human safety, if different regulatory bodies harmonize their requirements so that the same company does not have to perform different but very similar tests to satisfy, for example, the European, the Japanese, and the U.S. authorities. Such harmonization seems to be slowly on the way now.[17]

Also, the demand for harmful animal experiments can be limited, if authorities change their guidelines when scientists find methods which are less harmful to the animals or involve smaller numbers of animals. An example is the LD_{50} test for toxicity, which was required until recently by all the major regulatory bodies. In the test 50% of the animals have to die before the test can be concluded, but toxicologists have for a long time been able to get reliable results by means of tests which are much less harmful to the animals.

Another way of limiting the demand for animal experiments is by means of so-called alternatives. Here it is important to point out that often alternatives cannot fully replace experiments on live animals, but will rather help to cut down the number of these experiments. For example, by screening potential irritants on isolated tissue, it may be possible to reduce the number of substances which have to be tested on conscious rabbits.[18] Viewed from an egalitarian point of view, this should be considered as a step in the right direction.

The aim of cutting down the number of animals used in experiments need not run counter to the aim of conducting experiments in accordance with the highest standards of scientific inquiry — quite to the contrary. A careful consideration of why an experiment is conducted, of how many animals are really needed, and of the severity of the procedures to which the animals are exposed, will in most cases improve the quality of the results found in the experiment. Careful thinking rather than mindless repetition of traditional experimental procedures seems to be the most efficient way to achieve rapid scientific progress. Forcing researchers to think of ways to limit the demand for animal experiments may therefore not only improve the lot of the animals but also the quality of the research.

To illustrate the latter point, I can mention that over a period of ten years a major Danish pharmaceutical company has managed to reduce the number of animals used to less than half, while at the same time intensifying its efforts in research and development.

Last, but not least, the demand for animal experiments can be limited if humans accept and enforce the following three principles:

- If it is possible to replace a harmful animal experiment with one where humans are caused only limited pain or inconvenience, this should be done by means of human volunteers.
- If it is possible to replace a harmful animal experiment with one using organs or tissue from dead humans, aborted human fetuses, or the like, this should be done.
- If doing without a harmful animal experiment involves only a slight risk or loss to humans, we should do without it.

I am aware that these suggestions run counter to a strong tendency in the Western world to become more and more sensitive about what we are doing to humans in biomedical research.[19] Often this sensitivity is presented as an ethical concern. But if the price for this concern is to be paid for by suffering animals, there is a moral problem.

However, even if it is possible to get some way of limiting the demand for animal experiments, it is realistic to assume that in the foreseeable future a considerable number of animal experiments will still be conducted. Therefore, it is also important to consider how the conditions for animals used in experiments may be improved.

IMPROVING THE CONDITIONS OF ANIMALS USED IN EXPERIMENTS

One way of improving the conditions of animals used in experiments is by means of legislation. Laws for the protection of animals used in research may specify minimum standards for the accommodation and care of research animals, they may prescribe the use of anesthetics and pain-killers, they may prescribe that animals involved in potentially harmful experiments should be killed as soon as possible, and they may in various other ways aim to limit the suffering and other kinds of harm inflicted on the animals.

Such legislation is certainly an important element in bringing ethical standards to bear on the conditions of animals used in experiments. What I would like to focus on here, however, is not so much the conditions which these laws prescribe for the animals, but the way in which the laws are enforced.

In most cases animal legislation is enforced by a public office giving researchers licenses to conduct animal experiments and controlling that the law and the conditions of the licenses are complied with. Such a system is good as far as it goes. The system may, however, have the shortcoming of not forcing the researchers to engage in a constant dialogue about how to improve the conditions of the animals. Rather, it may serve as a pretext for doing nothing: when the legal requirements are fulfilled, everything is assumed to be as good as it should be.

As a supplement to, and partly a replacement of, a centralized system of licensing and control, a system of local animal experimentation ethics committees may be considered. Such committees are already at work in Finland, Sweden, Australia, and to some extent in the U.S.[20–22] Such an ethical committee can be made up of both scientists and lay people, for example, members of moderate animal welfare groups. The committee must weigh the scientific or other value of an experiment against the harm inflicted upon the animals and decide whether an experiment should be allowed, modified, or rejected. Ideally, prior to decision, a dialogue must take place between the scientist and members of the committee. The committee must also monitor the care and use of animals in the area or the institution that it covers.

The advantages of such a system, when it functions well, are several: those taking the decisions have a first-hand knowledge of the people affected by them and may therefore be less bureaucratic and more flexible than a central office. Members of the committee are able to engage in ethical reflections. The scientists are forced to consider thoroughly the pros and cons of their proposed experiments, and must argue for their views. This may improve both scientific quality and ethical standards. Finally, the fact that lay people are members of the committees may help to improve the often highly polarized public debate about the use of animals in research. The public may be less skeptical about what scientists do to animals when they know that the experiments have been endorsed by lay people.

It may be noted that a system similar to the one proposed here is functioning in many countries for biomedical research involving human subjects. The system is based on the Declaration of Helsinki,[6] according to which: "The design and performance of each experimental procedure involving human subjects should be clearly formulated in an experimental protocol which should be transmitted to a specially appointed independent committee for consideration, comment and guidance. ... The research protocol should always contain a statement of the ethical considerations involved ...".

At the beginning of this chapter I mentioned several reasons why scientists ought to engage in moral reflections concerning the use of animals in biomedical research. I can now conclude by stating what may be seen as the most important reason: if before embarking on an animal experiment a scientist thoroughly considers the ethical consequences involved, this will in most cases be to the advantage of the animals.

ACKNOWLEDGMENTS

I want to thank Stian Erichsen, Nils Holtug, Klemens Kappel, Bo Petersson, and Jesper Ryberg for helpful comments to earlier versions of this chapter. Thanks are also due to the Danish Research Council for the Humanities for financial support.

REFERENCES

1. Riesman, D., *The Lonely Crowd*, Yale University Press, New Haven, CT, 1961.
2. Regan, T., *The Case for Animal Rights*, Routledge, London and New York, 1984.
3. Singer, P., Killing humans and killing animals, *Inquiry, 22, 145, 1979.*
4. Lockwood, M., Singer on killing and the preference for life, *Inquiry, 22, 157, 1979.*
5. Petersson, B., Etik og kohlhydrater: En forskningsetisk studie om Vibeholmsundersökningarna, *Vest, Tidsk. Vetenskabsst., 5, 3, 1991.*
6. *Declaration of Helsinki,* Recommendations guiding medical doctors in biomedical research involving human subjects, Adopted by the 18th World Medical Assembly, Helsinki, Finland, 1964, and revised by the 29th World Medical Assembly, Tokyo, Japan, 1975.

7. *Research Involving Human Subjects, Ethics/Law*, Ministry of Health, Copenhagen, 1989.
8. Petersson, B., Etik og kohlhydrater: En forskningsetisk studie om Vipeholmsundersökningarne, *Vest, Tidsk. Vetenskabsst., 5, 6, 1991*.
9. Singer, P., *Animal Liberation*, 2nd. ed., Review/Random House, New York, 1990.
10. Narveson, J., Animal rights, *Can. J. Philos., 7, 161, 1977*.
11. Frey, R. G., Vivisection, morals and medicine, *J. Med. Ethics, 9, 95, 1983*.
12. Frey, R. G., *Rights, Killing & Suffering*, Basil Blackwell, Oxford, 1983.
13. Singer, P., *Practical Ethics*, Cambridge University Press, Cambridge, 1979.
14. Smith, J. A. and Boyd, K. M. (eds.), *Lives in the Balance. The Ethics of Using Animals in Biomedical Research*, Oxford University Press, Oxford, 1991.
15. Regan, T., *The Case for Animal Rights*, Routledge, London and New York, 1984.
16. Sapontis, S. F., *Morals, Reasons, and Animals*, Temple University Press, Philadelphia, 1987.
17. D'Arcy, P. F. and Harron, D. W. G. (eds.), *Proceedings of the First International Conference on Harmonisation, Brussels 1991*, The Queen's University of Belfast, 1992.
18. Rodd, R., *Biology, Ethics and Animals*, Clarendon Press, Oxford, 1990, p. 153.
19. Rodd, R., *Biology, Ethics and Animals*, Clarendon Press, Oxford, 1990, p. 145.
20. Anderson, W., A new approach to regulation of the use of animals in science, *Bioethics, 4, 45, 1990*.
21. Rollin, B., *The Unheeded Cry*, Oxford University Press, Oxford, 1990, p. 177.
22. Finsen, L., Institutional animal care and use commitees: A new set of clothes for the emperor?, *J. Med. Philos. 13, 145, 1988*.

Chapter 2

European Legislation on the Use of Live Animals for Scientific Research

Stian Erichsen

CONTENTS

INTRODUCTION

The use of live animals for experimental purposes in Europe is regulated both on the international and the national levels, involving European intergovernmental organizations and national governments. The international bodies that are involved are two different organizations, the Council of Europe (CE) and the European Communities (EC), which have both adopted supranational or international rules or laws to regulate the use of live animals for experimental and other scientific purposes in the member states. The aims of these initiatives have been to assist the member countries in their efforts to modernize their legislation in this particular field and, not the least, to harmonize it so that the differences between them will be minimal. As the enforcement of legislation is the responsibility of each independent country, it follows that they must adopt national laws and regulations in this particular field as in many other fields. In the following it will therefore be necessary to present both sets of supranational or international rules as well as the laws of the individual member countries. In addition, the situation in those countries that are not members of the relevant European organizations, but which might still be considered to be European by some criterion, will be dealt with.

0-8493-4378-X/94/$0.00+$.50
© 1994 by CRC Press Inc.

INTERNATIONAL RULES

THE COUNCIL OF EUROPE CONVENTION FOR THE PROTECTION OF VERTEBRATE ANIMALS USED FOR EXPERIMENTAL AND OTHER SCIENTIFIC PURPOSES

These rules were adopted by the CE Committee of Ministers in Strasbourg and opened for signature by the member states on March 18, 1986. The member states are now: Austria, Belgium, Cyprus, Czechoslovakia, Denmark, Finland, France, Germany, Greece, Hungary, Iceland, Ireland, Italy, Liechtenstein, Luxembourg, Malta, the Netherlands, Norway, Poland, Portugal, San Marino, Spain, Sweden, Switzerland, Turkey, and the United Kingdom, 26 countries in all. The convention has been signed by 14 countries (Belgium, Denmark, Finland, France, Germany, Greece, Ireland, the Netherlands, Norway, Spain, Sweden, Switzerland, Turkey, and the United Kingdom) and by the EC. It has been ratified by Belgium, Finland, Germany, Greece, Norway, Spain, and Sweden and is legally binding for all these countries as of July 1, 1992.

The Convention comprises 37 articles and two appendices, "Appendix A — Guidelines for accommodation and care of animals", and "Appendix B — Statistical tables, etc". It applies to any live non-human vertebrate animal used or intended for use in any experimental or other scientific procedure where that procedure may cause pain, suffering, distress, or lasting harm. The fundamental provision is that any such procedure may only be performed for the following purposes and subject to the restrictions laid down in the convention itself:

- Avoidance or prevention of disease, ill-health or other abnormality, their effects, in man, vertebrate or invertebrate animals or plants, including the production and quality, efficacy and safety testing of drugs, substances or products
- Diagnosis or treatment of disease, ill-health or other abnormality, or their effects, in man, vertebrate or invertebrate animals or plants
- Detection, assessment, regulation or modification of physiological conditions in man, vertebrate and invertebrate animals or plants
- Protection of the environment
- Scientific research
- Education and training
- Forensic inquiries

However, such procedures may not be performed for any of these purposes if another scientifically satisfactory method, not entailing the use of an animal, is reasonably and practicably available.

These basic conditions for conducting procedures in live animals are then deepened and supplemented by a number of provisions covering these subjects: care and management; conduct of procedure; authorization; breeding, supplying and user establishments; education and training; supervision and control; record keeping and statistics; recognition of procedures carried out in the territory of another party; multilateral consultations and the legal formalities that apply to the Convention itself. A detailed examination of all the articles covering these sections lies beyond the scope of this presentation, but some important points must be mentioned.

The first requirement that must be met before one can conduct any procedure is that the establishment, that is the animal house or rooms, is registered and approved by the responsible authority and is operated in conformity with the rules set for care and management. Also breeding and supplying establishments must be registered and satisfy the same rules. Further, all such registered establishments should have named, competent administrative and professional management and trained staff. Then follows that a procedure as defined above may be carried out only by persons authorized, or under the direct responsibility of a person authorized, or if the experimental or other scientific project concerned is authorized in accordance with provisions of national legislation. Such authorization will only be granted to persons deemed to be competent by the responsible authority. This authority may also grant permission to conduct procedures outside registered establishments when necessary.

Animals of the species most used in procedures must be acquired directly or indirectly from registered breeding establishments, unless a general or special exemption has been granted by the responsible authorities. This provision applies to the mouse, rat, guinea pig, golden hamster, rabbit, dog, cat, and quail. However, no exemption may be made for stray dogs and cats. All categories of experimental animal establishments are obliged to keep such records of animal movements and of animals in stock and use as are further specified in various articles. Cats and dogs must be individually marked and recorded.

Various aspects of the conduct of procedures are dealt with in detail in several articles, such as the use of anesthesia and analgesia, procedures where the use of such drugs is incompatible with the aim of the procedure, procedures which will or may cause severe pain that is likely to endure, the killing of an animal at the end of a procedure, and the conditions for the reuse of animals in procedures, or their release after the close of the procedure.

The Convention puts restrictions on the conduct of procedures in live animals when the purpose is education and training. Such procedures are only permitted in education, training or further training for professions or other occupations, including the care of animals used or intended for use in procedures, and not for any other purpose. The procedures must be restricted to what is absolutely necessary for the curriculum. They must also be notified to the authorities beforehand and be supervised by a competent person.

The articles dealing with statistical information direct the authorities to collect the information from the users that is necessary to prepare and publish statistical information on the use of animals in procedures. This must be done annually according to detailed specifications in Appendix B. The material thus collected shall then be made available to the general public and the CE administration.

The Convention requests that the authorities in the signatory countries try to avoid unnecessary repetition of procedures required by law on health and safety and to recognize, where practicable, the results of procedures carried out in the territory of another signatory country. The Convention also prescribes that multilateral consultations be held at five-year intervals to examine the application of the Convention, and the advisability of revising it or extending any of its provisions.

It is also important to notice that no provision in the Convention prevents the signatory countries from adopting stricter measures for the protection of animals used in procedures or for the control and restriction of the use of animals in procedures.

THE EUROPEAN COMMUNITIES COUNCIL DIRECTIVE REGARDING THE PROTECTION OF ANIMALS USED FOR EXPERIMENTAL AND OTHER SCIENTIFIC PURPOSES

This Directive, (86/609/EEC), the full title of which is "The Council Directive on the approximation of laws, regulations and administrative provisions of the Member States regarding the protection of animals used for experimental and other scientific purposes", was adopted by the EC Council in Brussels on November 24, 1986 and became binding for the member states as of November 24, 1989. The EC member states are Belgium, Denmark, France, Germany, Greece, Ireland, Italy, Luxembourg, the Netherlands, Portugal, Spain, and the United Kingdom, 12 countries in all.

The EC Directive consists of 27 articles and two annexes of which Annex I comprises a list of the species covered by the Directive, and Annex II is identical to Appendix A of the CE Convention. Briefly, the state of affairs is now that there are two sets of international rules in Europe that cover the field of experiments or procedures conducted in live animals, viz., the CE Convention and the EC Directive. The former applies to the 26 CE member states and the latter to the 12 EC member states. The situation is somewhat complicated by the fact that the 12 EC states are also members of the CE. The important question that inevitably arises from this is whether or not there is agreement between these two sets of rules?

The wish to achieve harmonization of the relevant legislation in the member states and to tighten the conditions for and the control of the use of live animals for experimental purposes is emphasized by both organizations. However, the EC Directive has the further aim of preventing national legislation from leading to unfair trade and trade restrictions that would be contrary to the implementation and function of the EC common market. A further examination of the two documents nevertheless reveals that there is, with some exceptions, a high degree of agreement between them.

There is a semantic discrepancy on a central point in that the CE Convention uses the word "procedure" where the EC Directive uses the word "experiment". When the Convention was drafted it was emphasized that the word "experiment" was often understood to mean only an action undertaken to discover something not yet known. This interpretation or use of the word would mean that many, perhaps a majority, of the actions undertaken with live animals for various scientific purposes or by the use of scientific methods would not be covered by the Convention. To avoid any misunderstanding, it was decided to use the neutral word "procedure", which would cover any use of live animals for true experimental purposes as well as other uses where the outcome might be more or less known or anticipated in advance, such as in efficacy and safety testing, demonstrations, training, etc. In the EC

Directive the word "experiment" is thus used with the same meaning as "procedure" in the CE Convention.

Just like the CE Convention, the EC Directive applies to any live non-human vertebrate animal used or to be used for experimental or other scientific purposes which may cause pain, suffering, distress, or lasting harm. The fundamental provision in the Directive is that it applies only to the use of animals in experiments which are undertaken for one of the following purposes:

- The development, manufacture, quality, effectiveness and safety testing of drugs, foodstuffs and other substances
- For the avoidance, prevention, diagnosis or treatment of disease, ill-health or other abnormality or their effects in man, animals or plants
- For the assessment, detection, regulation or modification of physiological conditions in man, animals and plants
- The protection of the natural environment in the interests of the health or welfare of man and animal.

The EC Directive deviates from the CE Convention on an important point here, in that it does not apply to scientific research, education and training, and forensic inquiries, purposes that are all covered by the CE Convention. This means that the EC member states that have not signed and ratified the CE Convention are not legally bound to adopt legislation on the use of live animals for experimental purposes within these three important fields, and they may not do it. The EC Directive is, however, in accordance with the CE Convention in that it does not allow experiments when another scientifically satisfactory method of obtaining the result sought, not entailing the use of an animal, is reasonably and practicably available.

There are also differences on other points, although it is only a question of phrasing and editing in many cases. In substance, there is a high degree of agreement between the two documents. Like the CE Convention, the EC Directive contains articles that cover the following subjects: care and management; conduct of experiments; authorization; breeding, supplying, and user establishments; supervision and control; record keeping and statistics; recognition of experiments carried out in the territory of another member state; consultations; and legal and administrative formalities. Here one will notice that, for reasons explained above, there are no provisions in the Directive about the conduct of experiments in live animals for education and training, although it is stated in several articles that responsible persons and staff should be trained for their respective tasks.

Certain other points must also be mentioned because they deviate more than a trifle from the provisions of the CE Convention. One such case is the Directive requirement that the member states establish procedures whereby the experiments or the details of the person conducting them, are notified in advance to the authorities. Authorization of experiments by the authorities is only prescribed when it is planned to subject an animal to an experiment in which it will, or may, experience severe pain which may endure. However, elsewhere it is stressed that the member states may require prior authorization of experiments or programs of work in place of advance notification only.

The Directive list of the species of animals that must originate from registered breeding or supplying establishments includes, in addition to those listed in the EC Convention, also non-human primates. It is further required that non-human primates be individually recorded and marked like cats and dogs. The use of animals considered as endangered according to international conventions and EC regulations is prohibited unless it is done in conformity with the basic conditions of the Directive and the objects of the experiment are (1) research aimed at preservation of the species in question, or (2) essential biomedical purposes where the species in question exceptionally proves to be the only one suitable for the purposes. The CE Convention does not contain a direct parallel to this provision.

The Directive articles covering the use of anesthesia and analgesia conform broadly with the corresponding articles in the CE Convention, but stress more explicitly the obligation to use analgesia to relieve any pain caused by an experiment.

Both the EC Directive and the CE Convention prescribe that the authorities in the member states shall collect statistical information on the use of live animals for experimental purposes and make this information periodically available to the general public, subject to the restrictions in national legislation. Both documents require that the number and species of animals used for experimental purposes are stated, but because the two documents differ somewhat in their scope, the Directive not covering scientific research, education and training, and forensic inquiries, the lists of items on the returns will differ. Another difference between the two systems is that the CE Convention requires that the member states submit the statistical information annually to the Secretary General of the Council of Europe in order that it may be published as joint European statistics. The EC have no corresponding joint statistics, the publication of this sort of information being left to the responsibility of the authorities in the member states.

Just like the CE Convention, the EC Directive does not restrict the right of the member states to apply or adopt stricter measures for the protection of animals than those prescribed in the Directive itself.

Finally, the Directive requires that the member states adopt the measures necessary to ensure that the authorities responsible for the administration, control and supervision of the activities covered by the Directive, may have the advice of experts competent in the matters in question. The CE Convention contains no corresponding provision.

NATIONAL LEGISLATION IN COUNCIL OF EUROPE MEMBER STATES

AUSTRIA

Austria has not yet signed the CE Convention. It may become a member of the European Communities before the end of the century. The use of live animals for experimental purposes is regulated through a federal law, *Bundesgesetz vom 27 September 1989 über Versuche an lebenden Tieren*, which came into force on January 1, 1990. This law conforms in its substance fully with the CE Convention in its most important provisions. However, some fields comprised by the Convention are only superficially covered or not covered at all. This applies to the use of analgesia, disposal after close of procedure, the control of breeding and supplying establishments, regulation of the procurement of animals, bans on the use of stray animals, and education and training.

The authorities responsible for control and supervision are the Ministry of Science and Research (for universities and Austrian Academy of Science institutes) and the *Landeshauptmann* (for industry and other users). The handling of such matters should be carried out by civil servants holding specialized knowledge. All procedures are subject to an advance approval by one or the other of these authorities. Exceptions are made only for procedures authorized by law or court, and for inoculations, bleedings or similar interventions performed using recognized methods for diagnostic purposes, or for the production and control of sera and vaccines. Permission to carry out procedures involving surgical interventions is only granted to persons holding a university degree in biomedicine or related fields who in addition, have specialized knowledge. The Ministry of Science and Research may prohibit procedures which have become outdated.

Inspection of authorized premises and the activities there are carried out by qualified personnel acting on behalf of the Ministry or the *Landeshauptmann*. Each place should be subjected to at least one unannounced inspection annually.

BELGIUM

Belgium has signed and ratified the CE Convention. It is a member of the European Communities and is bound by Directive 86/609/EEC.

Regulations on the use of animals for experimental purposes in Belgium have their legal basis in a law covering animal protection in general, *Loi du 14 Aout 1986 relative à la protection et au bien-être des animaux*, in which Chapter 8 deals with experiments on animals. In accordance with the provisions in this law a royal decree on the protection of experimental animals *(Arrêté royale relatif à la protection des animaux d'expérience)* has been adopted by the Government but not yet by the State Council. This decree contains supplementary and more detailed provisions.

An animal experiment is defined in the law as any intervention or observation on a live animal for the purpose of confirming a scientific theory, collecting information, testing or harvesting certain products, maintaining stocks of microorganisms and tumors, establishing the reactions of an animal, or conducting demonstrations in education and training. This definition seems to have a much wider scope than the corresponding parts of both the CE Convention and the EC Directive in that it covers all animals, not only vertebrates. However, in the royal decree it appears that its provisions in principle apply only to vertebrates. The decree conforms with the CE Convention in that it lists scientific research, education and training as acceptable purposes, but like the EC Directive, not forensic inquiries. Concerning the remaining acceptable purposes, they seem to conform broadly in substance with those listed in the Directive although the wording differs. It is explicitly stated that it is forbidden to conduct experiments on animals for any other purpose.

Otherwise, the Belgian legislation regulating experiments in live animals conforms almost entirely with the EC Directive, but a few deviations occur. For example, provisions about the conditional setting free of animals after the close of an experiment are missing.

The legislation provides for the establishment of ethical committees in all user establishments where experiments that may cause pain, suffering, or lasting harm are conducted. The committee must have at least six members representing the management, staff, independent externals, and the Ministry of Agriculture. The tasks of the committee are to evaluate experiments in advance and retrospect, and to give advice to the various parties involved in matters of an ethical nature. This local ethical committee must not be confused with the Deontological Committee established in conformity with the Directive, Article 6. 2., whose task it is to advise the Ministry of Agriculture in matters relating to experiments in animals in general.

DENMARK

Denmark has signed but not ratified the CE Convention. It is also a member of the European Communities and is bound by Directive 86/609/EEC.

The Danish law regulating experiments on animals, *Lov om dyreforsøg*, is dated April 1, 1987. It states in Chapter 1 that the conduct of procedures or experiments on vertebrates can only be carried out with the permission of the Controlling Body, *Dyreforsøgstilsynet,* appointed by the Ministry of Justice, which is the responsible authority. Permissions can only be granted for the purposes specified in the CE Convention to named, educated and skilled persons on further conditions specified in each individual case. Chapter 2 contains the essential rules for the conduct of procedures which conform with both Convention and Directive in substance. The composition and rules of procedure for the Controlling Body are covered in Chapter 3. Wide powers are also given to the Body to set conditions for the conduct of procedures, the care and management of animals, and the design and equipment of user establishments. In Chapter 4 the Ministry of Justice is authorized to lay down further rules to comply with those provisions of the Convention and Directive which are not covered in the law itself. In accordance with this the Ministry has issued three ordinances, one dated December 6, 1988 covering the keeping of records in user establishments, one dated May 18, 1990 on breeding and supplying establishments and the acquisition of animals, and another, also dated May 18, 1990, dealing with care and management.

FINLAND

Finland has signed and ratified the CE Convention. It may become a member of the European Communities before the end of the century.

Legislation in Finland regulating animal experimentation is based on an animal protection law, *Djurskyddslag*, dated January 27, 1971. It authorizes the regulation of activities in this field through decrees and defines an animal experiment as any procedure where an intervention on an animal is necessary, and in education unavoidable, for the pursuit of health in animals and man, and for scientific research, and is conducted by scientific methods at the responsibility of a qualified person. The ensuing decree, (*Förordning om försöksdjurverksamhet*), is dated December 20, 1985 and came into force January 1, 1986.

The substance of the decree, which applies only to vertebrates, conforms with the CE Convention in the basic parts, but with some deviations. Missing is a specified list of permissible purposes. So also are provisions concerning the acquisition, recording, and marking of animals, and their use in education and training.

The decree has a provision that distinguishes between two categories of procedures that may cause pain or suffering. Category One comprises procedures which may cause severe pain or suffering, or serious disease, while Category Two includes procedures that cause only trifling and/or transitory pain or suffering, or which are conducted under anesthesia. The conduct of a Category One procedure requires the permission of county authorities, whereas Category Two procedures only need the approval of the local committee on animal experiments. Such committees are found in all authorized user establishments. The members are representatives of the personnel and at least two other people with insight into animal experimentation. Their main task is the advance appraisal and approval of all experimental protocols without which no procedure may be conducted.

FRANCE

France has signed, but not ratified the CE Convention. At the time of signature it made a reservation concerning the articles dealing with statistical information. It is also a member of the European Communities and is bound by Directive 86/609/EEC.

Animal experimentation is regulated through *Décret no 87-848 relatif aux expériences pratiquées sur les animaux* of October 19, 1987 and three supplementing *Arrêtés* of April 19, 1988. The provisions conform to a high degree with both the CE Convention and the EC Directive, primarily the latter. The regulations cover any experiment on a live vertebrate that will involve any suffering for the animal. Such procedures may only be carried out by individuals holding a personal license, or working under the direct control of someone holding such a license. Establishments, whether user, breeding, or supplying, must be approved.

There seem to be some deviations from the CE and EC documents, but this is only because the matters concerned are covered by earlier legislation: breeding and supplying establishments for cats and dogs must keep records of the origin of their animals and to whom they have been sold (*Arrêté* of June 2, 1975); the same applies to establishments producing and selling other species for use in experimental procedures. The use of stray cats and dogs for such purposes is forbidden (*Décret* of June 27, 1987). Furthermore, all cats, dogs, and non-human primates must be individually and permanently marked and recorded in official registers. The list of animals that must be procured from authorized sources includes a few little used or protected species, viz., the South African clawed toad (*Xenopus laevis*), the Mexican axolotl (*Ambystoma mexicanum*), the Spanish newt (*Pleurodeles waltlii*), and the Chinese hamster (*Cricetulus griseus*). User establishments may accept animals donated for use in experiments, provided that no compensation is paid.

The authority responsible for the implementation of the regulations and the supervision and control of the whole field is usually the Ministry of Agriculture, but in certain matters of a military nature the Ministry of Defence is the responsible authority. In conformity with the Directive, Article 6. 2., it is prescribed that a 20 member strong National Committee on Animal Experimentation shall be established. The purpose of this committee is to advise the ministries in all matters related to legislation and regulation, education and training of personnel, and development of non-animal methods, as well as breeding, care and management of experimental animals. Provisions dealing in great detail with the submission and handling of applications for authorization (licensing) of personnel and establishments are also given. The same applies to such fields as supervision and control, training curricula, and design and function of facilities.

GERMANY

Germany has signed and ratified the CE Convention, but with reservations regarding articles dealing with statistical information. It is also a member of the European Communities and is bound by Directive 86/609/EEC.

In Germany the legislation covering experimental procedures on animals is found in the federal animal protection law, *Tierschutzgesetz*, as amended on August 18, 1986. Section V, *Tierversuche*, contains the essential provisions in this field, but relevant articles are also found in Sections II, III, VI, and X. All sections in this law apply to animals in general, but vertebrates are given special protection in several articles of Section V. There is full conformity both with the CE Convention and the EC Directive on almost every point, the deviations being very few and mostly restrictive in nature.

The list of acceptable aims agrees for most items with that of the Directive. It is noteworthy that purposes like the testing of weapons, ammunition and similar equipment are totally forbidden. The testing of tobacco, washing-powder, and cosmetics is also forbidden, but for such substances the ban may be lifted by the Federal Ministry of Food, Agriculture and Forestry in special cases. Very detailed and comprehensive rules are given about the course that must be followed both by applicants and responsible authorities in the handling of applications for licenses. There is a very elaborate notification system. It applies also in those cases where the procedures, in accordance with the law, can be conducted without a license. An ordinance, *Allgemeine Verwaltungsvorschrift zur Durchführung des Tierschutzgesetzes,* of July 1, 1988, issued by the Federal Ministry of Food, Agriculture and Forestry covers it all.

Only vertebrates bred for experimental purposes in licensed breeding establishments may be used for experimental procedures, but the competent authorities may grant exemptions from this provision, which aims both at the protection of animals in general and at the conservation of endangered species.

The responsibility for the implementation of the law and any ordinance issued in accordance with it, rests with the administrative authorities in the respective Länder. The consequence is that there may be regulatory differences between the various Länder. Each Länd must also appoint one or more committees to advise the authorities in the handling of applications for licenses to conduct procedures.

GREECE

Greece has signed and ratified the CE Convention. It is a member of the European Communities and is bound by Directive 86/609/EEC. National legislation which covers experiments on live animals has been adopted by an act of Parliament dated April 12, 1991. This law conforms almost entirely with the Directive both in substance and in wording. Most articles are identical to the corresponding articles in the Directive; the drafting is different or more detailed in a few cases only. The Annexes I and II to the Directive are also included in the law itself.

ICELAND

Iceland has not signed or ratified the CE Convention. It is not a member of the European Communities.

In accordance with provisions in the law on protection of animals of April 13, 1957, the Ministry of Culture and Education has issued regulations dealing with the use of animals for scientific purposes, *Reglugerò um notkun dyra í vísindalegum tilgagni*, dated March 7, 1973. The six articles of this regulation deal with licensing and licensing conditions, use of anesthesia, killing procedure, qualification requirements for licensees and other personnel, and keeping of records and statistics. The authority responsible for licensing and supervision is the Chief Veterinary Officer. These provisions conform with corresponding provisions in the CE Convention, but other parts of the Convention are not covered.

IRELAND

Ireland has signed, but not yet ratified, the CE Convention. It is a member of the European Communities and is bound by Directive 86/609/EEC.

In Ireland experiments and other scientific procedures on animals are performed under the Cruelty to Animals Act, 1876, and the EC Directive. Apparently the Directive works as common law supplemented by the provisions of the Act where they are stricter, or deal with fields that are not covered by the Directive, and details concerning implementation, licensing, control, and supervision.

No procedure can be carried out without a personal license granted by the Ministry of Health, which is also the authority responsible for inspection. Accepted purposes are the advancement of physiological knowledge or of knowledge useful for the saving of life or alleviating suffering. Procedures may be conducted for teaching purposes under anesthesia and only if considered essential. Public procedures are prohibited.

ITALY

Italy has not signed or ratified the CE Convention. It is a member of the European Communities and is bound by Directive 86/609/EEC.

The legislation on animal protection, including experimental procedures on animals, dated May 1, 1941, was replaced by a new law on the protection of all animals used for experiments and other scientific purposes, which was adopted by decree on January 27, 1992. In substance this new law conforms with the EC Directive on almost every point. It is noteworthy that this law also covers the use of animals in basic research and teaching, fields that are not mentioned in the Directive. It also gives special protection to non-human primates, cats, and dogs, although it is not necessary for animals of such species to be bred for the purpose. The devocalization of animals and the use of devocalized animals are explicitly forbidden.

All experiments that are planned and carried out for an acceptable purpose have to be notified to the responsible authority, which is the Ministry of Health. Copies of letters of notification have to be sent to the regional and local authorities. The use of animals for diagnostic purposes in human or veterinary medicine would only need to be notified to the local health authorities. Procedures to be carried out on endangered species, non-human primates, cats, and dogs, for teaching purposes, or without anesthesia when anesthesia is incompatible with the object of the experiment, must be approved by the Ministry.

User establishments must be authorized by the Ministry, while breeding and supplying establishments only need the authorization of local councils. The councils must, however, keep updated lists of all such establishments within their area and submit copies to the Ministry and also to the Regions and Prefectures. Supplementary regulations that will give effect to various provisions in the law are in preparation.

LUXEMBOURG

Luxembourg has not signed or ratified the CE Convention. It is a member of the European Communities and is bound by Directive 86/609/EEC.

The existing law covering animal protection and welfare, including experimental procedures, was adopted in 1983, but no amendments have been made since then. The reason is probably that experiments in live animals are very rare in this country with no user, breeding, supplying, or training establishments in this particular field

THE NETHERLANDS

The Netherlands have signed, but not ratified, the CE Convention. They are a member of the European Communities and are bound by Directive 86/609/EEC.

In the Netherlands the conduct of experiments on live animals is regulated by an act of January 12, 1977, *Wet op de Dierproeven*, supplemented by a royal decree dated May 31, 1985 concerning the implementation of certain articles of this law. Although this legislation precedes the CE Convention by several years, it conforms in substance to a high degree with that of the Convention. This applies in particular to such basic parts as the scope (only vertebrates are covered), definition of a procedure, list of acceptable purposes, use of other methods, licensing, user establishments, qualification requirements for licensees, auxiliary personnel and competent persons, record keeping, and care and management. As matters stand, there are inevitably some differences. It is compulsory to appoint animal welfare officers wherever experiments on animals are conducted. The protection of the environment and forensic inquiries are not mentioned as acceptable purposes; nor are breeding and supplying establishments mentioned. The handling and disposal of animals post-procedure are among matters that are sparsely dealt with.

The authority responsible for licensing is the Minister of Public Health and Environmental Hygiene. No experiment may be carried out without a license issued by the Minister. Licenses may be granted to juridical persons (institutions, commercial firms, etc.), in which case the head of the establishment is the legally responsible person, or to individual persons, who are only responsible for their own experiments. Limitations and conditions may be set for any type of license. It is also provided that no procedure may be carried out under any type of license unless the protocol has been approved by an expert authorized by administrative order. The control and supervision function is vested in the governmental health inspectorate, *Staatstoezicht op de Volksgezondheid, Veterinaire Hoofdinspectie*, and the local animal welfare officer. An animal experiments advisory committee is appointed to advise the Minister and other authorities in all matters concerning animal procedures.

A proposal for a revision of the legislation to bring it in line with the EC Directive and to ratify the CE Convention is now before the Parliament.

NORWAY

Norway has signed and ratified the CE Convention. It may become a member of the European Communities before the end of the century.

The basic legislation regulating the use of live animals for experimental purposes is found in the animal protection law, *Lov om dyrevern*, dated December 20, 1974. In accordance with articles 21 and 22 in this law the Ministry of Agriculture on November 19, 1976 issued an ordinance, *Forskrifter om biologiske forsøk med dyr*, which contains the existing legislation regulating the use of animals for experimental purposes, notwithstanding the fact that Norway ratified the CE Convention as early as 1986. The consequence is that there are obvious shortcomings and gaps which must be filled to attain the standard set in the Convention. Missing are primarily provisions dealing with acceptable purposes, general care and accommodation, breeding and supplying establishments, marking and acquisition of specified species, education and training, and more detailed rules for the treatment of animals during and after experiments. In other fields there exists a reasonable conformity with the Convention in substance.

The responsible authority is the Experimental Animal Board, a body appointed by the Ministry of Agriculture and composed of legal, biomedical, and animal welfare expertise. This Board certifies establishments, issues licenses to conduct procedures, scrutinizes all planned procedures and projects, and inspects facilities and their activities. Personal licenses may be granted to individuals meeting certain qualifications, but in most cases licenses are granted to university or health service institutes, hospitals or other bodies operating within the same or related fields. In such cases the license is granted on condition that the applicant can nominate a person whom the Board finds qualified to be responsible for compliance with legislation and other conditions set for the experimental activity at the particular establishment. No procedure or project involving the use of animals for experimental purposes can be carried out without the consent of this responsible person who acts as an advisor, supervisor, and referee, reporting back to the Board. A revision of the ordinance is in progress to bring it in line with the CE Convention.

PORTUGAL

Portugal has not signed or ratified the CE Convention. It is a member of the European Communities and is thus bound by Directive 86/609/EEC. National legislation conforming with the Directive is in preparation.

SPAIN

Spain has signed and ratified the CE Convention. It is also a member of the European Communities and is bound by Directive 86/609/EEC.

A royal decree, *Sobre proteccíon de los animales utilizados para experimentacíon y otros fines científicos*, of March 14, 1988, regulates the field of animal experimentation. This legislation conforms in great measure with the EC Directive of November 24, 1986, with appendices with regard to both substance and wording, but with one important amendment. The list of acceptable purposes also includes scientific research, education and training, and forensic inquiries. This means that the Spanish legislation, broadly speaking, conforms with the CE Convention.

The implementation of the provisions in the royal decree is delegated to the 17 autonomous local governments which must register all breeding, supplying, and user establishments within their territories and also authorize the use of animals for experimental purposes. However, in the case of state ownership the authority responsible for these functions is the Ministry of Agriculture, Fisheries and Nutrition. In any case, the user establisments are under obligation to notify the responsible authority quarterly about experiments that are being planned. Moreover, the autonomous governments must inform the Ministry each quarter about the establishments registered, with particular emphasis on such details as their names and activities, name and qualifications of the responsible person, species and number of animals bred, supplied or used, and, when relevant, procedures conducted including information on their nature, the species and number of animals used and their final fate, method of killing and possible exceptions conceded within their competence.

SWEDEN

Sweden has signed and ratified the CE Convention. It may become a member of the European Communities before the end of the century.

The basis for the legislation regulating the use of live animals for experimental purposes in Sweden is the common animal protection act, *Djurskyddslag*, of June 2, 1988. In this law articles 19, 20, 21, 22, and 23 deal with the use of animals for scientific and similar purposes. It should be noticed, however, that these articles do not cover all parts or articles of the CE Convention. However, what is prescribed in this law is that procedures carried out for certain specified purposes and involving certain interventions or suffering, may only be carried out with the permission of the responsible authorities, which are the Government or the Swedish Board of Agriculture. The list of acceptable purposes is so worded that it includes all such listed in the CE Convention even if they are not explicitly mentioned. Only purpose-bred animals may be used for procedures. Breeding and user establishments must be approved; the latter must also have an approved responsible head. A further requirement is that the experimenter should be competent and that he and all auxiliary personnel should have such training as may be appropriate. A final condition which must be satisfied before any procedure can be carried out is that it should be subjected to an ethical evaluation. Authority is given to the Government and the Swedish Board of Agriculture (SBA) to issue supplementary ordinances and make exceptions from certain provisions.

In accordance with the authority given, two ordinances dated June 2, 1988 may be mentioned, namely the Animal Protection Ordinance and the Central Experimental Animal Board Ordinance. The former provides for the establishment of regional ethical committees to make the prescribed ethical evaluation of planned procedures, sets certain rules about the use of anesthesia, and the keeping of records and journals, and authorizes the SBA to issue licenses to conduct procedures and make exceptions from certain general rules; the latter provides for the establishment of a central body whose task it is to coordinate and prepare matters concerning experimental animals, and draws up its terms of reference. Briefly, the tasks of this Central Experimental Animal Board are to promote improvement on all levels and within all aspects of the particular field, including the promotion of so-called alternative methods, the issue of codes of practice and recommendations regarding education and training, and compilation of statistics.

SWITZERLAND

Switzerland has signed, but not ratified, the CE Convention. It may become a member of the European Communities before the end of the century.

The Federal Act on Animal Welfare, *Tierschutzgesetz*, of March 9, 1978, with amendments enforced as from November 1, 1991, lays down the basic provisions for experiments on live animals. In accordance with an article in this law the Federal Council has further issued a statutory regulation, *Tierschutzverordnung*, of May 27, 1981, also with amendments enforced as from November 1, 1991. Supplementary and detailed provisions regarding experiments in live animals are found in its Chapter 7. This whole legislation conforms to a very high degree both in scope and substance with the CE Convention, although the wording is not identical. The most notable fact is that it goes further than the Convention on several points. Thus, it applies not only to vertebrates, but also to decapods and cephalopods. The definition of a procedure is general and covers virtually any type of experimental use of a live animal. The responsible authorities, which are cantonal, are also given powers to limit or set conditions for the conduct of procedures.

All procedures must be notified to the cantons, and if they may cause pain, suffering, distress, or lasting harm, a license is needed from the cantonal authorities. These authorities are also responsible for control and supervision. Licenses are only granted to the scientific head of an institute or undertaking and this person is responsible for compliance on all levels with legislation, and conditions and orders set. Each canton must appoint an independent experimental animal committee whose task it is to advise and assist the cantonal authorities in the appraisal of applications for licenses and other matters concerning animal procedures. A federal committee of experts must be appointed by the Federal Council to advise the Federal Veterinary Office and the cantonal experimental animal committees. The former is responsible for a documentation unit for animal procedures and alternative methods, as well as the publication of annual statistical information for the federation.

TURKEY

Turkey has signed, but not ratified, the CE Convention. It is not a member of the European Communities. There is as yet no legislation covering the use of animals for experimental purposes in Turkey.

THE UNITED KINGDOM

The United Kingdom has signed, but not ratified, the CE Convention. It is a member of the European Communities and is bound by Directive 86/609/EEC.

In the United Kingdom (U.K.), experimental procedures on live animals are regulated by the Animals (Scientific Procedures) Act 1986, effective from January 1, 1987. The provisions of this law conform broadly with those of the CE Convention although the wording may be different. Deviations exist; in some cases they are definitely of a restrictive nature, in other cases seemingly more lenient, but these are compensated for by the fact that several articles authorize the Minister of State (Home Office) to set special conditions when issuing licenses and certificates. Further, general guidances and codes of practice are issued, some of them in cooperation with external bodies or persons. An example is the "Home Office Code of Practice for Housing and Care" prepared at the initiative of the Royal Society and the Universities Federation for Animal Welfare (UFAW). Other guidances include permitted procedures for killing animals.

A more important aspect of the U.K. law is that it goes much further than the Convention on several points. This applies in particular to the licensing system. Three conditions must be met before a procedure can be performed: the establishment must be certified, the person who is to perform it must be licensed, and finally, the program or project must also be licensed by the Home Office. Inspectors appointed by the Home Office advise the authority on such matters and also visit and supervise establishments, licensees, and the procedures authorized. It is further prescribed that there shall be an Animal Procedures Committee appointed by the Secretary of State to advise him (the Home Office) on matters concerning the law. The composition of the committee will be such that biomedical, juridical, as well as animal welfare expertise is adequately represented. All laboratory animal facilities are required to appoint a "Named Veterinary Surgeon" who must ensure maximal welfare of the animals.

Among the other more restrictive provisions one notices that the breeding of animals for use in procedures requires a project license, that the elimination of pain and suffering by analgesia, anesthesia or any other method for any experimental or other scientific purpose is defined as a regulated procedure, that non-human primates are listed as animals that must be acquired from a designated breeding or supplying establishment, and that the use of cats, dogs, non-human primates, and equidae may only be licensed if no other species are suitable or practically available. It is explicitly prohibited to use neuro-muscular blocking agents instead of anesthetics, or to display procedures in any place or by any method in public.

COUNCIL OF EUROPE MEMBER STATES WITH NO NATIONAL LEGISLATION

Among the member states are several small countries or sovereign states, i.e., Cyprus, Liechtenstein, Malta, and San Marino. None of them has signed and ratified the CE Convention and, with one exception, none of them has any legislation on the use of animals for experimental purposes, possibly because it would have no relevance. The exception is Lichtenstein, which has adopted a total ban on the use of animals for experimental procedures within its territory.

Czechoslovakia, Hungary, and Poland have recently become members of the CE and have not yet signed and ratified the Convention. National legislation, if such exists, is either fragmentary or outdated. However, sources report that new legislation is being initiated in these countries.

EUROPEAN COUNTRIES OUTSIDE THE COUNCIL OF EUROPE

Albania, Bosnia-Hercegovina, Bulgaria, Croatia, Estonia, Latvia, Lithuania, Macedonia, Romania, Slovenia, and Yugoslavia are all European countries, although they are today not members of the Council of Europe. The same can be said about several of the states that today make up the Commonwealth of Independent States (CIS). None of them is known to have any legislation protecting animals used for experimental purposes of any kind.

Chapter 3

North American Legislation and Regulation of the Use of Live Animals for Scientific Research

Melvin B. Dennis, Jr. and Gerald L. Van Hoosier, Jr.

CONTENTS

LEGISLATION AND REGULATION OF ANIMAL RESEARCH IN THE UNITED STATES

The U.S. Congress has enacted a series of laws to ensure the humane and proper use of animals in teaching, testing, and research. Regulation and enforcement has been delegated to different agencies, i.e., the United States Department of Agriculture (USDA) for the Animal Welfare Act and the Department of Health and Human Services (DHHS) for the Health Research Extension Act. This has resulted in a complex array of different regulations which often seem conflicting. As an example, the Public Health Service (PHS) Policy[1] requires a minimum of three persons on the Institutional Animal Care and Use Committee (IACUC); while the USDA regulations[2] require five persons. Institutions or individuals which are required to comply with more than one set of regulations face a challenge, since no one document addresses all aspects of animal care and use.

Depending upon the species of animals used, the studies being conducted, and the agency providing the funding, institutions may need to comply with some or all of the regulations and guidelines discussed below. An institution using only laboratory mice and rats and funded internally is not subject to the USDA regulations or the PHS policy. If the institution receives funds from the National Institutes of Health (NIH), however, it is subject to the PHS policy and the provisions of the *Guide For The Care And Use Of Laboratory Animals (Guide)*. If the institution uses species other than mice or rats, such as hamsters, guinea pigs, nonhuman primates, dogs, or cats, it is subject to USDA regulations. Since most U.S. research institutions are subject to both the PHS policy and the USDA regulations, this chapter will present the procedures necessary in order for institutions, their IACUCs, and research investigators using animals to comply with the PHS Policy,[1] USDA regulations,[2] and *Guide*.[3] The reference listed after various requirements refers to the applicable regulation.

LEGISLATION, GUIDELINES, AND POLICIES

The primary laws and regulations governing the use of animals in research in the United States are listed below.

ANIMAL WELFARE ACT
(Public Law 89-544, 1966; amended in 1970, 1976, and 1985) — The 1985 amendment directed the Secretary of the USDA to promulgate regulations to ensure that animals used in research, teaching, and testing receive humane care and treatment. The regulations are enforced by Regulatory Enforcement and Animal Care (REAC), a unit of the Animal and Plant Health Inspection Service (APHIS), which is under the USDA. The regulations apply to warm-blooded animals, alive or dead, except that the USDA has, by policy, exempted rats, mice, birds, and "farm" species when used in food and fiber research.

U.S. GOVERNMENT PRINCIPLES FOR THE UTILIZATION AND CARE OF VERTEBRATE ANIMALS USED IN TESTING, RESEARCH, AND TRAINING
The principles (Figure1) were developed by the Interagency Research Animal Committee (IRAC) and endorsed by the PHS. They must be considered whenever government agencies perform or sponsor procedures involving vertebrate animals.

GUIDE FOR THE CARE AND USE OF LABORATORY ANIMALS[3]
The *Guide* was prepared by the Committee on Care and Use of Laboratory Animals of the Institute of Laboratory Animal Resources (ILAR) Commission on Life Sciences, National Research Council. It was first published in 1963 as the *Guide for Laboratory Animal Facilities and Care*. The current edition was published in 1985 to "...assist institutions in caring for and using laboratory animals in ways judged to be professionally and humanely appropriate." It is considered to be the *"Bible"* for laboratory animal programs.

HEALTH RESEARCH EXTENSION ACT OF 1985
(Public Law 99-158, November 20, 1985) — This is an amendment to the Public Health Service Act originally enacted in 1944. It required the Director of the NIH to establish guidelines for the proper care and treatment of animals to be used in biomedical and behavioral research, and for the organization and operation of the IACUC. The provisions of this law are enforced by DHHS.

PHS POLICY ON HUMANE CARE AND USE OF LABORATORY ANIMALS[1]
The amended policy was published in 1986 to incorporate changes required by the Health Research Extension Act. It applies to institutions that apply to PHS for awards for activities involving animals, including both intramural and extramural NIH research. Institutions in foreign countries receiving PHS

The development of knowledge necessary for the improvement of the health and well-being of humans as well as other animals requires *in vivo* experimentation with a wide variety of animal species. Whenever U.S. Government agencies develop requirements for testing, research, or training procedures involving the use of vertebrate animals, the following principles shall be considered; and whenever these agencies actually perform or sponsor such procedures, the responsible Institutional Official shall ensure that these principles are adhered to:

   I.   The transportation, care, and use of animals should be in accordance with the Animal Welfare Act (7 U.S.C. 2131 et.seq.) and other applicable Federal laws, guidelines, and policies.

  II.   Procedures involving animals should be designed and performed with due consideration of their relevance to human or animal health, the advancement of knowledge, or the good of society.

 III.   The animals selected for a procedure should be of an appropriate species and quality and the minimum number required to obtain valid results. Methods such as mathematical models, computer simulation, and *in vitro* biological systems should be considered.

  IV.   Proper use of animals, including the avoidance or minimization of discomfort, distress, and pain when consistent with sound scientific practices, is imperative. Unless the contrary is established, investigators should consider that procedures that cause pain or distress in human beings may cause pain or distress in other animals.

   V.   Procedures with animals that may cause more than momentary or slight pain or distress should be performed with appropriate sedation, analgesia, or anesthesia. Surgical or other painful procedures should not be performed on unanesthetized animals paralyzed by chemical agents.

  VI.   Animals that would otherwise suffer severe or chronic pain or distress that cannot be relieved should be painlessly killed at the end of the procedure or, if appropriate, during the procedure.

 VII.   The living conditions of animals should be appropriate for their species and contribute to their health and comfort. Normally, the housing, feeding, and care of all animals used for biomedical purposes must be directed by a veterinarian or other scientist trained and experienced in the proper care, handling, and use of the species being maintained or studied. In any case, veterinary care shall be provided as indicated.

VIII.   Investigators and other personnel shall be appropriately qualified and experienced for conducting procedures on living animals. Adequate arrangements shall be made for their in-service training, including the proper and humane care and use of laboratory animals.

  IX.   Where exceptions are required in relation to the provisions of these principles, the decisions should not rest with the investigators directly concerned but should be made, with due regard to Principle II, by an appropriate review group such as an institutional animal care and use committee. Such exceptions should not be made solely for the purposes of teaching or demonstration.

Figure 1. U.S. government principles for the utilization and care of vertebrate animals used in testing, research, and training.

support for activities involving animals must comply with the Policy or provide evidence to PHS that acceptable standards for humane care and use of animals will be used in PHS-conducted or supported activities. The policy applies to live, vertebrate animals used in research, research training, experimentation, or biological testing or for related purposes.

MISCELLANEOUS LAWS AND REGULATIONS

Additional laws, regulations, and guidelines may be applicable to particular animal uses when they are funded by private agencies, involve protected species, or are performed to meet the requirements of a regulatory agency. These are not concerned with humane care and use of animals and will not be discussed in this chapter. Examples of these regulations are

- *Good Laboratory Practice (GLP)* Regulations. The U.S. Food and Drug Administration (FDA) published the regulations in 1978 and amended them in 1984 and 1989. They apply to non-clinical studies used to request research or marketing permits preparatory to approval of drugs for human use. They require standard operating procedures, a quality assurance unit, and well documented records.

- *Endangered Species Act* 4 (Public Law 93-205, 1973). The law delegates authority to regulate the importation and use of endangered species to the Fish and Wildlife Service of the Department of the Interior.

- *Marine Mammal Protection Act.* Administered by the Department of Commerce.
- *Food, Drug and Cosmetic Act.* Administered by the FDA.
- *Toxic Substance Control Act.* Administered by the Environmental Protection Agency.

ACCREDITATION OF ANIMAL USE PROGRAMS

Accreditation by the American Association for Accreditation of Laboratory Animal Care (AAALAC) is a voluntary program for institutions that use animals in teaching, testing, or research. Site visits by peers and annual reports submitted by the institution are used to evaluate animal care and use programs and accreditation is granted based on meeting requirements in the *Guide*.

INSTITUTIONAL COMPLIANCE WITH REGULATIONS

REGISTRATION

USDA — Research facilities using regulated animal species must register with the Secretary of Agriculture by submitting a form available from the REAC Sector Supervisor of APHIS. The registration must be signed by the "Institutional Official", who is defined as the individual at the facility, such as the president or chief executive officer, who is authorized to legally bind the institution and commit the institution to meet the requirements of the regulations. It must be updated every three years.[2]

PHS Assurance Statement — In order to apply for PHS grants and contract awards, institutions must have an approved assurance statement signed by the Institutional Official on file with the Office for Protection from Research Risks (OPRR), NIH.[1] The *Guide*[3] should be used as the basis for developing the animal use program and the PHS Policy[1] provides instructions for drafting and submitting the assurance document. The institution must provide assurance either that it is accredited by AAALAC and its IACUC evaluates the program every 6 months, or that its IACUC will evaluate its programs and facilities every 6 months using the *Guide* as a basis for evaluation. An assurance can be approved for up to 5 years.

IACUC

The institution must have an IACUC which is appointed by the Institutional Official.[1-3] It should have not less than five members, including:

- Doctor of Veterinary Medicine with training or experience in laboratory animal science and medicine, who has program responsibility[1-3]
- practicing scientist with experience in research involving animals[2,3]
- non-scientist[1]
- person unaffiliated with the institution other than as a member of the IACUC[1-3]

One individual can serve to fulfill more than one category, for example, the unaffiliated member can also be the non-scientist. Not more than three members can be from the same administrative unit of the facility.[2]

TRAINING

It is the responsibility of the research facility to ensure that all personnel involved in animal care, treatment, and use are qualified to perform their duties. Training and instruction must be made available and qualifications of personnel reviewed by the IACUC.[2,3] Training must include:

- Information on humane methods of animal maintenance and experimentation; handling and care; pre- and post-procedural care; aseptic surgical methods; and the proper use of anesthetics, analgesics, and tranquilizers[1-3]
- Research or testing methods that minimize the number of animals required to obtain valid results or minimize animal distress[1,2]
- Methods to report deficiencies in animal care and treatment[2]
- Special training for people using hazardous agents[3]
- Services available to provide information on appropriate methods of animal care and use, alternatives to use of live animals in research, methods to prevent unintended and unnecessary duplication of research involving animals, and the intent and requirements of the Animal Welfare Act[2]

OCCUPATIONAL HEALTH

An occupational health program is required for personnel having substantial animal contact. In establishing a program, the institution should consider documenting the person's medical history, performing physical examinations, treating bites and allergies, giving appropriate immunization, and monitoring hazardous agent exposure. Zoonosis surveillance for diseases such as tuberculosis, toxoplasmosis, and Q fever should also be considered.[3]

Shower facilities should be available and clean clothing which is not worn outside the facility should be provided. In some situations, accessories such as shoe covers, head covers, safety glasses, or masks may be necessary. It may also be necessary to decontaminate clothing following use. Eating, drinking, and smoking should not be allowed in animal rooms, but separate areas should be provided.[3]

HAZARDOUS AGENTS

When hazardous agents are administered to animals within the animal facility, the institution has a responsibility to develop a safety program to assess hazards and determine necessary safeguards. A biosafety committee should be established to ensure that personnel are properly trained and that the program is in compliance with Federal, state, and local regulations. Animal housing and use should be separated from other areas for the protection of personnel and animals. Use of safety hoods, specialized caging systems, negative air pressure chambers or rooms, air filters, and protective clothing should be considered.[3]

RECORDS

Regulations require that research institutions maintain certain records for a period of at least 3 years after completion of the activity. They must be accessible for inspection and copying by authorized APHIS, OPRR, or Federal funding agency representatives at reasonable times and in a reasonable manner.[1,2] The required records include:

- An assurance statement that has been approved by the PHS.[1]
- Minutes of IACUC meetings.[1,2]
- Applications, proposals, and proposed significant changes in the care and use of animals and records stating whether IACUC approval was given or withheld.[1,2]
- Reports and recommendations, including minority views, of the IACUC's semi-annual evaluation of the animal use program as forwarded to the institutional official.[1,2]
- Records of accrediting body determinations.[1]
- Records of each live dog or cat purchased or acquired, including the name and address of the source and either the USDA license or registration number of licensed or registered sources, or the vehicle license number, driver's license number, and state of an unlicensed or unregistered source. In addition, the records must contain the date of acquisition, USDA tag or tattoo number, identification number or mark assigned by the research facility, and a description of each dog or cat.[2]
- Records of the transport, sale, or disposal of any live dog or cat. The record must include the name and address of person to whom conveyed; the date of transportation, sale, euthanasia, or other disposal; and the method of transportation.[2]
- Individual clinical records for larger animals, including dogs, cats, and non-human primates.[3]

ANNUAL REPORT TO THE USDA

On December 1 of each calendar year, each research facility must submit a report of animal use to the USDA.[2] The report is submitted to the APHIS, REAC Sector Supervisor for the state where the facility is located. It must be signed and certified by the Institutional Official. The report covers the previous Federal fiscal year (October 1 through September 30), and shall:

- Assure that professionally acceptable standards governing the care, treatment, and use of animals were followed.
- Assure that each Investigator considered alternatives to animal use before employing painful procedures.
- Assure that the facility adhered to the Animal Welfare Act and required that any exceptions be specified and explained by the Investigator and approved by the IACUC.
- State the location of all facilities where animals were housed, used, or held for use.

- State the numbers of animals used involving (1) no pain, distress, or use of pain-relieving drugs; (2) pain or distress to the animals for which appropriate anesthetic, analgesic, or tranquilizing drugs were used; (3) pain or distress to the animals for which the use of appropriate anesthetic, analgesic, or tranquilizing drugs would have adversely affected the procedures, results, or interpretation.
- State the numbers of animals being bred, conditioned, or held for use, but not yet used.

SITE VISITS AND INSPECTIONS

USDA — During business hours, APHIS officials can enter registered research facilities to examine records required to be kept by the Animal Welfare Act and USDA regulations.[2] They are authorized to examine facilities, property, or records. They may make copies of the records and document areas of non-compliance by taking photographs and other means. APHIS officials can confiscate and euthanize animals not being used to carry out research, testing, or experimentation and found to be suffering as a result of the failure of the research facility to comply with the provisions of the regulations. The APHIS official must make a reasonable effort to notify the facility of the condition of the animals and request that the condition be corrected. If the facility refuses to comply, the official may confiscate the animal(s) for care, treatment, or euthanasia if in the opinion of the Administrator, circumstances indicate the animal's health is in danger. APHIS inspectors will maintain confidentiality of information and will not remove it from the premises unless there has been an alleged violation.[2]

PHS — Awardee institutions are subject to review, which may include a site visit at any time by PHS staff and advisors in order to assess adequacy or accuracy of the institution's compliance or assurance of compliance with the PHS Policy.[1]

Others — Law enforcement authorities can enter an animal facility to inspect animals and records for the purpose of seeking animals that are missing.[2] However, the authorities must provide a written description of the missing animal and abide by all security measures required by the research facility.

FACILITY DESIGN

Animal facilities should be of smooth, impervious, easily cleaned construction. It is desirable to site them near, but separated from, laboratories and they should be separated from personnel areas such as offices and conference rooms.[3]

Requirements for facilities to perform survival surgery on non-rodent species include a separate surgical suite, surgery support area, prep area for animals, surgeon's scrub area, and recovery area. Rodent survival surgery can be performed in a laboratory that is readily sanitized and not used for any other purpose during the time of surgery.[3]

ANIMAL PROCUREMENT AND IDENTIFICATION

Procurement of all animals must be from lawful sources. Animal quality should be evaluated by quality control data from the vendor and by a health surveillance program to screen incoming animals. An appropriate quarantine and stabilization program should be in place.[3]

Research facilities that obtain dogs and cats from sources other than dealers must hold the animals for 5 full days, not including the day of acquisition, before they may be used by the facility.[2] When imported into the U.S., dogs, cats, and non-human primates are inspected by a PHS quarantine officer at the port of entry. Only those with no evidence of communicable disease can enter the country. Dogs must have a rabies vaccination unless they are less than 3 months old or originate from a rabies-free area. Non-human primates must be free from signs of yellow fever and have departed any yellow fever area at least nine days before entry, have been in a mosquito-proof structure for at least 9 days, or have been vaccinated against yellow fever. Laboratory rodents must be free of ectoparasites and evidence of diseases communicable to humans.[2]

Each dog and cat delivered to an animal facility by a USDA licensed dealer must have an official USDA tag or tattoo and the identification number must be listed in records of purchase, acquisition, euthanasia, or sale. All dogs and cats in a research facility must be identified by a tag, tattoo, or collar which individually identifies the animal by number. The official USDA tag or tattoo affixed to the animal at the time it was acquired may be used or the facility can use its own system. After the animal is euthanized or dies, the research facility shall remove and retain the tag until called for by an APHIS official or for a period of 1 year.[2]

All animals in a facility should be identified individually by number and/or by room, rack, or cage cards. Identifying cage cards should include the source of animals, strain or stock, name and location of investigator, and any pertinent dates, such as birth or arrival.[3]

TRANSPORTATION

Rats and mice are not regulated by the USDA and therefore can be readily imported into the U.S. A courtesy import permit can be obtained from the Administrator of APHIS to facilitate clearance through customs by USDA. Most carriers also require a health certificate executed by a veterinarian.

Dogs, cats, or nonhuman primates transported in commerce must be accompanied by a health certificate executed by a veterinarian, stating that the animal was inspected not more than 10 days prior to transport and appeared to the veterinarian to be free of any infectious disease or physical abnormality which would endanger the animal, other animals, or the public health. The Secretary of Agriculture may provide exceptions on an individual basis for animals shipped for purposes of research, testing, or experimentation when the research facility requires animals not eligible for certification. Requests for exceptions should be sent to the Administrator of APHIS.[2]

Dogs, cats, and nonhuman primates must not be delivered to an intermediate carrier more than 4 hours prior to the scheduled departure of the conveyance vehicle. The consignor must sign and attach to the outside of the primary container a document giving: (1) the consignor's name and address, (2) identity of the animal(s), (3) the date and time the animal(s) were last fed and watered, and (4) certification that the animal(s) were offered water within 4 hours prior to delivery to the intermediate carrier.[2] The animals must not be exposed to temperatures below 45°F (7.2°C) or above 85°F (29.5°C) for more than 4 consecutive hours. Containers must be cleaned and well ventilated, animals housed together must be compatible, and animals shipped by air must be in pressurized cargo space if flying at over 8,000 ft. Animals must be fed at least once every 24 hours (12 hours for dogs and cats under 16 weeks or nonhuman primates under 1 year of age) and watered every 12 hours. The animal(s) must be observed at least every 8 hours.

The intermediate carrier must attempt to notify the consignee of arrival of the animal(s) at least once every 6 hours until notified. If the consignee cannot be notified within 24 hours or if the consignee does not pick up the animal(s) within 48 hours of notification, the carrier must return the animal(s) to the consignor or his designate. The carrier must provide proper care, feeding, and housing until the animal(s) are picked up or returned.[2]

ANIMAL CARE

Institutions using animals are charged with providing for the basic needs of the species being housed. In deciding how to house animals, interspecies and intraspecies disease transmission should be considered, as well as anxiety from housing animals near natural enemies. Generally, housing should provide for physical separation of animals by species and also by source or health status. Group housing should be considered, weighing the potential for transmission of viruses, communal and territorial needs of the animals, and conflict between animals of the same species.[3]

Caging must be of adequate size, be secure, have no sharp edges, and keep the animals clean and dry. Animals should have adequate headroom to stand and be allowed to have normal activity. When bedding is provided, it should be absorbent, uncontaminated, and non-palatable.[2,3]

Cages and utensils must be cleaned and sanitized with sufficient frequency to keep the animals clean, dry, and free from harmful contamination. This means cleaning cages housing rodents 1 to 3 times weekly and cages housing larger animals daily. Solid bottom cages and accessories should be sanitized once or twice weekly by washing in water at 82.2°C (180°F), or by appropriate chemical disinfection. Wire bottom cages should be sanitized every 2 weeks and cage racks, monthly. Cleaning utensils should not be transported between animal rooms. There should be a vermin control program.[3]

Farm animals can be housed in conventional laboratory animal facilities or on suitable farms. When housed on farms, the animals must be maintained in their thermocomfort zone and protected against environmental extremes, of wind, rain, and sun. They must have sufficient space and access to feed and water.[3]

Food should be provided which is palatable, uncontaminated, and nutritionally adequate for the species. It should be stored under conditions and for periods that ensure prevention of the loss of nutritional quality. Animals should also be provided with continuous access to fresh, potable, uncontaminated drinking water.[3] Animal rooms should have adequate ventilation to provide for 10 to 15 changes per hour, keep relative humidity between 40 and 70%, and sufficient temperature control to maintain the animals in their thermocomfort zone. Air should not be recirculated unless it is filtered. In areas where hazardous agents are present, exhaust air treatment may be required. Air pressure in rooms used to house animals is generally adjusted to be positive to hallways, except when used for quarantine, isolation, or hazardous materials use.[3]

Lighting levels should be determined to accommodate the needs of both the people working in rooms and animals being housed. It is recommended that 75 to 100 footcandles (fc) of light be provided for people working in animal rooms. However, 30 fc of light is recommended to prevent retinal damage in albino rodents, so variable intensity controls are often used. Timers are also useful to control light and dark cycles for species requiring a regular diurnal lighting cycle.[3]

Noise should be minimized in laboratory animal facilities. Levels above 85 decibels have been shown to cause hearing loss and other effects. Containment of dog noise is important both for other species being housed and for people in the area.[3]

A plan must be developed and approved by the attending veterinarian to provide dogs with the opportunity for exercise. This requirement can be met for dogs caged individually if they are provided with twice the floor space required for individual housing. It can be met for group-housed dogs by providing at least 100% of the space required if the dogs were housed individually. If a dog has no sensory contact with another dog, it must be provided with positive human contact daily.[2]

A plan must be developed to provide environmental enhancement adequate to promote the psychological well-being of non-human primates housed in research facilities. The plan must address the social needs of the animals and provide for housing with compatible animals when possible. Primary enclosures must provide methods of expressing non-injurious species-typical activities, such as perches, swings, mirrors, etc.[2]

Dogs and non-human primates can only be exempted from these requirements by the attending veterinarian due to considerations of health or well-being, or by the IACUC for scientific reasons set forth in the research proposal.[2]

IACUC COMPLIANCE WITH REGULATIONS

FUNCTIONS

The required functions of the IACUC are as follows:

- To meet not less than annually.[3]
- To inspect all institutional animal facilities and review the institution's program for the humane care and use of animals every 6 months using the *Guide*[1] and the USDA regulations[2] as the basis. The IACUC may use subcommittees of at least two committee members for the inspections and may invite ad hoc consultants to assist; however, no committee member wishing to participate in any evaluation may be excluded.[2]
- To prepare and submit a report of IACUC evaluations to the Institutional Official every 6 months. The report must describe the institution's adherence to the *Guide*[1] and specify departures from provisions of CFR Title 9, Parts 1, 2, and 3.[2] It must describe the reasons for the departures.[1,2] The report must be reviewed and signed by a majority of IACUC members and must contain any minority views.[2] The report must distinguish significant (may be a threat to health or safety of animals as determined by IACUC and Institutional Official) from minor deficiencies. It must have a plan and schedule for correcting each deficiency.[1,2] Any failure to adhere to the schedule that results in a significant deficiency remaining uncorrected shall be reported within 15 days by the IACUC, through the Institutional Official to APHIS and any Federal agency funding the activity.[2]
- To review concerns involving care and use of animals at the institution resulting from public complaints received and from reports of non-compliance received from laboratory or research personnel.[1,2]
- To make recommendations to the Institutional Official regarding the program, facilities, or training.[1,2]
- To review, approve, require modifications in, or withhold approval of activities related to care and use of animals or significant changes (undefined) in ongoing activities.[1-3]

- To be authorized to suspend an activity it previously approved but determines is not being conducted in accordance with the Animal Welfare Act, the *Guide*, the institution's PHS assurance, or as proposed and approved. If the IACUC suspends an activity, it and the Institutional Official must review the reasons for the suspension, take corrective action, and report the action to APHIS, any Federal agency funding the activity, and OPRR.[1,2] The IACUC can suspend an activity only after review of the matter at a convened meeting of a quorum of the IACUC and with the suspension vote of a majority of the quorum present.[2]
- The IACUC is not permitted to prescribe methods or set standards for the design, performance, or conduct of actual research or experimentation.[2]

PROJECT REVIEW

Each animal use activity must be reviewed annually.[2] In reviewing a proposed activity, the IACUC is charged to confirm that the activity conforms with the Animal Welfare Act and is consistent with the *Guide*, unless acceptable justification for departure is presented in writing by the investigator.[1,2] The IACUC must determine that the proposed use conforms with the institution's PHS assurance and that:

- Procedures avoid or minimize discomfort, distress, and pain to the animals. Procedures causing more than momentary or slight pain or distress will employ appropriate sedation, analgesia, or anesthesia, unless justified for scientific reasons by the investigator in writing. Animals that would experience severe or chronic pain or distress that cannot be relieved, will be euthanized.[1,2]
- Living conditions will be appropriate for the species and contribute to their health and comfort.[2] Animals will get proper care and medical attention[1] by a qualified veterinarian.[2] Housing, feeding, and non-medical care of animals will be directed by the attending veterinarian.[2] Use of food or water deprivation to train, work, or otherwise handle animals is discouraged. It must be scientifically justified in writing by the investigator.[2] Personnel conducting procedures are trained and qualified.[1,2]
- Any euthanasia method must be consistent with the recommendations of the American Veterinary Medical Association's Panel on Euthanasia[4] unless departure is justified for scientific reasons in writing by the investigator.[1,2] Procedures should be performed only by trained personnel. Killing should be rapid and painless. Physical methods should be scientifically justified and approved by the IACUC.[3]
- The Principal Investigator has considered alternatives for procedures that may cause more than momentary or slight pain or distress. The Investigator must provide a written narrative description of the methods and sources used to determine that alternatives were not available.[2] The Principal Investigator must provide written assurance that the proposed activities do not unnecessarily duplicate previous experiments.[2]
- When there will be more than momentary or slight distress to the animals, the attending veterinarian must be involved in planning the project.[2]
- Paralytic drugs will not be used without anesthesia with procedures that can cause more than momentary or slight pain.[2]
- Survival surgery must employ aseptic procedures, including sterile surgical gloves, gowns, masks, sterile instruments, and aseptic technique. Major survival surgery (i.e., surgery that penetrates a body cavity or has potential for producing a permanent handicap in an animal that is expected to recover) can be conducted only in facilities intended for that purpose. Minor and rodent surgeries do not require a dedicated facility, but must employ aseptic procedures.[2,3] Field studies do not require a dedicated facility, but must employ aseptic procedures.[2]
- No animal may be used in more than one major operative procedure from which it is allowed to recover unless justified for scientific reasons by the Principal Investigator in writing,[2,3] required as a veterinary procedure to protect the health or well-being of the animal,[2] or under other special circumstances as determined by the APHIS Administrator.[2] Multiple procedures are justified if they are related components of a research project, but cost savings is not an adequate justification.[3]
- Surgery procedures must include proper pre- and post-operative care. Appropriate records should be maintained.[3]
- Handling of animals must be done as expeditiously and carefully as possible in a manner that does not cause trauma, overheating, excessive cooling, behavioral stress, physical harm, or unnecessary discomfort. There can be no physical abuse used to train, work, or otherwise handle the animals.[2] When studies require use of prolonged physical restraint, including the chairing of non-human primates, the restraint must have IACUC approval. Prolonged restraint should be avoided unless essential to the research objectives, and when it is necessary, animals should be conditioned to the restraint apparatus.[3]

The IACUC members must be provided with a list of projects to be reviewed at each meeting and written descriptions must be available. Any member can call for full committee review of any project and approval of such projects can only be granted after review at a convened meeting of a quorum by a majority of the quorum present. A quorum is a majority of the members.[1-3] The IACUC can invite consultants to assist in such reviews, but they cannot vote.[1,2]

If full IACUC review is not called for, at least one IACUC member designated by the chair and qualified to conduct the review, must review and can approve, require modifications in, or request full committee review of the project. No member can participate in review of a project in which she or he has a conflict of interest except to provide information, nor can such a member contribute to a quorum for a vote on that project.[1,2]

The IACUC must notify investigators in writing of results of the review. If approval is withheld, it shall include written notification of the reasons and give the investigator the opportunity to respond.[1,2]

Approved activities and significant changes in ongoing activities can be subject to further appropriate review and approval by the institution, but the institution cannot approve an activity involving care and use of animals unless approved by the IACUC.[1,2]

REPORTING REQUIREMENTS

At least once every 12 months, the IACUC, through the Institutional Official, must report in writing to OPRR whether there are any changes in the institution's program or facilities which would place the institution in a different category than specified in its assurance, in the description of the institution's program for animal care and use, or in IACUC membership. The report must include the dates the IACUC conducted its semi-annual evaluations of the institution's programs and facilities and submitted the evaluations to the institutional official. In addition, the report must provide OPRR with a full explanation of the circumstances and actions taken with respect to any serious or continuing non-compliance with the PHS Policy, any serious deviation from the provisions of the *Guide*, or any suspension of an activity by the IACUC. The report must include minority views filed by IACUC members.[1]

ATTENDING VETERINARIAN AND ADEQUATE VETERINARY CARE

Each animal facility must have an attending veterinarian who is a voting member of the IACUC, has appropriate authority to ensure provision of adequate veterinary care, and oversees the adequacy of other aspects of the animal care and use program. He or she must be certified by the American College of Laboratory Animal Medicine or have training or experience in laboratory animal science and medicine. If the attending veterinarian is employed on a part-time basis, arrangements must include a written program of veterinary care and regularly scheduled visits to the facility.[2]

Each facility must establish and maintain a program of adequate veterinary care that includes the availability of appropriate facilities, equipment, personnel, and services to comply with USDA regulations. There must be appropriate methods to prevent, control, diagnose, and treat diseases and injuries, as well as a mechanism for communication of animal health problems to the veterinarian. The program must provide for daily observation of all animals to assess their health and well-being, as well as emergency, weekend, and holiday care.[2,3]

There should be an appropriate surveillance program that includes quarantine, evaluation of health, stabilization of new arrivals, and isolation of animals with contagious diseases. The program should also include surveillance of any transplantable tumors used.[3]

Guidance must be provided to investigators and other personnel regarding adequate pre- and post-procedural care programs, handling, immobilization, anesthesia, analgesia, tranquilization, and euthanasia of animals.[2,3]

INVESTIGATOR COMPLIANCE WITH REGULATIONS

APPROVAL OF ANIMAL USE

IACUC approval must be obtained prior to using animals in teaching, testing, or research and prior to making a significant change in an approved activity.[1-3] Regulations require that a proposal to the IACUC must contain the following:

- A complete description of the proposed use of the animals.[2] The investigator should ensure that the IACUC is provided with sufficient information to conduct its project review as described above.
- The species and the approximate number of animals to be used. The rationale for using animals in the proposed activity and the appropriateness of the species and numbers of animals to be used.[2]
- A description of procedures designed to assure that discomfort and pain to animals will be limited to that which is unavoidable for the conduct of scientifically valuable research, including provision for the use of analgesic, anesthetic, and tranquilizing drugs where indicated and appropriate to minimize discomfort and pain to the animals.[2]
- Description of any euthanasia method to be used.[2]

PHS AWARD PROPOSALS

In applications for PHS awards involving animal use, the investigator must include the four items listed above that are required for local IACUC approval. In addition, verification of approval of the animal use by the IACUC is required to be submitted to the funding agency within 60 days of the submission of the application. Applications for renewal of awards must state if there are significant changes to the previous application.[1]

LEGISLATION AND REGULATION OF ANIMAL RESEARCH IN CANADA

Canada has no specific Federal legislation relating to the care and use of experimental animals. They employ a voluntary control program with regulation by the local institution. Cruelty to animals is prohibited by Section 402 of the Criminal Code of Canada, and transportation of animals is regulated by the "Animal Disease and Protection Act" of 1975.

CANADIAN COUNCIL ON ANIMAL CARE (CCAC)

In 1966, a study by the National Research Council made recommendations regarding the regulation of experimentation using animals in Canada. The report recommended that regulation of animal use be voluntary and under the control of the local university or research institution. It also recommended that Provincial advisory boards be established to regulate procurement of experimental animals. Some provinces have passed legislation concerned with procurement of animals, including Alberta, Ontario, and Saskatchewan, which give universities the right to use unclaimed dogs from pounds for research. The National Research Council asked the Association of Universities and Colleges to establish the CCAC to serve as an outside advisory body to ensure uniform application of guidelines for the care and use of experimental animals. The CCAC was established in 1968 as a standing committee of the Association of Universities and Colleges of Canada. It is an autonomous, non-governmental advisory and supervisory body charged with making recommendations and improvements in the procurement, production, housing and care of laboratory animals and in the control over experiments involving laboratory animals.

The CCAC is financed by grants from the National Research Council and the Medical Research Council. It has representatives from 16 academic, government, foundation, and industrial agencies, and 2 representatives from the Canadian Federation of Humane Societies. The CCAC has a Secretariat composed of an Executive Director, a Director of Assessments, and Committees. It also has assessment panels.

The CCAC serves as a resource and information center which offers assistance to persons responsible for the care and use of laboratory animals. It has published the two-volume series *Guide to the Care and Use of Experimental Animals*[5] in both French and English. Adherence to this guide is required by all major national funding agencies in Canada. The CCAC also publishes a semi-annual newsletter and periodic information bulletins.

ANIMAL CARE RESOURCES PANEL

The Animal Care Resources Panel is an advisory group made up of professionally trained laboratory animal scientists experienced in laboratory animal care and research working in government and academia. They review programs and advise the CCAC.

ASSESSMENT PROGRAM

The CCAC Assessment Panels consist of scientists from Universities, government, and industry, with representatives from the Canadian Federation of Humane Societies. They perform site visits to research facilities every 3 years to ensure uniformity of nationwide standards. They meet with the local Animal Care Committee and review the animal care and use program. They recommend improvements in the program and submit a report of their findings to the CCAC.

LOCAL ANIMAL CARE COMMITTEE.

Formulation and implementation of policy regarding the care and use of animals in research in Canada is vested in the local institution through the Animal Care Committee. It must, however, respond to the recommendations of the CCAC Assessment Panels. The Animal Care Committee must have senior scientific personnel experienced in the care and use of animals in teaching, testing, and research as well as a veterinarian, biologist, or animal scientist experienced in the care and use of experimental animals. The institution must have a "Director of Animal Care", who has overall responsibility for the care of experimental animals, is an *ex officio* member of the Animal Care Committee, and is directly responsible to the senior administrative official. The institution must ensure that adequate veterinary care is provided. The Animal Care Committee must meet at least annually; and, through the chair or other delegated person, must approve all projects and major changes to projects.

The review must include the ethical aspects of the procedures and the acceptability of methodologies. It must ensure that unnecessary pain is alleviated, personnel are properly trained, adequate veterinary care is provided, and that any euthanasia method is suitable. All facilities, equipment, and care must meet the standards.

The Animal Care Committee is empowered to stop any objectionable procedure and euthanize animals in distress that cannot be alleviated.

GUIDE TO THE CARE AND USE OF EXPERIMENTAL ANIMALS

All applicants for Federal grants involving animals in Canada must indicate that the animals will be cared for in accordance with *The Guide for the Care and Use of Experimental Animals*[5] published by the CCAC. The *Guide* presents principles of ethics to provide guidance for animal experimentation. It also prescribes facility and husbandry standards, health and safety responsibilities, and standards for surgery and anesthesia.

REFERENCES

1. Office of Protection from Research Risk, Public Health Service Policy on humane care and use of laboratory animals. Revised 1986.
2. CFR (Code of Federal Regulations), Title 9; Parts 1, 2, and 3, (Docket No. 89-130). Federal Register, vol. 54, No. 168, August 31, 1989, and 9 CFR Part 3, (Docket No. 90-218). Federal Register, vol. 56, No. 32, February 15, 1991.
3. Committee on the Care and Use of Laboratory Animals of the Institute of Laboratory Animal Resources, Guide for the Care and Use of Laboratory Animals. NIH Publ. No. 86-23, Public Health Service, U.S. Department of Health and Human Services, Bethesda, Maryland, 1985.
4. American Veterinary Medical Association, 1986 report of the AVMA Panel on euthanasia. *J. Am. Vet. Med. Assoc., 188, 252, 1986.*
5. Canadian Council on Animal Care, *Guide to the Care and Use of Experimental Animals.* 2 vols. CCAC, Ottawa, Ontario, 1980-1984.

GLOSSARY OF ACRONYMS

AAALAC	American Association for Accreditation of Laboratory Animal Care
APHIS	Animal and Plant Health Inspection Service (a unit of USDA)
CCAC	Canadian Council on Animal Care
DHHS	Department of Health and Human Services
FDA	Food and Drug Administration
GLP	Good Laboratory Practices (regulations by FDA)
Guide	*The Guide For The Care And Use Of Laboratory Animals*
IACUC	Institutional Animal Care and Use Committee
ILAR	Institute of Laboratory Animal Resources
IRAC	Interagency Research Animal Committee
NIH	National Institutes of Health (a unit under PHS)
OPRR	Office for Protection from Research Risks (a unit in NIH)
PHS	Public Health Service (a unit under DHHS)
REAC	Regulatory Enforcement and Animal Care (a unit of APHIS)
USDA	United States Department of Agriculture

Chapter 4

Good Laboratory Practice

Bodil Lissau

CONTENTS

INTRODUCTION

If your animal studies are of a basic scientific nature, you may think that this chapter on Good Laboratory Practice (GLP) is of no concern to you. In a sense you would be right. Most scientists, however, aim at performing high-quality experiments, so if you are one of them, an overview of these guidelines may be of some help, and will certainly not do any harm, because quality is what GLP is all about.

If, on the other hand, the experimental data you generate in *in vivo* or *in vitro* studies are to be submitted to a governmental authority for the assessment of potential hazards of a chemical, you may already know that you are obliged to comply with GLP, as set down by your national regulatory authorities in legislation governing the particular type of chemical you are working on, whether it is a pharmaceutical (drug), a pesticide, or a food additive.

HISTORICAL BACKGROUND

The history of GLP dates back to the mid-1970s. During a critical assessment of documentation submitted for new drug applications, the U.S. Food and Drug Administration (FDA) found several examples of malconduct and, in some instances, even fraudulence. To examine the matter further, "The Senate Health Committee" was formed in 1974, and in 1976 the FDA launched a "Bioresearch Monitoring Program" employing more than 600 people. A "Toxicology Laboratory Task Force" was set up with the responsibility of assuring the quality of data submitted for new drug applications and for this purpose proposed regulations for GLP.[2,3] The FDA GLP proposals became effective from June 20, 1979.[4]

Subsequently the Organisation for Economic Cooperation and Development (OECD) Principles of GLP were formally recommended by the OECD Council in 1981 for application in Member Countries.[1]

OECD GUIDELINES

PURPOSE

The purpose of the Guidelines is stated as follows:

> "The purpose of these Principles of Good Laboratory Practice is to promote the development of quality test data. Comparable quality of test data forms the basis for the mutual acceptance of test data among countries."

> "If individual countries can confidently rely on test data developed in other countries, duplicative testing can be avoided, thereby introducing economies in test costs (animals) and time. The application of these Principles should help avoid the technical barriers to trade, and further improve the protection of human health and the environment.[1]"

DEFINITION

The Guidelines define GLP as follows:

> "Good Laboratory Practice (GLP) is concerned with the organisational process and the conditions under which laboratory studies are planned, performed, monitored, recorded, and reported.[1]"

Thus, GLP does not describe the "science" of a study; one could say that it is orientated towards the process rather than the product. The underlying philosophy is that by controlling the process by which data are collected, quality can be achieved while allowing for a high degree of flexibilty (scientific judgement and/or innovation) in the design of the study.[2] In other words: if a properly qualified scientist has made clear the aim of the study and the reasons for the choice of animal species and study design, the scientific rationale behind the decision should not come up for discussion in a GLP context.

SCOPE

The scope of the Guidelines is described as follows:

> "These principles of GLP should be applied to testing of chemicals to obtain data on their properties and/or their safety with respect to human health or the environment. Studies covered by GLP also include work conducted in field studies. These data should be developed for the purpose of meeting regulatory requirements.[1]"

Most countries only require GLP for safety studies.

GLP PRINCIPLES ACCORDING TO OECD GUIDELINES

The GLP principles of the OECD guidelines fall under the ten main headings given below. The notes under each heading place special emphasis on the animal work. But anyone whose work in any way involves GLP should study the national regulations closely, as there may be some modifications of the OECD Guidelines, depending on the country, and consequently the regulatory authority to which the data are submitted.

The OECD Guidelines must be followed within the European Communities (EC). Japanese and U.S. guidelines do not differ in essential ways.

TEST FACILITY ORGANIZATION AND PERSONNEL

The management holds the final responsibility for ensuring GLP compliance. An appropriately qualified study director must be appointed for each study and an adequate number of well-trained personnel employed to ensure that the operations are carried out as required.

University laboratories where GLP has not been implemented may face problems with GLP compliance if they work as subcontractors on safety studies. In a case of this kind, it would be wise to leave a decision on the matter to the quality assurance unit of the sponsoring company and the GLP inspectors of the regulatory authorities.

QUALITY ASSURANCE PROGRAM

The test facility must have a documented quality assurance program which should be carried out by a quality assurance unit (QAU) composed of one or more persons that are responsible for monitoring each study to ensure that facilities, equipment, personnel, operations, etc. meet the requirements of GLP. The QAU must check that the protocol and the Standard Operating Procedures (see below) are followed, that raw data are present, and that the final report reflects conclusions drawn from the raw data. The QAU is independent of the study director, reports directly to management, and has to certify that the study has been inspected and that the report has been revised by the QAU.

FACILITIES

The premises and operational units must be of a suitable construction and location and provide an adequate degree of separation of different activities. This means that animals used for different projects must be housed separately and there must be separate facilities for reception of new animals, for storage of feed, for storage and preparation of test substances, for archival purposes, and for waste disposal.

APPARATUS, MATERIALS, AND REAGENTS

Equipment must be appropriate to the function, periodically cleaned, maintained, and calibrated. Qualification and instructions for use of critical apparatus must exist. Reagents must be appropriately labeled (e.g., concentration, manufactoring date, expiry date, initials of technician, etc.).

TEST SYSTEMS

"Test system" refers to "any animal, plant, microbial, as well as other cellular, subcellular, chemical, or physical system or a combination thereof".[1] For instance, in a carcinogenicity test, the test system would be the animals (rats or mice), whereas in an "Ames Test" the test system would be the bacteria.

Suitable conditions, in accordance with current knowledge on animal behavior and welfare and with national regulations on laboratory animal welfare, must be established for housing, handling, and taking care of the animals. Newly received animals must be isolated and acclimatized to the environment before a study is initiated, and records of source, date of arrival, and arrival conditions must be kept. Cages must be furnished with a label identifying the animals inside.

TEST AND REFERENCE SUBSTANCES

Homogeneity and stability of substances must be assured throughout the study. Records, including substance characterization (batch number and concentration), date of receipt, and quantities received and used in studies, must be kept.

STANDARD OPERATING PROCEDURES

The laboratory must have written Standard Operating Procedures (SOPs) covering all phases of standard in-house operations. Procedures mentioned under the headings "Quality Assurance Program", "Apparatus, Materials and Methods" and "Test and Reference Substances" above, procedures for record keeping, data collection, including computerized systems, and reporting belong to this category.

A considerable proportion of SOPs in most *in vivo* toxicology laboratories concern the animals. The following list gives some examples of the contents of animal SOPs:

- *General data on animals* (separate SOPs for each species), e.g., species, supplier, documentation of health status
- *Receipt of animals,* e.g., transportation, health check, quarantine
- *Housing facilities,* e.g., location, cage type; temperature, humidity, and air change (how this is checked and acceptable limits)
- *Randomization of animals,* at receipt and before entering into a study
- *Identification of animals,* e.g., ear tag, tattoo; labeling of cages
- *Approval of animals before entering into a study,* e.g., who examines the animals
- *Food supply,* e.g., manufacturer, supplier, ingredients, quality control, and acceptable limits
- *Water supply*
- *Bedding,* e.g., manufacturer and supplier, quality control, and acceptable limits
- *Cleaning and disinfection,* e.g., animal rooms, cages, water bottles; specification of chemicals used
- *Weighing of animals,* e.g., balance type (special SOP for apparatus), handling of data
- *Dosing of animals,* e.g., orally, intraperitoneally; maximum volumes allowed, needle gauge
- *Blood sampling,* e.g., anticoagulant, equipment

- *Killing and disposal of dead animals,* disposal according to local regulations
- *Necropsy*

PERFORMANCE OF THE STUDY

A written protocol, indicating objectives and methods to be employed, must exist before initiation of the study. Changes are accepted when justified and agreed to by the study director. All data must be recorded directly, promptly, accurately, and legibly, and all entries must be signed and dated.

REPORTING OF STUDY RESULTS

The final report must include all information and data required in the study plan, together with the results, including calculations and statistical methods, and a conclusion.

STORAGE AND RETENTION OF RECORDS AND MATERIAL

Protocols, raw data, reports, samples, and specimens should be retained in archives for a period specified by the relevant authorities.

FINAL COMMENTS

To someone who has never worked with GLP, this system may seem very difficult to comply with. Those scientists who have worked with the system for a number of years still recall the tremendous amount of work it took to implement the system, their own and their colleagues' reluctance to spend time on what they saw as non-productive work, and the reluctance of technicians to cooperate in working out SOPs and finally having to adhere to them. In fact, at the beginning, many people felt that they were under suspicion when the QAU came around to inspect work routines.

Now that GLP has become routine in many laboratories, however, all the advantages of the system have begun to emerge. For example: a laboratory technician need no longer be unjustly accused of giving the wrong compound to an animal, because everything is recorded and a look at the raw data will quickly unravel the matter; when you are asked for details of a particular study several years later the task is easy, because each step has been written down and accounted for.

REFERENCES

1. Decision of The Council concerning Mutual Acceptance of Data in the Assessment of Chemicals. *OECD Principles of Good Laboratory Practice. C(81)30(Final) Annex 2.*
2. Van Houweling, C. D., An overview of Good Laboratory Practices, *Clin. Toxicol., 15, 5, 1979.*
3. U.S. Food and Drug Administration, Non-Clinical Laboratory Studies, Good Laboratory Practice Regulations, *U.S. Federal Register.* Vol. 41, No.225, 19 November 1976, pp. 51206-51226.
4. U.S. Food and Drug Administration, Non-Clinical Laboratory Studies, Good Laboratory Practice Regulations, *U.S. Federal Register.* Vol. 43, No.247, 22 December 1978, pp. 59986-60020.

Chapter 5

Classification of Animal Experiments

Karl Johan Öbrink

CONTENTS

INTRODUCTION

Animal experiments have, throughout history, been a matter of concern for many individuals as well as for society. While some people feel that animal experiments should be abandoned altogether, others are more moderate and accept them but find that certain limitations are necessary. Evidently there exists some kind of gradation or scale distinguishing between different types of animal experiments. They are classified in different ways, e.g., those of immediate application to medical practice as opposed to those performed out of pure scientific curiosity, or those that cause no harm or distress to the animals as opposed to those inflicting a severe strain.

DEFINITION OF ANIMAL EXPERIMENTS BY THE COUNCIL OF EUROPE

In order to classify animal experiments it is necessary to define what an *animal experiment* is. One might think that this would offer no difficulty, but it does politically and judicially. The meaning of *animal experiment* has been thoroughly discussed by the Council of Europe in its preparation of the *European Convention for the Protection of Vertebrate Animals Used for Experimental and Other Scientific Purposes*.[1] In Article 1 of the convention it is stated: "The Convention applies to any animal used or intended for use in any experimental or other scientific procedure where that procedure may cause pain, suffering, distress or lasting harm". Procedure is then defined as "any experimental or other scientific use of an animal which may cause it pain, suffering, distress or lasting harm, including any course of action intended to, or liable to, result in the birth of an animal in any such condition, but excluding the least painful methods accepted in modern practice (that is, "humane" methods) of killing or marking an animal".

Consequently, *in vitro* experiments with organs or cells are not animal experiments according to the European Convention. This definition has a great impact on the statistics concerning the number of animals used for scientific experiments, as a substantial number of laboratory animals will be excluded because they are humanely killed in order to deliver material for *in vitro* experiments on organs or cells. More than 20% of the total number of laboratory animals used belong to this "organ donor" category (statistics from Uppsala University). In some countries these animals are included in their statistics, but in others they are not. It is obvious that in a discussion of the classification of animal experiments it is important whether or not this large group of animals is included. The reasons for including them, however, seem convincing, namely: prior to being killed these animals are treated and cared for in the same way as other laboratory animals. This means that breeding, genetic precautions, husbandry, feeding, microbiological protection, etc. are identical for all animals, whether used for long-lasting experiments or killed at the beginning of an experiment. Consequently, in the following text all work with laboratory animals, also with those killed for organs or cells, are included in the discussion of the classification of animal experiments.

0-8493-4378-X/94/$0.00+$.50

THREE WAYS OF PERFORMING ANIMAL EXPERIMENTS

Laboratory animals are used for biomedical research in acute experiments, in chronic experiments, and as organ donors. Acute experiments are usually those where the animals are anesthetized, the experiments carried out under anesthesia, and the animals killed while still unconscious at the end of the experiment. These procedures should not cause pain or distress.

In chronic experiments the animals either survive a surgical procedure under anesthesia as an introduction to further use and observation for some varying length of time, or they are investigated directly without sedation (the most common type). The experiments may vary from simple observations of the animal's behavior to procedures involving significant distress or discomfort.

Many of the chronic experiments will cause few or no ethical problems, whereas others may give rise to serious concern. Evidently experiments involving a severe burden to the animal must always be thoroughly planned and the animals cared for especially well. These experiments place a heavy responsibility not only on the researchers but also on the caretakers and animal departments to provide optimal husbandry. No efforts must be spared in trying to improve the experimental techniques so as to minimize pain and distress.[2]

In donor experiments the animals are anesthetized or humanely killed and organs or tissues are removed for experimentation. Provided the animals are properly handled they experience no pain or distress. "Donor experiments" are, in fact, "acute" experiments. It would be practical and recommendable to categorize them as such, were it not for the fact that "donor experiments" are not considered "animal experiments" by the Council of Europe if the animals have been killed prior to removal of the tissue.

CLASSIFICATION OF EXPERIMENTS ACCORDING TO THE DEGREE OF HARM TO THE ANIMAL

Most ethical judgements follow the utilitarian principle, i.e., a comparison between the degree of cost (pain or distress inflicted on a sentient creature) and the value of the expected results, in other words a cost-benefit evaluation. The social benefit derived from animal experiments may be evident but difficult to quantify. A scale for costs can, however, be established. An example is a scheme worked out by E. Bárány in the late 1970s for the Swedish Medical Research Council[3] consisting of the following five groups:

1. Experiments which, with or without surgery, are expected to cause only negligible pain or agony (injections, blood sampling, tube feeding, behavioral experiments without significant restraint of the animal, anesthesia to make the animal manageable)
2. Experiments carried out on anesthetized animals which do not recover from anesthesia (blood pressure measurement, removal of organs for histological or biochemical investigation or experiments on surviving organs or parts of organs)
3. Experiments involving painful stimulation of unanesthetized animals which cause the animal short-lasting light pain, or operations carried out under general or local anesthesia, after which the animal recovers or experiences the cessation of the action of the analgesic (behavioral experiments with flight or avoidance reactions, exposure of blood vessels, implantation of chronic catheters, simple central nervous system lesions, extensive surgical operations, burns)
4. Experiments on unanesthetized animals of whom some can be expected to become seriously ill or suffer significant pain or agony (toxicity testing, production of radiation sickness, certain infections, stress and shock experiments, production of pain clearly above the threshold level, behavioral experiments with significant restraint of the animal, e.g., fixation)
5. Experiments on unanesthetized and curarized animals (certain physiological and pharmacological experiments on the nervous system)

This scale system was taken up by the United States for their "Animal Use and Care Committees" and today has the following classification,[4] which seems useful for many purposes:

Category A: Experiments involving either no living materials or the use of plants, bacteria, protozoa or invertebrate animal species (studies on tissues from slaughter-house or embryonated eggs)

Category B: Experiments on vertebrate animal species that are expected to produce little or no discomfort (holding animals, injections, blood sampling, acute experiments (according to the definition above), standard methods of euthanasia)

Category C: Experiments that involve some minor distress or discomfort (short-duration pain) to vertebrate animal species (exposure of blood vessels or implantation of chronic catheters under anesthesia, behavioral experiments on awake animals that involve stressful restraint, food/water deprivation for short periods, and surgical procedures under anesthesia that may result in minor post-surgical discomfort)

Category D: Experiments that involve significant but unavoidable distress or discomfort to vertebrate animal species (deliberate induction of behavioral stress in order to test its effect, major surgical procedures under anesthesia that result in significant post-operative discomfort, induction of an anatomical or physiological deficit that will result in pain or distress, application of noxious stimuli from which escape is impossible, prolonged periods of physical restraint, induction of aggressive behavior leading to self-mutilation or intra-species aggression, painful procedures in which anesthetics are not used, toxicity testing with death as an end point, production of radiation sickness, pain approaching the pain tolerance threshold)

Category E: Experiments that involve inflicting severe pain near, at, or above the pain tolerance threshold of unanesthetized conscious animals (use of muscle relaxants or paralytic drugs without the use of anesthetics, severe burn or trauma infliction on unanesthized animals, attempts to induce psychotic-like behavior)

The gradation according to degree of harm to the animals may be a practical tool for promoting and evaluating "refining" of experimental procedures, "refining" being one of the three Rs in the definition of "Alternative Methods".[2] "Refining" means an improvement of the experimental procedure so as to minimize the possible distress and suffering of the animals.

CLASSIFICATION ACCORDING TO PHYLOGENESIS

The phylogenetical classification of animals is reflected in most animal protection laws. All regulations include the vertebrates, whereas invertebrates are usually not protected by law. This is a result of classifying animals in higher and lower species, where higher animals are those with the best-developed associative brain function or those with the largest brain cortex. This classification of laboratory animals reflects the conviction that higher animals are more likely to suffer than lower ones. There is no doubt that people are more concerned about experiments on higher animals than on lower ones. However, also among higher animals like mammals, people care more about certain species than others. Apart from cost problems, apes and monkeys are not used unless absolutely necessary from a scientific point of view. Similarly, experiments on pets, especially dogs and cats, are frequently avoided. This is due to irrational feelings more than logical thinking, as experiments on pigs, rabbits, and other highly developed animals are more easily accepted. This is also one of the reasons why small rodents are the most used species today. Consequently the choice of animal species is mostly a result of compromise. In theory scientific judgement should be decisive, but in practice several other variables outweigh it, e.g., availability, cost, lowest possible phylogenetic species, and public concern.

Life sciences are concerned not only with the intact animal but also with the function of its organs and cells.[5] A full understanding of life mechanisms necessitates research on every level of biological organization. No level can be a substitute for another. Biomedical science covers the span from molecules to intact organisms, and biomedical researchers study at all these levels. Even though the material used in cell biology and molecular biology originates from living animals (or man), the ethical problems of these experiments are much smaller than of those related to work with whole animals. However, several shortcomings of the work with the expression of foreign genes in isolated cells and cell cultures may be overcome by studying the cell functions in the intact body, and this has led to the creation of transgenic animals.

FUNDAMENTAL AND APPLIED RESEARCH

A common classification of animal experiments is according to scientific purposes:

1. To search for new knowledge
2. To diagnose diseases

3. To test new therapeutic techniques and new medicines
4. To detect and analyze drugs, hormones, and other biological compounds
5. To produce and test vaccines, sera, and other biological compounds
6. To test for toxicity, carcinogenicity, and teratogenicity of new and old drugs and chemical compounds

Other systems of categorization may differ in details; in the European Convention groups 3–5 are conjoined into one group, and in other instances experiments are categorized into further and slightly deviant groups, e.g., in the statistics of Great Britain.[6] Besides using animals for the above purposes, laboratory animals are also used in teaching.

Several kinds of experiments mentioned above aim at immediate application of the results. Tests of new drugs are good examples of applied research and so are safety tests for side effects of drugs and chemicals. Search for new knowledge, however, may have no apparent or immediate application. The experiments are entirely aimed at increasing our level of understanding. Experience tells us, however, that these experiments, which are called fundamental or basic research, are the most important for later practical developments. For instance, in a detailed investigation into the most spectacular advances in the treatment of heart-lung disorders, it was shown that the advances mostly resulted from fundamental research, of which more than 50% was carried out without any application in mind and was certainly not intended for use in heart-lung therapy.[7] The recognition of basic research as a prerequisite for biomedical progress is vital in ethical evaluations of animal experiments for the very reason that inexperienced laymen may not always realize the beneficial effects of such experiments when applying the utilitarian principle to their judgements.

We may, however, condense the six categories of animal experiments above into the following two groups:

1. Fundamental or basic research (number 1 above)
2. Manufacturing and testing (numbers 2 to 6 above)

The reason for using this condensed form of classification is its usefulness in discussing "alternative methods" and more precisely the component "replacing".[2] In order to be able to replace an animal experiment with some other technique, basic biological knowledge must first be available. For instance, it would not be possible to detect a carcinogenic effect in a cell culture if we did not already know what a cancer cell looks like. It would not be possible to produce a vaccine in a cell culture if we did not already know which compound and which properties we were looking for. If, however, a biological problem is approached for the first time, and it is formulated so that the question may be answered by means of an animal experiment, there can theoretically be no alternative to the animal experiment that would not change the basic question.

REFERENCES

1. Council of Europe, No 123, *European Convention for the Protection of Vertebrate Animals Used for Experimental and Other Scientific Purposes*, Strasbourg, 1986.
2. Russel, W. M. S. and Burch, R. L., *The Principles of Humane Experimental Technique*, Charles C. Thomas, Springfield, IL, 1959.
3. Öbrink, K.J., Swedish law on laboratory animals, In *Scientific Perspectives on Animal Welfare*, Dodds, W.J. and Orlans, F.B., Eds., Academic Press, New York, 1982, 55.
4. Orlans, F. B., Classification system for degree of animal harm, *Scand. J. Lab. Anim. Sci.*, 13, 93, 1986.
5. Smyth, D.H., *Alternatives to Animal Experiments*, Scolar Press in association with the Research Defence Society, London, 1978.
6. Home Office, *Statistics of Scientific Procedures on Living Animals*, Great Britain. The Government Statistical Service, Cm 1574, Her Majesty's Stationery Office, London, 1990.
7. Comroe, J. H. and Dripps, R. D., Scientific basis for the support of biomedical science, *Science*, 192, 105, 1976.
8. Öbrink, K. J., Basic research in physiology and pharmacology; some introductory remarks, in *Animals in Biomedical Research: Replacement, Reduction and Refinement: Present Possibilities and Future Prospects*, Hendriksen, C. F. M. and Koëter, H. B. W. M., Eds., Elsevier, Amsterdam, 1991, 79.

Chapter 6

Laboratory Animal Science and Service Organizations

Otto Kugelberg and Lars Wass

CONTENTS

0-8493-4378-X/94/$0.00+$.50

INTRODUCTION

The expansion of biomedical research after World War II resulted in a rapid increase in the use of laboratory animals. Much pioneer work was done within the field and associations or federations for laboratory animal science were formed.

Demands for healthy and later on genetically and microbiologically defined animals, education and training of scientists and technicians, housing and care of the animals, and relations to antivivisectionists were issues that early became main interests in the associations.

Laboratory animal science is a young discipline created to help the users of animals and therefore it has been the intention to stress the science/service combination.

INTERNATIONAL COUNCIL FOR LABORATORY ANIMAL SCIENCE; ICLAS

ORGANIZATION AND MEMBERSHIP

ICLA, the International Committee on Laboratory Animals, forerunner of ICLAS, was founded in 1956 in Paris. Today ICLAS is formed by national members, scientific members, and union members. A general assembly is convened every four years. The governing board (GB) consists of the President, the Vice-President, the Secretary General, the Treasurer, and five representatives from the national members, two from the scientific members and one from the union members.

AIMS

According to its constitution the aims of ICLAS are

- To promote and coordinate the development of laboratory animal science throughout the world
- To promote international collaboration in animal science
- To promote quality monitoring and definition of laboratory animals
- To collect and to disseminate information on laboratory animal science
- To promote the humane use of animals in research through recognition of ethical principles and scientific possibilities

MEETINGS

International scientific meetings are organized by a national member or a regional scientific member in connection with an ICLAS general assembly every fourth year. Regional scientific meetings are organized by local scientists in connection with GB meetings. Other meetings of ICLAS experts may also occur irregularly.

PUBLICATIONS

The *ICLA (ICLAS) Bulletin* was published twice yearly from 1957 to 1990. Today ICLAS informs via the newsletter *ICLAS News* from its sectretariat.

Over the years ICLAS has also been responsible for many different publications, such as special reprints, guidelines and recommendations, proceedings of scientific meetings, manuals, etc.

SCHOLARSHIPS

ICLAS has always been very much oriented towards establishing laboratory animal science in developing countries. A number of individual training scholarships have been created, making it possible for students from developing countries to carry out studies, mostly in the U.K. and Germany.

There are also student travel fellowships for young scientists to support active participation in scientific congresses and Visiting Expert Scientist Scholarships to provide training on the spot in developing areas.

GENERAL COMMENTS

Further information about ICLAS is available through Prof. Osmo Hänninen, Secretary General, Dept. of Physiology, University of Kuuopio, P.O. Box 1627, SF-70211 Kuopio, Finland.

48

AMERICAN ASSOCIATION FOR LABORATORY ANIMAL SCIENCE; AALAS

ORGANIZATION AND AIMS

The American Association for Laboratory Animal Science, AALAS, was founded in Chicago in 1950. AALAS is an organization of individuals, affiliated organizations, and approximately 45 branches that carry out the program of AALAS at the local level. The purpose of AALAS is the improvement of animal care and use through education and information exchange. One of the aims of AALAS is to collaborate with analogous organizations throughout the world and currently has members appointed as liaison to both the Federation of European Laboratory Animal Science Associations (FELASA) and ICLAS.

MEMBERSHIP

AALAS has approximately 6000 members, including:

- scientists who design and conduct biomedical research
- clinical veterinarians who supervise the care of animals
- animal technicians or technologists who monitor the animals' health and provide daily care
- representatives of companies that sell products and services used in laboratory animal facilities
- educators who train animal caretakers, technicians, and related personnel
- research and animal care and use program administrators

MEETINGS

The AALAS Annual Meetings are the world's largest gatherings of people concerned with producing, caring for, and studying laboratory animals.

PUBLICATIONS

AALAS supports its educational objectives by publishing two journals: *Laboratory Animal Science (LAS),* and *Contemporary Topics in Laboratory Animal Science.* In addition, the AALAS Bulletin section advises members about upcoming meetings and activities, provides information about AALAS programs, and gives updates on other issues related to laboratory animal science. AALAS publishes and distributes technician training manuals and instructional guides which are the basis for preparing applicants for the certification examination.

The *Guide for the Care and Use of Laboratory Animals,* a document identifying proper animal care, was conceived as an AALAS project and is now sponsored by the National Institutes of Health.

GENERAL COMMENTS

To help ensure the quality of the care and handling of laboratory animals, AALAS administers a certification program for the technicians and technologists who provide direct animal care. The AALAS Animal Technician Certification Program certifies three levels of knowledge: Assistant Laboratory Animal Technician, Laboratory Animal Technician, and Laboratory Animal Technologist. An AALAS program for voluntary accreditation of laboratory animal facilities in the United States and Canada is now conducted by a separate sister organization, the American Association for the Accreditation of Laboratory Animal Care (AAALAC).

The address of AALAS and of the LAS editorial office is AALAS, 70 Timber Creek Drive, Suite 5, Cordova, TN 38018.

AMERICAN COLLEGE OF LABORATORY ANIMAL MEDICINE; ACLAM

ORGANIZATION

The officers of the American College of Laboratory Animal Medicine are President, President-Elect, Immediate Past President, and Secretary-Treasurer. They are elected by the ACLAM Diplomates via mail ballot and serve for one year.

Standing committees exist for Credentials, Examination, and Nominations. Other committees are appointed if necessary to accomplish the aims and implement the policies of the College.

AIMS

The American College of Laboratory Animal Medicine was founded in 1957 for the following reasons:

- To encourage education, training and research in laboratory animal medicine
- To establish standards of training and experience for veterinarians professionally concerned with the care and health of laboratory animals
- To recognize qualified persons in laboratory animal medicine by certification examination and other means

It is a specialty recognized by the American Veterinary Medical Association (AVMA). The basic policies and concepts of the College have not changed since its formation. The testing and certification of qualified veterinarians in this specialty continue to have the highest priority.

MEMBERSHIP

Membership is open to all veterinarians who are graduates of a college or school of veterinary medicine accredited or approved by the AVMA, or who possess an Educational Commission for Foreign Veterinary Graduate (ECFVG) certificate, or are qualified to practice veterinary medicine in some state, province, territory, or possession of the United States, Canada, or other country; have satisfactory moral character and impeccable professional behavior; and have been certified as Diplomates in accordance with Article II of the bylaws.

Diplomates: Diplomates are those veterinarians who have satisfactorily completed the prerequisites prescribed by the constitution and bylaws of the College. They have fulfilled the experience and training requirements; have contributed to the advancement of knowledge in some aspect of laboratory animal medicine; have satisfactorily completed the certifying examination; and have been elected to membership by a majority of the Board of Directors of the College.

Retired Members: Permanently retired Diplomates, upon request, may be removed from active Diplomate status and placed on the retired roster. Retired members do not have the right to vote and are not required to pay dues.

Honorary Members: Individuals who have made outstanding contributions to laboratory animal medicine may be elected to honorary membership. Honorary membership is not limited to veterinarians. The College now numbers over 430 Diplomates.

EDUCATIONAL PROGRAMS AND PUBLICATIONS

ACLAM has been actively involved in continuing education for its members and other interested scientists since its formation. ACLAM conducts a semi-annual continuing education forum and various symposia on different topics to keep Diplomates informed of new discoveries and innovations in laboratory animal medicine. ACLAM also has programs for postdoctoral education in laboratory animal medicine. The purpose of these programs is to provide broad basic training for veterinarians desirous of teaching or studying laboratory animal medicine or acting as professional directors of laboratory animal facilities.

In addition, a series of autotutorial materials has been sponsored by ACLAM for veterinarians, biomedical scientists, students, and technicians. The educational endeavors have also resulted in a great number of handbooks and other scientific papers in laboratory animal medicine.

GENERAL COMMENTS

Additional information about postdoctoral education, etc. may be obtained from the ACLAM Secretary-Treasurer: Charles W. McPherson, American College of Laboratory Animal Medicine, 200 Summerwinds Drive, Cary, NC 27511.

CANADIAN ASSOCIATION FOR LABORATORY ANIMAL SCIENCE; CALAS

ORGANIZATION

The Canadian Association for Laboratory Animal Science (CALAS) was originally founded in 1962 as the Canadian Society for Animal Care. CALAS is composed of individuals and institutions concerned with the care and use of laboratory animals, including veterinarians, physicians, researchers, administrators, technicians, and others interested in the proper care and use of animals in research, teaching, and testing.

Committees are formed to manage specific areas of concern, such as education, membership, promotion, publication, and convention. As an extension of the Association members are encouraged to form

Regional Chapters with their own administrative officers, bylaws, and activities, for promoting regional advancement of good standards of animal care.

AIMS

The Association is dedicated to the elimination of inhumane and unnecessary use of animals in research and to the improvement of their standard of care.

The aims can be summarized as follows:

- To advance the knowledge, skills and status of those who care for and use laboratory animals
- To improve the standards of animal care and research
- To provide a forum for the exchange and dissemination of knowledge of sound animal care and research

MEMBERSHIP

CALAS membership is at several levels, as follows: *Institutional Membership* is intended for institutions that are concerned with the care and use of laboratory animals and wish to participate in efforts to improve the scientific quality of animal research and the educational standards of animal care personnel. The organization obtaining such membership is issued two membership cards for named representatives who carry full National Membership rights. In addition, one copy of each issue of *Laboratory Animal Science* magazine is forwarded, as are copies of the *CALAS Newsletter* and announcements from CALAS.

National Membership in the National Association carries full voting rights and the entitlement to be elected to the Board of Directors or selected as an *ex officio* member of the Board. There is also an option to purchase a subscription to *Laboratory Animal Science,* the journal of AALAS. Each National member receives the bimonthly issues of the *CALAS Newsletter.*

MEETINGS

Each year CALAS hosts a national convention in a different part of Canada to provide a forum for the exchange and dissemination of knowledge in the areas of sound animal care and research. Technical papers and workshops are complemented by exhibits mounted by commercial firms to display their products. The Annual General Meeting is held at the National Convention, giving voting members of the organization a chance to discuss CALAS business.

PUBLICATIONS

Every member of CALAS receives a bimonthly newsletter which is intended to keep members informed of CALAS events and to provide information on pertinent topics. The newsletter also includes scientific and technical articles presented at annual CALAS conventions, as well as articles on continuing education. All members are encouraged to submit items of interest to the newsletter editor and Regional Chapters are expected to contribute by advising of current events in their areas.

EDUCATION AND EDUCATIONAL PROGRAMS

The Education Council of CALAS is concerned with all aspects of education pertaining to the field of laboratory animal science. To advance the knowledge and skills of those who care for and use laboratory animals, the Education Council of CALAS has established a Registry for Laboratory Animal Technicians. The Registry represents a national standard for Canada. The Registry uses as it base graduation from a recognized formal program in animal health/care/science/technology, combined with practical experience in a laboratory animal facility.

GENERAL COMMENTS

Various awards are presented annually in conjunction with the national convention. Further information about CALAS and membership can be obtained from the CALAS National Office: c/o Dr. Donald McKay, Executive Secretary, CALAS, M524 Biological Science Building, Bioscience Animal Service, University of Alberta, Edmonton, Alberta T6G 2E9, Canada.

JAPANESE ASSOCIATION FOR LABORATORY ANIMAL SCIENCE; JALAS

ORGANIZATION AND MEMBERSHIP

The Japan Experimental Animal Research Committee founded in 1951 became the Japan Experimental Animal Research Association in 1980, and the name was changed to the Japanese Association for Laboratory Animal Science (JALAS). The organization consists of 15 to 20 directors, including one president and five managing directors, 2 auditors, and 50 to 100 trustees. There are 1680 regular members, 145 organizations as supporting members, and 1 honorary member.

AIMS

The aims of JALAS are to contribute to the development of laboratory animal science and related academic fields by means of publication of basic and applied research, exchange of knowledge, and supply of information on laboratory animals.

MEETINGS

A General Meeting is held once a year and the Board of Directors meets twice a year.

PUBLICATIONS

The *Bulletin of the Experimental Animals,* published since 1952, became *Experimental Animals* in 1968. It is the official publication of JALAS. It is published quarterly and has titles, summaries, and some papers in English.

GENERAL COMMENTS

Further information about JALAS can be obtained from The Director, T. Nomura, Central Institute for Experimental Animals, 1430 Nogowa, Miyamae, Kawasaki 216, Japan.

INSTITUTE OF ANIMAL TECHNOLOGY; IAT

ORGANIZATION AND AIMS

The Institute of Animal Technology was formed in 1965 and was originally named the Institute of Animal Technicians. The aims of the Institute are

- To advance and promote excellence in the technology and practice of laboratory animal care and welfare
- In furtherance of these objectives, alone or in collaboration with others, to issue books, journals, slides, films, video and audio tapes, and other means of communication, to organize lectures and meetings, to mount and accredit courses and examinations, to establish and maintain registers of those professionally engaged in the care and management of animals used for scientific and educational purposes, to give evidence to select committees concerned with welfare and well-being of laboratory animals, and by grant, scholarship or other bursaries assist in training, both nationally and internationally
- To form branches in the United Kingdom or wherever deemed necessary, who under supervision of the Council would promote the Institute's objects locally

MEMBERSHIP

The main activities of the Institute are education and examination of animal technicians. Members and Fellows of the Institute are eligible to apply to be entered into a Register for Animal Technicians. This involves a serious interview before members of the Board of the Institute, and the applicant has to agree to abide by the "code of conduct". Registered animal technicians may use the letters R.An.TECH. in addition to M.I.A.T. or F.I.A.T. after their name.

MEETINGS

Since 1965 there has been an annual three-day IAT Congress during the Easter vacation that is hosted in turn by the Universities of England, Scotland, and Wales. There is also a one-day symposium in September each year, and workshop meetings are envisaged.

PUBLICATIONS

The Institute publishes a journal, *Animal Technology*, a bulletin, and training material. *Principles of Animal Technology I,* leading to the first examination of the Institute has replaced the early IAT Manual. Parts II and III leading to the higher examinations are in preparation. The Institute has produced videos dealing with the handling of and the techniques used on laboratory and farm animals.

EDUCATION

Courses leading to the Institute's examinations take place in many colleges and elsewhere. The examination qualification system is outlined below.

The Certificate in Animal Technology is taken after one year of part-time study. Students who achieve in the Animal Technology components and attend but do not succeed in the background science are awarded the Certificate in Animal Husbandry. The Membership Examination (MIAT) is taken after a further two years of part-time study. The Fellowship Examination (FIAT) is taken after another two years of part-time study.

Under preparation are also the Post-Graduate Diploma in Animal Technology (one year part time), a Master of Science Degree (M.Sc.) in Animal Technology and Management (a further two years part time), and by extension of the project unit of the M.Sc., the degree of Doctor of Philosophy (Ph.D.).

GENERAL COMMENTS

Further information on IAT is available through Dr. K.G. Millican, Chairman of IAT. Registered Office: 5, South Parade, Summertown, Oxford OX2 7JL, U.K.

LABORATORY ANIMAL SCIENCE ASSOCIATION; LASA

ORGANIZATION AND AIMS

LASA was founded in 1963 by scientists and technologists from industry, universities, ministries, and research councils. LASA, which has just over 400 members, is the only U.K. organization for senior workers in all aspects of laboratory animal science — provision, care, and use. It represents British interests in Europe through FELASA and worldwide through ICLAS.

The aims of LASA are

- To share with other professionals the difficulties inherent in using laboratory animals
- To improve knowledge of the latest and best methods
- To make personal contributions to progress by presenting papers to meetings, by taking part in discussions, and by publishing papers in its journal

MEMBERSHIP

Detailed information is available from the Membership Secretary at the LASA Registered Office: 20 Queensberry Place, London SW7 2DZ, U.K.

MEETINGS

The main scientific meetings of LASA consist of a one-day meeting in the spring and a two-day residential meeting in the autumn or winter, at various loocations in the U.K. Within LASA, there are four Scientific Sections for the discussion of specialist interests: animal health and nutrition; management; pathology; toxicology and safety evaluation. These Sections each meet once or twice a year.

PUBLICATIONS

LASA Newsletter, which is sent free to members, contains notices of forthcoming meetings, reports on conferences, news items on the animal science field throughout the world, and correspondence from members.

Laboratory Animals is published quarterly. Its scope is original papers, reviews, and short articles on all aspects of laboratory animal science, technology, and education. LASA now shares *Laboratory Animals* as its official journal with the corresponding German and Dutch associations. Since the journal is provided to the three associations at a greatly reduced price, LASA is able to include the cost in its membership fee. The address of the registered office of Laboratory Animals Ltd. is the same as that of LASA.

Special study groups are often set up to prepare guidelines. One has recently published guidelines on "The assessment and control of the severity of scientific procedures on laboratory animals" (Laboratory Animals (1990), 24, 97-130) and another is formulating guidelines on the transport of laboratory animals. Two more groups are working on guidelines for the education and training of those working with laboratory animals. In connection with the Animals (Scientific Procedures) Act 1986, LASA contributed significantly to guidelines that were subsequently used by the Home Office as the basis for its "Code of Practice on the care and housing of laboratory animals". LASA has also published, with the Universities Federation for Animal Welfare (UFAW), further guidelines on "Surgical procedures" (1989) and "Planning and design of experiments" (1990).

In addition, LASA has recently established the practice of inviting major U.K. bodies to workshops on issues of current interest. Recent workshops have dealt with education and animal health monitoring.

GESELLSCHAFT FÜR VERSUCHSTIERKUNDE — SOCIETY FOR LABORATORY ANIMAL SCIENCE; GV-SOLAS

ORGANIZATION AND MEMBERSHIP
Representatives from different interest groups within the laboratory animal field in West Germany decided to form this society for Laboratory Animal Science in 1964. Today GV-SOLAS has about 500 members from many European countries, mainly from central Europe. Full membership of GV-SOLAS applies only to university graduates. The General Assembly elects the Governing Board, which also has an Advisory Board.

Important activities of GV-SOLAS are the working parties for hygiene, for standardizing the methods for maintenance of laboratory animals, and for nutrition and feeding.

AIMS
The aims of GV-SOLAS are to:

- Produce standardized methods for maintenance and care of laboratory animals that accord with the welfare and well-being of the animals
- Optimize the experimental conditions for animal experiments
- Ensure the performance of animal experiments according to medical, biological, and animal welfare principles

MEETINGS
The General Assembly of GV-SOLAS is held yearly in connection with its scientific meeting. Every third year the scientific meeting can be combined with the FELASA symposium.

PUBLICATIONS
GV-SOLAS has no journal of its own, but it shares *Laboratory Animals* with the English and Dutch associations. The journal is distributed free to the members.

The results of the working parties (see above) are usually published in a series of reports, *Veröffentlichungen*. Up till now 12 reports have been published. Most of them are edited both in German and English.

Widely used by, but not linked to, GV-SOLAS is the *Journal of Experimental Animal Science*, (until 1991 known as *Zeitschrift für Versuchstierkunde*). This journal publishes original articles, short communications, and reviews related to comparative medicine and experimental animal science. The address of the editor is Dr. H. J. Hedrich, Zentralinstitut für Versuchstierzucht, Hermann-Ehlers-Allee 57, P.O. Box 910345, D-W-3000 Hannover 91, Germany.

GENERAL COMMENTS
Awards may be given by GV-SOLAS for studies in the furtherance of laboratory animal science. The address of GV-SOLAS is c/o Dr. U. Märki, Institut für Biologisch-Medizinische Forschung (B.R.L.Ltd), Wölferstr. 4, CH-4414 Füllinsdorf, Schweiz.

SCANDINAVIAN FEDERATION FOR LABORATORY ANIMAL SCIENCE; SCAND-LAS

ORGANIZATION AND MEMBERSHIP

To establish laboratory animal services in the northern European countries a federation was formed in 1970 with board members from Denmark, Norway, and Sweden. Today the federation has about 400 members, mainly from Denmark, Norway, Finland, and Sweden. Membership is open to everyone working within the laboratory animal field.

AIMS

The aims are to increase knowledge of laboratory animal science and service among the members. To achieve this Scand-LAS has established working parties on education, health monitoring, and pain, stress and discomfort.

MEETINGS

A symposium is held every year in connection with the general assembly. Following a fixed order, Denmark, Norway, Finland, and Sweden are the host countries for these meetings.

PUBLICATIONS

Scand-LAS publishes a quarterly journal, *Scandinavian Journal for Laboratory Animal Science,* with papers on basic and applied laboratory animal science. The journal is sent free to the members of Scand-LAS. The address of the editorial office is c/o Margareta Bertram, National Food Agency, Mörkhöj Bygade 19, DK-2860 Söborg, Denmark.

EDUCATIONAL PROGRAM

Scand-LAS has contributed to the production of a number of audiovisual programs, including slides, texts, and tapes about the handling of and basic techniques used on different species of laboratory animals. A number of computerized educational programs are being produced.

GENERAL COMMENTS

The address of the Scand-LAS Secretariat is c/o Barbro Salomonsson, MFR, P.O. Box 7151, S-10388, Stockholm, Sweden.

SOCIÉTÉ FRANCAISE D'EXPÉRIMENTATION ANIMALE; SFEA

ORGANIZATION AND MEMBERSHIP

The Société Francaise d'Expérimentation Animale, SFEA, was founded in 1972. In 1982 it merged with ATAL (Association des Techniciens d'Animaux de Laboratoire, founded in 1970) under the name of "SFEA". In 1992 the Association counted about 800 members: scientists, laboratory and animal technicians, specialists in laboratory animal science, breeders, and suppliers. In 1986 the SFEA created a "daughter association" called GEFA (Groupe des Eleveurs et Fournisseurs d'Animaleries/Breeders and Animal House Suppliers Association).

The Association is a member of FELASA and is a permanent member of ICLAS.

MEETINGS

The association organizes two annual national meetings: a three-day scientific meeting (usually in the spring), and a one-day technical meeting (usually in the autumn).

PUBLICATIONS

The Association publishes four regular issues a year of its journal, *Sciences et Techniques de l'Animal de Laboratoire*, STAL, plus additional special issues.

GENERAL COMMENTS

The SFEA Prize is awarded each year at the Scientific Meeting to a student or professional in recognition of his/her work. The office of SFEA is at: Centre d'Expérimentation Animale et de Recherches Chirurgicales,

Université de Paris, Val de Marne, Faculté de Médecine, 6 rue de Général Sarrail, 94010 Créteil cedex, France.

NEDERLANDSE VERENIGING VOOR PROEFDIERKUNDE; NVP

ORGANIZATION AND AIMS

The Nederlandse Vereniging voor Proefdierkunde (NVP; Dutch Association for Laboratory Animal Science) was founded in 1971. NVP is a scientific society with the aim to promote a responsible use of laboratory animals in biomedical sciences.

Through working groups an opinion is formulated on subjects like housing and care of laboratory animals, surgical interventions, assessment of discomfort, anesthesia, euthanasia, etc.

MEMBERSHIP

In 1992 NVP had about 200 members. Everybody who sympathizes with the aims of NVP may become a member. Membership includes a subscription to the journals *Biotechniek* and *Laboratory Animals*.

MEETINGS

NVP organizes national symposia/meetings in the spring and the fall for its members and other persons interested in the field of laboratory animal science.

PUBLICATIONS

NVP is a co-publisher of the scientific journal *Laboratory Animals*. Information on issues dealing with laboratory animal science is also published in the Dutch journal *Biotechniek*.

GENERAL COMMENTS

The address of NVP is Dr. J. Ritskes-Hoitinga, Secretary NVP, Unilever Research Laboratory Vlaardingen, P.O. Box 114, 3130 AC Vlaardingen, The Netherlands.

BELGIAN COUNCIL FOR LABORATORY ANIMAL SCIENCE; BCLAS

ORGANIZATION AND MEMBERSHIP

The Belgian Council for Laboratory Animal Science, BCLAS, was founded in 1970. Today the association is composed of a little more than 100 ordinary members, plus sponsoring and honorary members. The council of the Society is composed of 20 members from universities, scientific institutions, and pharmaceutical firms. BCLAS is a member of FELASA.

AIMS

The aims of the association are included in the statutes. They are

- To promote and to develop the proper use of laboratory animals in scientific research and education
- To better the understanding of the ethics and legislation within this field
- To develop the relations between the different branches of laboratory animal science
- Through symposia, working groups, courses, exhibitions, etc., to regularly exchange all kinds of information about laboratory animals
- To encourage research into and promote knowledge about laboratory animals

MEETINGS

During the last four years BCLAS has organized four symposia on problems related to laboratory animals, e.g., in Brussels in 1992 on the topic: New Animal Models and Alternative Methods.

EDUCATION

BCLAS has organized courses for animal technicians and for animal caretakers.

GENERAL COMMENTS

BCLAS has organized working groups on problems related to laboratory animals, with the main interest upon education, health, pathology, alimentation, and ethical problems. The present address of the BCLAS secretariat is J. Vankerkom, VITO, Départment de Biologie, Boertang 200, B-2400 Mol, Belgium.

COMITATO ITALIANO PER LE SCIENZE DEGLI ANIMALI DE LABORATORIO; CISAL

ORGANIZATION

Since 1991 Comitato Italiano per le Scienze degli Animali de Laboratorio (CISAL; Italian Committee for Laboratory Animal Science) has been the official Italian member of FELASA. The Italian Committee is a dual organization, in which GISAL, the Italian Group for Laboratory Animal Science, joins forces with AIMAS, the Italian Association for Experimental Animal Models.

AIMS

Since its foundation in 1986 GISAL has been working to improve the knowledge and skills of people working with laboratory animals. The main aims are

- To improve the quality of use of animals in biomedical research so as to meet international standards and guidelines
- To educate and up-date researchers, students and technicians in the field of laboratory animal sciences, through educational programs at all necessary levels
- To promote and coordinate contacts with parallel organizations working in Italy, Europe, and the United States

MEETINGS AND EDUCATION

Since its foundation GISAL has organized a number of minisymposia, study days, and basic and advanced courses in laboratory animal science and technology.

PUBLICATIONS

GISAL has published proceedings of the mini-symposia and study days, a teaching manual for the basic course and a textbook on ethical, scientific, technical, and legislative aspects of the use of laboratory animals. All publications are in Italian.

GENERAL COMMENTS

The address of the CISAL secretariat is A. Guaitani, GISAL Coordinator, Istituto di Ricerche Farmacologiche "Mario Negri", Via Eritrea 62, 20157 Milano, Italy.

SCHWEIZERISCHEN GESELLSCHAFT FÜR VERSUCHSTIERKUNDE; SGV

ORGANIZATION AND MEMBERSHIP

Eligible as ordinary members in the Schweizerischen Gesellschaft für Veresuchstierkunde (SGV), Swiss Laboratory Animal Science Association are persons who hold appropriate qualifications in biological, veterinary, or medical sciences or who, by their experience and attainments, qualify as respected specialists in laboratory animal science. Eligible as institutional members are persons or organizations intending to support the activities of the association. SGV is a member of FELASA.

AIMS

SGV was founded in 1987 and aims at promoting laboratory animal science and furthering animal protection and ethical considerations in animal experiments by organizing education and the flow of information within the scientific community. The association represents the views of its members vis-à-vis the authorities and the general public, and cooperates with other scientific associations both in Switzerland and abroad.

MEETINGS AND EDUCATION

An annual scientific meeting is organized, usually together with the Swiss Union of Societies for Experimental Biology, as well as a two-day training course on a selected topic.

PUBLICATIONS

An informal Newsletter appears twice a year; the official journal of the association is *Laboratory Animals*.

GENERAL COMMENTS

Each year the association awards a prize to a young scientist for an outstanding contribution to laboratory animal science in the field of Russel and Burch's "3Rs". Further information may be obtained from the secretary of SGV: Mr Ludwig Ullmann, RCCF, Landstrasse 33, 4452 Itingen, Switzerland.

UNIVERSITIES FEDERATION FOR ANIMAL WELFARE; UFAW

ORGANIZATION AND AIMS

The Universities Federation for Animal Welfare was founded over 65 years ago. It is concerned with the welfare of all animals. UFAW adopts an objective and realistic approach to animal welfare by looking at the behavior and needs of animals, making rational judgments based on the facts available, and giving expert advice on how particular species should be cared for and managed. UFAW accepts that animals are used in scientific experiments, taking the view that "the three Rs" of animal experimentation should be applied.

The Federation holds annual symposia and occasional workshops; carries out and sponsors scientific research into many aspects of the biology and welfare of farmed, companion, wild, zoo, and laboratory animals; produces standard texts on animal care and management, and publishes technical reports on animal welfare matters.

PUBLICATIONS

UFAW has been particularly concerned with the housing and breeding of laboratory animals. The *UFAW Handbook on the Care and Management of Laboratory Animals* is regarded by many as the standard work in the field.

UFAW has recently established a scientific quarterly journal *Animal Welfare*; bringing together original research and technological advances in the field, it acts as a focus and output for research. The journal also accepts critical reviews and interpretative articles concerned with the subjects of animal welfare.

GENERAL COMMENTS

In 1992 UFAW founded the International Academy of Animal Welfare Sciences (IAAWS) to promote humane treatment of animals on a global scale. Further information on UFAW can be obtained from the Secretary, UFAW, 8 Hamilton Close, South Mimms, Potters Bar, Herts EN6 3QD, U.K.

FEDERATION OF EUROPEAN LABORATORY ANIMAL SCIENCE ASSOCIATIONS; FELASA

ORGANIZATION

FELASA was founded in 1978 by GV-SOLAS, LASA, and Scand-LAS. It was later joined by NVP, SFEA, BCLAS, CISAL, and SGV. FELASA has a Board of Management consisting of two authoritative representatives from each constituent association. The Board of Management elects from its members a President, a Vice-President, a Secretary, and a Treasurer.

AIMS

The objects of the Federation are

- as an international body to represent common interests of constituent associations in the furtherance of all aspects of laboratory animal science by:

- coordinating the development of education, animal welfare, health monitoring and other aspects of laboratory science in Europe by such means as meetings, study groups and publications
- acting as a focus for the exchange of information on laboratory animal science among European states
- establishing and maintaining appropriate links with international or national bodies as well as other organizations concerned with laboratory animal science
- promoting the recognition and consultation of FELASA as the specialist federation in laboratory animal science and welfare throughout Europe
- promoting a triennial joint scientific meeting of constituent associations

ACTIVITIES AND POLITICAL ROLE

Within Europe, FELASA sees as its role not only to respond rapidly to EC and Council of Europe developments, but also to guide the thinking of these bodies by offering them timely and authoritative advice. In a wider context, FELASA is strengthening its links with laboratory animal science in the U.S. and Canada and is also looking at developments in this field in Eastern Europe. With the purpose of establishing a common European standard for laboratory animals, working parties for education, health monitoring and pain, stress and discomfort have been formed.

In November 1991 FELASA achieved observer status in the Council of Europe for the sector of laboratory animals.

MEETINGS

Triennial joint scientific meetings are arranged by the member societies.

GENERAL COMMENTS

The address of the present secretary of FELASA is Dr. V. Baumans, Rijksuniversiteit Ütrecht, Bureau Proefdierkundige, Postbus 80.166, 3508 TD Ütrecht, the Netherlands.

Chapter 7

Allergy to Laboratory Animals

Steinar Hunskaar and Richard T. Fosse

CONTENTS

INTRODUCTION

Allergy to laboratory animals (ALA) is a well-known occupational disease in personnel engaged in work with these animals. Several authors have reviewed this topic.[1-8]

Allergic or hypersensitivity reactions can be divided into four types — types I, II, III, and IV.[9] Type I reactions (immediate reactions) are predominant in allergy to laboratory animals. This type of reaction occurs most frequently in individuals who are predisposed to develop increased amounts of immunoglobulin E (IgE) class antibodies in response to antigenic stimuli. Common examples of this reaction are hay fever, urticaria, and asthma. People who have a hereditary predisposition to IgE reactions are said to be atopic. The mechanism of atopy is based on the fact that atopic persons have a hereditary disposition to produce IgE. They have a much greater risk of developing specific allergic diseases, but also to react "hypersensitively" to many different irritants, for example cigarette smoke.

Employees in biomedical research laboratories come into contact with organic material from the animals in many ways. Injections, testing, training, operations, killing, feeding, or blood sampling are examples of tasks where a person will be exposed to allergens. Allergens from animals have traditionally been generally mentioned as fur, hairs, or dander. These allergens are present in most urine-contaminated organic waste materials from the animals, and to some extent, because of circulation, in tissues. Using modern immunological techniques it has been possible to characterize the allergens. In mice, the main allergen is a urine molecule, possibly prealbumin. Serum albumin is also an important allergen candidate.[10-12] In rats, serum albumin, α_2-globulin, and prealbumin are the predominant allergens.[12] There is no significant cross-reaction between species,[2,12-14] but cross-reactivity between strains seems likely because of an almost identical structure of proteins.[14,15] The allergens are present in hair, skin, feces, urine, and other material from the animals when measured by skin-prick tests.[7] This probably reflects the fact that allergenic serum proteins are present in organic material from the animals and that urine proteins will be found due to contamination. Air in laboratory rooms will also show a significant loading of allergens.[16,17] In conclusion, the allergens are widespread wherever the animals are kept, and it is not possible to be in contact with the animals without having contact with allergenic material.

EPIDEMIOLOGY

PREVALENCE: HOW MANY HAVE ALA?

Pooled data from the studies of 4988 persons at risk indicate a prevalence of ALA of about 20%.[7] Some of the studies do not distinguish between different species, and some record allergy to "small laboratory animals". The studies are heterogeneous according to how the population is defined, but we think they represent the best studies available.

INCIDENCE: THE RISK OF GETTING ALA

The median time for development of ALA suggests that 50% of the persons who will subsequently develop ALA, do so within less than two years.[7] There is great variation in exposure time in the persons investigated and also great variation in the length of the period before allergy is clinically present. Some experience almost immediate reactions, while others may have contact with the animals for 15 to 20 years before they react.[18-23]

In one report, a one-year incidence of ALA was determined in all individuals who entered employment to work with laboratory animals during a two-year period. One hundred and forty-eight persons entered the study. Five reported the development of allergic symptoms within one year of employment and another 17 reported symptoms at an anniversary interview, giving a total incidence of 15%. The overall incidence of asthma specifically due to ALA was 2% or one of seven (14%) of those with symptoms.[24] In another study, 383 individuals occupationally exposed to rodents and rabbits were examined during their first three years of exposure at the research facilities. These people were assigned to one-year cohorts and symptoms were graded according to severity. In the first year, the total incidence of symptoms was 28%, 12% had mild, while 16% had moderate or severe symptoms. A maximum was reached in the second and third years of the study, when 37% of the employees got ALA during their first year of employment.[25]

Lutsky et al.[26] studied the severity of symptoms ranging from mild (rhinitis) to severe (asthma). This study revealed that the prevalence of asthma was significantly higher among laboratory animal house workers, compared to a matched control group. However, there seems to be a greater prevalence of ALA among scientific personnel than among animal handlers.[2]

One well-designed study found a significant relationship between ALA and smoking.[27] If the association proves true, smoking cessation could reduce the development of ALA. Employers could offer education and courses on stopping smoking not only because of health in general, but for specific occupational reasons.

Atopy defined from personal history or by skin prick tests increases susceptibility to ALA. These results have important implications for pre-employment screening. There has been some suggestion that atopic persons should be excluded from working with animals,[28-30] while others claim that too many atopics never develop ALA.[31] The exclusion of about one third of the population from employment would therefore not be justified. However, some subgroups may be defined and the answers need not be the same for all positions, persons, or types of atopy.

WHAT IS THE REAL RISK OF GETTING ALLERGY?

An applicant to a position where contact with laboratory animals is part of the work, expects to be given a clear answer to the headline question. The answer is neither quantitative (% risk) or qualitative (great/ little). We must first know something about the working conditions. From the incidence and prevalence studies we can say that there is a general risk of about 10–15% of getting ALA within the first year of employment. Two percent could get asthma each year. The prevalence is about 20%. The median time (the time span until half of those who will get ALA have actually got it) is less than two years. However, these numbers were collected some years ago when modern ventilation and equipment were not frequently used. In new buildings with good animal rooms and a clean working environment, the risk is possibly less.

Second, we must know something about the job. Although exposure per se does not influence the risk, persons with different jobs seem to be at different risks.[22,26,28,32-34] Third, we must know something about the person. Is there a family history of allergy? Does the person have a personal history of allergic disease? Does he or she smoke? Does he or she react hypersensitively to irritants or smoke? Is there enough information to diagnose the applicant as atopic, and by which definition?

Based on collected information an answer to the question of the personal risk may vary from slight to large. Whether or not the person has been tested or screened prior to employment, each applicant has the right to know his/her estimated risk of getting ALA.

CLINICAL MANIFESTATIONS

SYMPTOMS

For practical reasons we shall consider three groups of symptoms: eye and nose symptoms, chest symptoms, and skin manifestations. Eye and nose symptoms are characterized by rhinoconjunctivitis with red and itching eyes, sneezing, nasal stenosis or watery discharge, and a strong feeling of irritation. The main chest symptom is bronchial obstruction or asthma with periodic wheezing sounds, cough, mucoid sputum and dyspnea. Skin rashes are either general or contact urticaria.[35] In the general form itching wheals occur all over the body. In contact urticaria the wheals occur only at the contact area, usually on the face, hands, and underarms.[36] Occasionally angio-neurotic edema occurs. The symptoms develop very shortly after exposure. In a series of 102 cases inhalation of allergens produced symptoms immediately or within 5 minutes in 71% and within 10 minutes in 95% of the workers. Anaphylactic reactions with severe systemic effects like hypotension and shock seem to be an extremely rare manifestation of ALA.[37]

SYMPTOM DISTRIBUTION

Eye and nose symptoms are the most frequent; some studies report that every person with ALA experiences rhinoconjunctivitis.[19,21] Immediate-type asthma and skin reactions are less common, about 40% of patients develop such symptoms. Rhinoconjunctivitis is found in 53–100%, asthma in 13–71%, and skin reactions in 13–70%.[7] The pooled data, however, give a rather consistent picture of symptom distribution. Of 10 persons with ALA, 8 will have rhinoconjunctivitis, 4 will have asthma, and 4 will have urticaria.[7] When prevalence studies are performed in a "steady-state" population of persons exposed to laboratory animals, some patterns of overlap are found. These patterns are results of the sequence of development, the risk of getting each allergic manifestation, and the selection of workers that endure working conditions despite their illness. Figure 1 describes the symptom overlap as pooled from two well-performed studies.[32,34]

SYMPTOM SEVERITY

The symptoms of ALA may be experienced very differently by different people. Slight discomfort can be the result of rhinorrhea or nasal congestion. Bronchial obstruction and asthma can be experienced as an unbearable condition accompanied by fear and frustration.

DIAGNOSIS

The diagnosis of ALA is mainly clinical. A proper history will identify an allergic disease. The physician must look for the connection between allergic symptoms and contact with the specific allergens. The type of allergic reaction and the symptom group(s) the patient belongs to should be identified by history in typical cases. For therapeutic purposes only this may be enough, but as medico-legal aspects often will be involved, examinations and laboratory tests should also be performed.

In rhinoconjunctivitis, a profuse watery nasal discharge and nasal obstruction, together with conjunctival infection, may be observed. In bronchial asthma, a hyperresonant percussion note and pathological breath sounds may be noticed, together with prolonged expiration. Urticaria is easily recognized.

Pulmonary function tests are indicated when bronchial obstruction is suspected. The tests can also be used to determine whether, and to what extent, it can be relieved by drugs. The tests thus have an important place in the diagnosis.

Skin prick tests with allergenic material may be performed, mainly by dermatologists and allergologists. Physicians can send blood for determination of specific IgE antibodies against commercially available highly purified mouse or rat allergens. More than 60% will be positive by immunoassay. Almost all asthmatic individuals react positively.

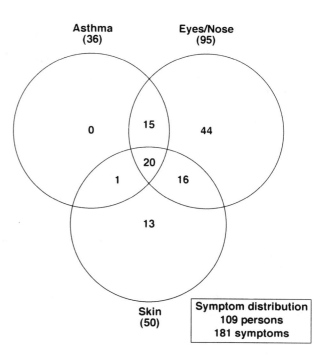

Figure 1. Symptom overlap and frequency among 109 persons with ALA, having 181 symptoms. All numbers refer to the number of persons with the actual symptom. (Reproduced from Hunskaar, S. and Fosse, R.T., *Lab. Anim.*, 24, 358, 1990. With permission.)

PROGNOSIS

Medical consequences of rhinoconjunctivitis or urticaria in itself are few or absent. No long-term complications or lasting injury are expected, but side effects from treatment may occur. Subclinical but significant bronchospasm remains for days to weeks after an acute attack of asthma. However, the long-term consequences of asthma are few, but may be serious. There is no evidence that it leads to permanent pulmonary parenchymal damage in the form of chronic bronchitis or emphysema. While the overall mortality for all forms of asthma is less than 0.1% per year, the rate increases markedly (2–4%) for patients with episodes of status asthmaticus. These remarks presuppose that the allergen has been identified, that any known allergens or irritants have been avoided when possible, and that the condition has been properly treated.

The social consequences of ALA are many and affect quality of life. Some persons are forced to resign and perhaps leave an occupation they like and for which they are qualified. For those who endure working, daily symptoms, effects of drugs or the use of personal protection may, in some cases, reduce well-being only slightly, but for many people this can reach unacceptable levels. The endurance threshold varies considerably between individuals and, as such, is subjective and cannot be predicted.

MEDICAL THERAPY

Avoidance of exposure by removal of an ALA sufferer from the animal environment results in a fairly rapid recovery from symptoms. As discussed elsewhere in this chapter this preferred action is in many cases not possible. However, depending on the severity of symptoms, many are able to continue their working if provided with adequate personal protection. Medical therapy will often be appropriate for those who want to continue working with animals. Drugs are, however, palliative measures only. Drugs can also be used as prophylaxis. Use of antihistamines, theophylline, and maintenance bronchodilator therapy can help curb the frequency and severity of attacks. Likewise topical steroid therapy is efficacious. Cromolyn sodium is a unique and important prophylactic agent that works by preventing degranulation of mast cells. Allergic rhinitis may be treated with intramuscular depot injections of steroid. A single depot injection has a prolonged duration of action that may produce benefits for a period of up to three months.[8] Such injections should be avoided, however, because of the high risk of side effects when the need for therapy is chronic. It may be a good choice for seasonal rhinitis, or for persons with short periods of exposure only.

PERSONNEL ISSUES

The health and safety issues which require clarification cover personnel matters such as recruitment policy, pre–employment selection, health screening, and the working practices of the staff. Companies should have a general policy statement on this subject which includes attitude to pre–employment selection and medical screening, medical surveillance during employment, relocation and dismissal. There is a general responsibility to provide information to all relevant people at a place of work, that they might risk developing ALA as a consequence of work. This information should cover the basic facts about prevalence, symptoms, protection, reporting procedures, screening, investigation and management and may also refer to policy on issues such as relocation. Table 1 describes an education program that is offered to employees at the University of Bergen in Norway.

Individuals who already have allergic symptoms from exposure to animals, including pets, are more susceptible to ALA, and these people should be assessed by a physician regarding their suitability for work with laboratory animals. Where there is a history of allergy to relevant laboratory animals or where candidates are suffering from chronic skin diseases or asthma, consideration should be given to recommending rejection. Monitoring of exposed staff is advisable at annual intervals. Health surveillance protects the health of individual workers and assists in evaluation of control measures. Early detection of ALA will enable precautionary measures to be adopted, and may prevent progression to severe symptoms. In many countries regulations do not require employers to provide health surveillance for non–employees (e.g., students and some researchers), but in higher education or research facilities, these non–employees may be exposed in the same way as employees and may constitute a major part of the exposed persons. In these circumstances it is recommended that employers should voluntarily extend their health surveillance schemes to cover such non–employees.

The employee should report any symptoms of ALA, if necessary in confidence, to the employer, the safety representative and/or the occupational health department. It should be kept in mind that in many cases it is possible to reduce the severity of symptoms by a combination of precautionary measures and, should needs be, limiting exposure to particular species or procedures. Table 2 lists several precautionary measures that should be considered when planning a policy for an individual with recently developed ALA.

THE ROLE OF THE LABORATORY ANIMAL FACILITY MANAGER

The facility manager with responsibility for the building and its activities, will play a major part in identifying potential problem areas. A person in contact with most of the different categories of staff engaged in the facility will be able to play a role in information and giving advice. The manager can recommend prophylaxis and, if necessary, take action in the event of allergy developing in an individual. The manager should plan all work routines that could be associated with the development of allergy, and can institute protective measures together with the institution's safety/medical service. He or she will also serve in an advisory capacity to the institution's safety/medical service in the event of relocation and should preferentially participate in pre-employment interviews, since first contact plays an important role in the type of information that a person receives and his/her subsequent motivation for the job.

ANIMAL HOUSE PLANNING

The design of buildings housing laboratory animals is an important element in attempts to reduce the incidence of allergy in persons working with these animals. There is a general consensus of opinion that certain measures will reduce exposure and thereby contribute to an improvement in symptoms in afflicted individuals, or possibly reduce the incidence to a minimum.

One of the problems associated with evaluating building design is that there is relatively little evidence that specific building (ventilation or architect design) systems actually protect from allergy. There is a general assumption that ventilation design contributes to reductions in particle counts and thereby leads to less allergy (particle counts are related to the level of development of allergy), but there is little published evidence regarding the significance of the various forms of technology. Despite the development of complex technology aimed at reducing allergy, sooner or later individuals will inevitably be exposed to allergens in the course of their work with animals and allergy will result in some of them. It is possible to measure the levels of environmental allergens using radio allergo sorbent test (RAST)

Table 1. The Contents of an Education Program Given Yearly at the University of Bergen, Norway

1. Facts about ALA, including prevalence, symptoms and medical treatment
2. Demonstration of prick and patch testing
3. Lung function testing
4. Atopy
5. Working routines in the animal facility
6. How and where to seek medical advice
7. Where to obtain and how to use personal protecting clothing
8. How to use control measures
9. Details of health surveillance arrangements
10. Legal rights
11. Worker's compensation

Table 2. Precautionary Measures to be Considered for an Individual with ALA

1. Limit the hours of exposure
2. Withdraw the individual from those procedures most likely to put him/her at risk
3. Use respiratory protection and other personal equipment
4. Use a safety cabinet where possible
5. Increase periodic monitoring to assess the efficacy of protective measures
6. Monitor any possible progression of the disease
7. Assess periodically to determine continuing fitness for work

technology.[38,39] Such measurements reveal that there are variations in antigen concentration at different times of the day and associated with differing work operations.[16,17,40] There is, however, a lack of documented correlation between antigen concentration and the effectiveness of the various ventilation systems studied and the incidence of allergy or symptom severity.

Apart from design considerations directed to animal housing, care must be taken to include facilities that contribute to reductions in exposure when not directly working with animals. These should include adequate washing and showering facilities that are located within the animal unit. Change rooms should be provided with lockers specifically designed to reduce contamination of everyday clothing. Cage cleaning and bedding management should be done in dedicated areas. These areas should be provided with specific ventilation extractor systems. Offices and rest rooms (lunch room, meeting/seminar rooms) should be segregated from areas in which animals are handled or experiments with animals carried out.

Table 3 shows various factors that should be taken into consideration when planning an animal house.

PERSONAL PROTECTIVE EQUIPMENT

The primary objective should always be that building and room design coupled to working routines should be seen as the first line of defense against ALA. Personal protective measures should only be relied upon after these measures have failed or an individual has developed signs of ALA. The use of personal protective equipment can be divided into two categories, general protection consisting of general hygiene (hand washing) and specific equipment (face masks, overalls, gloves, shoe covers).

PROTECTIVE CLOTHING

Most modern laboratory animal facilities require personnel to use special clothing while working in the facility. The objective of this is to prevent microbiological contamination of the animals within the facility. The type of clothing will vary according to the degree of protection required and may consist of full surgical clothing with gown, cap, mask, and shoe covers to conventional changes of laboratory coat. The design of protective clothing is important. Coat or coverall arms should be designed such that allergens are not trapped inside the arm surface, thereby increasing the risk of contact urticaria on the forearm. Clothing arms should be closed by an elastic hem or other suitable closure mechanism. Alternatively, coverall arms should be rolled back so as to allow personnel to wash both hands and

Table 3. Factors that Influence the Animal House Environment

General principles Animal rooms should be ventilated so that the flow of allergens towards the workers is reduced. There should be a slight negative pressure in the animal room in relation to the outer-lying corridor or adjacent procedure rooms unless special stock protection requirements dictate otherwise. Recirculation of extracted air should be avoided. Interleading doors, doors to animal rooms and personnel areas should be kept closed to prevent the spread of allergens, and facilitate correct and efficient operation of the ventilation system.

Air humidity There is a negative correlation between the relative humidity in an animal room and the number of particles suspended in the air. A high relative humidity will reduce the effect of static charges on dust particles. Animal room humidity should be maintained at 50% ± 10% (relative humidity). Increased relative humidity may induce fungal growth on wall surfaces and in the ventilation system.

Air changes General reductions in particle counts have been achieved by increasing the rate of room air exchange to above 15 changes per hour, in a room in which animals are kept in open caging.

Cleaning routines Human activity will increase free particle counts during the day. Forced ventilation systems will tend to produce air currents and draughts which aerialize particles and increase contamination, while passive diffusion ventilation systems will permit particles to remain on surfaces and thereby be available for cleaning. Cleaning should usually be performed by means of moist mopping or vacuum cleaning. Centralized vacuum units should be used and not vacuum cleaners that blow exhaust air into the room.

Ventilation design Attempt to reduce the flow of particles directed from the animal or dust-laden air zone of a room towards the worker. Provide a clean (cleaner) air working zone for the worker. Direct air gradients away from the worker towards the animal. In rooms with plastic curtains hung in front of the animal racks, workers will stand in the center of the room in a stream of filtered clean air and draw back a narrow opening in the curtaining when working with the animals. In rooms with perforated walls air is drawn from the room into the wall for extraction, ensuring even distribution of air throughout the animal room. Depending on design, particles will inevitably collect behind the perforated section, representing a risk when cleaning and renovating.

Filter management The placement of inlet and outlet filters plays an important role. Modern room ventilation systems specify individual outlet filters for each room and in a large animal facility there will be a considerable number of filters that need maintenance. Service staff (engineering/ventilation) can be exposed to high levels of allergens. Filters should be withdrawn into sealable plastic containers as a new filter slides in to replace the old one, thereby protecting the operator.

Ventilated cabinets Ventilated cabinets draw filtered air into a closed cabinet (Figure 2). Filtered exhaust air is extracted from the cabinet. The efficiency of such cabinets is maintained as long as the cabinet remains closed. The filters themselves will represent a significant source of allergens when changed. Ventilated cubicles or ventilated racks with individually ventilated cage placement are other forms of ventilated caging. Efficiency drops significantly as soon as the cage is removed from its place in the rack.

Filter hoods Filter hood systems allow housing of animals in cages that are individually covered by hoods or caps that contain filter material. Air passes through the cap, while particles are retained (Figure 3). The filter represents a concentrated source of allergens. Symptoms in allergy sufferers are effectively prevented as long as the animals remain in the cage under the filter hood and the cage is not opened. Such cage hoods could be combined with clean bench technology. Cage changes could be performed in air-flow benches. Filter caps for cages can be used when animals are removed from dedicated animal rooms and are kept in laboratories or other working areas.

Down-ventilated benches In down-ventilated benches air flows past the operator and passes though a perforated bench plate placing the animal in an airstream that passes away from the operator (Figure 4). The efficiency of the perforated surface is dependent on the velocity of the air that passes through. The efficiency of the system can be enhanced by extracting all the exhaust air of the room through the bench. High air-flow rates past the animal must be weighed against cooling and possible hypothermia of the animal.

Other factors The entire building should be designed so that surfaces are accessible and finished and cleaning is facilitated. Rough surfaces (unfinished concrete) should be avoided wherever possible.

Data presented in this table are collected from Hunskaar and Fosse.[7,8]

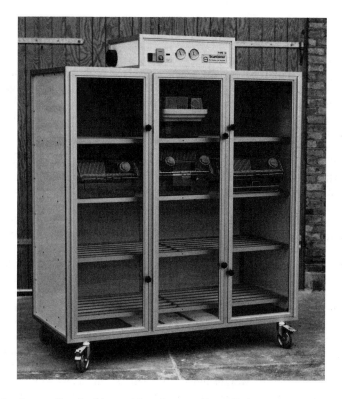

Figure 2. An example of a ventilated cabinet with an integrated ventilation system and built-in filters. (Picture supplied by Scanbur ApS.)

forearm. The role played by clothing in the transport of allergens has been demonstrated by analyzing allergen particles in school rooms. Here one finds significant concentrations of cat, dog, and small rodent (guinea pig and hamster) allergens, which must have been carried in on the clothes worn by school children.[41-43] Clothing will subsequently be handled by other personnel (laundry staff, porters) and they must be considered as potential candidates for allergy.

VENTILATED HELMETS

Air-stream respirator helmets have been shown to alleviate occupational asthma due to ALA.[44] Several types of ventilated masks and helmets have been developed in which filtered air is delivered to the operator. A major drawback with this type of helmet is that it does not easily facilitate working close up to the animal (surgery, microscopy, etc.). Adequate filter changing procedures must also be taken into account, since the filter itself will represent a major source of allergens.

FACE MASKS

When working in animal facilities, it is not uncommon to see users wearing paper or synthetic textile surgical masks primarily designed to protect the surgery subject from contamination and not allergy. Such masks should be avoided. A more efficient tool would be the use of fine dust masks used in spray painting which cover the nose and mouth in a tight-fitting, face-conforming design. The drawback is that fitted face masks are uncomfortable to use over extended periods of time.

PERSONAL HYGIENE

Closely connected to the use of protective clothing, face masks, shoe covers and hoods is the role played by personal hygiene in the spread of allergens and degree of personal exposure. Persons who work with animals may often choose to work without gloves and it is not common practice for animal caretakers and technicians to use gloves when handling animals or changing cages. This is not advisable seen from an allergological viewpoint. If gloves are used, care must be taken to ensure that allergens do not contaminate the skin by entry via the open arm end of the glove or through puncture holes. The material

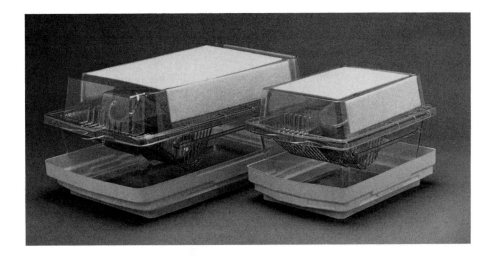

Figure 3. An example of a filter hood used in conjunction with standard macrolon rat or mouse cages. (Picture supplied by Scanbur ApS.)

used in gloves may in itself be allergenic. It is also common to wash hands repeatedly during the course of a working day. Care must be taken to prevent small skin fissures from developing, since these will increase the risk of allergen exposure and contribute to the development of contact urticaria on the hands and wrists.

WORK ROUTINES

Work routines in the animal facility should be planned such that allergen contamination of the area surrounding the individual worker is kept to a minimum.[45-48] Routines must also be designed to prevent the spread of allergens into the environment and transfer to adjacent areas – corridors, offices, lunch room, etc., not to mention to adjacent buildings (laundry, technical support areas). Work should be planned in a way that prevents the spread of allergens within the room. Cages should not be emptied in the animal room but removed to the cleaning area, where they should be emptied into closed transport systems that deliver the bedding to sealed containers. The container is then transported and emptied, usually by renovation staff. It is important to develop handling routines that afford protection similar to that for laundry staff handling potentially contaminated clothing. Empty soiled cages should be moistened before transport from the room. This can be best done by spraying the soiled cages with water or a neutral soap solution. Transport of soiled cages from the animal room to the cleaning area should be done using a closed transport trolley. Should this not be possible, cages should be draped with a cover cloth or plastic sheet.

Animal rooms and other potentially contaminated areas should be cleaned using dust-reducing methods. Examples of this are the use of closed vacuum cleaners that deliver dust into a closed pipe conveyor with deposition into a sealed container, the use of moist mopping, or damp sweeping. High-pressure hosing should be avoided since this type of cleaning causes contaminated aerosols in the room which are easily inhaled and contribute to sensitization.

Animals should be transported in suitable transport cabinets equipped with filter material that prevents the spread of allergens along corridors and in lifts (Figure 2). Single cages with animals should be transported using a filter top (Figure 3). Cages with animals should be kept in suitable ventilated cabinets when in procedure rooms (Figure 4). Single cages should likewise be covered with a filter top when standing freely in laboratory or procedure rooms.

Soiled bedding is possibly the most significant single source of allergens in the animal facility. Care must be taken to reduce allergen spread from this source at all points of handling. Cage changing and transport has been mentioned above.

Workers should spend as little time as possible in rooms containing animals and at no time should workers be allowed to eat, drink, or smoke in such areas. Separate facilities should be provided for this type of activity and for report writing.

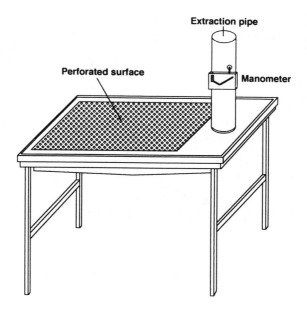

Figure 4. An example of a down-ventilated bench showing the perforated plate mounted in the center of the working area. (Picture supplied by B&K Universal.)

LEGAL ASPECTS

Several countries have enacted general legislation regarding aspects of health and safety at work that would also cover ALA as an occupational disease. Examples of these are the Health and Safety at Works act of 1974 in the United Kingdom, the Health and Safety at Work act of 1977 in Sweden, and the Worker Health and Environment Act of 1977 in Norway. Allergy resulting from work with laboratory animals would therefore entitle an affected worker to free medical assistance. The worker would also be entitled to an extra disablement pension and industrial injury compensation. Sweden has legislation similar to the Norwegian, with the exception that ALA is defined as an occupational disease in its own right. In the United Kingdom occupational allergy to laboratory animals is defined under the Control of Substances Hazardous to Health Regulations of 1988.[49] Furthermore, occupational asthma resulting from work with laboratory animals must be notified to the Health and Safety Executive under the Reporting of Injuries, Diseases and Dangerous Occurrences Regulations of 1985.

REFERENCES

1. Lutsky, I. and Toshner, D., A review of allergic respiratory disease in laboratory animal workers, *Lab. Anim. Sci.*, 28, 751, 1978.
2. Lutsky, I., Occupational asthma in laboratory animal workers, in *Occupational Asthma*, Frazier, C. A., Ed., Van Rostrand-Reinhold Co., New York, 1980, 193.
3. Newman Taylor, A. J., Laboratory animal allergy, *Eur. Respir. Dis.*, 63, 60, 1982.
4. Longbottom, J. L., Occupational allergy due to animal allergens, *Clin. Immunol. Allerg.*, 4, 19, 1984.
5. Olfert, E. D., Allergy to laboratory animals: An occupational disease, *Lab. Anim.*, July/August, 24, 1986.
6. Poulsen, O. M., A general introduction to allergy to laboratory animals (ALA), *Scand. J. Lab. Anim. Sci.*, 4, 155, 1990.
7. Hunskaar, S. and Fosse, R. T., Allergy to laboratory mice and rats: A review of the pathophysiology, epidemiology and clinical aspects, *Lab. Anim.*, 24, 358, 1990.
8. Hunskaar, S. and Fosse, R., Allergy to laboratory mice and rats: a review of its prevention, management, and treatment, *Lab. Anim.*, 27, 206, 1993.
9. Gell, P. G. H. and Coombs, R. R. A., *Clinical Aspects of Immunology*, Blackwell, Oxford, 1968.

10. Schumacher, M. J., Characterization of allergens from urine and pelts of laboratory mice, *Mol. Immunol.*, 17, 1087, 1980.
11. Finlayson, J. S., Asofsky, R., Potter, M., and Runner, C. C., Major urinary protein complex of normal mice: origin, *Science*, 149, 981, 1965.
12. Longbottom, J. L., Purification and characterization of allergens from the urines of mice and rats, in *Advances in Allergology and Immunology*, Oehling, A., Ed., Pergamon Press, New York, 1980, 483.
13. Wahn, U., Peters, T., and Siraganian, R. P., Studies on the allergenic significance and structure of rat serum albumin, *J. Immunol.*, 125, 2544, 1980.
14. Walls, A. F. and Longbottom, J. L., Quantitative immunoelectrophoretic analysis of rat allergen extracts. II. Fur, urine and saliva studied by crossed radio-immunoelectrophoresis, *Allergy*, 38, 501, 1983.
15. Lutsky, I., Fink, J. N., Kidd, J., Dahlberg, M. J., and Yunginger, J. W., Allergenic properties of rat urine and pelt extracts, *J. Allerg. Clin. Immunol.*, 75, 279, 1985.
16. Davies, G. E., Thompson, A. V., and Rackham, M., Estimation of airborne rat-derived antigens by ELISA, *J. Immunol.*, 4, 113, 1983.
17. Platt-Mills, T. A. E., Heyman, P. W., Longbottom, J. L., and Wilkins, S. R., Airborne allergens associated with asthma: Particle sizes carrying dust mite and rat allergens measured with a cascade impactor, *J. Allerg. Clin. Immunol.*, 77, 850, 1986.
18. Böhm, W. and Braun, W., Beruftsbedingte Sensibilisierungen der Atemwege durch Haare von Labortieren, *A. S. A.*, 7, 94, 1972.
19. Lutsky, I. and Neuman, I., Laboratory animal dander allergy. I. An occupational disease, *Ann. Allerg.*, 35, 201, 1975.
20. Neuman, I. and Lutsky, I., Laboratory animal dander allergy. II. Clinical studies and the potential protective effect of disodium cromoglycate, *Ann. Allerg.*, 36, 23, 1976.
21. Gross, N. J., Allergy to laboratory animals: epidemiological, clinical, and physiological aspects, and a trial of cromolyn in its management, *J. Allerg. Clin. Immunol.*, 66, 158, 1980.
22. Slovak, A. J. M. and Hill, R. N., Laboratory animal allergy: a clinical survey of an exposed population, *Br. J. Ind. Med.*, 38, 38, 1981.
23. Hook, W. A., Powers, K., and Siraganian, R. P., Skin tests and blood leukocyte histamine release of patients with allergies to laboratory animals, *J. Allerg. Clin. Immunol.*, 73, 457, 1984.
24. Davies, G. E., Thompson, A. V., Niewola, Z., Burrows, G. E., Teasdale, E. L., Bird, D. J., and D.A.P., Allergy to laboratory animals: a retrospective and a propective study, *Br. J. Ind. Med.*, 40, 442, 1983.
25. Botham, P. A., Davies, G. E., and Teasdale, E. L., Allergy to laboratory animals: a prospective study of its incidence and of the influence of atopy on its development, *Br. J. Ind. Med.*, 44, 627, 1987.
26. Lutsky, I., Baum, G. L., Teichtahl, H., Mazar, A., Aizer, F., and Bar-Sela, S., Respiratory disease in animal house workers, *Eur. J. Respir. Dis.*, 69, 29, 1986.
27. Venables, K. M., Upton, J. L., Hawkins, R., Tee, R. D., Longbottom, J. L., and Newman Taylor, A. J., Smoking, atopy, and laboratory animal allergy, *Br. J. Ind. Med.*, 45, 667, 1988.
28. Schumacher, M. J., Tait, B. D., and Holmes, M. C., Allergy to murine antigens in a biological research institute, *J. Allerg. Clin. Immunol.*, 68, 310, 1981.
29. Patterson, R., The problem of allergy to laboratory animals, *Lab. Anim. Care*, 14, 466, 1964.
30. Lincoln, T. A., Bolton, N. E., and Garret, A. S., Occupational allergy to animal dander and sera, *J. Occup. Med.*, 16, 465, 1974.
31. Newill, C. A., Evans, R., and Khoury, M. J., Pre-employment screening for allergy to laboratory animals: epidemiologic evaluation of its potential usefulness, *J. Occup. Med.*, 28, 1158, 1986.
32. Cockcroft, A., Edwards, J., McCarthy, P., and Andersson, N., Allergy in laboratory animal workers, *Lancet*, 1, 827, 1981.
33. Agrup, G., Belin, L., Sjøstedt, L., and Skerfving, S., Allergy to laboratory animals in laboratory technicians and animal keepers, *Br. J. Ind. Med.*, 43, 192, 1986.
34. Venables, K. M., Tee, R. D., Hawkins, R., Gordon, D. J., Wale, C. J., Farrer, N. M., Lam, T. H., Baxter, P. J., and Newman Taylor, A. J., Laboratory allergy in a pharmaceutical company, *Br. J. Ind. Med.*, 45, 660, 1988.
35. Agrup, G. and Sjøstedt, L., Contact urticaria in laboratory animal technicians working with animals, *Acta Derm. Venereol. (Stockholm)*, 65, 111, 1985.

36. Rudzki, E., Rebandel, P., and Rogozinski, T., Contact urticaria from rat tail, guinea pig, streptomycin and vinyl pyridine, *Contact Dermatitis*, 7, 186, 1981.

37. Teasdale, E. L., Davies, G. E., and Slovak, A., Anaphylaxis after bites by rodents, *Br. Med. J.*, 286, 1480, 1983.

38. Agarwal, M. K., Yunginger, J. W., Swanson, M. C., and Reed, C. E., An immunochemical method to measure atmospheric allergens, *J. Allerg. Clin. Immunol.*, 68, 194, 1981.

39. Twiggs, J. T., Mahendra, K. A., Dahlberg, M. J. E., and Yunginger, J. W., Immunochemical measurement of airborne mouse allergens in a laboratory animal facility, *J. Allerg. Clin. Immunol.*, 69, 522, 1982.

40. Edwards, R. G., Beeson, M. F., and Dewdney, J. M., Laboratory animal allergy: the measurement of airborne urinary allergens and the effects of different environmental conditions, *Lab. Anim.*, 17, 235, 1983.

41. Dybendal, T., Vik, H., and Elsayed, S., Dust from carpets and smooth floors. II. Antigenic and allergenic content of dust vacuumed from carpeted and smooth floors in schools under routine cleaning schedules, *Allergy*, 44, 401, 1989.

42. Dybendal, T. and Elsayed, S., Dust from carpeted and smooth floors. V. Cat (Fel d I) and mite (Der p I and Der f I) allergen levels in school dust. Demonstration of the basophil histamine release induced by dust from class rooms, *Clin. Exp. Allergy*, In press, 1992.

43. Elsayed, S., Personal communication, 1992.

44. Slovak, A. J. M., Orr, R. G., and Teasdale, E. L., Efficacy of the helmet respirator in occupational asthma due to laboratory animal allergy (LAA), *Am. Ind. Hyg. Assoc. J.*, 46, 411, 1985.

45. Bland, S. M., Evans, R. E., and Rivera, J. C., Allergy to laboratory animals in health care personnel, *Occup. Med.*, 2, 525, 1987.

46. Dewdney, J. M., Johnson, R. D., Skidmore, I. F., Slovak, A., Teasdale, E. L., and Williams, G. A., Eds., *Advisory Note on Allergy to Laboratory Animals*, The Association of the British Pharmaceutical Association, London, 1987.

47. Education Services Advisory Committee, *What You Should Know About Allergy to Laboratory Animals*, Her Majesty's Stationery Office, Sheffield, U.K., 1990.

48. Andersson, S., Baneryd, K., and Lindh, G., *Working with Laboratory Animals*, Arbeteskyddstyrelsen, Publikasjonsservice, Rep. no: AFS 1990:11, Stockholm, 1990.

49. COSHH, *Control of Substances Hazardous to Health Regulations*, Her Majesty's Stationery Office, Report. no: 1988/1657, 1988.

Chapter 8

Zoonoses

Ann Detmer

CONTENTS

INTRODUCTION

A zoonosis is a disease that is transmittable between animals and man. Zoonoses are caused by many different agents, including viruses, bacteria, and parasites. More than 200 zoonoses are recognized today.[1] The transmission from animal to man can occur in a number of different ways. The most important are via food, direct contact with an infected animal, or indirect transmission through insects. In many cases the animal is only a carrier of the zoonotic agent and does not develop a disease. The distribution of zoonotic diseases around the world changes with ecological factors like climate, hygiene, and socioeconomic factors. The risk of becoming infected with a zoonotic disease is normally small when working with defined laboratory animals.

The best way to avoid zoonotic infections is knowledge, both of the potential disease panorama (Tables 1 and 2) and through careful monitoring of research animals. The minimum requirement for a laboratory animal is absence of zoonoses. This can only be achieved by thorough health monitoring programs carried out by the breeder and the research premises.

0-8493-4378-X/94/$0.00+$.50

Table 1. Diseases Transmittable from Monkey to Man

Disease or disease agent	Modes of transmission
Amebiasis (*Entamoeba histolytica*)[2]	Via feces
B-virus (*Herpes virus simiae*)	Bites and scratches contaminated by saliva
Chikungunya fever	Mosquitoes
Hepatitis A	Via feces
Marburg	Direct contact with body fluids and organs
Monkeypox	Direct contact, inhalation
Oropouche fever (*Bunyaviridae*)	Midge and mosquito bites
Rabies	Bites or saliva in contact with wounds
Salmonella/shigella	Via feces
Tuberculosis	Direct contact, inhalation
Yellow fever (*Togaviridae*)	Mosquito bites
Zika fever (*Togaviridae*)	Mosquito bites

Data from Reference 1.

Table 2. Diseases Transmittable from Laboratory Animals (Other than Monkeys) to Man

Disease or disease agent	Risk animal
Lymphocytic choriomeningitis	Hamsters, mice, rats
Haanthan-virus	Mice, rats, voles
Rat bite fever	Rats, mice
Hymenolepsis spp.	Mice, rats
Ringworm	Guinea pigs, cats
ß-Hemolytic streptococci	Guinea pigs, dogs, pigs
Yersiniosis	Pigs, guinea pigs, rats
Encephalitozoonosis	Rabbits, guinea pigs
Pasteurella sepsis	Bite wounds from dogs, cats
Chlamydiosis	Sheep, birds
Leptospirosis	Dogs, sheep, rats
Orf	Sheep
Q fever	Sheep, goats, cattle
Listeriosis	Sheep, goats
Rabies	Dogs, cats, bats
Salmonella spp.	All species
Visceral larva migrans (Toxocara)	Cats, dogs
Toxoplasmosis	Cats
Campylobacter jejuni/coli	Cats, dogs, chicken

Diseases may also be transmitted through products derived from animals, like blood, body fluids, tumors, soiled bedding, and other waste products. This chapter briefly reviews selected zoonotic agents and diseases in animals. It should, however, also be noted that diseases and disease agents in humans can cause considerable problems among susceptible animals, e.g., measles, herpes simplex, respiratory syncytial virus, and pyogenic cocci.

PRIMATES

Particular attention should be paid to the risk of zoonotic infections from primates because they often carry diseases infective to humans. Primates should be handled under anesthesia only, and protective clothing including eye glasses should always be used. All new monkeys should be isolated in a quarantine even if they have completed quarantine elsewhere. Serological tests are good supplements, but are not available for all disease agents. Diseases transmittable from monkey to man are listed in Table 1. Some of these will be described below.

HERPES SIMIAE

B virus infection, also called *Herpes simiae* virus infection, is a major threat to humans working with primates.[3-5] The causative agent is a herpes virus and the monkeys remain infected for their entire lifetime. The only visible signs in the monkeys (usually macaques) are small and inconspicuous vesicles in the mouth or on the genital organs which resemble lesions caused by *Herpes simplex* infection in man. During quarantine the monkeys should be inspected under anesthesia and animals with lesions should be eliminated. Using serology, reactants can be found and eliminated. The criterion for seronegative status is that the animal has had a negative test for B virus antibody on two occasions with an interval of two months, during which it has been kept isolated from other monkeys who may harbor the virus. Purpose-bred monkeys should also be checked on a regular basis, since many breeding colonies are infected. Monkeys from a group of animals where known reactants to B virus have been found should always be treated as B virus-positive.

Humans can be infected by bites and scratches, and by contamination of the skin with monkey saliva. The incubation time is 1–5 weeks. Clinical signs of B virus infection in humans are fever, headache, muscle pain, abdominal pain, and in the final stage an ascending flaccid paralysis. In most cases death occurs within three weeks.

MARBURG DISEASE

Marburg disease is a rare but often fatal hemorrhagic fever.[4] In 1967 an outbreak among laboratory workers in Germany caused the loss of several human lives.[6] African green vervet monkeys (*Cercopithecus aethiops*) recently imported from Uganda were used without prior quarantine. Serology is available as a diagnostic method, but it is probably only vervet monkeys that survive the disease. A quarantine period of 6–8 weeks should be adequate for other monkeys caught in the wild.[4]

The incubation time for humans is 3–9 days. Symptoms include fever with rigor, headache and pain, anorexia, vomiting, diarrhea, and jaundice. Between the third and eighth day a rash appears, lasting for 3–4 days. Death usually occurs at the beginning of the second week.

TUBERCULOSIS

Tuberculous monkeys are a hazard to man and other animals. Monkeys are susceptible to all three varieties of tuberculosis: human, bovine, and avian. Simians are free from tuberculosis in their natural habitat and acquire the disease by contact with man. Rhesus monkeys are especially sensitive. To control tuberculosis, skin tests and chest X-rays should always be performed. Animal caretakers and other staff should be screened on a regular basis.

SHIGELLOSIS AND SALMONELLOSIS

Bacterial enteritis is the most common disease and cause of death in primates. Enteritis in primates is frequently caused by infection with *Shigella flexneri* or *Salmonella typhimurium*. The symptoms may be acute, with death occurring after a few days, or chronic, with hemorrhagic diarrhea and dehydration.

The pathological signs are ulcerations and necrosis of the gastric and intestinal mucosa. Diagnosis is secured by isolation of the bacteria in feces.

Humans may be infected via contact with feces from infected primates.

BITE WOUNDS

Bite wounds from monkeys can be very dangerous both because of the risk of B virus and due to bacterial infection of the wounds, which are often deep. Careful handling and a thorough knowledge of animal behavior is necessary to avoid taking unnecessary risks. Some laboratories remove the sharp canine teeth.[7] Bite wounds should be cleaned immediately and proper medical treatment should always be carried out.

RODENTS

LYMPHOCYTIC CHORIOMENINGITIS

Lymphocytic choriomeningitis virus (LCM) is mainly a mouse virus, but hamsters may also carry the infection. The causative agent is an Arenavirus, which occurs worldwide. The natural reservoir is the domestic mouse. The infection is congenital, and virus is excreted in saliva, urine, and feces throughout the life of the animal. The disease usually remains subclinical following natural infection, whereas experimentally infected mice develop convulsions and often die. Dead animals show glomerular nephritis and meningitis.

Laboratory staff are infected from contaminated bedding, handling of dead mice, and from mouse bites. Symptoms of LCM in man are influenza-like, lasting for up to two weeks. Meningitis, paralysis and coma may occasionally follow. During convalescence joint pains frequently occur.

The disease is prevented by using only mice and hamsters from breeders who maintain a proper health monitoring system. Scientists working with wild mice should maintain strict hygienic standards, including the use of protective gloves and face masks.

KOREAN HEMORRHAGIC FEVER

Korean hemorrhagic fever (KHF) has occurred in laboratory personnel in Korea, Japan, and Belgium.[8,9] The causative agent is Hanthaan virus. The natural reservoir is wild rodents, especially the house rat, but antibodies to Hanthaan virus have also been found in laboratory rats. The disease has a subclinical course in rats, but virus is excreted in urine and saliva. Screening for Haanthan virus is now included in the standard health monitoring carried out by most commercial breeders.

The mode of transmission to humans has not been clearly defined, but contact with infected rat urine and saliva is a definite possibility. In humans the incubation time is 1–5 weeks. KHF is a febrile disease with renal complications, and symptoms are high fever, headache, muscle pain, vomiting, diarrhea, and an affected kidney function. The fatality rate is about 5%, and the pathological findings are congestion and hemorrhages in the kidneys and other organs.

The disease is prevented by using animals from recognized breeders who can guarantee the health of their animals. When working with wild rats, strict hygienic precautions should be followed, including the use of protective gloves and face masks.

RAT BITE FEVER

Rat bite fever[10] is an infection that occurs worldwide. The causative agents are *Streptobacillus moniliformis* and *Spirillum minus*. Rats are the natural reservoir and excrete organisms in their urine and saliva. The symptoms in rats are subclinical. Laboratory personnel can be infected by rat bites. *S. moniliformis* causes fever for a few days combined with headache, nausea, joint pains, and an erythematous rash on hands and feet. The infection may occasionally lead to endocarditis. Infection with *S. minus* causes ulceration at the site of the bite, regional lymphadenitis, fever, and a rash on chest and arms.

The disease can be treated with penicillin. Barrier-bred rats are usually screened for these agents, and if laboratory rats are protected from contact with wild rats this disease should not cause any problems.

YERSINIOSIS

Yersinia pseudotuberculosis is a disease agent which can infect several species, including man. Among laboratory animals, yersiniosis occurs spontaneously in guinea pigs, non-human primates, and rabbits. Small rodents can be silent carriers. Symptoms in animals are subacute and acute enteritis and severe diarrhea and weight loss. Enlarged lymph nodes can sometimes be palpated in the abdomen. Death occurs in 2–12 weeks in 5–7% of affected guinea pigs.

In humans the symptoms are acute onset of fever, abdominal pain, and diarrhea. The infection is usually self-limiting, but non-suppurative arthritis and skin lesions complicate the course.

STREPTOCOCCOSIS

Streptococcus zooepidemicus is a commonly occurring bacterium in retropharyngeal abscesses in guinea pigs.[11] Humans can be infected by contact with infected material from guinea pigs. The symptoms are cervical adenitis and pneumonia. The infection may be complicated by endocarditis and nephritis.

RINGWORM

Ringworm is a fungal skin disease caused by various species of *Tricophyton* and *Microsporum*. Guinea pigs, cats and dogs are the most frequently affected laboratory animals. The lesions appear as hairless, circular plaques, which gradually enlarge. Cats, however, often show no lesions. The diagnosis is made by mycological culturing of hairs from the edges of a lesion. Examination of cats with Wood's lamp reveals fluorescence from *Microsporum* species.

The symptoms in humans are characterized by ring-shaped, scaly skin lesions with loss of hair. The disease is prevented by avoiding contact with infected animals and by hand washing. Treatment with oral griseofulvin or topical antifungal agents is effective.

HYMENOLEPSIASIS

Hymenolepsis nana (dwarf tapeworm) and *Hymenolepsis diminuta* can be transmitted to humans. The natural reservoir of *H. nana* is the house mouse, and the main reservoir of *H. diminuta* is the rat. Both parasites require arthropods as intermediate hosts, although *H. nana* may cause infection directly. Moderate infection is asymptomatic, whereas heavy infestation may cause a mild catarrhal enteritis with diarrhea.

Humans are infected by ingestion of infected insects or by ingestion of *H. nana* eggs excreted by affected mice. The infection is usually asymptomatic in humans unless very heavy, when it causes anorexia, diarrhea and anal itching. Diagnosis is secured by identifying eggs in feces. The infection can be prevented in laboratory personnel by using barrier-derived animals, by eradication of arthropods, and by avoiding contact with soiled bedding.

RABBITS

PASTEURELLOSIS

Pasteurella multocida is common among rabbits with respiratory disease, but the risk for staff here is small, since the main mode of transmission is through bite wounds, which rarely occur when handling rabbits. *Pasteurella pneumotropica,* which mainly infects small rodents, can also cause upper respiratory disease in rabbits and has been cultured from animal caretakers with upper respiratory and middle-ear infections.

SHEEP

A number of diseases, including brucellosis, chlamydiosis, leptospirosis, orf (parapox virus), Q fever, and Rift Valley fever (only in Africa), are transmittable from sheep to man via direct contact. New sheep should be kept in quarantine before being introduced into the laboratory.

BRUCELLOSIS

Brucellosis in sheep is caused by *Brucella ovis.* Infection in sheep causes abortion, and since sheep are frequently used for research in fetal physiology, laboratory personnel may be infected following contact with fetal membranes, amniotic fluid, or fetuses.

The incubation time in humans is 1–6 weeks. The symptoms are undulating fever, pains, weakness, and weight loss. The condition may persist for months unless treated with antibiotics.

The disease is prevented by acquiring animals from tested herds only.

CHLAMYDIOSIS

Chlamydia psittaci can be found in feces of healthy adult sheep, and a large concentration of the infective agent is present in the placentas of ewes that have aborted (enzootic abortion of ewes). Infection with *C. psittaci* of ovine origin has caused several cases of abortion in pregnant women in Great Britain.[12,13] The disease agent can be difficult to diagnose.

Q FEVER

Q fever is caused by a rickettsia, *Coxiella burnetii,* transmitted via feces or placentas and fetal membranes. *C. burnetii* is distributed worldwide and can survive for months outside animals. No evident disease has been seen in farm animals except for the rare occurrence of abortions in sheep and goats, although experimental infection in guinea pigs produces a febrile non-fatal pneumonia.

Symptoms of Q fever in humans are persistent high fever, headache, pneumonia, and hepatitis. It spreads to humans very easily, mainly through aerosols, but the greatest risk to laboratory personnel is contact with fetal material. Bernard et al.[14] have published recommendations for research facilities using sheep.

PIGS

Bacteria like *Streptococcus suis, Erysipelotrix rhusiopatiae,* and *Yersinia enterocolitica* can infect humans, but the risk for animal caretakers is small.

CARNIVORES

Bite wounds are a major risk when working with dogs and cats. The normal oral flora of both dogs and cats contains *Pasteurella multocida,* which can cause very rapid and serious infections in man after bite wounds. *Cytocapnopha canimorsus,* a newly found normal inhabitant in the canine oral flora, can also cause wound infections. Immediate and thorough cleaning of bite wounds with physiological saline helps to prevent infection. Both of the above-mentioned bacteria are normally sensitive to penicillin, and a person bitten by a cat or dog should always contact a doctor immediately for proper treatment.

RABIES

Rabies is a viral infection of the central nervous system. The disease is present in all continents except Australia. Certain countries, including the United Kingdom, Sweden, Norway, Japan, and New Zealand, are rabies-free. The virus can infect all warm-blooded animals and birds, and is transmitted by bites. Rabies occurs in two clinical forms: the furious and the paralytic forms. In both forms the first symptom is abnormal behavior. In the furious form the dog becomes aggressive, salivation is profuse due to lack of the swallowing reflex, and gradually the animal develops convulsions and paralysis ending in death. In the paralytic form the animal rapidly becomes paralyzed and dies.

The disease poses a serious risk to laboratory personnel working with dogs, cats, and wild animals in areas where rabies is common, especially in Africa. The incubation time is from a few days to a year, depending on where the bite wound is located. The closer to the head the shorter the incubation time. The disease is fatal unless treated immediately. The wound should be cleaned and disinfected and the surrounding tissue infiltrated with rabies antiserum. Because of the long incubation time postexposure vaccination is effective. There is no effective treatment once the disease has developed.

Pre-exposure vaccination is highly recommended for laboratory personnel working in enzootic areas. Dogs and cats should be kept vaccinated, and always handled safely.

LEPTOSPIROSIS

Leptospirosis is a bacterial disease occurring worldwide and with a great variety of serotypes. It is transmitted via urine. *Leptospira ichterohaemorrhagie* and *L. canicola* are common species in dogs. Symptoms in dogs are gastroenteritis, jaundice, and nephritis. The presence of leptospires can be established by a serological test. Vaccine is available for dogs and streptomycin can be used for treatment.

The incubation time for humans is 3–20 days. The symptoms include fever, vomiting, jaundice, hemolytic anemia and nephritis.

TOXOPLASMOSIS

Toxoplasmosis is caused by the protozoan *Toxoplasma gondii.* The definitive host is the cat, which hosts the parasite in its intestinal tract. Intermediate hosts are a number of animals and birds, and humans, in which the parasitic cyst is present in the muscle tissue. The protozoa can also be present in the placenta of pregnant ewes. The disease is usually subclinical in animals. Humans are infected either by eating raw meat from infected sheep or cattle, or by ingestion of oocysts from cat's feces. There are usually no symptoms, but fever and headache may occur. The greatest risk is congenital infection of the fetus if a pregnant woman is infected during the second trimester. Congenitally infected children may become mentally retarded and blind.

Pregnant women should avoid contact with cat's feces and lambing ewes.

CAT SCRATCH DISEASE

The causative agent of cat scratch disease is unknown. A Gram-negative bacillus is often found on histological examination, but it has not been cultured.

The incubation time for humans is 3–14 days following a bite or a scratch from a cat. The clinical manifestation of cat scratch disease in man is lymphadenopathy, which may persist for months. Infection can be prevented by washing cat scratches immediately.

PARASITES

Parasites constituting a potential risk are *Echinococcus granulosus, Toxocara canis et cati, Strongyloides stercoralis,* as well as dog hookworm. They can be controlled by good sanitation and antiparasitic treatment.

BIRDS

CHLAMYDIOSIS

Chlamydiosis can be a risk when working with birds, especially budgerigars, parrots, and pigeons. Birds dying in quarantine with respiratory distress less than 3 months after arrival should be autopsied with psittacosis (ornithosis) in mind. The pathological findings include edema of the lungs and fibrous exudate in the pleural and peritoneal cavities.

Clinical manifestation of chlamydiosis in humans is very often an atypical pneumonia which persists unless treated with antibiotics.

This is only a short review and further reading is recommended.[17–19] Finally, however, after listing possible diseases, both common and rare, it deserves to be said that if health-monitored animals are used, the risk of being infected with a zoonotic disease is very small during work in the animal house.

REFERENCES

1. Bell, J. C., Palmer, S. R., and Payne J. M., *The Zoonoses: Infections Transmitted from Animals to Man,* Edward Arnold, London, 1988.
2. Detmer, A., Infektion med Entamoeba histolytica i en koloni med Macaca fascicularis, *Sv. Vet. Tidn.* *42, 699, 1990.*
3. *The Management of Simians in Relation to Infectious Hazards to Staff,* Medical Research Council, London, 1985.
4. Kalter, S. S. and Heberling, R. L. J., Primate viral diseases in perspective, *Med. Primatol., 19, 519, 1990.*
5. Hazards of handling simians, *Laboratory Animals Handbook,* Vol. 4., Laboratory Animals Ltd., 1969.
6. Martini, G. A. and Siegeit, K. (Eds.), *Marburg Virus Disease,* Springer-Verlag, Berlin, 1971.
7. Schofield, J. C., Alves, M. E. A. F., Hughes, K. W., and Bennett, B.T., Disarming canine teeth of nonhuman primates using the submucosal vital root retention technique. *Lab. Anim. Sci. 41, 128, 1991.*
8. Tsai, T. F., Hemorrhagic fever with renal syndrome: mode of transmission to humans, *Lab. Anim. Sci. 37, 428, 1987.*
9. Quimby, F., Zoonotic implications of haanthan-like viruses: an introduction, *Lab. Anim. Sci. 37, 411, 1987.*
10. Anderson, L. C., Leary, S. L., and Manning P. J., Rat-bite fever in animal research laboratory personnel. *Lab. Anim. Sci. 33, 292, 1983.*
11. Murphy, J. C., Ackerman, J. I., Marini, R. P., and Fox, J. G., Cervical lymphadenitis in guinea pigs: infection via intact ocular and nasal mucosa by Streptococcus zooepidemicus. *Lab. Anim. Sci. 41, 251, 1991.*
12. Buxton, D., Potential danger to pregnant women of Chlamydia psittaci from sheep, *Vet. Rec. 118, 510, 1986.*
13. Chlamydia psittaci: zoonotic potential worthy of concern. *Clin. Microbiol. Newslett., 9, 1, 1987.*
14. Bernard, K. W., Parham, G. L., Winkler, W. G., and Helmick C. G., Q fever control measures: recommendations for research facilities using sheep, *Infect. Contr., 3, 6, 1982.*

15. Fox, J. G., Campylobacteriosis — A "new" disease in laboratory animals, *Lab. Anim. Sci., 32, 625, 1982.*

16. Bhatt, P. N., Jacoby, R. O., and Barthold, S. W., Contamination of transplantable murine tumors with lymphocytic choriomeningitis virus, *Lab. Anim. Sci., 36, 136, 1986.*

17. Fox, J. G., Cohen, B. J., and Loew, F. M. (Eds.), *Laboratory Animal Medicine,* pp. 613-648. Academic Press, New York, 1984.

18. Melby, E. C., Jr. and Altman, N. H., *Handbook of Laboratory Animal Science,* Vol. 2, pp. 243-269. CRC Press, Boca Raton, FL, 1974.

19. Acha, P. N. and Szyfres B. (Eds.), *Zoonosis and Communicable Diseases Common to Man and Animals.* Pan American Health Organisation.

Chapter 9

Laboratory Animal Facilities

Dag R. Sørensen

CONTENTS

INTRODUCTION

Laboratory animals should be housed under conditions where their basic etiological needs can be fulfilled, where infectious diseases can be prevented, and where environmental factors can be controlled. In this way experimentation can be performed without the risk of harming the animals, without the risk of exposing the staff to allergens and infections, and at the same time ensuring reliable experimental results.

The planning and building of laboratory animal facilities is a complicated and time-consuming task that may take several years. Compared with other kinds of buildings, the cost may be up to two to three times more per square meter, the ventilation system being responsible for an essential part of this cost.

When planning the construction of a laboratory animal facility, close cooperation between the academic and technical staff, the users, the administrators, and the constructors is essential. The basic interests of the different groups usually differ. For professional reasons the staff responsible for the keeping of the animals will prefer a centralized animal facility. The administration tends to have the same preference for economical reasons, whereas the users often prefer a departmental or individual animal facility.

A centralized unit should be headed by a veterinarian who is responsible for the health and welfare of the animals, for advising the experimenters, and for performing complicated procedures like anesthesia and experimental surgery. A sufficient number of well-trained animal technicians should be available for the daily care of the animals, including cleaning of animal rooms and cages, feeding and watering, and assistance in experimental procedures. The number of technicians required depends on the number of animals, the species, and the involvement in experimental procedures. As a general rule one technician can manage 4000 mice, 1400 rats, or 250 rabbits. It should also be taken into consideration that animals must be cared for during weekends and holidays.

It should also be realized that up to 80% of the working time in an animal house is used for cleaning rooms, cages, and equipment. Even the technically most advanced animal facility will become a failure if this fact is not accepted.

Table 1. Area Requirements for Different Animal Species

Animal species	Area requirement (animal/m²)
Mice	40
Rats	15
Guinea pigs	17
Hamsters	17
Rabbits	0.8
Cats	0.8
Dogs	0.2
Primates	0.5
Small ruminants	0.2
Pigs	0.2

TYPE AND SIZE OF FACILITY

There are distinct differences between a university animal facility and a facility needed in the pharmaceutical industry. Universities will have to cater for many different small projects that run over a limited period and involve several species, whereas the pharmaceutical industry tends to perform uniform experiments with large numbers of animals of the same or limited number of species.

Consequently the university facility should be designed with a sufficiently large number of relatively small animal rooms to allow each project its own individual animal room. The design of the rooms should allow for a great degree of flexibility, so that different species can be accomodated, or the room can be used for experimental purposes.

In the pharmaceutical facility the animal rooms should be designed for a specific species of animals. Since experiments for safety testing are often prolonged, it is important to secure the animals against infections and environmental variations. Making a barrier system is necessary.

The size of the facility depends on the numbers and species of animals used, the microbiological quality required and on whether animals are bred on site or acquired from a commercial breeder.

THE NUMBERS AND SPECIES OF ANIMALS

In multidisciplinary establishments, such as universities and medical schools, a relatively small number of animals of different species is used. The types of projects vary constantly and with this variation the numbers and the preferred species. As a general rule clinical research tends to use larger species like pigs, dogs, and small ruminants, whereas basic and preclinical research tend to use small rodents and rabbits. The area requirements for the different animal species are shown in Table 1.

Besides animal rooms, laboratory space, service rooms and office space is required. In a basic science/preclinical animal facility the total area should be divided approximately as follows:

Animal rooms: 55%
Laboratory space: 20%
Service rooms (cage washing, feed and bedding stores, etc.): 20%
Office space: 5%

Since clinical research mainly uses large animals in single experiments, the area requirements are different and should be approximately as follows:

Animal rooms: 35%
Laboratory space, including surgical facilities: 40%
Service rooms: 20%
Office space: 5%

When planning the actual size of the animal facility the total number of animals required at any one time is the important factor. This number, however, is difficult to estimate. Most scientists will have a relatively precise idea of the total number of animals they plan to use per year, whereas it appears much more difficult to predict when they are to be used, and how many at a time. There is a tendency to concentrate most of the activities at certain periods of the year and reduce activity at other periods. This

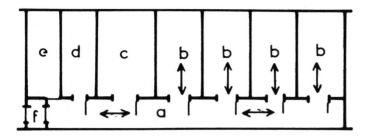

Figure 1. A single-corridor system. a: supply/disposal corridor; b: animal rooms; c: cage cleaning; d: store; e: staff. (From G. Clough.)

has to be taken into consideration when planning the size of the animal facility and the working routines of the animal technicians.

MICROBIOLOGICAL STATUS OF THE ANIMALS

There is an increasing trend toward using high-quality animals of defined microbiological and genetic quality. There is, however, a potential conflict of interests when evaluating quality requirements. Animal facilities that serve homogeneous research environments, e.g., safety testing, immunology or oncology, can be restrictive when it comes to quality and, even more important, the mixing of animals of different quality backgrounds. The issue becomes more complicated when designing a facility for a heterogeneous university or faculty. Here there will be needs for several species, not all of which will be of the same quality standard. This has implications for the types of barriers that are designed and even more important for the staffing requirements of the building. The solution to this problem could be the "two corridor system" that allows the individual animal room to be serviced from either a "clean" area or a "dirty" area (Figure 3).

PROCUREMENT OF ANIMALS

The overall cost of institutionally bred animals is considerably higher than the cost of commercially bred animals. Breeding animals in a research facility should only be considered when there are scientific reasons for doing so, e.g., if the protocol demands newborn animals or if the specific strain of animals is not available commercially.

Breeding for whatever reason demands that barrier facilities be established. These can be in the form of a zone barrier, a flexible film isolator, or similar isolation technology. Newborn animals represent a potential source of contamination in that they are sensitive to infection.

LOCALIZATION

Ideally the animal facility should be at the ground level in a separate building. For security reasons some institutions prefer to accomodate laboratory animals in existing buildings far from the main entrance. This, however, causes substantial transport problems considering the large amounts of materials (feed, bedding, waste, etc.) that have to be moved to and from an animal facility.

The disadvantage of a separate building is the problem of moving animals to different laboratories for experimental procedures. Whenever possible experiments should be performed in the animal facility. If it becomes necessary to move the animals to laboratories outside the animal facility, closed, movable ventilated cabinets should be used to protect the animals against infection and stress, and staff against allergens. As a general rule live animals should not return from outside laboratories to the animal facility.

DESIGN PRINCIPLES

Two basically different designs of laboratory animal facilities have been developed: the single-corridor system and the dual-corridor system.[1]

A single-corridor system has animal room doors leading to a single corridor. Traffic flow may be either bidirectional or unidirectional relative to the flow of cages between the animal room and the cage sanitation facility (Figure 1). The most significant advantage of a single-corridor system is that it allows more efficient use of space. The primary concern with a single-corridor system is the potential risk of cross-contamination in the corridor when clean and soiled cages share circulation space. In addition, the congestion caused by moving animals, cages, and supplies through a single corridor is greater than if two corridors are used.

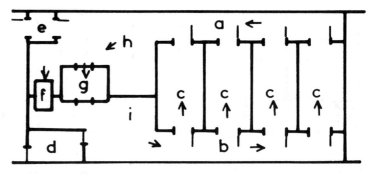

Figure 2. A dual-corridor system. a: "dirty" disposal corridor; b: "clean" supply corridor; c: animal rooms; d: "clean" staff entry; e: "dirty" staff entry; f: autoclave; g: formaldehyde fumigation. (From G. Clough.)

A dual-corridor system has animal-room doors leading to two separate corridors, one designated for clean cages and the other for soiled cages. The flow of cages is generally unidirectional (Figure 2). The primary advantage of this system is the elimination of the necessity of mixing clean cages and supplies in the same corridor with soiled cages and refuse, thereby reducing the risk of cross-contamination. A dual-corridor system also facilitates the movement of supplies and equipment through the facility. The primary disadvantage of a dual-corridor system is its high cost in terms of space utilization. Another disadvantage is that labor costs are significantly greater than with a single-corridor system if the dual-corridor facility is managed to maintain true separation between the clean and soiled sides.

When the major objective is to protect the animals from infections, i.e., in a breeding colony or in laboratories where the use of microbiologically defined animals is essential, a barrier system designed and managed to keep out contaminants is necessary. The barrier includes an entrance for personnel which allows complete separation of daily clothes and working clothes, and showering, an entrance for animals which allows complete separation between transport cages and permanent cages, an autoclave for decontamination of bedding, working clothes and other autoclavable materials, and facilities for formalin treatment of non-autoclavable materials (plastic cages, water bottles, etc.). Feed should be irradiated rather than autoclaved to avoid destruction of essential nutritional components. The barrier, furthermore, includes a ventilation system with sufficient filters to protect against microorganisms.

When the objective is to control naturally occurring or experimentally induced contaminants that may be shed by the animals, a containment animal housing system designed and managed to retain contaminants is used.

Between the barrier (keep out) and the containment (keep in) housing systems there is the conventional animal housing system designed and managed to accomplish both, but at a lower level of intensity and dedication. An improvement of the conventional system is the "two corridor" system, which allows barrier separation between adjacent animal rooms without maintaining a permanent barrier housing system (Figure 3). In this system the animal rooms can either be serviced from a "dirty" corridor (conventional system) or from a "clean" corridor (barrier system). The advantage is flexibility, as the status of the rooms can be changed simply by locking or opening a door and disinfecting the room. This system is most useful in a heterogeneous university or faculty animal facility.

Air balancing is a critical element in the control of airborne contaminants. The basic objective is to direct the movement of air from the least contaminated area to the most contaminated area. This is accomplished by carefully balancing the ventilation system to create air pressure differentials between connecting spaces, forcing air to move in the desired direction.

Effective control of airborne contaminants requires control of airflow at multiple sites and the use of multiple barriers. The more barriers that exist, the more effectively airborne contaminants can be controlled. Multiple barriers may be provided at the facility level or to an area within the facility, with entry and/or exit vestibules, at the room level with anterooms, within the animal room at the rack level with animal cubicles or ventilated racks, or at the cage level with microisolation cages that can be individually ventilated. Each system has significant advantages and disadvantages and each offers a different degree of efficiency in controlling airborne contaminants.

The major risk of infection in an animal colony, however, is not airborne microbes, but rather new animals and other biological material brought into the facility. If animals are procured from different sources or the microbial status of the animals cannot be guaranteed sufficiently by the breeder a quarantine procedure may be necessary. Separate animal rooms, efficiently isolated from the rest of the facility, should be available for this purpose.

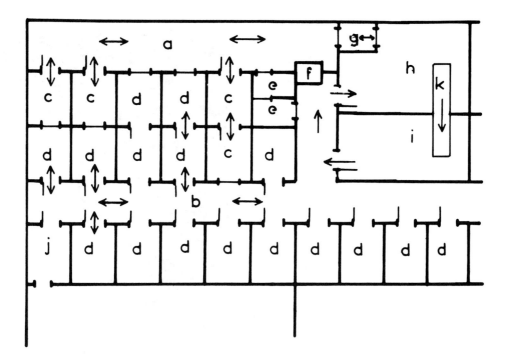

Figure 3. A dual-corridor system, which allows barrier separation between adjacent animal rooms without maintaining a permanent barrier system. a: "clean" supply/disposal corridor; b: "dirty" supply/disposal corridor; c: "clean" animal rooms; d: "dirty" animal rooms; e: "clean" staff entry; f: autoclave; g: formaldehyde fumigation; h: cage cleaning; i: store; j: anesthesia room; k: washing machine. (Odense University.)

SERVICE FACILITIES

Service facilities in the animal unit include a refrigerated feed storage room, storage space for bedding material, and facilities for cage cleaning and waste disposal. Since soiled bedding is the major cause of allergy, the disposal system should be designed to reduce the amount of dust released. This is efficiently done by a closed vacuum system (Figure 4), which can conveniently be placed in connection with a tunnel cage washing machine.

Storage facilities for temporarily vacant equipment (cages, etc.) is essential. In university animal facilities, temporary storage space for scientific equipment is also important.

LABORATORY FACILITIES

As a minimum the animal department should have laboratory facilities for performing autopsies and other diagnostic procedures to secure the health of the colony. The animal facility does, however, represent a research resource in its own right, and facilities for research should also be available. In heterogeneous university or faculty animal facilities a substantial part of the experimental work can preferably be carried out in laboratories associated with the animal unit.

In the case of clinical and physiological research, facilities for performing extensive surgical operations and microsurgical procedures are necessary. These include preparation and anesthesia rooms, operation rooms, X-ray facilities, post-operative care rooms, and facilities for disinfection and storage of equipment. Laboratory facilities should also include good facilities for performing post-mortem examinations, including histopathology, and facilities for performing basic clinical laboratory tests.

STAFF FACILITIES

The staff area should have the required number of offices, a common room, a room for communication including environmental monitoring, facility management and security systems.

TECHNICAL INSTALLATIONS

Laboratory animals are easily influenced by changes in light intensity and duration, and consequently the animal rooms should be without windows. Ventilation, temperature regulation, and illumination are

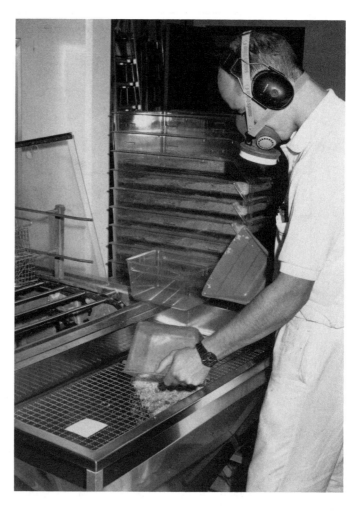

Figure 4. Closed vacuum system for removal of soiled bedding material.

therefore dependent on artificial systems. Walls, floor and ceiling should have surfaces that allow frequent washing down with hot water and disinfection with formaldehyde. Doors should be made of metal and designed to allow pressure above the atmosphere in the animal rooms.

VENTILATION SYSTEMS
The efficiency of the ventilation system sets the limits for the maximum animal density in the animal rooms. The more air changes per hour the more animals can be kept in a given area. The cost of the ventilation system vs. the construction costs determines how efficient the system should be. In practice a ventilation system that allows for approximately 20 air changes per hour appears to be the best choice. Air should enter the animal room from pipes under the ceiling, and be removed at several points, for instance from vertical pipes along the walls (Figure 5).

Temperature and humidity of the incoming air should be regulated so that room temperature can be maintained within ±2°C and humidity within ±5%.

Incoming and outgoing air should pass filters to reduce or prevent the entrance of pollutants from the external environment to the animals and prevent allergens from entering other parts of the building.

LIGHT AND SOUND
The light intensity in the animal rooms should be ajusted to give between 60 and 250 lux in the cages. Light/dark periods are usually 12 hours, but the possibility of changing the ratio is very useful. Some animal species are nocturnally active, and in some types of experiments a reversal of day and night is important. To make the change between day and night less abrupt, a twilight period of about half an hour is useful, in which half the lights are switched off.

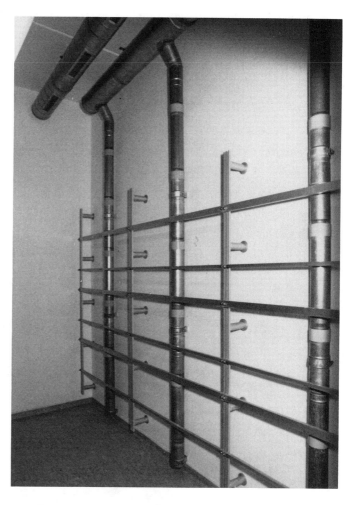

Figure 5. Ventilation system in animal room. Air enters through a pipe under the ceiling, and is removed via vertical pipes along the walls.

The animal rooms should be constructed to prevent excessive noise from the environment (bells, slamming of doors, etc.). While the human ear will register sound in the range from 20 to approximately 16,000 Hertz, most animals can hear sound up to 30,000–40,000 Hertz. Animal rooms should thus be checked for ultra high sound frequencies to prevent stress to the animals and interference with their metabolism and consequently experimental results.

CAGES

Cages should be standardized, and the number of types reduced as much as possible. Small rodents are caged in standard macrolon cages (Figure 6). Four sizes are available, allowing for specific numbers of the different rodent species (Table 2). The cage tops are made from stainless steel and designed as a feed hopper and support for the water bottle.

Rabbits are usually kept in single cages made of plastic or metal with a floor area between 2500 and 3500 cm^2 and a height between 35 and 40 cm (Figure 7).

Cats should be kept in pens with a floor area of not less than 2 m^2 per animal. Temporarily they can be kept in cages with a minimum floor area between 2000 and 6000 cm^2, depending on the body weight.

Dogs should also be kept in pens with floor areas ranging from 0.5 to 2 m^2 per animal depending on body size. Temporary caging with floor area between 0.75 and 1.75 m^2 is also possible.

Non-human primates are kept in cages with a floor area between 0.25 and 1.5 m^2 and a height between 60 and 125 cm, depending on the body size. Pigs and small ruminants are kept in pens.

Minimum requirements for cages are published in the EC Directive 86/609[3] and in the Council of Europe Convention on the use of Live Animals for Experimental Purposes.[4]

Table 2. Species and Maximum Numbers in Standard Cages for Small Rodents

| Cage type | Size (l x w x h cm) | Maximum number of animals in cage | | | |
		Mice	Hamsters	Rats	Guinea pigs
Type 1	20 × 10 × 13	1	1	—	—
Type 2	23 × 17 × 14	5	4	1	—
Type 3	38 × 22 × 15	10	6	3	—
Type 4	55 × 33 × 20	20	10	5	2

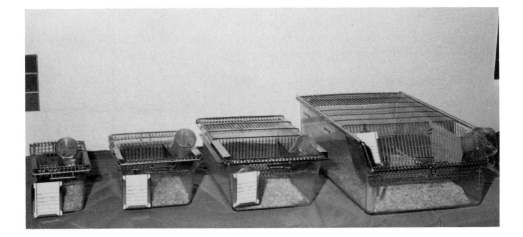

Figure 6. Cages for small rodents.

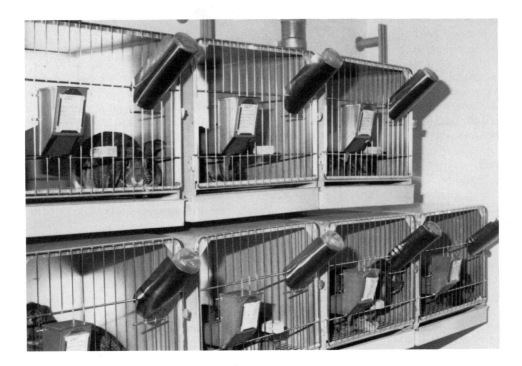

Figure 7. Cages for rabbits.

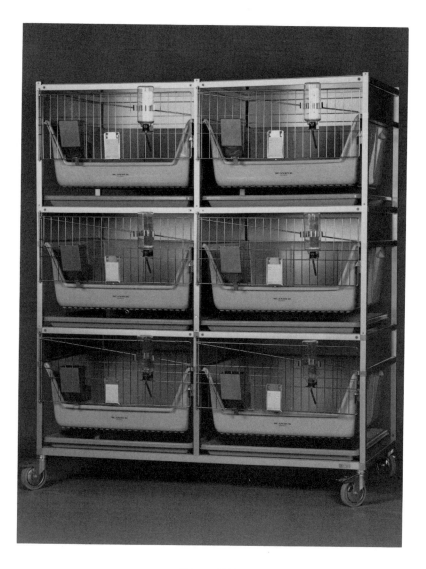

Figure 7 B.

REFERENCES

1. Reus, T. The effect of animal species and types of design of animal facilities, in *Handbook of Facilities Planning,* Vol. 2, *Laboratory Animal Facilities,* Ed. Reus, New York, 1991, chap. 1.3.
2. Clough, G. The animal house: design, equipment and environmental control, in *The UFAW Handbook on the Care and Management of Laboratory Animals.* Trevor Pole, Ed., Sixth Edition, 1989, chap. 8.
3. Retningslinier for anbringelse og pasning af dyr. *European Community Directive 86/609.*
4. The use of Live Animals for Experimental and Industrial Purposes. Council of Europe Convention.

Chapter 10

Laboratory Animal Genetics and Genetic Monitoring

Frederik Dagnæs-Hansen

CONTENTS

0-8493-4378-X/94/$0.00+$.50
© 1994 by CRC Press Inc.

INTRODUCTION

Due to the increased use of inbred laboratory animals, a greater concern with respect to the genetic quality of the laboratory animals has emerged.[1-4] Considerable improvement in the declaration of strains and stocks, using a correct nomenclature, has been seen in more recent literature, although numerous examples of the use of vague definitions still appear.[5-7] Examples of the use of non-authentic or genetically contaminated laboratory mice in biomedical research have been listed.[5,7-12] The best known example was reported by Kahan et al.,[10] who found inbred "BALB/c" mice, supplied by a commercial breeder in the U.S., to exhibit discrepancies with respect to histocompatibility and to an isoenzyme marker. Two congenic strains of mice examined by Lowell and Festing[11] were found not to be isogenic, and Gubbels et al.[12] found that nude mice, backcrossed three to four times on an inbred strain, were not congenic. Genetic contamination has also been observed in inbred rat colonies. More surprising, however, was the report by Festing and Bender, in which they found differences in two identically denominated inbred strains of Sprague-Dawley rats.[13]

This illustrates that the proper definition of a strain/stock must include a description of the origin. What has been described as genetic contamination in some cases, may have been an incorrect use of nomenclature or a vague definition, rather than a mixture of different inbred strains.

The discussion of laboratory animal genetics should concern those characteristics which are inherited and describe how animals with such characteristics are obtained and maintained. Genetic monitoring should ascertain that a particular laboratory animal strain or stock has the expected genetic constitution, and secure its preservation through continued breeding.

GENERAL ASPECTS

The gene is defined as the basic unit of inheritance by which hereditary characteristics are transmitted from parent to offspring. At the molecular level a single gene consists of a length of DNA which exerts its influence on the form and function of the organism by encoding and directing the synthesis of a protein. The two (or more) forms of a gene are called alleles, and the position which a gene occupies on the chromosome is called a locus. If there are more than two alternative choices known for a gene they are called multiple alleles. The combination of alleles of a particular locus comprises the genotype. A group of loci closely situated on the chromosome constitutes a linkage group. If a trait clearly diverging from the normal type or wild type is discovered in an animal, the animal is called a mutant. The gene causing the trait is called a mutated gene or mutated allele. The genes or alleles of a chromosome pair are represented by letter symbols. A gene can be located on the X or Y chromosome and is said to exhibit sex linkage. Genes placed on the other chromosomes are autosomal. If the alleles of an autosomal locus

Table 1. Mating Types Considering One Locus and the Alleles s (Mutant Allele) and + (Wild Type)

Mating type	Autosomal	X-linked	matings of
Incrosses	+ / + x + / +	+ / + x + / Y	Like homozygotes
Crosses	+ / + x s / s	+ / + x s / Y	Unlike homozygotes
	s / s x + / +	s / s x + / Y	
Backcrosses	+ / + x s / +		
	+ / s x + / +	s / + x + / Y	Homozygotes and
	+ / s x s / s	s / + x s / Y	heterozygotes
	s / s x s / +		
Intercrosses	+ / s x + / s		Heterozygotes

on a chromosome pair are alike, the animal is said to be homozygous, if different heterozygous. The same term applies to X-linked loci in females, while males are hemizygous.

A single gene consists of a string of DNA characterized by the specific sequence of the bases. The genome is the total number of genes carried by an animal. The genes and other specific base sequences, for instance minisatellites, may be detected by probes, which are fragments of DNA having nucleic acid sequences complementary to the sequence in the gene or minisatellite. When two complementary DNA strands are reassociated to form a double helix, they are said to hybridize. Hybridization is a technique for determining the similarity of two strings of DNA by reassociating single strands from each DNA molecule and determining the extent of double helix formation.

In the breeding of animals, matings are denominated according to the genotype of animals involved. Four groups are used (Table 1): matings between homozygotes are denominated incrosses, while crosses are matings between homozygotes differing with regard to a particular gene. Backcross is mating between a homozygote and a heterozygote with respect to one gene pair, and intercrosses are matings between individuals that are heterozygotic concerning a particular gene.[14-16]

The combination of alleles in all loci in an individual comprises its genotype. The genetically inherited characteristics may be modified by the environment. The interaction of the genes and the surrounding environment results in the phenotype (Figure 1). It is important to realize that although a laboratory animal is genetically well defined, the environment may greatly influence its phenotypical appearance.

Table 2. Categories of Laboratory Animals

Random-bred, outbred, non-inbred
Inbred
F1 hybrids
Recombinant inbred
Coisogenic and congenic
Segregating inbred

CATEGORIES OF LABORATORY ANIMALS USED IN BIOMEDICAL RESEARCH

BREEDING SYSTEMS

There are two main genetic types of laboratory animals: outbred stock and inbred strains. They can be further subdivided into six categories (Table 2). The purpose of all breeding systems is to preserve or restrict the genetic cause of variability in traits of interest. Theoretically, in large populations under specified environmental conditions, random mating in the absence of selection or mutations will keep the means and variances of all qualitative traits constant. Inbreeding will subdivide a population and increase or decrease the means and decrease the genetic variability. Outcrosses (matings between populations, in

GENOTYPE ⟷ ENVIRONMENT = PHENOTYPE

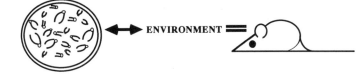

Figure 1. The phenotypical appearance of an animal is a result of the interaction of the genes and the environment.

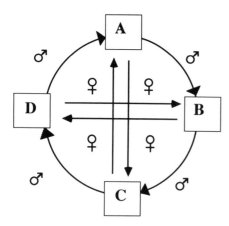

Figure 2. The principles of rotation breeding for avoidance of inbreeding. Males from colony A are mated with females from colony D in colony B, etc.

this context strains or stocks) will usually change the means and increase the genetic variance of the resulting population.[14-16]

RANDOM-BRED, OUTBRED STOCK
Breeding of Outbred Stock

In a large population, theoretically, random breeding will preserve the gene and genotype frequencies generation after generation. In a population of a small size the results of a random breeding system will be slightly different. The rate of random fixation, or loss of alleles at each locus, will be determined by the effective breeding number. If this is large the rate of appearance of homozygosity will be slow, if small, homozygosity will follow rapidly. This effect is known as the "inbreeding effect". Furthermore, selection, mutations, and varying nongenetic or environmental causes of variation are impossible to avoid and all of these factors will cause the population to change in time. In finite populations random breeding has been replaced by breeding systems to avoid inbreeding. A better term for these stocks would therefore be non-inbred. Systematic mating of cousins may preserve heterozygosity better than random mating in smaller populations. Other systems have been devised for maintaining heterozygosity, such as circular, circular pair, and circular subpopulation mating systems.[17-21] The principles of rotation breeding are illustrated in Figure 2.

Use of Random-Bred Animals

Random-bred animals are useful in biomedical research. They may serve as a base population for a selection experiment, in which case it is especially desirable to perpetuate a random-bred line as a control. They may furthermore serve as a population harboring deleterious mutations. In multiple recessive stocks used in radiation or mutagenesis experiments, random breeding may be necessary for maintaining sufficient hybrid vigor in the presence of the many deleterious mutations.[22]

However, there are many reasons for not using random-bred or non-inbred laboratory animals, if suitable inbred, defined strains are available. Well-designed experiments on the responses of laboratory animals to the effects of physical and chemical agents require at least two matched sets of animals, one for treatment and one for control. Ethical reasons and economy demand that the size of the samples be reasonably small, but if the two samples drawn are from a non-inbred or random-bred stock of animals, their responses may not be comparable, thus invalidating the conclusions of the experiment.

Traditionally random-bred laboratory animals have been used extensively in toxicological studies, because they have been said to have a degree of variance similar to what would be expected in the human population. However, outbred stocks are genetically variable to the extent that all individuals are genetically unique, but they tend to be relatively uniform in comparison with the variability within the species. The toxicological testing of a compound in a single stock of outbred animals can be said to be equivalent, genetically, to doing clinical trials in an isolated human population. An alternative strategy for testing would be to use a number of different inbred strains of the same species, the so-called factorial experiment. This could be done by carrying out the animal tests on a sample of five to ten inbred strains. The advantages of this strategy would be that the factorial experiment, still using the same number of animals as in the classical design, would include a wider range of phenotype variations within the test species, thus indicating whether the response to the drug is under genetic control. In this way the test

Table 3. Summary of the Characteristics of Outbred Stock

Characteristics:
    Heterozygosity undefined
    Genetic profile unknown
    Random-mated, closed colonies
Examples:
    Mice: NMRI, OF, CD-1, SWISS-WEBSTER mice
    Rats: Sprague-Dawley
    Beagles, rabbits, guinea pigs
Research use:
    Genetics irrelevant, toxicological testing
    Selection experiments
    For the maintenance of multiple recessive stocks
Advantages:
    Often easy to obtain, cheap
    High reproductive performance and high vigor
    Only type available for some species (dogs, cats)
Disadvantages:
    Unknown genetic make-up
    Phenotypically variable
    Not identifiable — not defined by a genetic profile
    Demands a higher number of animals to achieve high accuracy
    Accuracy of experiment is decreased due to genetic variability
Maintenance:
    "Random breeding"
    Systems for avoidance of inbreeding, i.e., rotation, circular breeding

would be statistically more powerful.[2,4,23,24] The characteristics of outbred stocks are summarized in Table 3.[22]

INBRED STRAINS AND DERIVED STRAINS
Inbred Strains
Inbreeding and the Effect of Inbreeding

Inbred strains, isogenic strains, are laboratory animals produced by inbreeding. By definition, an inbred strain is produced by 20 or more consecutive generations of brother-sister matings. This definition was approved by The Committee on Standardised Genetic Nomenclature for Mice in 1952, but is more or less also accepted as the standard for other laboratory animals, although lower levels of inbreeding are accepted for higher species such as the chicken, rabbit, and pig.

The objective of inbreeding is to reduce the genetic variability towards zero. Animals with certain characteristics of interest may be selected in order to fix the character or characters along with the inevitable selection for viability and fertility. Inbreeding depression, i.e., loss of reproductive fitness as inbreeding progresses, is impossible to avoid; however, selection for more vigorous animals in each generation may prevent reproductive failure. Inbreeding depression is a result of "uncovering" deleterious recessive genes by making them homozygous.[15,16,25]

The extent of inbreeding may be quantified in terms of the coefficient of inbreeding, which is the probability that the two genes at any locus are identical by descent, i.e., that the two genes in one individual originate from one of its ancestors.[15] The coefficient of inbreeding will increase in a population at different rates depending on the degree of relationship between the individuals mated. The closest relationship which may be obtained is between brother and sister, and the coefficient of inbreeding should theoretically reach 99.8% after continued brother-sister mating for 20 generations. Other systematic mating systems would also lead to a high level of inbreeding, such as half-sib and cousin matings. Repeated backcrossing to an inbred strain increases homozygosity as rapidly as self-fertilization (Figure 3). One hundred percent inbreeding can never be reached and the coefficient of inbreeding is calculated under the assumption that the reproductive performance of homozygotes is equal to that of heterozygotes, and that no mutations occur. None of these assumptions can be fulfilled and the level of inbreeding must

94

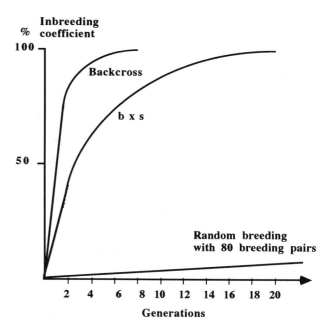

Figure 3. The effect of inbreeding on the inbreeding coefficient. The coefficient of inbreeding should theoretically reach 98.6% after continued brother-sister matings for 20 generations. Repeated backcrossing to an inbred strain increases homozygosity as rapidly as self-fertilization. In small populations, random breeding will result in inbreeding.

be considered overestimated. When a population is inbred to the point where all animals are homozygous (apart from the residual heterozygosity) the population/strain is said to be isogenic, which is a more correct term for describing the genetic constitution of the population/strain.

The inbred strains have a long-term stability. Although an inbred strain does not remain absolutely constant due to residual heterozygosity and mutations, many inbred strains of mice that were developed in the 1920s are still very similar to the original strains even after a period of more than 70 years.[1-3,16,25] This can best be explained by the fact that selection within an inbred strain is ineffective in causing genetic changes. Subline differences do occur, however, as a result of mutations and residual heterozygosity and this sort of divergence may be of practical importance in some experiments. Subline differences have been intensively studied, but for the majority of laboratory animal users, the differentiation is unlikely to be of significant importance, as the main characters (histocompatibility, spontaneous tumor incidence, etc.) for which the animals are used are still the same as in the strain originally developed.

Systems of Inbreeding

During continued inbreeding it is necessary to select two or more single pairs from the offspring of each fertile couple of the preceding generation. Basically this can be done in two ways, either as a continuation of several parallel lines or by selecting one pair in the preceding generation as the ancestor couple (Figure 4). The first system will produce many substrains, as a mutation at any locus that has not been fixed in the former generation or has occurred later has a high probability of becoming fixed within the next 20 generations. In the second system substrain divergence is minimized, as each generation is descended from a common ancestral pair, only two generations earlier.[2,14,25,26] However, if a deleterious mutation arises in one of the breeders later selected as an ancestor, it is likely that this mutation will be fixed, leading to reproductive failure and discontinuation of the strain. A system which is based on the continuation of parallel lines, tracing back to a common ancestor three to five generations earlier, has most often been used.

It has been recommended that all current generations should trace back to a common ancestor five to seven generations earlier and that the selection of future breeding pairs should be based on breeding performance in all breeding pairs within all sublines tracing back to the common ancestor. However, as it is not always possible to have several parallel lines within a small foundation stock, a selection for each three to five generations has been found to be most practical.

In case of an intended selection which might decrease fertility, inbreeding in parallel lines may be advisable, because arrest of a line is likely to occur (NOD mice, MRL/Mp-*lpr/lpr* mice). If decreased fertility causes a line to cease breeding, the characteristics of the strain may be continued in one of the other lines.

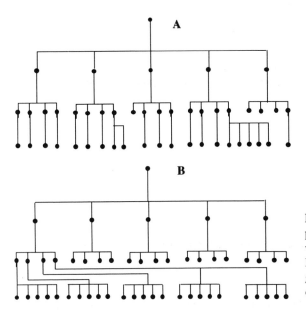

Figure 4. Selection of breeding pairs from the preceding generation can basically be done in two ways, either as a continuation of several parallel lines (A) or by selecting one pair in the preceding generation as the ancestor couple (B). The most often used system is a combination of the two.

Individuals within an inbred strain may not be absolutely identical. There may be some residual heterozygosity in excess of the amount expected, or there may be differences due to recent mutation, not yet fixed by inbreeding, or due to the inevitable selection for vigor in the course of inbreeding. Phenotypical variability of nongenetic causes may also be brought to expression due to the drastic reduction in genetic variability and higher sensitivity to environmental influences. It is important to realize that the relative genetic invariability of an inbred strain does not always imply less phenotypical variability. In fact, the opposite may often be true. MacLaren and Michie found the variability of the response to a given treatment to be three to four times higher among two inbred strains than in the hybrid strain. This was probably due to greater environmental sensibility among the inbred strains.[27]

Use of Inbred Strains
Inbred laboratory animals exhibit a high degree of uniformity in physiological traits. This makes them useful in a wide variety of experiments in which the effects of the experimental treatment may be relatively small and where precision of measurement of the effects is crucial. Since various inbred strains differ genetically, it is possible to improve the experimental setup by selecting specially suited strains.

A large number of inbred strains with genetically determined diseases have been developed. These are extensively used as models for the corresponding diseases in humans, for instance mice or rats with insulin-dependent juvenile diabetes mellitus (NOD mice, BB rats) or the various strains of rats with hypertension.[28-32]

Another valuable feature of inbred strains is the amount of background data that exist on the more common strains.[2,3] The characteristics of inbred strains are outlined in Table 4.[22]

F1 Hybrids
When animals of two different inbred strains are crossed, the resulting progeny are called F1 hybrids. They are heterozygous at all loci where the parental strains differed. The F1 hybrids are isogenic (not homozygous) but uniformly heterozygous, and therefore as genetically uniform as the inbred strains. F1 hybrids are valuable in biomedical research because of their isogenicity. They exhibit hybrid vigor, are genetically uniform and less sensitive to environmental influences, and therefore better suited for many experiments. Hybrid vigor is expressed in faster growth, higher rate of survival to maturity and longer life-span. Hybrid litters are often larger than inbred litters. Tumor grafts, skin and other tissues from either parental strain are usually accepted. Hybrids are reproducible as long as the parental strains exist and are recommended for use in the testing and evaluation of chemical carcinogenesis.[33]

Table 4. Summary of the Characteristics of Inbred Strains

Characteristics:
   Results of 20 or more consecutive generations of brother-sister matings
   An inbred strain may be regarded as an immortal clone of an almost constant genotype
Examples:
   Mice: CBA, NOD, AKR, C57BL
   Rats: F344, LEW
Research use:
   Almost all fields of biomedical research
Advantages:
   Isogenic
   Homozygous
   Genetic profiles known
   Histocompatible
   Phenotype uniformity (fewer animals needed in experimentation)
   Long-term stability (if fully inbred F >60)
   Background information available
   Identifiable (genetic profile available)
   Individuality — some strains have special characters of interest
Disadvantages:
   Poor breeding capacity
   Expensive
   Unsuitable for some experiments (e.g., selection)
   High sensitivity to environmental factors
Maintenance:
   Foundation colony or nucleus colony (NC)   ->
   Pedigree expansion colony (PEC)   ->
   Multiplication colony (MC)   -> research
      (traffic-light system)
   Foundation colony is maintained by brother-sister mating, pedigreed
   Quality control and good colony management essential
   In the multiplication colony random mating and simple records

Congenic and Coisogenic Strains

Two strains, identical except for a difference at a single genetic locus, are called coisogenic. Coisogenicity can only arise as a result of a mutation in an established inbred strain. Congenic strains are produced by a succession of backcrossings. In order to produce a congenic strain crosses are made between an inbred strain, donating the genetic background (background strain), and another strain or stock carrying the desired gene (the donor strain/stock). The donor strain/stock donates the chromosome segment or mutant gene. At every backcross with the inbred strain a selection is made for the donor-strain locus. Production of congenic mouse strains was started in the 1940s by George Snell, who worked with tissue transplantation. He produced strains of mice congenic with respect to their histocompatibility genes. Congenic lines that differ at a histocompatibility locus are resistant to each other's grafts and are therefore also called congenic resistant (CR).[34]

The procedure applicable for the production of a congenic strain, when the differential allele is dominant or codominant, is the backcross or NX system. This is exemplified in Figure 5. The original inbred partner is represented here by C57BL/6J, which is H-2 haplotype b/b. To obtain a C57BL/6J strain haplotype k/k, the AKR strain can be used as donor. The offspring of the mating of AKR and C57BL/6J is haplotype b/k; however, approximately half of the genome is from each of the parental strains. By backcrossing to C57BL/6J two kinds of offspring are produced: b/b and b/k. The b/b haplotype is discarded and the b/k genotype is used for further backcrossing. C57BL/6J k/k is produced by an intercross after backcrossing.

If the differential gene is recessive, a system of backcross-intercross (MX) must be used. The principles are outlined in Figure 6. For each backcross, the offspring have to be mated with each other in order to produce individuals homozygous with respect to the recessive gene.

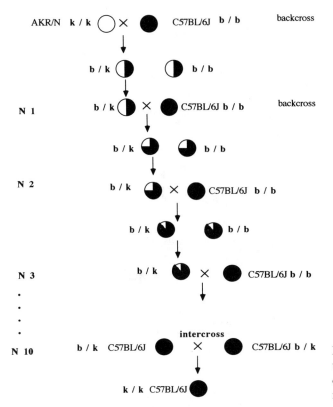

Figure 5. The backcross (NX) system is used for creating a congenic strain when the differential allele is dominant or codominant.

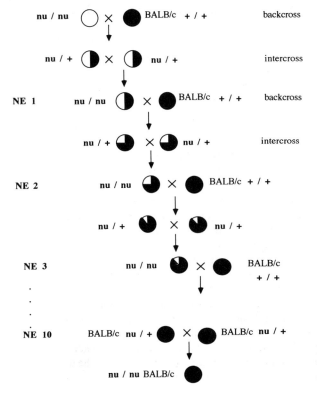

Figure 6. The backcross-intercross (MX) system is used for creating a congenic strain when the differential allele is recessive.

98

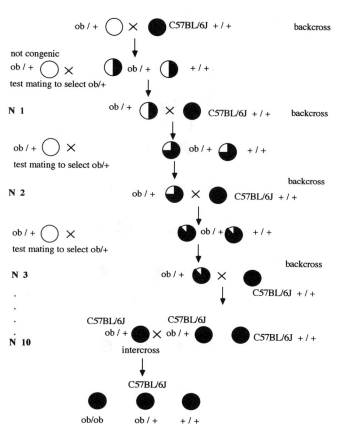

Figure 7. The backcross system with intervening intercross test matings is used for the production of a congenic strain, when the differential allele is recessive and the homozygotic animals are infertile, as in the case of the *ob* gene.

An even more complicated system is necessary if the recessive homozygous individuals are infertile, as is the case in mice carrying the *ob* gene. Backcrossing has to be performed with heterozygous individuals. Heterozygous individuals are found by test matings (Figure 7).

Each cycle of backcross, backcross-intercross is counted (N) to indicate the similarity between the background strain and the congenic strain. If more complex mating systems are employed, the generations should be expressed as N equivalents (NE). A strain developed by this method is regarded as congenic when a minimum of 10 backcrosses or backcross equivalents have been made (N = 10 or NE = 10), counting the first hybrid of F1 generation as generation 1 (N = 1).

Segregating Inbred Strains

Segregating inbred strains are similar to inbred strains except that heterozygosis is forced upon one or more named loci. The object is to produce two or more kinds of strains which are identical except for a difference at one or more loci. The two systems for producing segregating inbred strains are backcrossing and intercrossing. The breeding systems are shown in Figures 8 and 9. The motives for producing segregating inbred strains are similar to the motives for creating congenic strains; however, in the production of segregating inbred strains a higher degree of isogeneity is to be expected. In the segregating inbred strains, incrosses (development of homozygosity) follow with a speed equal to that obtained in normal inbreeding. Therefore, the probability of creating homozygosity in all loci, including those flanking the differential loci, is higher in the breeding system for segregating inbred strains than in that for congenic strains. In general, most strains carrying a mutation or a gene transferred from another strain are maintained by a combination of the systems for breeding congenic and segregating inbred strains. The resultant animals will have a very high degree of genetic similarity to mice of the background strain, because of the backcross or the cross-intercross, and they will have a relatively short segment of heterozygous chromosome bearing the differential allele, because of the brother-sister inbreeding with forced heterozygosity. The strain produced is denoted according to the number of backcrosses or the cross-intercrosses (N) and the number of succeeding inbred generations (F); for instance, the mouse strain denoted BALB/cA nu/+ N20F15 was created by 20 cycles of cross-intercross followed by 15 inbred generations.[14,26]

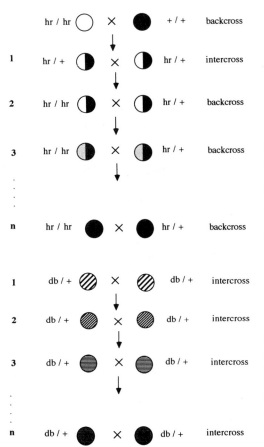

Figure 8. The backcross system for producing segregating inbred strains carrying the hairless (*hr*) mutation. Brother-sister inbreeding is continued by backcrossing. If backcrossing is started with two different strains, the segregating inbred strain will be different from both parental strains, as illustrated by the hatching.

Figure 9. The backcross-intercross system for producing segregating inbred strains carrying the diabetic (*db*) mutation. During continuous breeding, inbreeding will result in more homozygous animals. A fully inbred strain has been developed following 20 generations of brother-sister matings. If backcrossing is started with two different strains, the segregating inbred strain will be different from both parental strains, as illustrated by the hatching.

Recombinant Inbred Strains

Recombinant inbred strains or RI are produced by crossing two inbred strains, the progenitor strains. The F1 individuals are crossed, and from the F2 generation random pairs are selected for mating. The offspring from a number of these matings are perpetuated by brother-sister inbreeding. The lines that survive 20 or more generations of inbreeding comprise a collection of new inbred strains, all descending from a single pair of progenitor strains. Each recombinant inbred line is descended from a single F2 pair. RI strains are extremely useful for discovery of new hereditary traits and for detecting genetic linkage.[35,36]

Sublines

Sublines are not an intended product of a particular breeding system, but may be considered a side product in the process of continued inbreeding. The causes of subline development and the nomenclature are described later in this chapter.

Mutants and Transgenic Laboratory Animals
Mutant Strains

Mutants are animals in which a mutation has occurred or animals of strains to which a mutant gene has been transferred. If the mutation arises in an inbred strain, the strain is said to be coisogenic. If a mutation is transferred to an inbred strain, the strain so formed is called a congenic strain. Mutations may also be maintained in outbred strains as discussed earlier.

A particular mutation may then be passed on in the strain by continued inbreeding, if the mutation does not have deleterious effects on the viability or fertility of the animals. In some instances special husbandry procedures are necessary in order to secure the health of the animals; e.g., immune-deficient animals should be kept under germ-free or specific-pathogen-free (SPF) conditions in order to increase life-span and fertility.[30,31,37] If a mutant strain is bred by inbreeding, it may diverge from the non-mutant strain due to genetic drift. If isohistogeneity between the mutant and non-mutant control strain (apart from the mutation) is intended, crossing followed by intercrossing must be performed at regular intervals, similar to the breeding of congenic inbred strains.[14,26]

Some mutations are bred by backcrossing due to the reduced fertility of the homozygous mutant females.

Transgenic Laboratory Animals

Transgenic laboratory animals are laboratory animals produced by the introduction of foreign DNA into the genome, using recombinant DNA technology. The incorporated foreign DNA may be inherited by the offspring by normal Mendelian inheritance. Transgenic animals may be obtained by the introduction of DNA from the same species or from a foreign species. In all cases, the DNA introduced constitutes a new construction of DNA, contributing to the under- or overexpression of certain genes, or the expression of genes completely new to the animal species.[38-42]

There are many different techniques for the production of transgenic animals. The method mostly applied is micro-injection of small DNA constructs into the pronucleus of fertilized eggs. DNA may also be introduced by retroviral vectors into fertilized embryos or embryonic stem cells. The embryonic stem cells to which the DNA construct has been introduced by injection or by a viral vector are then transferred to blastocysts for the formation of chimeras. If the embryonic stem cells contribute to the formation of germ cells, the transgene may be transferred to the offspring, which then will have the transgene incorporated in all cells.

Transgenic animals may be compared to mutants with respect to the way in which they are bred. The principles in breeding transgenic animals will depend on the nature of the transgene, i.e., whether the expression of the transgene is recessive, dominant, or semidominant, and whether the transgene is lethal or causes reduced fertility when appearing homozygously.

The transgenic individual may express the foreign gene and may be able to transfer the transgene to the offspring, and is then called a founder. A founder animal may be of an inbred strain, it may be a hybrid or of an outbred strain, though in rats and mice the transgene is most often transferred to an inbred strain by backcrossing. By this process a transgenic strain is produced on a defined genetic background, and the original inbred strain may contribute a nontransgenic control strain.

The use and the techniques for the production of transgenic animals have been described in greater detail.[38-44]

GENETIC STABILITY OF STRAINS AND STOCKS OF LABORATORY ANIMALS

CAUSES OF PHENOTYPE VARIATION

The genotype may be modified by the environment, causing variations in the appearance of the animal, the phenotype. The causes of variation between laboratory animals may thus be divided into variation due to environmental causes, variation due to genetic causes, and variation due to the interaction between these two factors.

Although environmental conditions, such as circadian rhythms, temperature, light, humidity, noise, caging, bedding, ventilation, diet, animal housing personnel, social interaction between animals, infections, and health status are subject to further discussion elsewhere in this book, it is worthwhile to stress that animals may respond differently under different conditions. Even highly defined characteristics related to the genetic constitution of animals may be modified by environmental factors. The influence of the diet on the diabetes incidence in NOD mice illustrates this. The NOD mouse is an inbred mouse strain in which more than 70% of the females develop spontaneous diabetes between the ages of 80 and 200 days. The predisposition for development of diabetes has been found to be based on the inheritance of five or more genes.[45,46] However, it has been shown that feeding NOD mice a purified diet changes the incidence significantly (Figure 10).[47] The incidence of diabetes may also be changed drastically by viral infections.[48]

Numerous other examples of environmental influences may be cited, but in general it can be stated that polygenic traits, i.e., traits based on the collective effects of several or many different genes, may have a tendency to be more strongly influenced by the environment than monogenic traits.[2]

DEVELOPMENT OF SUBLINES

Inbred strains are bred by brother-sister mating, and the strains may be continued in one or more lines as discussed earlier. During continued inbreeding each line will become less and less related to the other

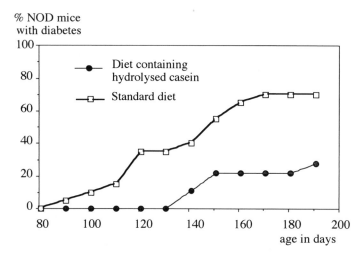

Figure 10. The effect of feeding NOD mice a purified diet. The diabetes incidence is significantly decreased.

lines, but not necessarily more different from the others. The lines so formed are denoted sublines. The extent to which one subline will deviate from the others will depend on several factors. The factors causing subline divergences are residual heterozygosity, mutations, and genetic contamination. These three factors are comprised under the term genetic drift.[49-53]

If separated lines have known differences, the term substrain is often used. Substrain development is caused by mutations or genetic contamination, but the development of substrains may also be a consequence of the separation of lines before inbreeding has been completed.

GENETIC DRIFT
Residual Heterozygosity

The number of heterozygotic genes in an inbred animal depends on the number of inbreeding generations. It has been estimated that the probability of the genome being completely homozygous after 60 generations is 99%, assuming that no mutation or selection has taken place.[14,15] This figure has been discussed and is considered highly overestimated.

Mutations

Mutations are changes in the sequences of DNA nucleotides and may occur in all cells. Only mutations which arise in the germ cells may be transferred to the offspring. If a mutation is fixed in the following generations, it might change the strain. Mutations are often difficult to detect, as many mutations have no or very little influence on the phenotype of the animals.

Genetic Contamination

Accidental crossing of an inbred strain with another strain or stock is probably the source of most existing major subline and substrain differences.[54-56] Genetic contamination will often be more obvious in an inbred strain than in an outbred stock. The number of contaminant genes fixed will be inversely proportional to the effective number of breeders maintained during the generations of random mating. Genetic contamination within a brother-sister mating system will either be very high (50%) or zero (0%).

Although genetic contamination is considered an undesired occurrence, some cases of genetic contamination have led to the development of new, interesting strains, as exemplified by the development of the non-obese diabetes resistant strain (NOR). The NOR arose from a genetic contamination between the NOD mice and another inbred strain, C57BL/KsJ. The NOR strain carries many diabetes susceptibility alleles in common with the NOD mice, yet it does not develop diabetes.[57]

NOMENCLATURE

THE CONTRIBUTION TO INTERNATIONAL STANDARDIZATION

The rules for designating mouse strains are issued by the International Committee on Standardised Genetic Nomenclature for Mice. The rules for the nomenclature of rats follow basically the rules for mice. The most recently published rules are found in the second edition of *Genetic Variants and Strains of the Laboratory Mouse*.[58] Changes or additions of new strains are updated periodically in the publication *Mouse Genome* (formerly *Mouse News Letter*). Rules for the nomenclature of outbred stocks have been proposed by Festing et al.[59] Rules for the nomenclature of genes, including the H-2 complex, have recently been presented.[58,60,61]

The most recent information of nomenclature on rats has been presented.[62–64] Rules for the nomenclature of genes and listing of gene symbols for rats are published periodically.[64]

RULES FOR NOMENCLATURE
Outbred Stock
Outbred stocks are denoted with the holder, followed by a colon and the name of the outbred stock. For instance Ssc: NMRI is the outbred NMRI stock, maintained at Ssc, Statens Serum Institut, Copenhagen. If the stock carries a mutant gene, e.g., the nude gene, the designation should be Ssc: NMRI-*nu/nu*.

Inbred Strains
Inbred strains should be designated by capital letters or Arabic numerals or a combination of capital letters and numerals, beginning with a letter. Strains with a common origin, separated before F20, should be regarded as related inbred strains and be given symbols indicating the relationship. Indication of inbreeding is given by an appending F, followed by the number of inbred generations in parenthesis. Example: C57BL/6J (F67). If information is incomplete, this is indicated by a question mark; example: C57BL/6J (F?+10).

Substrains
Inbred strains may be subdivided into substrains if known or probable genetic differences become established. This can happen because of residual heterozygosity at the time of branching, or because of later mutation, or contamination. Substrains are formed when (1) branches are separated after F20 and before F40, (2) a branch is known to have been maintained separately from other branches for >100 generations, (3) or when genetic differences from other branches are discovered. If the cause is contamination, which would lead to numerous genetic changes, the strain should be renamed.

Substrains are designated by the name of the parent strain followed by a slant line and an appropriate substrain symbol, whether a number, a person or laboratory at which the strain was maintained, or a combination of these. For instance C57BL/10ScN (line number 10 maintained by Scott at NIH). The substrain designations should be accumulated if successive genetic differences arise in an inbred strain.

Sublines
Sublines are inbred strains which are considered probably different from the parental strain due to environmental, maternal, or cytoplasmic differences. Sublines may be created by (1) manipulation: fostering (**f**), egg transfer (**e**), hand-rearing (**h**), ovary transplantation (**o**), or preservation by freezing (**p**); or by (2) the transfer of a strain to another holder. Subline designation is optional as the processes may not be relevant to the work being performed, and the subline symbols should not be accumulated, since environmental factors are unlikely to act cumulatively. Examples: C57BL/6J fostered on BALB/cJ are designated: C57BL/6JfBALB/c or C57BL/6JfC.

Subline designation due to the maintenance by another research laboratory should be the same as for a substrain, but the abbreviation of the research worker should be separated from the substrain designation by a double slanted line, e.g., C57BL/6J kept at Ssc, Statens Serum Institute, Animal Dept., Copenhagen, is C57BL/6J//Ssc. The complete story of the subline should be recorded in 'Mouse Genome'.

Hybrids
F1 hybrid strains are designated by the letters of the maternal strain followed by an x and the paternal strain with intervening spaces and in brackets, and appended by the letter F and the number 1. The maternal and paternal strains may be abbreviated if the full name is mentioned somewhere in the text. Recommended abbreviations for the most commonly used inbred strains of mice are given in Table 5. The offspring from crosses between F1 hybrids are designated in a similar way, substituting F1 with F2. Hybrids from backcrosses or other crosses are characterized similarly. For instance, the offspring from a mating between a C57BL/6J female and a DBA/2J male are described as: (C57BL/6J x DBA/2J)F1 or B6D2F1.

Recombinant Inbred
Recombinant inbred strains are denoted by an abbreviation of both parental strain names, separated by a capital X with no intervening spaces; CXB indicates a set of recombinant inbred strains, derived from a cross of BALB/c x C57BL. Different RI strains in the same series should be distinguished by numbers.

Table 5. Recommended Abbreviations of the Most Commonly Used Inbred Strains of Mice

AKR	AK
BALB/c	C
C3H	C3
C57BL	B
C57BL/10	B10
C57BL/6	B6
DBA/2	D2
NZB	ZB

Coisogenic, Congenic, and Segregating Inbred Strains

In general these strains are designated by the full or abbreviated symbol of the background strain followed by a period or hyphen next to the symbol of the differential locus and allele or an abbreviated symbol of the donor strain, or both of these; example: the coisogenic strain AKR/J-*nu*^{str} is an inbred strain in which the mutation *nustr* appeared in the nude locus. Heterozygotic animals are indicated by AKR/J-+/*nustr*. The gene symbols should be in italics in printed articles; example: the coisogenic strain C57BL/6J-*Thy-1ᵃ* or C57BL/6J.PL/J-*Thy-1ᵃ* or B6.P-*Thy-1ᵃ* is a congenic inbred strain in which the allele a in the locus Thy-1 has been transferred from the strain PL/J to C57BL/6J. If the strain is already widely known, a less complete symbol may be used, e.g., the designation A.SW is used for a congenic inbred strain in which the allele s in the locus H-2 has been transferred from the strain SWR/J to A/J (A/J.SWR/J-*H-2ˢ* or A.SW-*H-2ˢ*).

Transgenic Laboratory Animals

The nomenclature of transgenic animals should follow the rules described above for the background strain. The designation of the transgene is in principle similar to the designation of other gene symbols, i.e., locus and allele symbols; however, a general symbol, Tg, for this type of anomaly is used. The symbol is followed by the number of the chromosome into which the gene has been inserted. If unknown, the number zero should be used. Also enclosed in the brackets should be a detailed description of the gene and the species of origin (*Mus musculus:* MMU, *Rattus norvegicus:* RNO etc.). Following the brackets a serial number and the abbreviation of the laboratory should appear; example C57BL/6J-Tg(0HSAHba)As12 being a C57BL/6J mouse carrying a human gene for hemoglobin alpha-chain (Hba) in an unknown location (0), created by the 12th insertion performed at the University of Århus, Denmark (human: HSA, *Homo sapiens*; As, Århus). Other and more detailed information should be given in text or table form.

GENETIC CONTROL AND GENETIC MONITORING

Genetic control has two steps. The first step is to check the genetic constitution of the laboratory animal, either by obtaining the animal from a reference colony (origin) or by authenticity testing to ascertain that the genetic profile of the strain/stock is correct. In other words, to test whether or not the genetic profile is identical to the profile of the same strain/stock from other colonies or to the profile described in the literature.

The second step is to preserve this genetic constitution in further breeding by proper colony management and test sampling for the detection of contamination between the strains kept within the facility in which the animals are bred.

In long-term maintenance of the strain in the nucleus colony, there are two possibilities: either to test the breeding nucleus at regular intervals for its genetic authenticity, or to obtain a new breeding nucleus from a reference colony at regular intervals.

The genetic constitution refers to the population rather than to the individual. The outbred stock is thus attempted to be defined by the means, averages and deviations of a number of characteristics, i.e., the genotype spectrum. Testing for genetic heterogeneity has been done using biochemical markers and mandible shape.[64,65,73-76] As neither random matings nor rotation systems are quite sufficient for preserving the genotype spectrum of outbred populations, a system for monitoring and keeping the genotype spectrum largely constant has been described by Rapp and co-workers.[77,78] This system is based on the monitoring of reproductive data, mandible analysis, total body analysis, hematological data, and biochemical markers.[68,69] By use of DNA fingerprinting Hins and Gruber were able to quantify heterozygosity by the configuration of the DNA patterns. They suggested the use of this system for the characterization of outbred stocks.[79]

COLONY MANAGEMENT
The Nucleus Colony

The nucleus colony (NC) (stem colony, foundation colony, primary type colony) is the foundation of inbred strains. Any mistake that goes undetected will eventually be fixed and transferred to all descendant

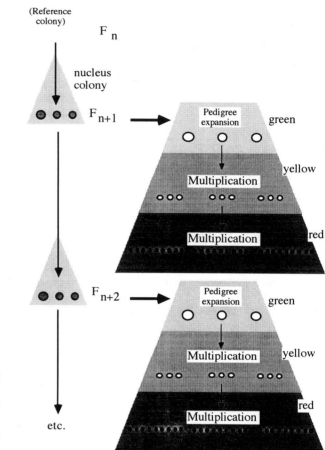

Figure 11. Organization of the traffic-light system in the pedigree expansion colony. Breeding animals from the nucleus colony are used in the pedigree expansion colony, which are bred for two generations in the traffic-light breeding system.

generations and colonies. Genetically the NC needs to be defined for a number of relevant characters, and it must be regularly monitored for the expression of specific markers. The NC can be physically isolated either in isolators or in separate breeding facilities.

Recording of all breeding data is of paramount importance in the maintenance of the nucleus colony and has to be undertaken carefully. Genetic supervision is especially needed, if the particular NC is not physically separated from other colonies.[2,14,25,26,80,81] Another possibility is to renew the NC at regular intervals from a reference colony where authenticity is controlled.

Pedigree Expansion Colony

The pedigree expansion colony (PEC) is a colony set up to meet a greater demand and is managed like a NC, except for the renewal of the breeding pairs, which are taken from the NC only. The PEC is structured like a pyramid with the nucleus at the top. The PEC follows directly beneath the NC and the base consists of up to three multiplication generations. Breeding animals are obtained from the colony above and all offspring from the base generation are used in experiments. The PEC is often organized according to the so-called traffic-light system. To meet an even greater demand for animals, a multiplication colony (MC) can be established with breeding animals from the PEC. There is no particular need to continue brother-sister mating in the MC. The PEC and MC systems ensure that animals used for research are only three or four generations from the breeding nucleus. The continuous renewal of breeding animals at the top of the pyramid also ensures that any possible contamination down the pyramid will be eliminated during further breeding and through renewal at the top of a new pyramid.

In the PECs and MCs several strains may be bred in the same facility; however, it is advisable only to keep phenotypically dissimilar strains together (Figure 11). Computerized systems have been developed for controlling breeding and production.[82-84]

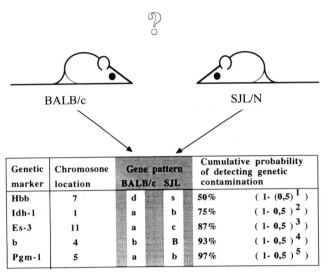

Genetic marker	Chromosone location	Gene pattern BALB/c	Gene pattern SJL	Cumulative probability of detecting genetic contamination	
Hbb	7	d	s	50%	$(1-(0,5)^1)$
Idh-1	1	a	b	75%	$(1-0,5)^2$
Es-3	11	a	c	87%	$(1-0,5)^3$
b	4	b	B	93%	$(1-0,5)^4$
Pgm-1	5	a	b	97%	$(1-0,5)^5$

Hbb; Hemoglobin beta-chain.   Idh-1; isocitrate dehydrogenase-1
Es-3; Esterase-3.   b/B; coat color brown.   Pgm-1; phophoglucomutase-1.

Figure 12. The principles of the critical subset. The testing is based on screening of five to six strategic non-linked genetic markers which are known to differentiate the inbred strains in question. For every single genetic marker included in the examination, the probability of detecting genetic contamination is increased. By testing five markers there is a 97% probability of detecting genetic contamination in the two strains in question.

GENETIC MONITORING
Authenticity Testing

The authenticity of any given strain is established by comparing the profile, with respect to a suitable set of genetic markers, with the published profile of the strain in question. Such a procedure will not always be able to detect a mutation or subline divergence.

Some markers are shared by many inbred strains, for instance the biochemical type of the amylase enzyme in mice. Examination for this marker would therefore be of limited value if inbred strains of mice were to be differentiated. Hence, it is obvious that genetic markers exhibiting high variability among strains are better suited for genetic monitoring, as is the case for markers within the H-2 complex in mice.

In breeding colonies it may be practical to test offspring from an animal, thus saving the animal itself for continued breeding. The markers should be evenly distributed over the entire genome since contamination may be located to one linkage group only.

In the monitoring of the NC, the test program should comprise a relatively large number of genes in order to assure the quality and integrity of the animals that will later give rise to the expansion colony.[68,85] Genetic monitoring has traditionally been based on analysis of biochemical markers, immunogenetic markers (including histocompatibility markers), coat color markers, morphological traits, mandible analysis, clinical chemical analysis, as well as other characteristics. For practical and economical reasons it has been proposed to examine two or three loci (biochemical, immunogenetic, or morphological) on each chromosome, as these markers would imitate random samples of the genome.[65,75] As isohistogeneity is a prerequisite for an inbred strain, skin transplantation should always be used.

Analysis of a total set of markers (two to three markers on all chromosomes) cannot be performed for each generation; however, it could be done for every four generations. Skin transplantation performed every second generation, and additional examination of the mandible every four generations might serve as criteria for the selection of new breeding pairs.[68,75] The test program preceding the selection of new common ancestors might typically include 11–14 biochemical markers, test matings, mandible analysis, skin transplantation, and an examination of reproduction data.

Critical Subset

It is often necessary to breed different inbred strains in the same animal room. In this case, it is advisable to keep only strains with differing phenotypes (coat colors) together. This is often not possible, and moreover, it may also be impossible to create physical barriers between the different strains within the animal room. Therefore it is necessary to have an efficient method for detecting unwanted matings between the different inbred strains maintained within an animal room. The most efficient way to check for genetic contamination is by examination for the single genetic markers which are known to differentiate the inbred strains in question. The testing is based on a screening of five to six strategic non-linked genetic markers (Figure 12). Such a set of markers is called a critical subset. The probability of detecting

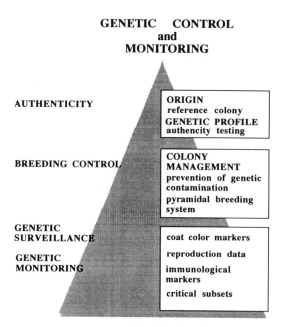

GENETIC CONTROL and MONITORING

AUTHENTICITY

ORIGIN
reference colony
GENETIC PROFILE
authencity testing

BREEDING CONTROL

COLONY
MANAGEMENT
prevention of genetic
contamination
pyramidal breeding
system

GENETIC
SURVEILLANCE

GENETIC
MONITORING

coat color markers

reproduction data

immunological
markers

critical subsets

Figure 13. Summary of genetic control and genetic monitoring. For further details see text.

genetic contamination by testing one marker is 50%. By testing more markers, the cumulative probability may be increased correspondingly, reaching 97% for five markers tested; however, any inbreeding subsequent to the genetic contamination further increases the probability of detecting genetic contamination. The monitored genes must be unlinked.[2,72]

Recommendations

The genetic analysis performed on a routine basis should include continuous registration of coat color markers and litter size, and periodically skin transplantation, serological examination for histocompatibility antigens, biochemical markers, and DNA fingerprinting should be used.

These monitoring systems would primarily be directed towards the detection of genetic contamination. Monitoring on a comparable basis for control of mutations and subline divergences, however, requires far more complicated systems, which are expensive to establish and are performed routinely only in very few laboratories. Moreover, the techniques available have not yet been internationally standardized, rendering direct comparison of results from different laboratories difficult (Figure 13).

LABORATORY PROCEDURES FOR GENETIC MONITORING
General Aspects

Laboratory procedures are available to detect differences among strains at all levels. DNA techniques can detect differences in the sequences of DNA, and biochemical methods can differentiate on the basis of differences in the composition of enzymes or other functional molecules. Immunological methods are used to differentiate between strains that differ with respect to their histocompatibility antigens. Phenotypically appearing traits are coat color, mandible shape, litter size, body weight, body fat content, and body size. Some of these characteristics may be modified by environmental factors.

Electrophoresis

Biochemical markers are analyzed by gel electrophoresis or electrofocusing. Traditionally, starch gel electrophoresis has been used; however, separation on various matrices such as polyacrylamide gel and cellulose acetate, has also been applied.[85-87] Proteins exposed to an electric field will migrate depending on the net charge (isoelectric point) and molecular weight of the protein at a certain pH. Hemoglobin, transferrin, seminal vesicle protein, enzymes and other proteins are found in different isotypes among strains. This means that the proteins are produced in alternating forms, coded for by one locus, and the differences in amino acid composition or secondary structure will cause the two forms to migrate differently in an electric field during electrophoresis. Alternating forms of proteins coded for by one locus are referred to as biochemical polymorphism. Enzymes generated by allelic differences are called allozymes.[87]

Table 6. Biochemical Markers of Three Inbred Strains of Mice, NOD, NON, BALB/c, and C57BL/6J

Genetic marker	Chromosome location	NOD	NON	BALB/c	C57BL/6J
Ahd-1	4	a	—	b	a
Akp-1	1	b	b	b	a
Amy-1	3	b	a	a	a
Amy-2	3	b	a	a	a
Apo-1	9	b	a	b	a
Car-2	3	a	b	b	a
Es-1	8	b	b	b	a
Es-2	8	b	b	b	b
Es-3	11	c	c	a	a
Es-10	14	a	a	a	a
Es-11	8	a	a	a	a
Glo-1	17	a	a	a	a
Got-1	8	b	b	b	b
Gpd-1	4	b	b	b	a
Gpi-1	7	a	a	a	a
Gpt-1	15	b	a	a	a
Gr-1	8	a	a	a	a
Gus-s	5	b	-	a	b
Hbb	7	s	s	d	s
Hc	2	o	o	1	1
Idh-1	1	a	b	a	a
Itp	2	b	-	a	b
Ldr-1	6	a	a	a	a
Mod-1	9	b	a	a	b
Mpi-1	9	b	b	b	b
Mup-1	4	new	new	a	b
Neu-1	17	b	b	b	b
Pep-3	1	b	b	a	a
Pgm-1	5	a	a	a	a
Pgm-1	4	a	a	a	a
Trf	9	b	b	b	b

The most common inbred strains of mice and rats have been characterized by 20 or more polymorphic biochemical markers.[88,89] An example of profiles of three inbred mouse strains is given in Table 6.[29] Biochemical methods are efficient in revealing when a strain and/or a subline diverges as a result of genetic contamination.[54-56] Simplified technical systems that make tests possible in only 1 hour have been described.[90,91]

When testing for biochemical markers, a tissue is taken from the animal and homogenized. The tissue needed and the buffer used are dependent on which protein has to be analyzed. Blood, either as erythrocyte lysate, plasma or serum, kidney, liver, and seminal vesicle fluid are the most often used tissues or body fluids. Figure 14 illustrates a possible outcome of a genetic analysis using biochemical markers. Technical details and the application of biochemical markers are described in detail elsewhere.[84,87,91-96]

Immunological Markers

Immunological markers are primarily detected by serological testing, cellular reactions (lymphocytes, erythrocytes), and transplantation (skin grafting). The immunological markers are cell surface antigens or soluble molecules which exist in different forms (alloantigens). In addition to the major histocompatibility complex (MHC), there are a number of other immunological markers, such as erythrocyte antigens,

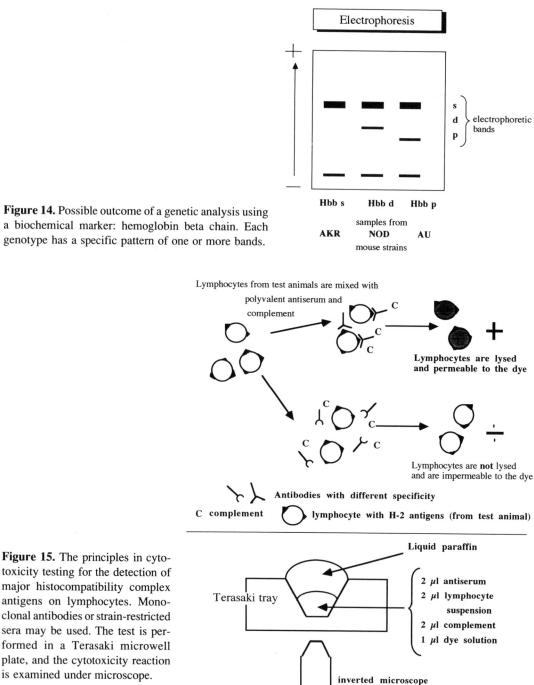

Figure 14. Possible outcome of a genetic analysis using a biochemical marker: hemoglobin beta chain. Each genotype has a specific pattern of one or more bands.

Figure 15. The principles in cytotoxicity testing for the detection of major histocompatibility complex antigens on lymphocytes. Monoclonal antibodies or strain-restricted sera may be used. The test is performed in a Terasaki microwell plate, and the cytotoxicity reaction is examined under microscope.

lymphocyte antigens, immunoglobulin allotypes, and minor histocompatibility antigens (minor histocompatibility complex).[97,98]

MHC regulates the synthesis of glycoproteins, which occur in many different forms among strains, i.e., the markers exhibit a high degree of polymorphism. The antigens are readily obtained from lymphocytes and peripheral blood cells, and may be used for testing. The antigens are highly immunogenic, i.e., animals confronted with alien histocompatibility antigens become specifically immunized against these antigens, and the MHC is of great importance in most immunological experiments. Many strains of laboratory animals are maintained just because of their MHC type (haplotype).[65,66,97,98] Genetic control using the MHC antigens may be based on *in vitro* or *in vivo* methods.

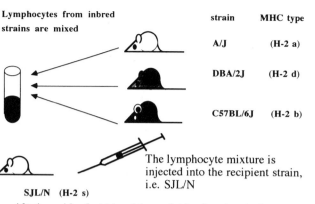

Lymphocytes from inbred strains are mixed

strain	MHC type
A/J	(H-2 a)
DBA/2J	(H-2 d)
C57BL/6J	(H-2 b)

SJL/N (H-2 s)

The lymphocyte mixture is injected into the recipient strain, i.e. SJL/N

After immunising 5 x (1 / week) serum is taken from the animals.
Serum (SRTS) is used in the genetic control.

EXAMPLE

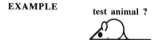

test animal ?

Is this mouse a SJL/J or ?

Lymphocytes are isolated from the animal and are mixed with polyvalent antiserum complement, and dye is added.

		polyvalent recipient serum produced in the following strains			
		C57BL/6J	DBA/2J	A/J	SJL/N
lymphocyte donor (test animal)	SJL/N	+	+	+	-
	A/J	+	+	-	+
	ASF1*	+	+	-	-

* A/J x SJL/N F1

Figure 16. The principles in producing strain-restricted sera for genetic control by immunizing animals of one strain with lymphocytes from other strains. The antiserum produced in the immunized animals is used in the testing.

In Vitro *Methods*

The *in vitro* procedures applied in genetic monitoring are complement-dependent cytotoxicity assay, hemagglutination, alloantiserum-binding analysis (flow cytometry), and mixed lymphocyte culture. In the cytotoxicity assay, lymphocytes from the test animal are exposed to antibodies against one or more antigen determinants. The antibodies may be monoclonal or polyclonal with more or less defined specificity. In the case of immunizing one strain in the colony with another strain, polyclonal polyspecific antisera are produced. Such sera are referred to as strain-restricted typing sera (SRTS).[99-102]

In cytotoxicity testing, lymphocytes from the test animals are mixed with antibodies directed against different MHC antigens. If specific antibodies directed against the MHC antigens of the test animal are present, the antigens and the antibodies will react and cause lysis, i.e., a destruction of the lymphocytes. The cell membrane of the lyzed lymphocytes will be permeable to a dye, which will make the lysis of the lymphocytes visible[103-105] (Figure 15).

In hemagglutination and alloantiserum binding analysis, the binding of the antibodies is visualized by agglutination of erythrocytes or by labeling with antiserum to the antibodies conjugated with fluorescent isothiocyanate (Figure 16). The amount of fluorescent antibody bound to each cell may be quantified by a technique known as flow cytofluorography, a procedure automated in a fluorescence-activated cell sorter.

In Vivo *Methods, Skin Grafting*

Skin grafting has been the standard method for testing isogeneity, whether or not a strain is inbred. Skin grafting can be used to detect genetic contamination in inbred strains and subline divergences. Apart from detecting differences within the MHC by acute rejection, differences in minor histocompatibility antigens are also detected (chronic rejection). The advantages of the method are that it is simple to perform, easy to assess, and that it is extremely sensitive in detecting minor differences between sublines, because

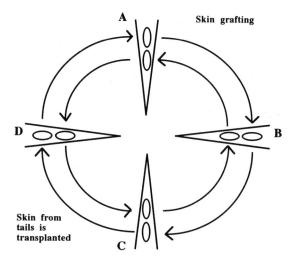

Figure 17. The principles of orthotopic tail skin graft in a reciprocal circle between the animals A, B, C, and D. The grafts are observed for at least 100 days. Technical failure causes graft loss within 1 week, while acute rejection, due to differences in the MHC, is seen within 2 to 3 weeks. Rejection of the skin graft after this period indicates differences in the minor histocompatibility antigens.

several hundred H genes monitored by this technique serve as markers distributed throughout the entire genome.[97,106] The disadvantages of skin grafting are the time and housing facilities which are required during the long observation period.

Skin from different parts of the body may be grafted, the most used technique, however, being orthotopic tail skin grafting in a reciprocal circle (Figure 17). Different methods for skin transplantations have been described.[106-111] Skin grafting is performed by anesthetizing the animals, removing a piece of the skin from one animal, and transferring it to another. The grafts are observed for at least 100 days. Technical failure causes graft loss within 1 week, while acute rejection, due to differences in the MHC, is seen within 2–3 weeks. Rejection of the skin graft after this period indicates differences in the minor histocompatibility antigens.

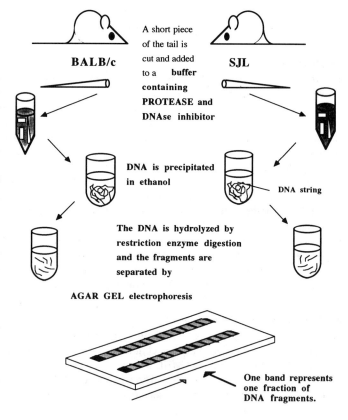

Figure 18. The principles in DNA fingerprinting. In the analysis of DNA from mice a piece of the tail is used. The freshly collected tissue is cut into small pieces and transferred to a buffered protease solution containing DNAse inhibitor. The protease digests the protein while the DNA is unharmed. The protein is removed by extraction and the DNA left is precipitated with ethanol. The DNA is hydrolyzed with a specific restriction enzyme and the fragments subjected to electrophoresis will separate on the gel according to the molecular weight of the DNA fragments. The DNA molecules are blotted (fixed) on a nitrocellulose filter. Minisatellite probes, containing radioactive or enzyme-labeled DNA, will hybridize to those bands on the blot containing fragments with minisatellite sequences. For each strain a specific pattern will be formed, depending on the kind of restriction enzyme used and the composition of the minisatellite probe.

DNA Technologies

The technologies have only been applied to genetic monitoring on an experimental basis and have not yet been established as routine methods for genetic control.[112-132]

Restriction Fragment Length Polymorphism (RFLP)

Restriction endonucleases (restriction enzymes) are enzymes that recognize short base sequences in the DNA string (five to seven base pairs) and hydrolyse the DNA string at these sites. Restriction fragment length polymorphism (RFLP) derives from the presence or absence of a cutting site for a particular restriction enzyme in DNA from different individuals. RFLP may be detected by comparing the DNA fragments generated by the action of a restriction enzyme on the genome. The total genome is hydrolyzed by a particular restriction enzyme, creating a number of fragments. Depending on the presence or absence of the restriction cutting sites, there will be differences in the size of the fragments. This difference is detected by hybridization with a probe for a particular gene. If polymorphism exists between two individuals, the hybridization will be allocated to fragments of different sizes in the two individuals.[112,113] As RFLP is based on differences in the DNA sequence in limited areas of the DNA string, it is likely that only a low degree of polymorphism exists. This has been confirmed by Knight and Dyson, who found that the incidence of RFLP, using single copy probes and 22 different enzymes, was relatively low.[112] This means that the variation within a species with respect to altered DNA sequences at the restriction sites is too low to be efficiently used in the differentiation of strains.

DNA Fingerprinting, Minisatellite DNA

Minisatellite DNA are DNA regions consisting of copies of short sequences, repeated and arranged in the same orientation. The minisatellite DNA may have a very variable appearance and demonstrate multiallelic variation.[114,115] Polymorphism is due to the varying number of copies in the different areas of the genome.[114-116]

In the analysis of DNA from mice only a minor amount of tissue is needed.[121] It is sufficient to take a blood sample, but often a piece of the tail is used. The freshly collected tissue is cut into small pieces and transferred to a buffered protease solution. The protease digests the protein, while the DNA is unharmed. The protein is removed by extraction and the DNA left is precipitated with ethanol. The DNA is now digested with a specific restriction enzyme and the fragments are separated by agarose electrophoresis. The fragments separate on the gel according to the molecular weight of the DNA fragments.

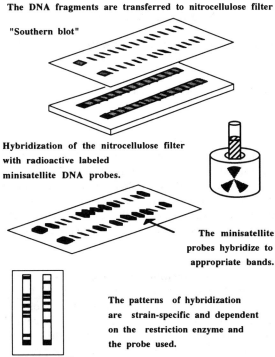

The DNA fragments are transferred to nitrocellulose filter

"Southern blot"

Hybridization of the nitrocellulose filter with radioactive labeled minisatellite DNA probes.

The minisatellite probes hybridize to appropriate bands.

The patterns of hybridization are strain-specific and dependent on the restriction enzyme and the probe used.

BALB/c SJL

The DNA molecules are blotted (fixed) on a nitrocellulose filter which is used for the hybridization. Minisatellite probes containing radioactively labeled DNA will hybridize to those bands on the blot containing fragments with minisatellite sequences. For each strain a specific pattern will be formed depending on the kind of restriction enzyme used and the composition of the minisatellite probe (Figures 18a and 18b).

As the minisatellite loci are scattered throughout the entire genome, each minisatellite locus represents a sample from the genome, and in one DNA analysis many loci representing different areas of the genome may be analyzed. Some minisatellite loci are linked, and for the purpose of differentiation of closely related strains or for contamination control, the analysis should be based on a number of different restriction enzymes and probes.[122] Moreover, differentiation of sublines is possible also by use of the DNA minisatellite analysis.[123] Hins and Gruber[79] used a single

Figure 18 B.

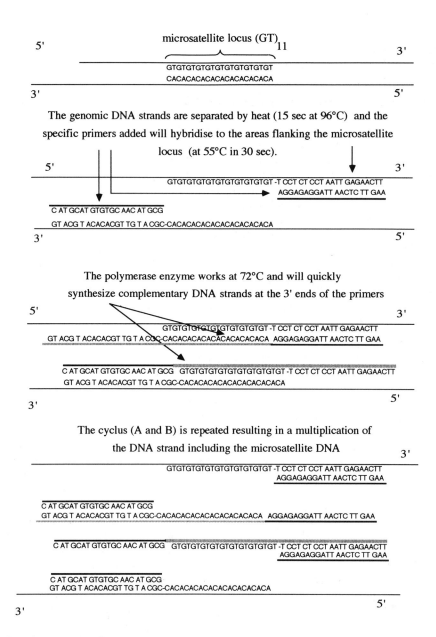

Figure 19. Genetic monitoring by means of a polymerase chain reaction and variable microsatellite loci. (A). The genomic DNA strands are separated by heat treatment. If a specific set of primers which is known to flank a microsatellite locus is added to genomic DNA, the primer will hybridize with the specific genomic DNA sequence homologous to the primer. A polymerase enzyme will synthesize the 3' flanking DNA sequence, containing the sequence of the microsatellite and the other primer. In the second cycle of the polymerase chain reaction, the newly synthesized DNA sequences will also hybridize primers and the polymerase will synthesize the 3' flanking DNA sequence containing the microsatellite sequence. The multiplication process will cause the multiplication of the DNA sequence containing the microsatellite.

probe and one restriction enzyme to set up a system for genetic monitoring of outbred stock and inbred strains of mice, and they found a good differentiation of the tested strains by this method.[79,124] Using a sequence in the M13 bacteriophage, Vassart et al.[125] were able to detect hypervariable minisatellites in different species. The M13 bacteriophage sequence simplified the technique, in that one probe could be used for a number of different species. Although specific DNA fingerprints may be established for each strain, some variation will always be present, as the minisatellites are considered hot spots for recombination because they are involved in the unequal crossing over during meiosis and mitosis.[117]

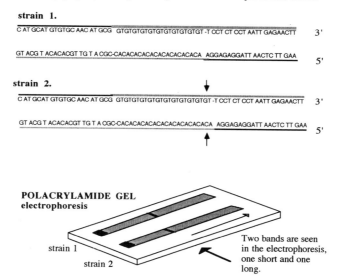

Size variation in the microsatellite locus, due to variations in the number of repeats, i.e. (GT)$_{11}$ or (GT)$_{12}$ is detected by polyacrylamide gel electrophoresis of the multiplied DNA strands

strain 1.

C AT GCAT GTGTGC AAC AT GCG GTGTGTGTGTGTGTGTGTGTGT -T CCT CT CCT AATT GAGAACTT   3'

GT ACG T ACACACGT TG T A CGC-CACACACACACACACACACACA AGGAGAGGATT AACTC TT GAA   5'

strain 2.

C AT GCAT GTGTGC AAC AT GCG GTGTGTGTGTGTGTGTGTGTGTGT -T CCT CT CCT AATT GAGAACTT   3'

GT ACG T ACACACGT TG T A CGC-CACACACACACACACACACACACA AGGAGAGGATT AACTC TT GAA   5'

POLACRYLAMIDE GEL electrophoresis

strain 1

strain 2

Two bands are seen in the electrophoresis, one short and one long.

Figure 19B. The multiplied products are separated by polyacrylamide electrophoresis, which separates the multiplied DNA fragments on the basis of size, and the gel is stained. The presence of one dinucleotide more or less is visualized on the polyacrylamide gel, as the one DNA fragment with an extra dinucleotide is longer than the other, and will show a separate band on the gel. The microsatellite loci often exhibit multiallelic variation, i.e. there are more than two different sizes of the microsatellite locus.

The method offers the advantage over the analysis of biochemical markers that the breeding animals to be tested do not have to be killed. When tested animals are used for breeding, the genetic status of the offspring is defined.[122]

Microsatellites

Microsatellites are dinucleotide repeats, i.e., (TG)n or (CG)n, which are dispersed all over the genome.[128-132] The dinucleotide repeats are polymorphic with respect to the number of repeats. The use of microsatellites as probes is based on the fact that the dinucleotide repeats are located in connection with other genes, and each dinucleotide sequence can be identified on the basis of the flanking gene sequences. In practice the microsatellites are identified by polymerase chain reaction (PCR) using the flanking DNA sequences as primers. PCR is a technical procedure by which a short sequence of a DNA molecule is multiplied (Figure 19). If specific pairs of primers which are known to flank a microsatellite locus are added to genomic DNA, the primers will hybridize with the specific genomic DNA sequence homologous to the primers and a polymerase will synthesize the 3' flanking DNA sequence, containing the sequence of the microsatellite and the other primer. In the second cycle of the PCR, the newly synthesized DNA sequences will also hybridize primers and a polymerase will synthesize the 3' flanking DNA sequence containing the microsatellite sequence. The multiplication process will result in the multiplication of the DNA sequence containing the microsatellite. The multiplied products are separated by polyacrylamide electrophoresis, which separates the multiplied DNA fragments on the basis of size. The presence of an extra dinucleotide is visualized on the gel, as a separate band. The examination of one dinucleotide sequence (one microsatellite locus) demands the use of a specific pair of primers, but only very little material is needed for the test. Love et al.[131] and Cornall et al.[132] demonstrated that the technique was usable to distinguish between inbred strains of mice. The use of microsatellites for the mapping of genes responsible for genetic diseases was demonstrated by Cornall et al.[46] and Todd et al.,[45] who were able to locate the insulin-dependent diabetes genes (Idd-3, -4, -5) to chromosomes 3, 11, and 1, respectively.

Table 7. Coat Color Variants of Inbred Mice, Some Commonly Used Hybrids and their Genotype

Strain/hybrid	A/a	B/b	C/c	D/d	P/p	Phenotype
A	a	b	c	D	P	Albino
AKR	a	B	c	D		Albino
BALB/c	A	b	c	D		Albino
CBA	A	B	C	D	P	Agouti (wild type)
C3H	A	B	C	D	P	Agouti (wild type)
C57BL/6	a	B	C	D	P	Black
C57BL/10	a	B	C	D	P	Black
DBA/2	a	b	C	d	P	Grey
BDP	a	b	C	d	p	Light yellow, pink eyed
MRL	a	B	c	D		Albino
NOD	A	B	c	D		Albino
NON	A	B	c	D		Albino
NZB	a	B	C	D		Black
NZW	A	b	c	D		Albino
PL	A	B	c	D		Albino
RF	a	B	c	D		Albino
RIII	A	B	c	D		Albino
SJL	A	b	c	D	p	Albino
129/Rr	A^w	B	c^{ch}	D	p	Light yellow
BALB/c x C57BL/6 F1	a/A	B/b	c/C	D	P	Agouti (wild type)
C57BL/6 x C3H F1	a/A	B/b	C	d/D	P	Agouti (wild type)
C57BL/6 x DBA/2 F1	a	B/b	C	d/D	P	Black
C3H x DBA/2 F1	a/A	B/b	C	d/D	P	Agouti (wild type)
C57BL/6 x CBA F1	a/A	B/b	C	d/D	P	Agouti (wild type)
BALB/c x DBA/2 F1	a/A	b	c/C	D	P	Light brown agouti

The gene symbols used are a, non-agouti; A, agouti (wild type); A^w, white-bellied agouti; b, brown; B, wild type at the b locus; c, albino; c^{ch}, chinchilla; C, wild type at the c locus; d, dilute; D, wildtype at the dilute locus; p, pink-eyed; P, wild type at the p locus.

Table 8. Coat Color Genotype and Phenotype of Some Commonly Used Inbred Strains of Rats

Strain	a	b	c	h	p	r	Phenotype
BB	a	B	c	h	P	R	Albino
BN	a	B	C	H	P	R	Albino
BUF	a	B	c	h	P	R	Brown
LE	a	b	C	h	P	R	Black-hooded
LEW	a	B	c	h	P	R	Albino
NEDH	a	B	c	h	P	R	Albino
PVG	a	B	C	h	P	R	Black-hooded
SHR	a	B	c	h	P	R	Albino
SPRD	a		c	h	P	R	Albino
WF	a		c		P	R	Albino
WKY	a	B	c	h	P	R	Albino

The gene symbols used are a, non-agouti; Am agouti (wild type); b, brown; B, wild type at the b locus; c, albino; C, wild type at the c locus; h, hooded; H, wildtype at the hooded locus; p, pink-eyed, dilute; P, wild type at the p locus; r, red-eyed, dilute; R, wild type of the r locus.

Table 9. Coat Color (phenotype) and Genotype of Offspring from the Crossing of Different Albino Mice with Multiple Recessive Coat Color Gene Carrying Mice; Detection of Hidden Coat Color Genes (Test Mating)

| Strains crossed | Locus | | | | | Phenotype |
	a	b	c	d	p	
A x DBA/2	a	b	c/C	d/D	P	Brown non-agouti
AKR x DBA/2	a	b/B	c/C	d/D		Black
BALB/c x DBA/2	a/A	b	c/C	d/D		Light brown agouti
MRL x DBA/2	a	b/B	c/C	d/D		Black
NOD x DBA/2	a/A	b/B	c/C	d/D		Agouti (wild type)
NZW x DBA/2	a/A	b	c/C	d/D		Light brown agouti
SJL x DBA/2	a/A	b	c/C	d/D	p/P	Light brown agouti

Coat Color and Pelage Variants

Coat color may be used for genetic control in species where color variations exist.[2,3,66-68,133] Some phenotypes may be more common than others in a species, e.g., albino (Tables 7 and 8). The albino gene, c, which is recessive, will in the homozygous state cause all other coat color genes not to be expressed. The unexpressed ("hidden") coat color genes can be detected by test mating with colored strains, carrying multiple recessive coat color genes. Table 9 gives examples of different strains of albino mice, and the results of test mating with colored animals. Genetic analysis using test mating is time-consuming and should not be performed in the breeding colony, due to possible risks of contamination of the breeding stock, although test mating may contribute to the genetic control performed in the laboratory.

Mandible Analysis

Among inbred strains there are differences in the dimensions of the skull, including the mandible. Measurements of the mandible shape are the most widely applied method. In mandible shape measurements, the size and shape of the mandible are determined by measuring the distance of 11 reference points of the mandible from the rectangular coordinates. The profile of the strain is calculated using a computer program.[2,134,135]

Other Polygenic Traits

A number of other traits have been proposed as markers for genetic monitoring, such as hematological data (erythrocyte count, leukocyte count, hemoglobin content, hematocrit), total body analysis (dry matter, total body fat), reproduction data (litter interval, live offspring born, weaned offspring, weight of offspring at a certain age), as well as inherited differences in the response to drugs.[20,21,77,78,136,137]

In the surveillance of the breeding nucleus and production colonies, a sudden increase in the reproductive performance could be an indication of outcrossing and genetic contamination.[2,22,70] In order to increase the accuracy of such tests, a considerable number of animals must be involved. Genetic monitoring using hematological data, total body analysis, and reproduction data has been applied for the genetic monitoring of outbred strains.[20,21,77,78]

Applicability of the Different Methods for Genetic Monitoring

Some of the methods are based on single genes: biochemical markers, some immunological markers, DNA restriction length polymorphism, microsatellites, coat color markers. Other methods are based on the monitoring of several genes simultaneously (multiple gene methods): skin grafting, strain-restricted typing sere (SRTS), DNA fingerprinting, osteometric traits, and other polygenic traits.[22,138,139]

The single gene methods are generally accurate, but as only one gene is examined per test, the methods are often laborious, and therefore less suited for the establishment of total genetic profiles. On the other hand, single gene methods are the methods of choice when the object is to discover genetic contamination and to set up a simple control system based on biochemical markers.

Multiple gene methods may often be suitable for detecting minor differences between sublines in one test, although some of the methods, e.g., litter size, may be too inaccurate to be used in differentiating closely related strains. Some of the multiple gene methods, e.g., skin grafting, DNA fingerprinting, and mandible shape analysis, are very suitable for the differentiation of sublines and substrains.

Table 10. Summary of the Application of the Laboratory Procedures for Genetic Monitoring

Genetic monitoring procedure	Outbred	Inbred	H-2 congenic	Sublines
Biochemical markers	0	+++	0	0
Coat color	0	+++	0	0
Strain-restricted typing sera	0	+++	+++	0
Skin grafting	0	+++	+++	++
Mandible shape	+++	+++	++	+++
Litter size	0	+++	0	0
RFLP	0	++	0	0
DNA fingerprinting	++	+++	?	+++
Microsatellites	?	+++	?	+++

0, not applicable; ++, applicable; +++, highly applicable; ?, unknown.

Table 10 summarizes the applicability of the methods for distinguishing within the different categories of laboratory animals.[22]

CRYOPRESERVATION OF EMBRYOS

BACKGROUND
Successful cryopreservation of mouse embryos was first described in 1972.[140,141] It became possible to secure the colonies against accidents caused by diseases, decreased fertility, genetic contamination, genetic drift, and environmental factors. Strains that were not used in research presently, but perhaps would be needed in the future, could be maintained in an easier and more economical way, and at the same time the previously mentioned risks of strains becoming extinct could be avoided. Transportation of the strain is also easier when the embryos are transported in deep-frozen state.[142,143]

The costs of maintaining strains by cryopreservation is considerably less than doing so by conventional breeding.[145-147]

STORAGE TIME AND POSSIBLE HARMFUL EFFECTS OF THE DEEP-FREEZING PROCEDURE ON THE EMBRYOS
Frozen embryos are usually stored at -196°C. At this temperature all chemical reactions dependent on molecular movements have stopped. Water exists only as crystals or in an amorphous form (vitrified) and in both cases the viscosity is so high that diffusion becomes very slow. The only type of reaction that may occur at this temperature is the development of free radicals and breakage of macromolecules as a result of background radiation. It has been suggested that over a prolonged period this radiation might destroy the DNA and harm the embryos. When embryos were exposed to a simulated long-term background radiation, no effects were found on the morphology of the thawed embryos, their development *in vitro*, nor on the number of implantations or live-born after transfer to pseudopregnant recipients.[149-151]

The freezing medium and the freezing procedure has no effect on the chromosomes, and cryoprotective compounds such as dimethylsulfoxide (DMSO) may protect against radiation. The mutation rate was not significantly changed after the exposure of embryos to DMSO, glycerol, or freezing.[152] Serum might decrease the extent of genetic and morphological damages in frozen embryos.[153]

Revitalization will always involve implantation in genetically different recipients. The maternal genotype may modify the fetuses with respect to their immunological constitution, and the incidence of, e.g., tumors may change.[154] It is therefore important to record the strain of the foster mother. The storage time and storage period have to be recorded as well, according to the rules for nomenclature.[58]

A number of institutions and laboratories have established embryo banks. Among these are Jackson Laboratory (U.S.), National Institutes of Health (NIH) (U.S.), Medical Research Council Laboratories (MRC) (U.K.), The Pasteur Institute (France), The Central Institute for Experimental Animals, Kawasaki (Japan), and the Central Institute for Laboratory Animals, Hannover, (BRD).[45,143,145,148,155] The traditional two-step freezing is the most used method. The number of embryos recommended to be stored depends on the breeding performance of the strain, and varies from 80 to 2000 embryos per strain.[145,157,158]

Table 11. Procedures for the Cryopreservation of Mouse Embryos

A. Traditional Two-Step Freezing Method Using Controlled Cooling Rate

Freezing:
a Collection of 8-cell embryos in superovulated and mated females.
b. Transfer of the embryos into freezing medium and equilibration for 20 minutes.
c. Transfer to -7°C for 10 minutes.
d. Seeding (induction of crystal formation) and holding for 10 minutes.
e. Slow cooling (-0.3 to -0,5°C/minute) to -35°C and holding for 30 minutes.
f. Transfer of the embryos to liquid nitrogen at -196°C and storage.
Thawing:
g. Thawing in water bath at 37°C.
h. Transfer of the embryos into thawing medium A.
i. Transfer of the embryos into thawing medium B.
j. Transfer of the embryos into cultivation medium.
k. Transfer of the embryos to a pseudopregnant female.
Media:
Freezing medium: 1,4 M glycerol in PBS with 20% FCS.Thawing A: 0,5 M saccharose 0,4 M glycerol in PBS with 20% FCS. Thawing medium B: 0,5 M saccharose in PBS with 20% FCS. Cultivation may be PBS with 10% FCS or M2.41.

B.The Quick-Freezing or Vitrification Method

Freezing:
a Collection of 8-cell embryos in superovulated and mated females.
b. Transfer of the embryos into equilibration (previtrification) medium.
c. Transfer of the embryos into vitrification medium.
d. Freezing directly in liquid nitrogen at -196°C and storage.
Thawing:
e. Thawing in water bath at 37°C
f. Transfer of the embryos into thawing medium.
g. Transfer of the embryos into physiological cultivation medium.
h. Transfer of the embryos to a pseudopregnant female.
Media:
Equilibration medium: 10% glycerol, 20% FCS in cultivation medium. Vitrification medium: 30% glycerol, 20% FCS, 50% 2 M saccharose in H_2O. Thawing medium: 0,5 M saccharose in cultivation medium. Cultivation may be PBS with 10% FCS or M2.41.

PBS, phosphate-buffered saline; FCS, fetal fetal serum.

TECHNICAL PROCEDURES FOR CRYOPRESERVATION

It is important when freezing mammalian cells to avoid ice crystal formation and too great osmotic gradients between intra- and extracellular compartments during the freezing and thawing procedures. The avoidance of crystal formation may be accomplished by adding a cryoprotective agent, such as glycerol, DMSO, propandiol, or ethyleneglycol. These substances seem to have a protective effect on proteins and lipids within the cell. An osmotically active substance such as saccharose is added to reduce the osmotic gradient between intracellular and extracellular compartments during thawing.[159-161]

The freezing is performed by adding a cryoprotective agent followed by cooling. The procedure for thawing is related to the freezing method used. Table 11 summarizes two methods for freezing mouse embryos. Freezing by controlled cooling rate (two-step freezing, rapid freezing) has been the method most often applied. Quick-freezing methods (vitrification) have gained wider use during the last 5 years, and will probably be the most applied method in the future, due to the simplicity of the procedure and the low cost of the equipment needed.[155,160,162-167,169]

REFERENCES

1. Morse, H. C., The laboratory mouse — a historical perspective, in *The Mouse in Biomedical Research*, Vol. 1, Foster, H. L., Small, J. D., and Fox, J. G., Eds., Academic Press, New York, 1981, 2.
2. Festing, M. F. W., *Inbred Strains in Biomedical Research*, MacMillan Press, London, 1979, 2.
3. Hedrich, H. J., Inbred strain in biomedical research, in *Genetic Monitoring of Inbred Strains of Rats*, Hedrich, H. J., Ed., Gustav Fischer Verlag, Stuttgart, 1990, 1.
4. Festing, M. F. W., Genetic factors in toxicology. Implication for toxicological screening. *Crit. Rev. Toxicol.*, 18, 1, 1987.
5. Festing, M. F. W., Genetic contamination of laboratory animal colonies: an increasingly serious problem. *ILAR News*, 25, 6, 1982.
6. Russell, E. S., The importance of animal genetics in biomedical research, in *Genetics in Laboratory Animal Medicine*, Proceedings of a symposium conducted at Boston, Massachusetts, July 22, 1968, National Academy of Science, Washington, D.C., 1969, 1.
7. Festing, M. F. W., Introduction to genetic monitoring. *Scand. J. Lab. Anim.*, 17, 119, 1990.
8. Lang, C. M., and Vesell, E. S., Environmental and genetic factors affecting laboratory animals: impact on biomedical research. *Fed. Proc.*, 35, 1123, 1976.
9. Pennline, K., Smith, J. P., and Bitter-Suermann, H., My kingdom for an inbred rat, *Transplantation*, 34, 70, 1972.
10. Kahan, B., Auerbach, R., Alter, B. J., and Bach, F. H., Histocompatibility, and isoenzyme differences in commercially supplied "BALB/c" mice. *Science*, 217, 279, 1982.
11. Lowell, D. P., and Festing, M. F. W., Relation among colonies of the laboratory rat. *J. Hered.*, 73, 81, 1982.
12. Gubbels, E., Poort-Keesom, R., and Hilgers, J., Genetically contaminated BALB/c nude mice. *Curr. Topics Microbiol. Immunol.*, 122, 86, 1985.
13. Festing, M. F. W., and Bender, K., Genetic relationships between inbred strains of rats. An analysis based on genetic markers at 28 biochemical loci. *Genet. Res. Cambridge*, 44, 271, 1984.
14. Green, E. L., Breeding systems, in *The Mouse in Biomedical Research*, Vol.1., Foster, H.L., Small, J. D., and Fox, J. G., Eds., Academic Press, New York, 1981, 91.
15. Falconer, D. S., *Introduction to Quantitative Genetics*, Oliver and Boyd, Edinburgh, 1970.
16. Falconer, D. S., Genetic aspects of breeding methods, in *The UFAW Handbook on the Care and Mangement of Laboratory Animals*, Fourth Edition, Churchill Livingstone, Edinburgh and London, 1972.
17. Kimura, M., and Crow, J. F., On the maximum avoidance of inbreeding. *Genet. Res.*, 4, 399, 1963.
18. Poiley, S. M., A systematic method of breeder rotation for non-inbred laboratory animals colonies. *Proc. Anim. Care Panel*, 10, 159, 1960.
19. Rapp, K. G., HAN-Rotation, a new system for rigorous outbreeding. *Z. Versuchstierkd.*, 14, 133, 1972.
20. Rapp, K. G., and Burow, K., Genetische Definition von Versuchstierpopulationen. *Tierlaboratorium*, 4, 16, 1977.
21. Rapp, K. G., and Burow, K., Genetische Standardisierung von Versuchstierpopulationen. *Tierlaboratorium*, 4, 109, 1977.
22. Festing, M. F. W., Introduction to laboratory animal genetics, presented at The Nordic Summer School in "Laboratory Animals in Biomedical Research", Kuopio, Finland, August 13–23, 1989, 1.
23. Shimkin, M. B., Section 2: Report of Discussion Group no. 1; Species and strain selection, in Carcinogenesis testing of Chemicals, from the Proceedings of the Conference on Carcinogenesis Testing in the Development of New Drugs, May 23-25, 1973, Washington, D.C., 1974.
24. Haseman, J. K., and Hoel, D. G., Statistical design of toxicity assays: role of genetic structure of test animal populations. *J. Toxicol. Environ. Health*, 5, 151, 1973.
25. Wolff, G. L., Some practical consideration for the inbreeding of laboratory mammals and their use in biological research. *Lab. Anim. Care*, 13, 49, 1963.
26. Green, E. L., Breeding systems, in *Biology of the Laboratory Mouse*, Green, E. L., Ed., McGraw-Hill, New York, 1966, 11.
27. MacLaren, A., and Michie, D., Variability of response in experimental animals: a comparison of the reaction of inbred, F1 hybrid and random-bred mice to a narcotic drug. *J. Genet.*, 54, 440, 1956.
28. Festing, M. F. W., A case for using inbred strains for laboratory animals in evaluation of the safety of drugs. *Food Cosmet. Toxicol.*, 13, 369, 1975.

29. Kornerup Hansen, A., and Dagnæs-Hansen, F., *An Introduction to the Use of Rodent Models in Diabetes Research*, Møllegård Ltd., Bomholtgård Ltd. 1990.

30. National Research Council, *Immunodeficient Rodents, A Guide to their Immunobiology, Husbandry, and Use,* National Academy Press, Washington, D.C., 1989.

31. Gershwin, M. E., and Merchant, B., *Immunologic Defects in Laboratory Animals*, Vols. 1 and 2. Plenum Press, New York, 1981.

32. Kolberg, R., Animals models point the way to human clinical trials. *Science*, 256, 772, 1992.

33. Rao, G. N., Birnbaum, L. S., Collins, J. J., Tennant, R. W., and Skow, L. C., Mouse strains for chemical carcinogenicity studies: overview of a workshop. *Fundam. Appl. Toxicol.,* 10, 385, 1988.

34. Snell, G. D., and Stimpfling, J. H., Genetics of tissue transplantation, in *Biology of the Laboratory Mouse*, Green, E. L., Ed., McGraw-Hill, New York, 1966, 457.

35. Bailey, D. W., Recombinant-inbred strains. *Transplantation*, 11, 325, 1971.

36. Swank, R. T. and Bailey, D. W., Recombinant inbred lines: value in the genetic analysis of biochemical variants. *Science*, 81, 1249, 1973.

37. Fortmeyer, H. P., *Thymusaplastische Maus, (nu/nu) Thymusaplastische Ratte (rnu/rnu), Haltung, Zucht, Versuchsmodelle,* Schriftenreihe Versuchstierkunde, heft 8, Paul Parey, 1981.

38. Jaenisch, R., Transgenic animals. *Science*, 240, 1468, 1988.

39. Gridley, T., Soriano, P., and Janisch, R., Insertional mutagenesis in mice. *Trends Genet.*, 3, 162, 1988.

40. Palmiter, R. D., and Brinster, R. L., Germline transformation of mice. *Annu. Rev. Genet.,* 20, 465, 1986.

41. Hogan, B., Costantini, F., and Lacy, E., *Manipulating the Mouse Embryo, a Laboratory Manual*, Cold Spring Harbor Laboratory, Cold Spring Harbor, NY, 1986.

42. Robertson, E. J., Ed., *Teratocarcinomas and Embryonic Stem Cells, a Practical Approach*, IRL press, Oxford, 1987.

43. Karlström, O., and Ågård Jensen, N., Transgenic mice: A powerful tool for basic research. *Scand. J. Lab. Anim. Sci.,* 16, 49, 1989.

44. Krypsin-Sørensen, I., The application of transgenic techniques to common domestic animals and fish. *Scand. J. Lab. Anim. Sci.,* 18, 81, 1991.

45. Todd, J. A., Aitman, T. J., Cornall, R. J., Ghosh, S., Hall, J. R. S., Hearne, C. M., Knight, A. M., Love, J. M., McAleer, M. A., Prins, J., Rodrigues, N., Lathrop, M., Pressey, A., DeLarato, N. H., Peterson, L. B., and Wicker, L. S., Genetic analysis of autoimmune type 1 diabetes mellitus in mice. *Nature*, 351, 542, 1991.

46. Cornall, R. J., Prins, J., Todd, J. A., Pressey, A., DeLarato, N. H., Wicker, L. S., and Peterson, L. B., Type 1 diabetes in mice is linked to the interleukin-1 receptor and Lsh/Ith/Bcg genes on chromosome 1. *Nature*, 353, 262, 1991.

47. Hoorfar, J., Buschard, K., and Dagnæs-Hansen, F., Prophylactic nutritional modification of the incidence of diabetes in autoimmune non-obese diabetic (NOD) mice, *Br. J. Nutr.,* in press.

48. Wilberz, S., Partke, H. J., Dagnæs-Hansen, F., and Herberg, L., Persistent MHV (mouse hepatitis virus) infection reduces the incidence of diabetes mellitus in non-obese diabetic mice, *Diabetologia*, 34, 2, 1990.

49. Bailey, D. W., Sources of subline divergence and their relative importance for sublines of six major inbred strains of mice, in *Origins of Inbred Mice*, Morse, H. C., Ed., Academic Press, New York, 1978, 197.

50. Papaioannou, V. E. and Festing, M. F. W., Genetic drift in a stock of laboratory mice. *Lab. Anim.*, 14, 11, 1980.

51. Bailey, D. W., How pure is inbred strains of mice. *Immunol. Today*, 3, 210, 1982.

52. Hedrich, H. J., Rapp, K. G., and Zschege, C., Untersuchungen zur genetischen Konstanz bzw. sublinien Drift von Mäuse- und Ratteninzuchtstämmen. *Z. Versuchstierk.,* 17, 263, 1975.

53. Morse, H. C., Differences among sublines of inbred mouse strains, in *Origins of Inbred Mice*, Morse, H. C., Ed., Academic Press, New York, 1978, 441.

54. Graff, R. J., Valeriote, F., and Medoff, G., Brief communication: marked histoincompatibility between and within sublines of AKR mice used in a syngeneic leukemia model. *J. Natl. Cancer Inst.,* 55, 1015, 1975.

55. Acton, R. T., Blankenhorn, E. P., Couglas, T. C., Owen, R. D., Hilgers, J., Hoffmann, H. A., and Boyse, E. A., Variations among sublines of inbred AKR mice. *Nature*, 245, 8, 1973.

56. Krog, H. H., and Moutier, R., Identification of inbred strains of mice. II. Characterisation of different substrains of the C3H strain. *J. Hered.*, 69, 66, 1978.

57. Prochazka, M., Serreze, D. V., Frankel, W. N., and Leiter, E. H., NOR/Lt mice: MHC-matched diabetes-resistant control strain for NOD mice. *Diabetes*, 41, 98, 1992.

58. Lyon, M. F. and Searle, A. G., Eds., *Genetic Variants, and Strains of the Laboratory Mouse*, Second edition, Oxford University Press, Oxford, 1989.

59. Festing, M. F. W., Kondo, K., Loosli, R., Poiley, S. M., and Spiegel, A., International standardized nomenclature for outbred stocks of laboratory animals. *ICLA Bull.*, 30, 4, 1972.

60. Klein, J., Bach, F. H., Festenstien, F., McDevitt, H. O., Shreffler, D. C., Snell, G. D., and Stimpfling, J. H., Genetic nomenclature of the H-2 complex of the mouse. *Immunogenetics*, 1, 184, 1974.

61. Shreffler, D. C., David, C., Gotze, D., Klein, J., McDevitt, H. O., and Sachs, D., Genetic nomenclature for new lymphocyte antigens controlled by the I-region of the H-2 complex. *Immunogenetics*, 1, 189, 1974.

62. Festing, M. F. W. and Staats, J., Standardized nomenclature for inbred strains of rats. Fourth listing. *Transplantation*, 16, 221, 1973.

63. Festing, M. F. W. and Greenhouse, D., Abbreviated list of inbred strains of rats. *Rat News Letter*, 26, 10, 1992.

64. Hoffman, H. A., Genetic quality control of the laboratory mouse (*mus musculus*), in *Origins of Inbred Mice*, Morse, H. C., Ed., Academic Press, New York, 1978, 216.

65. Hoffman, H. A., Smith, K. T., Crowell, J. S., Nomura, T., and Tomita, T., Genetic quality control of laboratory animals with emphasis on genetic monitoring, in *Animal Quality, and Models in Biomedical Research,* 7th ICLAS Symp., Utrecht, 1979, Spiegel, A., Erichsen, S., and Solleveld, H.A., Eds., Gustav Fischer Verlag, Stuttgart, 1979, 307.

66. Hsu, C. K., Genetic monitoring, in *Laboratory Animal Medicine*, Fox, J. G., Ed., Academic Press, New York, 1984, 73.

67. Hedrich, H. J., Aiming at genetic constancy of inbred strains via genetic monitoring, and cryopreservation, in *Animal Quality, and Models in Biomedical Research.* 7th ICLAS Symp., Utrecht, 1979, Spiegel, A., Erichsen, S., and Solleveld, H. A., Eds., Gustav Fischer Verlag, Stuttgart, 1973, 329.

68. Hedrich, H. J., Genetic monitoring, in *The Mouse in Biomedical Research*, Vol. 1., Foster, H. L., Small, J. D., and Fox, J. G., Eds., Academic Press, New York, 1981, 159.

69. Hedrich, H. J., Ed., *Genetic Monitoring of Inbred Strains of Rats,*. Gustav Fischer Verlag, Stuttgart, 1990.

70. Bailey, D. W. and Scott, O. C. A., Practices for controlling genetic quality of mice, in *Rodent Tumor Models in Experimental Cancer Therapy,* Kallman, R. F., Ed., Pergamon Press, New York, 1987, 57.

71. Ovejera, A. A. and Czerwinski, M., Genetic monitoring of laboratory animals, in *Rodent Tumor Models in Experimental Cancer Therapy*, Kallman, R. F., Ed., Pergamon Press, New York, 1987, 59.

72. van Zutphen, L. F. M. and Prins, J. B., *Genetic Monitoring of Inbred Strains; Some Practical Considerations.* 26th Scientific Meeting of the Society for Laboratory Animal Science. Basel, September 13-15, 1988, 125.

73. Eggenberger, E., Modellpopulationen zur Beurteilung von Rotationssystemen in der Versuchstierzucht. *Z. Versuchstierkd.,* 15, 297, 1973.

74. Groen, A. and Lagerwerf, A. J., Genetic heterogeneity and genetic monitoring of mouse outbred stocks. *Lab. Anim.,* 13, 81, 1979.

75. Hedrich, H. J., Eckwerte zur biologischen Charakterisierung einer Population. *Tierlaboratorium,* 4, 170, 1977.

76. Festing, M. F. W., Mouse strain identification by mandible analysis, in *Laboratory Animals in Drug Testing,* 5th ICLA Symp., Spiegel, A., Ed., Gustav Fischer Verlag, Stuttgart, 1973, 105.

77. Rapp, K. G. and Burow, K., Preservation of genetic homogeneity in outbred population by linear optimating, in *Animal Quality, and Models in Biomedical Research,* 7th ICLAS Symp., Utrecht, 1979, Spiegel, A., Erichsen, S., and Solleveld, H. A., Eds., Gustav Fischer Verlag, Stuttgart, 1980, 333.

78. Rapp, K. G., Kluge, R., and Sickel, E., Die Verwendung von ECV-Systemen in der Zucht von Auszuchtpopulationen. *Z. Verschstierkd.,* 32, 218, 1989.

79. Hins, J. and Gruber, F. P., Genetischen Fingerprinting von Inzuchtlinien, Auszuchten, transgene Individen und 3T3-Zellen von Mus musculus mit der sonde B.E.S.T. MZ 1.3. *J. Vet. Med. A.,* 38, 61, 1991.

80. Hedrich, H. J., Colony Management, in *Genetic Monitoring of Inbred Strains of Rats,* Hedrich, H. J., Ed., Gustav Fischer Verlag, Stuttgart, 1990, 11.

81. Festing, M. F. W., Production methods, in *The UFAW Handbook on the Care and Mangement of Laboratory Animals,* Fourth Edition, Churchill Livingstone, Edinburgh and London, 1972, 56.
82. Peters, A. G. and Festing, M. F. W., A computerised system for controlling breeding and production records of rat and mouse colonies. *Anim. Technol.*, 39, 21, 1988.
83. Frank, N., Riedesel, H., and Lenz, R., Das Versuchstierhaltungs-System (VTH) _ ein Tierhaus-Verwaltungs-DV-System. *J. Exp. Anim. Sci.*, 34, 140, 1991.
84. Kasai, N., Kasai, S., and Tsushima, Y., A computer program that draws pedigree charts for inbred strains of animals, *Exp. Anim.*, 38, 89, 1989.
85. Nomura, T., Kozaburo, E., and Tomit, T., *ICLAS Manual for Genetic Monitoring of Inbred Mice,* University of Tokyo Press, Tokyo, 1984.
86. Bulfield, G. and Bantin, G., Genetic monitoring of inbred strains of mice using electrophoresis and electrophocusing. *Lab. Anim.*, 15, 147, 1981.
87. Richardson, B. J., Baverstock, P. R., and Adams, M., *Allozyme Electrophoresis, A Handbook for Animal Systematics and Population Studies,* Academic Press, New York, 1986.
88. Roderick, T.H. and Guidi, J. N., Strain distribution of polymorphic variants, in *Genetic Variants and Strains of the Laboratory Mouse,* second edition, Lyon, M. F. and Searle, A. G., Eds., Gustav Fischer Verlag, Stuttgart, 1989, 76.
89. Festing, M. F. W., Polymorphic loci in inbred rat strains and stubstrains, a consolidated list for 71 loci. *Rat News Letter,* 26, 23, 1992.
90. Katoh, H. and Nomura, T., Genetic monitoring systems in the ICLAS coordinating monitoring center (Asia), in *Man and the Laboratory Animal: Perspectives for 1992,* Proc. 4th FELASA Symp., June 10-15, 1990, Foundation Marcel Merieux, Lyon, France, 1991, 467.
91. Moutier, R., Biochemical differences as a means of genetic control for inbred strains of laboratory mammals, in *Defining the Laboratory Animal,* National Academy of Science, Washington, D.C., 1971, 169.
92. Adams, M. and van Zutphen, B., Biochemical markers, in *Genetic Monitoring of Inbred Strains of Rats,* Hedrich, H. J., Ed., Gustav Fischer Verlag, Stuttgart, 1990, 36.
93. Hutton, J. J., Biochemical polymorphisms — detection, distribution, chromosomal location, and applications, in *Origins of Inbred Mice,* Morse, H. C., Ed., Academic Press, New York, 1978, 234.
94. Groen, A., Identification and genetic monitoring of mouse inbred strains using biochemical polymophisms. *Lab. Anim.*, 11, 209, 1977.
95. Czerwinski, M. J. and Crowell, J.S., Jr., Genetic monitoring of the rat (Rattus norvegicus): identification and genetic characterization. *Rat News Letter,* 17, 9, 1986.
96. Krog, H. H., Identification of inbred strains of mice, Mus musculus. I. Genetic control of inbred strains of mice using starch gel electrophoresis. *Biochem. Genet.*, 14, 319, 1976.
97. Demant, P., Histocompatibility genes and their use in genetic control of laboratory mice, in *Animal Quality, and Models in Biomedical Research.* 7th ICLAS Symp., Utrecht, 1979, Spiegel, A., Erichsen, S., and Solleveld, H. A., Eds., Gustav Fisher Verlag, Stuttgart, 1979, 299.
98. Günther, E., Immunological markers, in *Genetic Monitoring of Inbred Strains of Rat,* Hedrich, H. J., Ed., Gustav Fischer Verlag, Stuttgart, 1990, 23.
99. Hedrich, H. J., Strain-restricted typing sera, in *Genetic Monitoring of Inbred Strains of Rats,* Hedrich, H. J., Ed., Gustav Fischer Verlag, Stuttgart, 1990, 101.
100. Kendall, C., and Wagner, J. E., Characterization of strain specific typing antisera for genetic monitoring of inbred strains of rats. *Lab. Anim. Sci.*, 35, 364, 1985.
101. Arn, J. S., Riordan, S. E., Pearson, D., and Sachs, D. H., Strain restricted typing sera (SRTS) for use in monitoring the genetic integrity of congenic strains. *J. Immunol. Methods,* 55, 141, 1982.
102. Festing, M. F. W., and Totman, P., Polyvalent strain-specific alloantisera as tools for routine genetic quality control of inbred, and congenic strains of rats, and mice. *Lab. Anim.*, 14, 173, 1980.
103. Pincus, J. H., and Gordon, R. O., A microassay for the detection of murine H-2 antigens. *Transplantation*, 12, 509, 1971.
104. Shirosishi, T., Sagai, T., and Moriwaki, K., A simplified micro-method for cytoxicity testing using a flat-type titration plate for the detection of H-2 antigens. *Microbiol. Immunol.*, 25, 1327, 1981.
105. Fernandez, J. L., and Weeks, M., Genetic monitoring of rat strains using monoclonal antibodies specific for polymorphic class I and class II MHC antigens. *Lab. Anim.*, 22, 235, 1988.
106. Hedrich, H. J., Testing for isohistogeneity (skin grafting), in *Genetic Monitoring of Inbred Strains of Rats,* Hedrich, H. J., Ed., Gustav Fischer Verlag, Stuttgart, 1990, 102.

107. Brown, A. M., and Dinsley, M., Skin grafting and the homogeneity of inbred mouse strains. *Lab. Anim.*, 1, 81, 1967.

108. Brown, A. M., and Dinsley, M., Graft histocompatibility genes in sublines of inbred mice. *Nature*, 212, 1602, 1966.

109. Kindred, B., Skin grafting between sublines of inbred strains of mice. *Aust. J. Biol. Sci.*, 16, 863, 1963.

110. Gottfried, B., and Tadnos, M., A simple rapid method for skin grafting in mice. *Transplant. Bull.*, 6, 427, 1959.

111. Festing, M. F. W., and Grist, S., A simple technique for skin grafting rats. *Lab. Anim.*, 4, 255, 1970.

112. Knight, A. M., and Dyson, P. J., Detection of DNA polymorphisms between two inbred mouse strains — limitations of restriction fragment length polymorphisms (RFLPs), *Mol. Cell. Probes,* 4, 497, 1990.

113. Suzuki, M., and Hayashi, J.-I., Genetic monitoring of laboratory rat strains by restriction fragment length polymorphisms of mitochondrial DNA. *Exp. Anim.,* 36, 169, 1987.

114. Jeffreys, A. J., Wilson, V., and Thein, S. L., Hypervariable minisatellite regions in human DNA. *Nature*, 314, 67, 1985.

115. Jeffreys, A. J., Wilson, V., and Thein, S. L., Individual-specific "fingerprints" of human DNA. *Nature*, 316, 76, 1985.

116. Hill, W. G., DNA fingerprints applied to animal, and bird populations. *Nature*, 327, 98, 1987.

117. Jeffreys, A. J., Wilson, V., Kelly, R., Taylor, B. A., and Bulfield, G., Mouse DNA 'fingerprints', analysis of chromosome localization, and germ-line stability of hypervariable loci in recombinant inbred strains. *Nucleic Acids Res.*, 15, 2823, 1987.

118. Lewin, R., DNA fingerprints in health, and disease. *Science,* 233, 521, 1986.

119. Elliot, R.W., A mouse minisatellite. *Mouse News Letter*, 74, 115, 1986.

120. Kominami, R., Kohnosuke, M., and Masami, M., Nucleotide sequence of a mouse minisatellite DNA. *Nucleic Acids Res.*, 16, 1197, 1988.

121. Miniatis, T., Frisch, E. F., and Sambrook, J., *Molecular Cloning, a Laboratory Manual,* Cold Spring Harbor, NY, 1982.

122. Dagnæs-Hansen, F., The application of DNA-fingerprinting in the genetic monitoring, *Scand. J. Lab. Anim. Sci.,* 16 (Suppl. 1), 27, 1989.

123. Prins, J. B., Genetic Characterization of Inbred Strains of the Rat, Doctoral Thesis, 1990.

124. Thomann, R. E., Signer, E., Schelling, C. P., and Huebscher, U., DNA-fingerprinting for genetic quality assurance of inbred mice, in *Man and the Laboratory Animal: Perspectives for 1992*, Proc. 4th FELASA Symp., June 10–15, 1990, Foundation Marcel Merieux, Lyon, France, 1991, 423.

125. Vassart, G., Georges, M., Monsieur, R., Brocas, H., Lequarre, A. S., and Christophe, D., A sequence in M13 phage detects hypervariable minisatellites in human and animal DNA. *Science*, 235, 683, 1987.

126. Denny, A. A., and McDonald, B., DNA fingerprinting — a step forward in genetic monitoring. Abstract from LASA Winter Meeting, 28-29 November 1991. *Lab. Anim.*, 26, 141, 1992.

127. Knight, A. M., Simpson, E., Dyson, P. J., and Todd, J. A., Genetic analysis of the mouse genome using PCR-analysed microsatellites. Abstract from LASA Winter Meeting, 28-29 November 1991. *Lab. Anim.*, 26, 140, 1992.

128. Litt, M., and Luty, A., A hypervariable microsatellite revealed by in vitro amplification of a dinucleotide repeat within the cardiac muscle actin gene. *Am. J. Hum. Genet.,* 44, 397, 1989.

129. Tautz, D., Hypervariability of simple sequences as a general source for polymorphic DNA markers. *Nucleic Acids Res.*, 17, 646, 1989.

130. Weber, J. L., and May, P. E., Abundant class of human DNA polymorphisms which can be typed using the polymerase chain reaction. *Am. J. Hum. Genet.,* 44, 388, 1989.

131. Love, J. M., Knight, A. M., McAleer, M. A., and Todd, J. A., Towards construction of a high resolution map of the mouse genome using PCR-analysed microsatellites. *Nucleic Acids Res.,* 18, 4123, 1990.

132. Cornall, R. J., Aitman, T. J., Hearne, C. M., and Todd, J. A., The generation of a library of PCR-analyzed microsatellite variants for genetic mapping of the mouse genome. *Genomics*, 10, 874, 1991.

133. Wallace, M. E., *Learning Genetics with Mice,* Heinemann Educational Books Ltd., London, 1971.

134. Festing, M. F. W., Mouse strain identification. *Nature*, 238, 351, 1972.

135. Festing, M. F. W., and Lowell, D. P., Routine genetic monitoring of commercial, and other mouse colonies in the UK using mandible shape; five years of experience, in *Animal Quality, and Models in Biomedical Research.* 7th ICLAS Symp., Utrecht, 1979, Spiegel, A., Erichsen, S., and Solleveld, H. A., Eds., Gustav Fischer Verlag, Stuttgart, 1979, 341.

136. Meier, H., and Fuller, J. L., Responses to drugs, in *Biology of the Laboratory Mouse*, Green, E. L., Ed., McGraw-Hill, New York, 1966, 447.

137. Paigen, K., Genetic control of enzyme activity, in *Origins of Inbred Mice*, Morse, H. C., Ed., Academic Press, New York, 1978, 254.

138. Hedrich, H. J., and Crowell, J. S., Application of genetic monitoring techniques, in *Genetic Monitoring of Inbred Strains of Rats,* Hedrich, H. J., Ed., Gustav Fischer Verlag, Stuttgart, 1990, 71.

139. Hedrich, H. J., Principles of genetic monitoring, in *Genetic Monitoring of Inbred Strains of Rats,* Hedrich, H. J., Ed., Gustav Fischer Verlag, Stuttgart, 1990, 8.

140. Wilmut, I., The effect of cooling rate, warming rate, cryoprotective agent and stage of development of mouse embryos during freezing and thawing. *Life Sci.*, 11, 1071, 1972.

141. Whittingham, D. G., Leibo, S. P., and Mazur, P., Survival of mouse embryos frozen to -196°C and 269°C. *Science*, 178, 411, 1972.

142. Whittingham, D. G., Preservation of Embryos of the Laboratory Animals. 9th Int. Congress on Animal Reproduction and Artificial Insemination, June 16-20, 1980, 237.

143. Zeilmaker, G. H., Ed, *Frozen Storage of Laboratory Animals*. Gustav Fischer, Stuttgart, 1981.

144. Mobraaten, L. F., Embryo cryobanking. *J. In Vitro Fertil. Embryo Transf.*, 3, 28, 1986.

145. Mobraaten, L. F., The Jackson Laboratory genetic stocks resource repository, in *Frozen Storage of Laboratory Animals,* Zeilmaker, G. H., Ed., Gustav Fischer, Stuttgart, 1981, 1658.

146. Hedrich, H. J., and Reetz, I. C., Strain preservation of rodent embryos. Possibilities and limitations, in *New Developments in Biosciences; their Application for Laboratory Animal Science,* Beynen, A. C., and Solleveld, H. A., Eds., Martinus Nijhoff, Dordrecht, Holland, 1988, 163.

147. Glenister, P. H., and Lyon, M. F., Long-term storage of eight-cell mouse embryos at -196°C. *J. In Vitro Fertil. Embryo Transf.*, 3, 20, 1986.

148. Festing, M.W., Embryo banks in the production of genetically defined laboratory animals: a step toward the concept of type culture collections of defined laboratory animals, in *Frozen Storage of Laboratory Animals*, Zeilmaker, G. H., Ed., Gustav Fischer, Stuttgart, 1981, 149.

149. Glenister, P. H., Whittingham, D. G., and Lyon, M. F., Further studies on the effect of radiation during the storage of frozen 8-cell mouse embryos at -196°C. *J. Reprod. Fertil.*, 70, 229, 1984.

150. Whittingham, D. G., Lyon, M. F., and Glenister, P. H., Long term storage of mouse embryos at -196°C; the effect of background radiation. *Genet. Res. Cambridge*, 29, 171, 1977.

151. Lyon, M. F., Glenister, P. H., and Whittingham, D. G., Long term viability of embryos stored under irradiation, in *Frozen Storage of Laboratory Animals,* Zeilmaker, G. H., Ed., Gustav Fischer, Stuttgart, 1981, 139.

152. Ashwood-Smith, M. J., and Grant, E., Genetic stability in cellular systems stored in the frozen state, in *Freezing of Mammalian Embryos,* Elliot, K., and Whealan, J., Eds., Ciba Found Symp. no. 52., Elsevier, Amsterdam, 1977, 251.

153. Mizuno, A., and Hoshi, M., Frozen storage of mouse and rat embryos. *Rep. Res. Lab. Tech. Res. Inst.*, 83, 15, 1986.

154. Uphoff, D. E., Maternal influences; their immunologic aspects, in *Basic Aspects of Freeze Preservation of Mouse Strains*, Mühlbock, O., Ed., Gustav Fischer Verlag, Stuttgart, 1976, 85.

155. Hedrich, H. J., and Reetz, I., Cryopreservation of rat embryos, in *Genetic Monitoring of Inbred Strains of Rats*, Hedrich, H. J., Ed., Gustav Fischer Verlag, Stuttgart, 1990, 276.

156. Yokoyama, M., Wakasugi, N., and Nomura, T., An attempt to store inbred mouse strains, in *Frozen Storage of Laboratory Animals,* Zeilmaker, G. H., Ed., Gustav Fischer, Stuttgart, 1981, 113.

157. Whittingham, D. G., Lyon, M. F., and Glenister, P. H., Reestablishment of breeding stocks of mutant and inbred strains of mice from embryos stored at -196°C for prolonged periods. *Genet. Res. Cambridge*, 30, 287, 1977.

158. Yoshiki, A., Ohno, K., and Wakasugi, N., Cryopreservation of strain and mutant genes in mice. *Exp. Anim.*, 36, 279, 1987.

159. Leibo, S. P., and Mazur, P., Methods for the preservation of mammalian embryos by freezing, in *Methods in Mammalian Reproduction*, Daniel, J. C., Ed., Academic Press, New York, 1978, 179.

160. Rall, W. F., Factors affecting the survival of mouse embryos cryopreserved by vitrification. *Cryobiology*, 2, 387, 1987.

161. Whittingham, D. G., Low temperature storage of mammalian embryos, in *Basic Aspects of Freeze Preservation of Mouse Strains,* Mfhlbock, O., Ed., Gustav Fischer Verlag, Stuttgart, 1976, 45.

162. Scheffen, B., Van Der Zwalmen, P., and Massip, A., A simple and efficient procedure for preservation of mouse embryos by vitrification. *Cryoletters*, 7, 260, 1986.

163. Landa, V., and Tepla, O., Cryopreservation of mouse 8-cell embryos in microdrops, *Folia Biol.*, 36, 153, 1990.

164. Takahasihi, Y., and Kanagawa, H., Quickfreezing of mouse embryos by direct plunge into liquid nitrogen vapour; effects of sugars. *Jpn. J. Vet. Res.,* 33, 14, 1985.

165. Dubrinsky, J. R., Galise, J. J., and Robl, J. M., Development of vitrified rabbit embryos, *Theriogenology*, 33, 213, 1990.

166. Chupin, D., and DeReviers, M. M., Quickfreezing of rat embryos, *Theriogenology*, 26, 157, 1986.

167. Smorag, Z., Wieczorek, B., Gajda, B., and Jura, J., Vitrification of the rabbit embryos, 11th International Congress on Animal Reproduction and Artificial Insemination, University college, Dublin, June 26-30, 1988. Volume 2, Brief Communication.

168. Kobayashi, K., Nagashima, H., Yamakawa, H., Kato, Y., and Otawa, S., The survival of whole and bisected rabbit morulae after cryopreservation by the vitrification method. *Theriogenology*, 33, 777, 1990.

169. Tsunoda, Y., Soma, T., and Sugie, T., Frozen storage of rabbit and hamster embryos, in *Frozen Storage of Laboratory Animals*, Zeilmaker, G. H., Ed., Gustav Fischer, Stuttgart, 1981, 129.

Chapter 11

Health Status and the Effects of Microbial Organisms on Animal Experiments

Axel Kornerup Hansen

CONTENTS

INTRODUCTION

Since the beginning of the 1960s the microbiological status of rodents, especially rats and mice, has been highly improved. However, this does not mean that, although delivered from commercial breeders with long lists of absent microorganisms, rats and mice of today never suffer from disease caused by microorganisms or that the influence of microorganisms on research is a historical event. Microorganisms might influence experimental results, although disease symptoms are not observed. As health monitoring techniques have been improved, more and more microorganisms are found to be latently present in laboratory animals. Some of these, e.g., bacteria of human origin, are difficult to eliminate and other methods than elimination from the breeding colony must be used to avoid the influence on research.

GENERAL LABORATORY ANIMAL EPIZOOTIOLOGY

TERMS RELATING TO INFECTION IN ANIMALS
Health Status

Health status can be defined as the actual status of an individual animal concerning its clinical, pathological, and physiological appearance. The physiology of the animal organism attempts to maintain homeostasis, i.e., constant internal environment.[1] To achieve valid, significant and reproducible results animals must be standardized, i.e., the variation between animals must be kept at a minimum, both within the test group and between experiments. Differences in health status may counteract this aim.

Infection and Disease in the Individual and in the Population

The word *infection* designates the presence of a microorganism — *the agent* — in an animal host. *Disease* is the clinical manifestation of infection. Most infections are lacking clinical manifestations. Such infections are designated as *subclinical*, and may be divided into those cases in which the agent can be recovered — *dormant infections* — and those in which the presence of the agent can only be proved by indirect methods — *latent infections*.[2] The animal harboring a subclinical infection is called an *inapparent carrier*. Few diseases in which microorganisms are involved can be said to be *monofactorial*, i.e., the microorganism is the only factor influencing whether disease is observed or not. Most infectious diseases are *multifactorial*, i.e., the result of several factors, including the agent. All factors, the agent included, involved in the development of disease are designated *the determinants*. In all, the animal health status can be explained as a balance between, on the one hand, some determinants, the agent and the *inducers*, tending to disease the animal, and, on the other hand, some other determinants, the *protectors*, tending to prevent the development of disease.

The word infection may not only be used for individuals. Whole animal colonies or populations also may be said to be infected, although only some of the animals are actually infected with the agent in question. The fraction of animals infected with a certain microorganism at a certain point of time is termed the *instantaneous prevalence rate* or simply the *prevalence*.[3] When an infection is spreading, the prevalence will increase from day to day. To describe this increase one uses the term *incidence,* which is the fraction of new positives over a defined period. The ability of the microorganism to infect individuals is called *infectivity*. The ability of a certain microorganism to provoke disease is called *pathogenicity*. *Virulence* introduces the concept of degree, i.e., even small numbers of highly virulent microorganisms will provoke disease. Microorganisms always causing disease are said to be *obligate pathogens*, while organisms only causing disease in connection with inducers are *facultative pathogens* or *opportunists*. There can be no clear division between obligate and facultative pathogens. Very few examples of infections can be given where all cases result in disease. However, for certain microorganisms inducers and protectors play a very small part in the development of disease. If the host organism gains from their presence, microorganisms with no potential of causing disease are called *symbionts*, otherwise they are called *commensals.* Concerning symbionts the word *association* is used rather than the word infection. The absence of symbionts may serve as an inducer. A *copathogen* is a microorganism enhancing disease primarily produced by another agent.

Infections in Relation to Time

Some microorganisms only infect the animal temporarily, while others may infect it for life. This difference depends on the ability of the agent to persist in the organism. In Figure 1 an illustration is given of infections and immunological, physiological, and pathological changes related to time.

HEALTH STATUS AND ANIMAL EXPERIMENTS

It is essential to control the health status of each animal going to take part in the experiment, and the risk of a change in the animal's health status during the experiment.

If disease is diagnosed in the individual animal prior to experimentation, that particular animal will normally be excluded from the study; and whether the disease is caused by certain microorganisms or environmental factors may seem to be of minor importance. However, it is of major importance, because there may be a risk of disease development in the remaining healthy animals during the study, or these animals may be unsuitable for research although disease is not observed. Subclinical infection in the animal before the study may leave irreversible changes in the animal that will disturb the interpretation of the results later on, even though the agent has been eliminated from the animal. Thus, the ability of a certain microorganism to influence experiments is not only correlated to its ability to cause disease. Therefore, a health monitoring report from the supplying colony is essential.

If the study includes a test group and a control group and both are equally interfered with, the scientist may feel that infections are not of any importance. This is, however, not so, because the microorganisms may inhibit the induction of the animal model, and the infection may make it difficult to interpret the final results. If the test factor acts as an inducer, the effect of the microorganism may be dose-related, leading

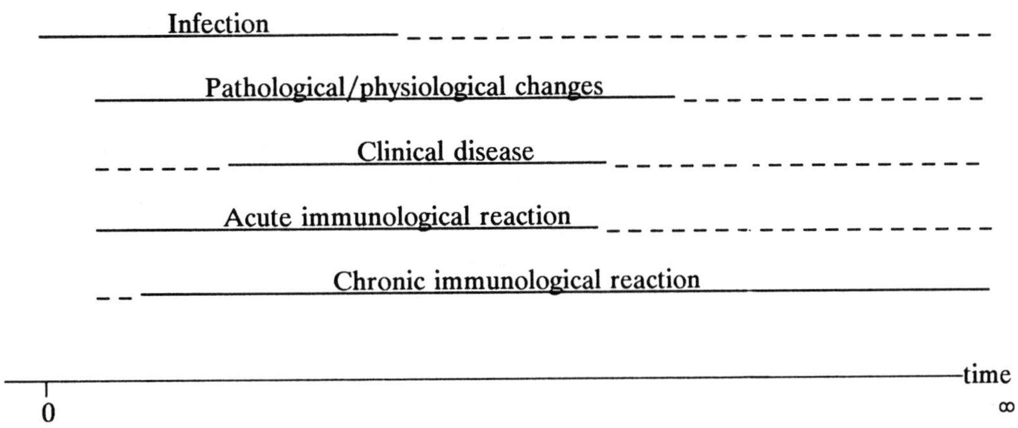

Figure 1. Infection and its consequences related to time. The full line indicates the normal relationship between infection and time. The agent enters the organism. After a period, *the incubation period*, pathological and physiological changes appear in the animal. Such changes may lead to the outbreak of clinical disease. The immune system may react with an acute reaction such as anaphylaxis, which normally disappears after elimination of the agent. Hereafter the lesions may regenerate and the animal recovers. However, T memory cells and antibodies may persist for life. The dotted lines illustrate that other reactions may persist for life, too. If the agent persists in the animal, the other events may either also persist, or disappear and reappear at intervals. Even if the agent is eliminated, it may have caused irreversible lifelong lesions, and in the worst cases such changes may debilitate the animal and make it chronically diseased.

to false conclusions in studies of pharmacology or toxicology. Microorganisms may also increase the variation inside the group, thereby leading to the use of a larger number of animals.

MICROBIAL INTERFERENCE WITH ANIMAL EXPERIMENTS

DETERMINANTS OF MICROBIAL RESEARCH INTERFERENCE AND LABORATORY ANIMAL HEALTH

In estimating the risk of a disease outbreak during an experiment, one has to consider several determinants. Although hazardous infections such as *Mycoplasma* and *Salmonella* are absent, infectious disease problems due to latent infections are commonly induced by environmental stress. The absence of disease symptoms cannot be interpreted as the absence of specific infections. A good environment, e.g., in the breeding facilities, may prevent such clinical symptoms. Transport stress and the new environment of the experimental facility may induce disease. As health monitoring results are always retrospective, knowledge of determinants is needed to evaluate experimental results which have been obtained from animals in which infection was not diagnosed early enough to avoid their use. Examples of such determinants are given below.

The Experiment

The experiment itself may be a stress factor. In surgery post-surgical infections are well known. Bacteria such as *Pseudomonas aeruginosa, Escherichia coli, Staphylococcus aureus*, and *Bacillus fragilis* may be responsible.[4-7] Aseptic surgical technique and adequate post-operative care should be applied to all surgical experiments to avoid complications. Experimental immunosuppression, which is commonly used in many experiments, may cause problems. Various bacteria and viruses, even the normal flora,[8] may cause disease and death in immunosuppressed animals. Examples are given in Table 1. A potent immunosuppressor may turn almost any apathogen bacteria into a pathogen.

The immune system may also be responsible for the damage caused to the animal, as is the case for e.g., of *Lymphocytic choriomeningitis*[42] and to some extent also for *Theiler's murine encephalomyelitis virus*.[43-45] In such cases immunosuppression may protect against the development of disease.

Table 1. Examples of Latent Infections which may be Activated by Immunosuppression

Agent	Effect	Species
Bacteria		
Bacillus piliformis[9-15]	Tyzzer's disease	Mouse, rat, hamster
Citrobacter freundii[14]	Ulcers in duodenum and ileum, enteritis	Mouse
Corynebacterium kutscheri[11]	Pseudotuberculosis	Mouse
Enterobacter cloacae[16-18]	Fatal neonatal diarrhea	Mouse
	Death	Mouse
Klebsiella pneumoniae[18]	Death	Mouse
Pseudomonas aeruginosa[19-20]	Bacteriemia, liver necrosis, lowered body weight	Mouse
Salmonella spp.[14]	Enteritis	Rat
Staphylococcus spp.[21-22]	Respiratory disease	Rat
Streptobacillus moniliformis[14]	Splenomegaly	Mouse
Yersinia enterocolitica[14]	Enteritis	Rat
Viruses		
Cytomegaloviruses[23-28]	Salivary gland inclusions	Mouse, rat
Kilham rat virus (HER strain)[29-31]	Hemorrhagic encephalopathy	Rat
Mouse hepatitis virus[32-40]	Hepatitis, enteritis, etc.	Mouse
Sendai virus[41]	Respiratory disease	Mouse

The induction of specific disease models often stresses the animals, making them more susceptible to disease; e.g., the induction of pulmonary edema is known to activate infections with *Streptococcus pneumoniae* in rats, resulting in different types of lung disease.[46]

The Environment

The environment may cause a certain stress on animals. Unintentional disease induction by stress may have similarities with experimental immunosuppression.[47] However, the mechanism seems to be more complex. Apart from having receptors capable of responding to glucocorticoids and catecholamines, lymphocytes and macrophages also have receptors for acetylcholine, endorphins, enkephalins, insulin, prolactin, somatotropin, estradiol, and testosterone.[48] Apart from causing a number of nonmicrobial side effects, stress may induce disease caused by opportunistic organisms harbored by the animal. To reduce stress one has to consider room temperature, relative humidity, noise, air change, movements within the room, diet, caging, other animals, etc. Extreme temperature and humidity may activate latent infections. The proper ventilation of the animal unit is essential. Reduced air exchange may lead to respiratory disease caused by bacteria with low pathogenicity, such as *Staphylococcus xylosus* and *P. aeruginosa*, especially in immune-deficient animals. Increased concentrations of NH_3 in the air may induce respiratory disease in rats latently infected with *M. pulmonis*.[49-51]

Nutrition and the quality of drinking water plays an essential part in the development of host defense against infectious disease.[52] Deficiency of vitamins A and E has been shown to induce respiratory disease in rats infected with *M. pulmonis*.[53] Deficiency of vitamin C in guinea pigs may be responsible for a high incidence of bacterial diseases caused by, e.g., *Streptococci* or *Klebsiella* spp.,[54] while iron deficiency has been described as an inducer of respiratory disease caused by *S. pneumoniae* in rats.[46] Several nutritional components are determinants for the development of Tyzzer's disease in *Bacillus piliformis*-infected mice. High contents of glucose and peanut oil seem to protect against the disease, while a high content of casein induces the disease.[10] The diet of the mother seems to influence the development of enzootic diarrhea of infant mice caused by mouse rotavirus.[55]

The Animal Host

Susceptibility to the development of disease is under the control of genetics, sex, sexual cycle, age, and other characteristics of the host. Immune-deficient rodents such as the nude mouse, the SCID mouse, and the nude rat are obviously more susceptible to the development of infectious diseases than immune-competent rodents. A frequently occurring problem is the high incidence of abscesses in the nude mouse caused by bacterial species such as *S. aureus*,[56,57] *Pasteurella pneumotropica*,[58,59] *Morganella morganii*,[58]

Table 2. Infection of Nude Mice and Rats with Various Microorganisms and the Differences Observed Compared to Infection in Immune-Competent Animals

Microorganism	Difference from immune-competent animals
The nude mouse (*nu/nu*)	
Mouse hepatitis virus	Mortality[60]
Sendai virus	Persisting infection[61]
Aspiculuris tetraptera	Lack of resistance[62]
Syphacia obvelata	Lack of resistance[62]
Hymenolepis nana	Lack of resistance[63]
The nude rat (*rnu/rnu*)	
Sendai virus	Persisting infection[64]
Sialodacryadenitis virus	Persisting infection[65]
Bacillus piliformis	Epizootic disease[66]
Listeria monocytogenes	No memory immunity[67]
	Increased nonspecific defense[67]
Eimeria nieschulzi	No memory immunity[68]

Table 3. Examples of Microorganisms for which Genetics of the Host Code for Differences in the Susceptibility to the Development of Disease as a Consequence of Infection

Agent	Clinical effect	Species	Susceptible strains/stocks
Bacteria			
Bacillus piliformis	Tyzzer's disease	Rat[13,69]	BB, LE, SHR, Sprague-Dawley
		Mouse[10]	ICR
Salmonella spp.	Salmonellosis	Mouse[70,71]	BALB/c, C57BL
Streptobacillus moniliformis	Streptobacillosis	Mouse[72]	C57BL/6J
Mycoplasmae			
Mycoplasma pulmonis	Mycoplasmosis	Mouse[73]	ddY
		Rat[74]	LEW
Viruses			
Ectromelia virus	Ectromelia	Mouse[75]	A, CBA, DBA, C3H, BALB/c
Lactic dehydrogenase virus	Paralysis	Mouse[76]	AKR, C58
Mouse hepatitis virus	Mortality	Mouse[77]	BALB/c, C57BL
Sendai virus	Mortality	Mouse[78]	DBA/2J, 129/J
Theiler's mouse encephalo-myelitis virus	Demyelinating disease	Mouse[79,80]	CD-1 (NMRI), DBA/2, SJL, SWR

Citrobacter freundii,[58] and *Streptococci*.[58] Some examples of differences in the behavior of infections in immune-deficient compared to immune-competent animals are given in Table 2.

Variation in susceptibility to infectious disease among inbred strains of rats and mice is known for several microorganisms (Table 3). Studies of *Sendai virus* in mice have shown that genetic susceptibility or resistance may be determined by a single autosomal locus and that resistance is dominant to susceptibility.[81] Studies of *B. piliformis* infection in rats indicate that the susceptibility may be linked to certain MHC-haplotypes.[13]

In most animals the immune system is not fully developed at birth, and neonatal animals are protected by maternal antibodies.[82,83] Animals no longer protected by maternal antibodies generally become infected shortly after weaning. Moreover, they are stressed by their new environment, and consequently their own immune system is depressed. For this reason infectious diseases are most common in young animals, e.g., Tyzzer's disease,[84,85] Sendai influenza,[86] sialodacryoadenitis,[87] etc. However, if the animal develops disease at a later age, either because it is infected with the agent for the first time late in life, or a persistent infection is reactivated by stress or immunosuppression, there is a tendency for the disease to be more severe than for younger animals, e.g., in the case of mycoplasmosis[88] and Sendai influenza.[89,90]

Differences between sexes in the susceptibility to the development of infectious disease may be observed. Female rats may be infected with *B. piliformis* earlier than males,[69] whereas no sex differences were observed in mice.[91] Infection with group C Streptococci in guinea pigs is more common in females than in males.[92] Colitis and rectal prolapse caused by *C. freundii* in mice are more common in males and may be prevented by castration.[58] The agent infecting a host organism enters into a balance with all other microorganisms present in the host. Some of these will act as protectors, others will act as inducers or copathogens, e.g., hepatitis as the result of infection with *Mouse Hepatitis Virus* is enhanced by coinfection with the blood parasite *Eperythrozoon coccoides*.[93] The parasite alone does not produce disease. Also splenomegaly caused by *Lactic dehydrogenase virus* may be enhanced by this parasite,[94] while *Lactic dehydrogenase virus* potentiates the pathogenicity of *Listeria monocytogenes* in mice.[95] Respiratory disease as a cause of *M. pulmonis* will be enhanced by the presence of other pathogens, such as *Sendai virus*,[96,97] *CAR bacillus*,[98,99] and *P. pneumotropica*.[100] The anaerobic intestinal flora is normally considered essential for digestion[101-103] and parts of the aerobic flora such as Enterococci, Lactobacilli, and Bacillus spp. may also have a symbiotic value for the animal.[104] From various farm animal species it is known that inoculation with such organisms reduces the incidence of enteric disease,[105,106] which may also be the case in rats.[107]

The Agent

Most viruses can be classified into different strains based on their antigenic structure, protein structure, RNA structure, etc. Virulence genes of these strains code for differences in virulence. Strains of *Mouse hepatitis virus* such as MHV-2, MHV-3, and MHV-A59 are more virulent than, e.g., MHV-1, MHV-S, MHV-Y, and MHV-Nu. A strain designated MHV-4 has a specific affinity for the nervous tissues.[108] In contrast to other strains of *Kilham rat virus*, the HER strain causes hemorrhagic encephalopathy in suckling or immunosuppressed rats.[109] Many strains of *Theiler's mouse encephalomyelitis virus* are known. However, the only pathogenic one may be GDVII.[110] The affinity for various tissues differs among strains of *Reovirus type 3*, a strain designated HEV being the most broad-spectered, producing encephalitis, pneumonia, hepatitis, as well as pancreatitis.[111-113] Infection in mice with the LDV-C strain of *Lactic dehydrogenase virus* is more likely to produce paralysis than other strains.[76]

Among bacteria strain variations are observed, and only one strain of *Citrobacter freundii*, named 4280, produces colitis in mice.[114,115] The difference in susceptibility to the development of Tyzzer's disease observed in different animal species may be connected with differences in the pathogenecity of the strains of *B. piliformis* infecting these species.[117-119] Some infections are eliminated totally by the immune system of the host and effects connected with the presence of the agent in the host organism are limited to a period of the animal's life. If the immune system is capable of eliminating the agent and keeping up a memory immunity, the host will only be infected for the period needed for the immune system to eliminate the agent. As the agent is no longer present in the organism to stimulate the immune system, reinfection may be possible after some time, e.g., reinfection with *Sialodacryoadenitis virus* is possible in rats about 6 months after the initial infection.[120]

Other infections are lifelong and in such cases the risk of research interference is much greater as the agent may cause contamination of biological products, immunomodulation, and to some extent also physiological modulation, microbiological competition, and oncogenic modulation.

Some interference risks may be totally eliminated by the use of animals above the age when infection is normally observed. An agent without the ability to survive in the environment may even eliminate itself from the colony. This principle is used in closed breeding colonies for the elimination of coronaviruses[121] or *Sendai virus*[122] by making a 6-week break in breeding. Persistence is a consequence of the ability of the agent to incorporate itself into the cells of the host, as is the case, e.g., for herpetoviridae or retroviridae, or of an insufficient immune response, e.g., against *Lymphocytic choriomeningitis virus*.[123]

Most bacteria, fungi, and mycoplasms persist in the animal. So do parasites, but a potent immune response is normally developed against parasite infections, thereby minimizing their number significantly in adult animals. Persistent infections should also be suspected from all DNA viruses and from the RNA viruses arenaviridae and retroviridae. The inability to establish persistent infections is characteristic of coronaviridae, paramyxoviridae, and picornaviridae.

Infectivity as well as virulence vary among microorganisms and normally there is a gap between the infective dose and the lethal dose, e.g., in guinea pigs the infective dose of *Bordetella bronchiseptica* has been found to be 4 colony-forming units, while the lethal dose has been found to be 1314 colony-forming units.[124] This means that the application of good hygienic principles will reduce the number of animals exposed to a lethal dose of bacteria. Some microorganisms of low infectivity only reach low prevalences in the population, e.g., *lymphocytic choriomeningitis virus*.[125] The fact that only a few animals in each group of the experiment are infected may lead to increased variation in the group, thereby leading to the need of a larger number of animals in order to reach statistical significance. On the other hand, microorganisms with a low infectivity may be eliminated from breeding or experimental colonies by frequent screening of the whole colony; e.g., the microsporidium *Encephalitozoon cuniculi* can be eliminated from rabbit breeding colonies by stamping out seropositive animals,[146] but serology can also successfully be used for selecting seronegative animals for experiments. A low pathogenicity of the agent may be used in the same way; e.g., low-grade Tyzzer's disease in rats is normally accompanied by very high titers against *B. piliformis* and the elimination of rats with such high titers will reduce the risk of incorporating animals with an abnormal liver function in the study.[66]

SPECIFIC EFFECTS OF MICROORGANISMS ON ANIMAL EXPERIMENTS
Contamination of Biological Products
Microorganisms present in the animal may contaminate samples and tissue specimens such as cells, sera, etc. This may interfere with experiments performed on cell cultures or isolated organs. Furthermore, the introduction of such products into animal laboratories will impose a risk to the animals kept in that laboratory. In theory all infections listed in Tables 4 to 9 may contaminate certain products from the animal. However, viruses and mycoplasmae are known to represent the major risk because of their ability to produce viremia in the animal and the ability of some viruses and all mycoplasmae to persist in specific organs. Some protozoans, e.g., *E. cuniculi*,[127] also have a potential of contaminating transplantable tumors.

Pathological Changes, Clinical Disease, and Mortality
Many microbial disease problems of today are caused by the combined effects of opportunistic bacteria and other determinants.[8,21] Thus, diseases can often be prevented by improving the environment. Tyzzer's disease in the rat is a good example of this. The majority of rats used in Europe have antibodies to the agent *B. piliformis*, but the disease is rare and mainly connected with stress, immunosuppression, etc., and most frequently observed in inbred strains.[13]

Some types of disease may resemble the animal model, but lack important characteristics of the model. For example, in a much-used model for testing antiarthritic drugs injection of different kinds of adjuvant results in polyarthritis in some inbred strains of rats. However, administration of adjuvant may also turn subclinical infection with *Mycoplasma arthritidis* into clinical disease, i.e., arthritis. As mycoplasmal arthritis is infectious, and experimental polyarthritis is rheumatic,[137-139] it may lead to an incorrect conclusion when screening drugs for their antirheumatic activity. Subclinical disease may also disturb essential parameters, e.g., subclinical sialodacryoadenitis reduces body weight in rats.[140] Additionally, behavior will often be changed during subclinical disease, e.g., leading to disturbances in the open field test, etc. The presence of some microorganisms may leave changes in the organs, resulting in difficulties in the interpretation of the pathological diagnosis included in, e.g., toxicological studies.

Immunomodulation
Many experiments depend on the function of the immune system, e.g., immunization and the development of insulin-dependent diabetes mellitus in the NOD mouse and the BB rat. Immunomodulation may be caused by microorganisms, also in the absence of clinical disease, and the effect can be divided into either *immune suppression* or *immune activation*. Some microorganisms even depress one part while activating another part of the system, e.g., *Toxoplasma gondii* is known to cause long-lasting suppression of T and B lymphocyte function,[141,142] but also nonspecific activation of macrophages[143] and enhanced protection against unrelated pathogens.[144-146]

Viruses are normally described as the most freqent immune modulators, one of the reasons being the viremic phase in the pathogenesis of many virus infections, during which cells of the immune system may be infected, lymphocytes by adenoviruses, cytomegaloviruses, leukemiaviruses, *Lymphocytic choriomeningitis virus, Thymic virus, Reovirus type 3, Minute virus of mice*, and *Mouse hepatitis virus;* and macrophages by *Cytomegalovirus*, leukemiaviruses, *Lymphocytic choriomeningitis virus, Lactic dehydrogenase virus*, and *Mouse hepatitis virus*.[149] The thymus itself may be infected by *Thymic virus*.[150] Leukemiaviruses even integrate themselves into the leukocytes by reverse transcription. Through various mechanisms such infection of the immune cells may suppress the immune system. One of the most

Table 4. Virus Infections and the Pathological Changes they Cause in Rodents and Rabbits

	Hosts	Organs with pathological changes
		DNA-Viruses
Adenoviridae		
Mouse adenovirus	M	Respiratory system, gastrointestinal tract, nervous system, urinary system, adrenal glands, skin, lymphatics
Rat adenovirus	R	Gastrointestinal tract
Guinea pig adenovirus	GP	Respiratory system
Herpetoviridae		
Mouse cytomegalovirus	M	Salivary glands, cardiovascular system, muscles, spleen
Rat cytomegalovirus	R	Salivary glands
Guinea pig cytomegalovirus	GP	Salivary glands
Virus III of rabbits	RB	Cardiovascular system, skin, male genitals, eyes
Thymic virus	M	Thymus
Guinea pig herpes-like virus	GP	0
Guinea pig X-virus	GP	0
Papovaviridae		
K virus	M	Respiratory system, cardiovascular system
Mouse polyoma virus	M	Respiratory system, nervous system, urinary system, salivary glands, adrenal glands, thyroid glands, skin, bones and joints
Rat polyoma virus	R	Salivary glands
Hamster papovavirus	H	Skin, blood and lymphatics
Rabbit kidney vacuolating virus	RB	0
Virus of oral papillomatosis	RB	Tongue
Rabbit papilloma virus	RB	Skin
Parvoviridae		
Kilham rat virus	R	Nervous system, male genitals, liver
Toolans H1 virus	R	Nervous system
Minute virus of mice	M	Nervous system
Rodent orphan parvovirus	M,R	0
Poxviridae		
Ectromelia virus	M	Skin, respiratory system, gastrointestinal tract, cardiovascular system, mouth and teeth, female genitals, liver, adrenal glands, blood and lymphatics
Mouse papule virus	M	Skin
Myxoma virus	RB	Skin, respiratory system, eyes

Shope's fibroma virus	RB	Skin, nervous system, male genitals, pleura & peritoneum, liver, thyroid and parathyroid glands
Rabbit pox virus	RB	Skin
Guinea pig pox-like virus	GP	Muscles

RNA Viruses

Arenaviridae		
Lymphocytic choriomeningitis virus	M,GP,H	Nervous system (M,GP), respiratory system (GP), cardiovascular system (H), urinary system (H), liver (M,GP)
Bunyaviridae		
Hantaan virus	R	0
Caliciviridae		
Rabbit hemorrhagic disease virus	RB	Cardiovascular system, liver
Coronaviridae		
Mouse hepatitis virus	M	Respiratory system, gastrointestinal tract, nervous system, liver, blood and lymphatics
Rat coronavirus	R	Respiratory system
Sialodacryaodenitis virus	R	Respiratory system, eyes, salivary glands, lacrimal glands, Harderian glands
Guinea pig coronavirus	GP	Gastrointestinal tract
Rabbit coronavirus	RB	Gastrointestinal tract, myocardium
Paramyxoviridae		
Sendai virus	M,R,H,GP	Respiratory system (M,R)
Pneumonia virus of mice	M,R,H,GP	Respiratory system (M,R)
Simian virus type 5	H,GP	Nervous system (H)
Guinea pig parainfluenza type 3	GP	Respiratory system
Picornaviridae		
Theiler's mouse encephalomyelitis virus		
Strain GDVII	M	Nervous system
Strain MHG	R	Nervous system
Encephalomyocarditis virus	M,R,GP,RB	Nervous system (M,R,GP,RB), heart (R,GP,R, RB), pancreas (M)
Guinea pig poliovirus*	GP	Nervous system
Reoviridae		
Reovirus type III	M,R,H,GP	Gastrointestinal tract (M), respiratory system (M), cardiovascular system (M), pancreas (M)
Mouse rotavirus	M	Gastrointestinal tract, nervous system, liver

Table 4. (continued) Virus Infections and the Pathological Changes they Cause in Rodents and Rabbits

	Hosts	Organs with pathological changes
Rat rotavirus	R	Gastrointestinal tract
Retroviridae		
Type A viruses	M	0
Type B viruses		
Mouse mammary tumor virus	M	Mammary glands
Type C viruses		
Leukemia viruses	M,R,H,GP**	Bone marrow and lymphatics (M,R,H,GP)
Sarcoma viruses	M,R**	Sarcomas in tissues of mesenchymal origin (M)
Togaviridae		
Lactic dehydrogenase virus	M	Macrophages, nervous system, spleen
		Unclassified viruses
Grey lung virus	M,R	Respiratory system

* Although the disease "guinea pig lameness," caused by guinea pig poliovirus is often clinically diagnosed in veterinary practice, the existence and importance of this virus has yet to be clarified.

** Although the species are written in common, leukemiaviruses and sarcomaviruses — of which several exist — are most likely to be species-specific.

Note: Virus infections observed in mice (M), rats (R), guinea pigs (GP), Syrian or Chinese hamsters (H), and rabbits (RB), and the pathological changes that they may cause in these species. Many virus infections only cause clinical disease under certain circumstances, although pathological changes may be present. Important exceptions from this are poxviridae and papovaviridae causing skin lesions, and rotaviruses giving rise to fatal diarrhea in newborn rats and mice. 0 designates that no pathological lesions are known to be caused by the virus in question. For further reading the following references are recommended: 2, 54, 125, 128-131.

Table 5. Infections Caused by Mycoplasmae, Chlamydia, Rickettsiae, and Fungi in Rodents and Rabbits

	Hosts	Disease
Mycoplasmae		
Mycoplasma pulmonis	M,R	Respiratory and genital disease (M,R), arthritis (R)
Mycoplasma neurolyticum	M	Lameness
Mycoplasma arthritidis	M,R	Arthritis (R)
Mycoplasma caviae	GP	0
Mycoplasma cricetuli	H	0
Mycoplasma collis	M	0
Mycoplasma muris	M	0
Chlamydia and Rickettsiae		
Chlamydia psitacci	M,R,GP,H,RB	Pneumonia (M,R,GP,H,RB), abortions (M,R,RB,GP), serositis (M,GP,RB), enteritis (GP,RB), keratoconjunctivitis (M,GP,RB), nephritis (RB), hepatitis (RB)
Chlamydia trachomatis	M	Pneumonia
Eperythrozoon coccoides	M	Anemia, splenomegaly
Hemobartonella muris	M,R,GP,H,RB	Anemia (R)
Rickettsia akari	M	Lymphadenopathy
Fungi		
Aspergillus spp.	R	Pneumonia
Candida albicans	M,GP	Candidiasis (GP)
Cryptococcus neoformans	M,GP,H	Wasting disease (H,GP)
Microsporum canis	GP,RB	Ringworm (GP,RB)
*Pneumocystis carinii**	M,R,GP,H,RB	Pneumonia (M,R,GP,RB)
Trichophyton mentagrophytes	M,R,GP,RB	Ringworm (M,R,GP,RB)

* In some taxonomic descriptions regarded as a fungus[133] in other descriptions as a protozoan.[134] Due to the fact that FELASA guidelines for health monitoring of laboratory rodents[135] lists it as a fungus, it is listed as a fungus in this text as well.

Note: Infections caused by Mycoplasmae, Chlamydiae, Rickettsiae and Fungi in mice (M), rats (R), guinea pigs (GP), Syrian or Chinese hamsters (H), and rabbits (RB), and the disease symptoms they may cause in these species. Note that the groups listed together in this table have no systematic relationship. 0 designates that no disease symptoms are known to be caused by the agent in question. For further reading the following references are recommended: 2, 54, 125, 128–130.

Table 6. Bacterial Infections

	Hosts	Disease
Gram-positive Cocci		Gram-Positive Bacteria
Staphylococcus aureus	M,R,GP,H,RB	Lymphadenitis (H,RB), mastitis (GP,RB), pododermatitis (GP,RB), pyodermia (M,GP, RB), generalized abscess formation (M,GP,H, RB)
Streptococcus group A/B/D/G	M,R,GP,H,RB	Lymphadenitis (M,R), generalized abscess formation (M), septicemia(RB),urolithiasis (GP)
Streptococcus group C	M,R,GP,H,RB	Lymphadenitis (GP,H), pyodermia (GP), generalized abscess formation (GP,H)
Streptococcus pneumoniae	M,R,GP,H,RB	Pneumonia (M,R,GP,H,RB)
Gram-positive Rods		
Corynebacterium kutscheri	M,R,GP,H	Pseudotuberculosis (M,R)
Erysipelothrix rhusiopathiae	R	Arthritis
Listeria monocytogenes	M,R,GP,H,RB	Listeriosis (GP,RB)
Obligate anaerobic Gram-positive bacteria		
Clostridium perfringens	M,RB	Fatal diarrhea (M)
Clostridium difficile	GP,H,RB	Wet tail (H), antibiotica-induced endotoxicosis (GP,H)
		Gram-Negative Bacteria
Enterobacteriaceae		
Citrobacter freundii		Colitis, rectal prolapse
Strain 4280	M	
Ocholi's isolate	GP	Enteritis, pneumonia
Escherichia coli	M,R,GP,H,RB	Enteritis (M,R,GP,H,RB), urogenital infections (M,R), abscesses (M,R), septicemia (RB), mastitis (H)
Klebsiella pneumoniae	M,R,GP,H,RB	Respiratory disease (M,GP,RB), septicemia (M,GP)
Salmonella spp.	M,R,GP,H,RB	Enteritis (M,R,GP), hepatitis (M,R,GP,H), septicemia (H,RB)
Yersinia pseudotuberculosis	M,R,GP,H,RB	Septicemia (GP), enteritis (GP,RB)
Pasteurellaceae		
*Pasteurella pneumotropica**	M,R,GP,H,RB	Abscesses (M), otitis (M), conjunctivitis (M), genital lesions (M), copathogen in respiratory disease of viral and mycoplasmal etiology (M,R)
Pasteurella multocida	M,R,GP,H,RB	Snuffles (RB), pneumonia (H,RB), septicemia (H,RB), otitis media (RB), genital infections (RB)

Species	Hosts	Disease
Haemophilus spp.	M,R,GP,H,RB	Suppurative lesions (M,RB), enteritis (M), pneumonia (R,RB), meningitis (RB)
Pseudomonadaceae		
Pseudomonas aeruginosa	M,R,GP,H,RB	Abscesses (M,R,GP,RB), pneumonia (M,R,GP,RB), septicemia (M,R,GP,H,RB), wound infection (M,R,GP,RB)
Other Facultative Anaerobic Gram-Negative Bacteria		
Bordetella bronchiseptica	M,R,GP,H,RB	Respiratory disease (GP,RB)
Francisella tularensis	R,RB	Septicemia (R,RB)
Streptobacillus moniliformis	M,R,GP	Lymphadenitis (M,GP), abscesses (GP), septicemia (M), polyarthritis (M)
Anaerobic Gram-Negative Bacteria		
Fusobacterium necrophorum	M,GP,RB	Necrobacillosis (RB)
Spirochaeltales		
Leptospira spp.	M,R	Subserosal hemorrhage (M,R)
Treponema cuniculi	RB	Rabbit syphilis (RB)
Spirillum minus	R	Lymphadenopathy (R)
Other Spiral Bacteria		
Campylobacter colijejuni	M,R,H,RB	0
Gram-Negative Bacteria of Uncertain Systematic Classification		
Bacillus piliformis	M,R,GP,H,RB	Tyzzer's disease (M,R,GP,H,RB)
CAR Bacillus	M,R,RB	Chronic respiratory disease (M,R)

* In modern taxonomy this species is rather to be regarded as an *Actinobacillus* spp.[124]

Note: Important bacterial infections observed in mice (M), rats (R), guinea pigs (GP), Syrian or Chinese hamsters (H), and rabbits (RB), and the desease symptoms they may cause in these species. Only infections which may influence research are mentioned, and it should be kept in mind that non-gnotobiotic animals harbor a great number of other bacterial species which are not mentioned here.[8] 0 designates that no disease symptoms are known to be caused by the agent in question. For further reading the following refernces are recommended: 2, 54, 125, 128-129.

Table 7. Protozoan Infections

	Hosts	Disease
Mastigophora (flagellates)		
Chilomastix spp.	R,H,RB	0
Giardia spp.	M,R,GP,H,RB	Enteritis (H)
Spironucleus muris	M,R,H	0
Tritrichomonas spp.	M,R,GP,H	0
Tetratrichomonas minuta	M,R,H	0
Pentatrichomas homonis	M,R,H	0
Trichomitis spp.	R	0
Hexamastix spp.	R,GP,H	0
Enteromonas spp.	R,GP	0
Retortamonas spp.	R,GP,RB	0
Monocercomonoides spp.	R,RB	0
Chilomitus spp.	GP	0
Octimitus spp.	R	0
Sarcodina (amebas)		
Entamoeba muris	M,R,H	0
Entamoeba cuniculi	RB	0
Sporozoa		
Microspora		
Encephalitozoon cuniculi	M,R,GP,RB	Encephalitozoonosis (Nosematosis) (RB)
Coccidia		
Eimeria falciformis	M	Large intestinal coccidiosis
Eimeria nieschulzi	R	Small intestinal coccidiosis
Eimeria miyarii	R	Small intestinal coccidiosis
Eimeria contorta	R	Small intestinal coccidiosis
Eimeria separata	R	Large intestinal coccidiosis
Eimeria caviae	GP	Large intestinal coccidiosis
Eimeria spp.*	RB	Intestinal coccidiosis
Eimeria stiedae	RB	Gall duct coccidiosis
Cryptosporidium spp.	R	Neonatal cryptosporidiosis
Toxoplasma gondii	M,R,GP,RB	Toxoplasmosis (M,GP,RB)
Sarcocystis muris	M,R	Sarcocystosis (M,R)
Sarcocystis cuniculi	RB	Sarcocystosis
Klossiella muris	M	Kidney coccidiosis
Klossiella cobayae	GP	Kidney coccidiosis
Ciliata		
Balantidium spp.	R,GP,H	0

* *E. irresidua, E. magna, E. media, E. perforans, E. exigua, E. intestinalis, E. matsubayishii, E. nagpurensis, E. neoleporis, E. piriformsis.*

Note: Some protozoan infections observed in mice (M), rats (R), guinea pigs (GP), Syrian or Chinese hamsters (H), and rabbits (RB), and the disease symptoms they may cause in these species. Mostly members of the class of Sporozoa seem to be pathogenic. However, members of the other classes may interfere with research in other ways. 0 designates that no disease symptoms are known to be caused by the agent in question. For further reading the following references are recommended: 2, 54, 125, 128-129, 132.

well-described viral infections suppressing the immune system is *Mouse Cytomegalovirus* infection,[151] in which the immunosuppressive effect is caused by the release of interferon and prostaglandins from the macrophages, resulting in the dominance of T suppressor cells.[152-158] A similar effect has been observed after infection with cytomegaloviruses in guinea pigs,[159,160] and *Lactic dehydrogenase virus*.[161,162] Depressed peripheral T cell mitogenesis has been described as an effect of *Sendai virus* infection in mice and rats[163] and after infection with *Minute virus of mice*.[164] The latter also depresses B cell mitogenesis.[164]

Table 8. Helminth Parasites

	Hosts
Nematodes	
Stomach worms	
Graphidium strigosum	GP,RB
Intestinal worms	
Trichostrongylus spp.	RB
Cecal Worms	
Paraspidodera uncinata	GP
Pinworms	
Aspiculuris tetraptera	M,R
Dermatoxys veligeria	RB
Passaluris umbiguus	RB
Syphacia muris	R,H
Syphacia obvelata	M,R,H
Bladder worms	
Trichosomoides crassicauda	R
Threadworms	
Strongyloides ratti	M,R,H
Capillaria hepatica	M,R,RB
Lungworms	
Protostrongylus spp.	RB
Cestodes	
Adult tapeworms	
Cittotaenia variabilis	RB
Hymenolepis nana	M,R,H
Hymenolepis diminuta	M,R,H
Cysticerci of tapeworms	
Cysticercus pisiformis	RB
Coenurus serialis	R
Strobilicercus fasciolaris	M,R
Trematodes	
Liver flukes	
Fasciola hepatica	GP,RB
Dicrocoelium dendriticum	GP,RB

Note: Some helminth parasites observed in mice (M), rats (R), guinea pigs (GP), Syrian or Chinese hamsters (H), and rabbits (RB). Normally helminth infestation does not cause disease. However, it may interfere with research by e.g., immunosuppression, retarded growth, changed digestion, changed hematological values, etc. For further reading the following references are recommended: 2, 54, 128, 132.

Table 9. Ectoparasites

	Hosts
Hair follicle mite	
Demodex aurata	H
Demodex caviae	GP
Demodex criceti	H
Demodex musculi	M
Demodex nanus	R
Ear mange mites	
Notoedres muris	R,GP,H
Psoroptes cuniculi	RB
Body mange mites	
Psorergates simplex	M
Notoedres cati	RB
Sarcoptes scabiei	M,R,GP, RB
Fur mites	
Cheyletiella parasitivorax	RB
Chirodiscoides caviae	GP
Myobia musculi	M
Myocoptes musculinus	M,GP
Listrophorus gibbus	RB
Radfordia affinis	M
Radfordia ensifera	R
Trichoecius romboutsi	M
Lice	
Haemodipsus ventricosus	RB
Polyplax serrata	M
Polyplax spinulosa	R
Gliricola porcelli	GP
Gyropus ovalis	GP
Ticks	
Haemaphysalis leporis-palustris	RB

Note: Some ectoparasites observed in mice (M), rats (R), guinea pigs (GP), Syrian or Chinese hamsters (H), and rabbits (RB). Of disease concern are the mange mites causing mange, and the hair follicle mites causing demodectic mange. Some ectoparasites together with some flea species not mentioned here may serve as vectors or intermediate hosts for endoparasites. For further reading reference No. 132 is recommended.

Thymic virus has an affinity for T helper cells and their precursors, which, apart from being depressive to the immune system by nature, also leads to the dominance of T suppressor cells.[165] Mice infected with murine leukemia viruses, may have the humoral and cellular immunity suppressed.[166,167]

Mycoplasma infections differ from viral immunosuppression as interferon production is impaired,[168] and the specific response to some antigens may be affected.[169-172]

Immunomodulatory bacteria include group A Streptococci, *P. aeruginosa*, *E. coli*, and *Salmonella* spp. The effect, which can be suppressive as well as stimulative, is often mediated through endotoxin production, the active component probably being lipid A.[167] The immunostimulating effect of cell walls of mycobacteria is well established, and brought to practical use in adjuvants for immunization purposes. Parasites with an influence on the immune system are protozoans such as *Toxoplasma gondii*,[141-148] helminths, such as *Syphacia* spp.,[181] and arthropods, such as *Demodex* spp.[167] Often an increased IgE production is observed, but the effect is mainly suppressive and varies among the parasite species. Some examples of immunomodulatory microorganisms are given in Tables 10 and 11.

Physiological Modulation

Some microorganisms have a specific effect on enzymatic, hematological, and other parameters. *Lactic dehydrogenase (LDH) virus* in mice inhibits the clearance of LDH and a number of other enzymes,[199,200] and *Mouse hepatitis virus* alters the hepatic enzyme activity,[201] which may lead to an altered response in toxicological testing.[202] Disturbances may be irreversible for some drugs, but reversible for others. In mice suffering from acute Tyzzer's disease the half-life of trimetophrim may be prolonged, but returning to normal in the recovered mice. However, the half-life of warfarin, also prolonged during acute Tyzzer's disease, never returns to the values observed in disease-free mice.[203] Infection with *Cytomegalovirus* in mice may be associated with a decrease in the P-450 microsomal fraction in the liver, resulting in a transient increase in parathion toxicity and in the sleeping time after phenobarbital administration. Interferon may be the mediator of this effect, as the heightened toxicity lasts longer than the duration of the viral replication in the liver.[204]

Interference with Reproduction

Infections with *Sendai virus*,[205,206] *Sialodacryoadenitis virus*,[207] and *Mouse hepatitis virus*,[208] giving rise to clinical disease in a major part of the population, are very likely to reduce the fertility. Infections with rotaviruses[209,210] or *Cryptosporidium* spp.[211] causes high mortality in neonates, abnormalities in sex hormones, pathological changes in the reproductive tract, and infection of the embryo, causing a high abortion rate. Several microorganisms may cross the placenta barrier, e.g., retroviruses, *Lymphocytic choriomeningitis virus*,[212] *H1 virus*,[213] *Kilham rat virus*,[214] and *Ectromelia virus*,[215] and some bacterial species, such as *B. piliformis*.[216,217] Uterine infections, probably without passage of the placenta barrier, have been observed for other bacteria, e.g., *Salmonella* spp.[218] and *P. pneumotropica*.[219] However, with the exception of the retroviruses and *Lymphocytic choriomeningitis virus*, spontaneous infections of fetuses are rare. *M. pulmonis* may alter a number of reproductive parameters, including spermatozoan motility, *in vitro* egg fertilization, embryo implantation, skeletal development and ossification of the fetus, and vaginal cytology, leading to an over-all reduction in fertility of up to 50%,[219-222] disturbing embryo transfer[223] and teratology.[224] Infection with purulent bacteria in the uterus and salpinx of the recipient mother is a risk in embryo transfer studies and the application of aseptic principles is essential. *E. coli* may ascend from the vagina to uterus in the early stages of progestational proliferation.[225]

Competition Between Microorganisms Within the Animal

In experimental infection studies the animals must be free of the infection in question. If an animal is used for propagation of viruses, it may be experimentally immunosuppressed to make it susceptible to the inoculated virus. However, some of the organisms mentioned in Table 1 may propagate instead. An example of this is a brain biopsy that was taken from a patient with encephalitis and inoculated into mice, which all died. Reinoculation was also fatal. The killing organism was identified as *Mouse hepatitis virus* and the patient was treated with an antiviral drug used for human hepatitis. The patient recovered, but in the recovery phase no antibodies were found to *coronavirus* (mouse hepatitis) while high titers against a togavirus were found. The patient had not been suffering from mouse hepatitis but from Western equine encephalitis.[226]

Some infections reduce the severity of disease caused by other agents, e.g., studies of experimental infection with *Kilham rat virus, Sendai virus,* and *Sialodacryoadenitis virus* failed due to natural infection with *Corynebacterium kutscheri*.[227] This effect may be expected from any infection altering the function of the immune system as described above.

Modulation of Oncogenesis

Infectious agents may either induce cancer, enhance the carcinogenic effect of certain carcinogens, or reduce the incidence of cancer in animals. Cancer is the most important implication in studies with aging animals or other long-term studies; e.g., 56% of female Sprague-Dawley rats develop mammary tumors before the age of 2 years.[228] Retroviruses are among the most important etiological factors, and certain strains or stocks of inbred mice or rats have high prevalences of tumors that are probably of retroviral origin. Other microorganisms that are not primary carcinogens may increase the incidence of specific tumors, either directly, e.g., *M. pulmonis*, which is known to increase the incidence of respiratory tract tumors,[229] or indirectly, e.g., *Mouse hepatitis virus*,[230] *Sendai virus*,[231] and *C. freundii*,[232] which may increase the susceptibility of the animal to some types of chemical carcinogenesis.

Table 10. Some Examples of Microorganisms Activating the Immune System

Effect	Agent	Species
Increased activity of natual killer cells	Sendai virus	Mouse[182,183]
Increased activity of B lymphocytes	E. rhusiopathiae	Rat[184]
Deposition of glomerular immune complexes	Sendai virus	Mouse,[185] hamster[186]
Reduced severity of disease caused by other infections	M. pulmonis	Mouse[187]
Increased humoral immune response	Lactic dehydrogenase virus	Mouse[188]

Table 11. Some Examples of Microorganisms Suppressing the Immune System

Effect	Agent	Species
Decreased severity of adjuvant arthritis	M. pulmonis	Rat[189]
	Sendai virus	Rat[190]
Increased susceptibility to experimental pyelonephritis	M. arthritidis	Rat[191]
Increased severity of other infections	Lactic dehydrogenase virus	Mouse[96,97]
	M. pulmonis	Mouse, rat[98]
Reduced incidence of diabetes mellitus type 1	M. pulmonis	Rat (BB)[192]
	Mouse hepatitis virus	Mouse (NOD)[193]
Various types of decreased cellular immune response	Lactic dehydrogenase virus	Mouse[194,195]
	M. arthritidis	Rat,[169,170] rabbit[171,172]
	M. pulmonis	Rat[196]
	Murine leukemiavirus	Mouse[166,167]
	Sendai virus	Mouse, rat[163,197,198]
	Mouse cytomegalo-virus	Mouse[152-158]
	Guinea pig cyto-megalovirus	Guinea pig[159,160]
Various types of decreased humoral immune response	M. arthritidis	Rat, rabbit[161,162]
	M. pulmonis	Rat[196]
	Streptococcus group A	Mouse,[167] rabbit[167]
	Murine leukemiavirus	Mouse[166,167]
	Syphacia spp.	Mouse[181]
	Minute virus of mice	Mouse[164]

Other agents have the ability to reduce the incidence of tumors; e.g., *Sendai virus* infection may decrease the incidence and delay the appearance of pulmonary adenomas,[233-235] *Reovirus type 3* may suppress pulmonary carcinogenesis due to urethan,[236] *Salmonella* may suppress the growth of transplantable tumors,[237] and *H1 virus* may have a general anticarcinogenic effect.[238-240] *Lactic dehydrogenase virus* enhances the growth of some tumor types, especially in the period shortly after infection.[2] Mice infected with *Mouse mammary tumor virus* are used as human cancer models, which may be obliterated by co-infection with *Lactic dehydrogenase virus*.[241]

PREVENTIVE PRECAUTIONS IN ANIMAL EXPERIMENTS

THE MICROBIOLOGICALLY DEFINED ANIMAL

Although germ-free animals may be preferable, most scientists have to use animals that are not of this quality. It is, however, important to use *microbiologically defined animals*,[242] i.e., animals that have been defined by the presence or absence of specified microorganisms according to a specified examination protocol. The production of such animals is carried out in three stages:

- Production of breeding animals for the upstart of a colony by rederivation techniques, e.g., hysterectomy or embryo transfer
- Breeding in a barrier-protected unit
- Regular health monitoring of animals from the colony

Production of microbiologically defined animals is usually the responsibility of the breeding centers, whereas the interpretation of the health status report, the introduction of precautions to reduce the influence of microorganisms already present in the animal, and the continuous protection and monitoring of the animals during the study are the responsibility of the users and their veterinary advisers.

HEALTH STATUS AND EXPERIMENTAL DESIGN
Protection Against Health Problems in Animal Experiments

The health monitoring report of the breeder should be studied carefully as part of the project planning. If tests for agents considered of importance for the experiment are missing, complementary tests should be required. It should be considered whether the microorganisms present in the breeding colony may influence the study in question or not. If interference can be expected, the study should be carried out using animals free from that particular microorganism. If such animals are not available, the second best choice is to avoid disease-inducing determinants during the experiment. One of the most essential improvements of the experiment may be the use of strains resistant to disease caused by the infection in question, if it is considered that the genetics of the alternative strain will not disturb the experiment. A high hygienic standard is also important to reduce the number of bacteria which the individual animal is exposed to. Probiotic treatment against enteric pathogens may be used, and stress should be minimized.

If all such measures are inadequate, the use of animals protected by vaccination may be considered. If vaccination is unavoidable, it may be an advantage to vaccinate the female breeding animals only, as passive immunization through maternal antibodies is less interfering with research than active immunization of the experimental animal itself. In this way, pneumonia due to *B. bronchiseptica* can be almost totally eliminated from breeding colonies of guinea pigs, although the agent still persists in the colony.[243,244] Vaccination of the experimental animals themselves has been used against *Sendai virus* pneumonia,[245] ectromelia,[125] mycoplasmosis,[246] and the various effects of infection with *Cytomegalovirus*.[247-250] However, with regard to infections that the animal colony can actually be kept free of, vaccination should be considered bad practice. Some of the unwanted microbial effects on research may be seen even in vaccinated animals, e.g., the immunosuppressive effect of *Sendai virus*.[252]

Finally, the possibility of using drugs to prevent infectious disease can be mentioned. However, this method should only be applied if all other possibilities have failed.

The health status of the animals should be included when publishing experimental results. Even though the author may consider the infections of the animals used unessential, others may have a knowledge which can explain some of the results obtained. *P. pneumotropica* was previously considered an essential respiratory pathogen in rats and mice, but since the development of methods for the diagnosis of infections with *M. pulmonis, Sendai virus,* etc., respiratory disease primarily caused by *P. pneumotropica* is only seldom diagnosed.

Retrospective Evaluation of the Health Status

Even a careful incorporation of the health status in the experimental design will not totally exclude infectious problems, as health monitoring results by nature are retrospective. When health monitoring in the breeding colony discloses new microorganisms, animals infected for some time already may have been used. Under such circumstances the same approach as in the experimental design should be used, i.e., the research influence potential of the microorganism as well as of the specific determinants associated with the experiment should be considered. One should never panic. A case in question is a study where antibodies to *E. cuniculi* were found in rabbits from nine out of ten suppliers, as well as in the serum products, such as complement and γ-globulin, of these rabbits.[252] Obviously, the absence of this infection would be ideal, but as long as these products are not used in tests for *E. cuniculi*, there is no reason to believe that these antibodies should be more interfering than any other of the numerous types of antibodies found in serum products. However, if the effects of the newly discovered microorganism on the specific experiment raise uncertainty about the results obtained, one should not hesitate to disregard the results of the experiment.

REFERENCES

1. Öbrink, K. J., Forsöksdjuren - våra okalibrerada instrument? *Läkartidningen*, 69(11), 1252, 1972.
2. National Research Council, *Infectious diseases of mice and rats*, National Academy Press, Washington, D.C., 1991.
3. Schwalbe, C. W., Riemann, H. P., Franti, C. E., *Epidemiology in veterinary practice*. Lea & Febiger, Philadelphia, 1977.
4. Edlich, R. F., Tsung, M. S., Rogers, W., Wangensteen, O. H., Studies in the management of the contaminated wound. 1. Technique of closure of such wounds together with a note on a reproducible animal model, *J. Surg. Res.*, 8, 585, 1968.
5. McRipley, R. J., Whitney, R. R., Characterization and quantification of experimental surgical wound infections used to evaluate topical antibacterial agents, *Antimicrob. Agents Chemother.*, 10, 38, 1976.
6. Moesgaard, F., Nielsen, M. C. L., Justesen, T., Experimental animal model of surgical wound infection applicable to antibiotic prophylaxis, *Eur. J. Clin. Microbiol.*, 2, 459, 1983.
7. Panton, O. N. M., Smith, J. A., Bell, G. A., Forward, A. D., Murphy, J., Doyle, P. W., The incidence of wound infection after stapled or sutured bowel anastomosis and stapled or sutured skin closure in humans and guinea pigs, *Surgery*, 98, 20, 1985.
8. Hansen, A. K., The aerobic bacterial flora of laboratory rats from a Danish breeding centre, *Scand. J. Lab. Anim. Sci.*, 19(2), 59, 1992.
9. Fujiwara, K., Takagaki, Y., Maejima, K., Tajima, Y., Tyzzer's disease in mice. Effects of corticosteroids on the formation of liver lesions and the level of blood transaminases in experimentally infected animals, *Jpn. J. Exp. Med.*, 34, 59, 1964.
10. Fujiwara, K., Tyzzer's disease, *Jpn. J. Exp. Med.*, 48, 467, 1978.
11. Takagaki, Y., Naiki, M., Ito, M., Noguchi, G., Fujiwara, K., Checking of infections due to Corynebacterium kutscheri and Tyzzer's organism among mouse breeding colonies by cortisone injection, *Exp. Anim.*, 16, 12, 1967.
12. Yamada, A., Osada, Y., Takayama, S., Akimoto, T., Ogawa, H., Oshima, Y., Fujiwara, K., Tyzzer's disease syndrome in laboratory rats treated with adrenocorticotropic hormone, *Jpn. J. Exp. Med.*, 39, 505, 1969.
13. Hansen, A. K., Svendsen, O., Møllegaard-Hansen, K. E., Epidemiological studies of Bacillus piliformis infection and Tyzzer's disease in laboratory rats, *Z. Versuchstierkd.*, 33, 163, 1990.
14. Juhr, N. C., Provocation of latent infections, in *New developments in biosciences: their implications for laboratory animal science*, Beynen, A. C., Solleveld, H. A., Eds., Martinus Nijhoff Publishers, Dordrecht, 127, 1988.
15. Boivin, G. P., Wagner, J. E., Besch-Wiliford, C. L., Use of cyclophosphamide in diagnostic provocation of Tyzzer's disease in hamsters, *Lab. Anim. Sci.*, 40(5), 545, 1990.
16. Banerjee, A. K., Angulo, A. F., Kong-A-San, J., Prevention of early deaths in mice contaminated with Gram negative enteric bacteria and fungus following irradiation. In *New developments in biosciences: their implications for laboratory animal science*, Beynen, A. C., Solleveld, H. A., Eds., Martinus Nijhoff Publishers, Dordrecht, 443, 1988.
17. Matsumoto, T., Early deaths after irradiation of mice contaminated by Enterobacter cloacae, *Lab. Anim.*, 14, 247, 1980.
18. Matsumoto, T., Influence of Eschericia coli, Klebsiella pneumoniae and Proteus vulgaris on the mortality pattern of mice after lethal irradiation with X rays, *Lab. Anim.*, 16, 36, 1982.
19. Taffs, L. F., Some diseases in normal and immunosuppressed animals, *Lab. Anim.*, 8, 149, 1974.
20. Urano, T., Maejima, K., Provocation of pseudomoniasis with cyclophosphamide in mice, *Lab. Anim.* 12, 159, 1978.
21. Detmer, A., Hansen, A. K., Dieperink, H., Svendsen, P., Xylose-positive staphylococci as a cause of respiratory disease in immunosuppressed rats, *Scand. J. Lab. Anim. Sci.*, 18(1), 13, 1990.
22. Brook, I., MacVilli, T. J., Walker, R. I., Recovery of aerobic and anaerobic bacteria from irradiated mice, *Infect. Immun.*, 46, 270, 1984.
23. Openshaw, H., Asher, L. V., Wohlenberg, C., Sekiazawa, T., Notkins, A. L., Acute and latent infection of sensory ganglia with herpes simplex virus: immune control and virus reactivation, *J. Gen. Virol.*, 44, 205, 1979.

24. Shanley, J. D., Jordan, M. C., Cook, M. L., Stevens, J. G., Pathogenesis of reactivated latent murine cytomegalovirus infection, *Am. J. Pathol.*, 95, 67, 1979.

25. Mayo, D., Armstrong, J. A., Ho, M., Activation of latent murine cytomegalovirus infection: cocultivation, cell transfer, and the effect of immunosuppression, *J. Infect. Dis.*, 138, 890, 1978.

26. Jordan, M. C., Takagi, J. L., Stevens, J. G., Activation of latent murine cytomegalovirus infection in vivo and in vitro: a pathogenic role for acute infection, *J. Infect. Dis.*, 145, 699, 1982.

27. Sekizawa, T., Openshaw, H., Encephalitis resulting from reactivation of latent herpes simplex virus in mice, *J. Virol.*, 50, 263, 1984.

28. Mayo, D. R., Rapp, F., Leukemia reactivates mouse cytomegalovirus, *J. Gen. Virol.*, 51, 410, 1980.

29. Nathanson, N., Cole, G. A., Santos, G. W., Squire, R. A., Smith, K. O., Viral hemorrhagic encephalopathy of rats. I. Isolation, identification, and properties of the HER strains of rat virus, *Am. J. Epidemiol.*, 91, 328, 1970.

30. Cole, G. A., Nathanson, N., Rivet, H., Viral hemorrhagic encephalopathy of rats. II. Pathogenesis of central nervous system lesions, *Am. J. Epidemiol.*, 91, 339, 1970.

31. Baringer, J. R., Nathanson, N., Parvovirus hemorrhagic encephalopathy of rats. Electron microscopic observations of the vascular lesions, *Lab. Invest.*, 27, 514, 1972.

32. Vella, P. P., Starr, T. J., Effect of X radiation and cortisone on mouse hepatitis virus infection in germ-free mice, *J. Infect. Dis.*, 115, 271, 1965.

33. Dupuy, J. M., Levey-Le-Blond, LeProvost, C., Immunopathology of mouse hepatitis virus type 3. II. Effect of immunosuppression in resistant mice, *J. Immunol.*, 114, 226, 1975.

34. Lavelle, G. C., Bang, F. B., Relationship of phagocytic activity to pathogenecity of mouse hepatitis virus as affected by triolein and cortisone, *Br. J. Exp. Pathol.*, 50, 475, 1969.

35. Ruebner, B. H., Hirano, T., Slusser, R. J., Electron microscopy of the hepatocellular and Kupffer-cell lesions of mouse hepatitis, with particular reference to the effect of cortisone, *Am. J. Pathol.*, 51, 163, 1967.

36. Datta, D. V., Isselbacher, K. J., Effect of corticosteroids on mouse hepatitis infection, *Gut*, 10, 522, 1969.

37. Willenborg, D. O., Shah, K. V., Bang, F. B., Effect of cyclophosphamide on the genetic resistance of C$_3$H mice to mouse hepatitis virus, *Proc. Soc. Exp. Biol. Med.*, 142, 762, 1973.

38. Weiner, L. P., Pathogenesis of demyelination induced by a mouse hepatis virus (JHM virus), *Arch. Neurol.*, 28, 298, 1973.

39. East, J., Parrott, D. M. V., Chesterman, F. C., Pomerace, A., The appearance of a hepatropic virus in mice thymectomized at birth, *J. Exp. Med.*, 118, 1069, 1963.

40. Sheets, P., Shah, K. V., Bang, F. B., Mouse hepatitis virus (MHV) infection in thymectomized C$_3$H mice, *Proc. Soc. Exp. Biol. Med.*, 121, 829, 1966.

41. Anderson, M. J., Pattison, J. R., Cureton, R. J., Argent, S., Heath, R. B., The role of host responses in the recovery of mice from Sendai virus infection, *J. Gen. Virol.*, 46, 373, 1980.

42. Thomsen, A. R., Bro-Jørgensen, K., Volkert, M., Fatal meningitis following lymphocytic choriomeningitis virus infection reflects delayed-type hypersensitivity rather than cytotoxicity, *Scand. J. Immunol.*, 17, 139, 1983.

43. Lampert, P. W., Rodriguez, M., Virus-induced demyelination, in *Concepts in viral pathogenesis*, Notkins, A. L., Oldstone, M. B. A., Eds., Springer, New York, 260, 1983.

44. Roos, R. P., Firestone, S., Wollmann, R., Variakojis, D., Arnason, B. G. W., The effect of short-term and chronic immunosuppression on Theiler's virus demyelination, *J. Neuroimmunol.*, 2, 223, 1982.

45. Lipton, H. L., Dal Conto, M. C., The contrasting effects of immunosuppression on Theiler's virus infection in mice, *Infect. Immun.*, 15, 903, 1977.

46. Weisbroth, S. H., Bacterial diseases, in *The Laboratory Rat*, Baker, H. J., Lindsey, J. R., Weisbroth, S. H., Eds., Academic Press, New York, Vol. 1, 194, 1979.

47. Gärtner, K., Büttner, D., Döhler, K., Firedel, R., Lindena, J., Trautschold, I., Stress response of rats to handling and experimental procedures, *Lab. Anim.*, 14, 267, 1980.

48. Terr, A. I., Dubey, P. D., Yunis, E. J., Slavin, R. G., Waldman, R. H., Physiologic and environmental influences on the immune system, in *Basic and clinical immunology*, Appleton & Lange, East Norwalk, 1991, chap. 16.

49. Lindsey, J. R., Davidson, M. K., Schoeb, T. R., Cassell, G. H., Murine mycoplasmal infections, diseases, and research complications, in *Complications of Viral and Mycoplasma Infections in Rodents to Toxicology Research*, Ham, T. E., Jr., Ed., Hemisphere Press, Washington, D.C., 91, 1985.

50. Broderson, J. R., Lindsey, J. R., Crawford, J., Role of environmental ammonia in respiratory mycoplasmosis of the rat, *Am. J. Pathol.*, 85, 115, 1976.

51. Schoeb, T. R., Davidson, M. K., Lindsey, J. R., Intracage ammonia promotes growth of Mycoplasma pulmonis in respiratory tracts of rats, *Infect. Immun.*, 38, 212, 1982.

52. Hoag, W. G., Strout, J., Meier, H., Epidemiological aspects of the control of Pseudomonas infection in mouse colonies, *Lab. Anim. Care*, 15(3), 217, 1965.

53. Tvedten, H. W., Whitehair, C. K., Langham, R. F., Influence of vitamins A and E on gnotobiotic and conventionally maintained rats exposed to Mycoplasma pulmonis, *J. Am. Vet. Med. Assoc.*, 163, 605, 1973.

54. Institute of Laboratory Animal Resources, *A guide to infectious diseases of guinea pigs, gerbils, hamsters and rabbits*, National Academy of Sciences, Washington, D.C., 1974.

55. Noble, R. L., Sidwell, R. W., Mahoney, A. W., Barnett, B. B., Spendlove, R. S., Influence of malnutrition and alterations in dietary protein on murine rotaviral disease, *Proc. Soc. Exp. Biol. Med.*, 173, 417, 1983.

56. Rygaard, J., Thymus & Self. *Immunobiology of the mouse mutant nude*, J. Wiley & Sons, London, 1973.

57. Custer, R. P., Outzen, H. C., Eaton, G. J., Prehn, R. T., Does the absence of immunological surveillance affect the tumour incidence in "nude" mice. First recorded spontaneous lymphoma in a nude mouse, *J. Natl. Cancer Inst.*, 51, 507, 1973.

58. Fortmeyer, H. P., Besondere gesundheitliche Risken der Mutante, in *Thymusaplastische Maus (nu/nu) Thymusaplastiche Ratte (rnu/rnu) Haltung, Zucht, Versuchsmodelle,* Paul Parey, Berlin and Hamburg, 1981, chap. 3.

59. Dagnæs-Hansen, F., Bisgaard, M., Biochemical characterization of P. pneumotropica subspp. and their clinical importance in mice. *GV-SOLAS Wissenschaftliche Tagung*, Hannover, 1989.

60. Fujiwara, K., Tamura, T., Taguchi, F., Hriano, N., Ueda, K., Wasting disease in nude mice infected with facultatively virulent mouse hepatitis virus, in *Proceedings of the Second International Workshop on Nude Mice*, Nomura, T., Ohsawa, N., Tamaoki, N., Fujiwara, K., Eds., University of Tokyo Press, Tokyo and Gustav Fischer Verlag, Stuttgart, 53, 1977.

61. Festing, M. F. W., Inherited immunological defects in laboratory animals, in *Immunodeficient animals for cancer research*, Sparrow, S., Ed., MRC Laboratory Animals Centre Symposium, 2, 1979, chap. 2.

62. Jacobson, R. H., Reed, N. D., The thymus dependency of resistance to pinworm infection in mice, *J. Parasitol.*, 60, 976, 1974.

63. Reed, N. D., Isaak, D. D., Jacobson, R. H., The use of nude mice in model systems, for studies on acquired immunity to parasitic infections, in *Proceedings of the Second International Workshop on Nude Mice*, Nomura, T., Ohsawa, N., Tamaoki, N., Fujiwara, K., Eds., University of Tokyo Press, Tokyo and Gustav Fischer Verlag, Stuttgart, 3, 1977.

64. Carthew, P., Sparrow, S., Sendai virus in rnu/rnu rats and germ-free AGUS rats, *Res. Vet. Sci.*, 29, 289, 1980.

65. Weir, E. C., Jacoby, R. O., Paturzo, F. X., Johnson, E. A., Ardito, R. B., Persistence of sialodacryoadenitis virus in athymic rats, *Lab. Anim. Sci.*, 40(2), 138, 1990.

66. Furuta, T., Kawamura, S., Fujiwara, K., Spontaneous Tyzzer's disease in nude rats, *Jpn. J. Vet. Sci.*, 46(6), 941, 1984.

67. Cheers, C., McKenzie, I. F. C., Pavlov, H., Waid, L., York, J., Resistance and susceptibility of mice to bacterial infection: course of listeriosis in resistant or susceptible mice, *Infect. Immun.*, 19, 763, 1978.

68. Rose, E. M., Ogilvie, B. M., Hesketh, P., Festing M. F. W., Failure of nude (athymic) rats to become resistant to reinfection with the intestinal coccidian parasite Eimeria nieschulzi or the nematode Nippostrongylus brasiliensis, *Parasite Immunol.*, 1, 125, 1979.

69. Hansen, A. K., Dagnæs-Hansen, F., Møllegaard-Hansen, K. E., Correlation between megaloileitis and antibodies to Bacillus piliformis in laboratory rat colonies, *Lab. Anim. Sci.*, 42(5), 449, 1992.

70. O'Brien, A. D., Rosenstreich, D. L., Scher, I., Campbell, G. H., MacDermott, R. P., Formal, S. B., Genetic control of susceptibility to Salmonella typhimurium in mice: role of the LPS gene, *J. Immunol.*, 124, 20, 1980.

71. Plant, J., Glynn, A. A., Genetics of resistance to infection with Salmonella typhimurium in mice, *J. Infect. Dis.*, 133, 72, 1976.

72. Wullenweber, M., Kaspareit-Rittinghausen, Farouq M., Streptobacillus moniliformis epizootic in barrier-maintained C57BL/6J mice and susceptibility to infection of different strains of mice, *Lab. Anim. Sci.*, 40(6), 608, 1990.

73. Saito, M., Nakagawa, M., Muto, T., Imaizumi, K., Strain differences of mouse in susceptibility to Mycoplasma pulmonis infection, *Jpn. J. Vet. Sci.*, 40, 697, 1978.

74. Davis, J. K., Cassell, G. H., Murine mycoplasmosis in LEW and F344 rats: strain differences in lesion severity, *Vet. Pathol.*, 19, 280, 1982.

75. Briody, B. A., Mouse pox (ectromelia) in the United States, *Lab. Anim. Care*, 6, 1, 1955.

76. Martinez, D., Wolanski, B., Tytell, A. A., Devlin, R. G., Viral etiology of age-dependent polioencephalomyelitis in C58 mice, *Infect. Immun.*, 23, 133, 1979.

77. Taguchi, F., Hirano N., Kiuchi Y., Fujiwara, K., Difference in response to mouse hepatitis among susceptible mouse strains, *Jpn. J. Microbiol.*, 20, 293, 1976.

78. Parker, J. C., Whiteman, M. D., Richter, C. B., Susceptibility of inbred and outbred mouse strains to Sendai virus and prevalence of infection in laboratory rodents, *Infect. Immun.*, 19, 123, 1978.

79. Lipton, H. L., Melvold, R. M., Genetic analysis of susceptibility to Theiler's virus-induced demyelinating disease in mice, *J. Immunol.*, 132, 1821, 1984.

80. Lipton, H. L., Rozhon, E. J., The Theiler's Murine Encephalomyelitis Viruses, in *Viral and Mycoplasmal Infections of Laboratory Rodents, Effects on biomedical research*, Bhatt, P. N., Jacoby, R. O., Morse, H.C., III, New, A. E., Eds., Academic Press, Orlando, 1986, chap. 14.

81. Brownstein, D., Genetics of natural resistance to Sendai virus infection in mice, *Infect. Immun.*, 41, 308, 1983.

82. Gruber, F., Ontogenese der Immunmechanismen, in *Immunologie der Versuchstiere*, Gruber, F., Ed., Verlag Paul Parey, Berlin, 46, 1975.

83. Brambell, F. W. R., Halliday, R., The route by which passive immunity is transferred from mother to fetus in the rat, *Proc. R. Soc. London, Ser. B.*, 145, 170, 1956.

84. Fujiwara, K., Hirano, N., Takenaka, S., Sato, K., Peroral infection in Tyzzer's disease in mice, *Jpn. J. Exp. Med.*, 43, 33, 1973.

85. Onodera, T., Fujiwara, K., Nasoencephalopathy in suckling mice inoculated intranasally with the Tyzzer's organism, *Jpn. J. Exp. Med.*, 43, 509, 1973.

86. Zurcher, C., Burek, J. D., van Nunen, M. C. J., Meihuizen, S. P., A naturally occurring epizootic caused by Sendai virus in breeding and aging rodent colonies. I. Infection in the mouse, *Lab. Anim. Sci.*, 27, 955, 1977.

87. Lai, Y. L., Jacoby, R. O., Bhatt, P. N., Jonas, A. M., Keratoconjunctivitis associated with sialodacryoadenitis in rats, *Invest. Opthalmol.*, 15, 538, 1976.

88. Jersey, G. C., Whitehair, C. K., Carter, G. R., Mycoplasma pulmonis as the primary cause of chronic respiratory disease in rats, *J. Am. Vet. Med. Assoc.*, 163, 599, 1972.

89. Sawicki, L., Influence of age on recovery from experimental Sendai virus infection, *Nature*, 192, 1258, 1961.

90. Sawicki, L., Studies on experimental Sendai virus infection in laboratory mice, *Acta Virol.*, 6, 347, 1962.

91. Kaneko, J., Fujita, H., Matsuyama, S., Kojima, H., Asakura, H., Nakamura, Y., Kodama, T., An outbreak of the Tyzzer's disease among colonies of the mice, *Bull. Exp. Anim.*, 9, 148, 1960.

92. Hardenbergh, J. G., Epidemic lymphadenitis with formation of abscesses in guinea pigs due to infection with hemolytic streptococci, *J. Lab. Clin. Med.*, 12, 119, 1926.

93. Gledhill, A. W., Dick, G. W., Andrewes, C. H., Production of hepatitis in mice by the combined action of two filterable agents, *Lancet*, 263, 509, 1952.

94. Riley, V., Persistence and other characteristics of the lactate dehydrogenase-elevating virus (LDH-virus), *Prog. Med. Virol.*, 18, 198, 1974.

95. Bonventre, P. F., Bubel, H. C., Michael, J. G., Nickol, A. D., Impaired resistance to bacterial infection after tumor implant is traced to lactic dehydrogenase virus, *Infect. Immun.*, 30, 316, 1980.

96. Saito, M., Nakagawa, M., Suzuki, E., Kinoshita, K., Imaizumi, K., Synergistic effect of Sendai virus on Mycoplasma pulmonis infection in mice, *Jpn. J. Vet. Sci.*, 43, 43, 1981.

97. Howard, C. J., Stott, E. J., Taylor, G., The effect of pneumonia induced in mice with Mycoplasma pulmonis on resistance to subsequent bacterial infection and the effect of a respiratory infection with Sendai virus on the resistance of mice to Mycoplasma pulmonis, *J. Gen. Microbiol.*, 109, 79, 1978.

98. Van Swieten, M. J., Solleveld, H. A., Lindsey, J. R., deGrott, F. G., Zurcher, C., Hollander, C. F., Respiratory disease in rats associated with a filamentous bacterium: a preliminary report, *Lab. Anim. Sci.*, 30, 215, 1980.

99. Ganaway, J. R., Spencer, T. H., Moore, T. D., Allen, A. M., Isolation, propagation and characterization of a newly recognized pathogen, cilia-associated bacillus of rats: an etiological agent of chronic respiratory disease, *Infect. Immun.*, 47, 472, 1983.

100. Brennan, P. C., Fritz, T. E., Flynn, R. J., The role of Pasteurella pneumotropica and Mycoplasma pulmonis in murine pneumonia, *J. Bacteriol.*, 97, 337, 1969.

101. Koopman, J. P., Janssen F. G. J., van Druten, J. A. M., The relation between the intestinal microflora and intestinal parameters in mice, *Z. Versuchstierkd.*, 19, 54, 1977.

102. Koopman, J. P., Kennis, H. M., Characterization of anaerobic caecal bacteria in mice, *Z. Versuchstierkd.*, 21, 185, 1979.

103. Koopman, J. P., Welling, G. W., Converting germ-free mice to the normal state with defined anaerobic bacteria. In *Animal Quality and Models in Biomedical Research*, Spiegel, A., Erichsen, S., Solleveld, H. A., Eds., Gustav Fischer Verlag, Stuttgart, 193, 1980.

104. Jawetz, E., Melnick, J. L., Adelberg, E. A., *Review of medical microbiology*, Lange Medical Publications, Los Altos, 1980.

105. Fuller, R., A review. Probiotics in man and animals, *J. Appl. Bacteriol.*, 66, 365, 1989.

106. Jørgensen, M., Probioticum (Streptococcus faecium Cernelle 68 - SF68) for improvement of health and well-being with mink and fox, *Scientifur*, 12, 250, 1988.

107. Tannock, G. W. R., Demonstration of epithelium-associated microbes in the oesophagus of pigs, cattle, rats and deer, *FEMS Microbiol. Ecol.*, 45, 199, 1987.

108. Barthold, S. W., Smith, A. L., Mouse hepatitis virus strain-related patterns of tissue tropism in suckling mice, *Arch. Virol.*, 81, 103, 1984.

109. ElDadah, A. H., Nathanson, N., Smith, K. O., Squire, R. A., Santos, G. W., Melby, E. C., Viral hemorrhagic encephalopathy of rats, *Science*, 156, 392, 1967.

110. Theiler, M., Gard, S., Encephalomyelitis of mice. I. Characteristics and pathogenesis of the virus, *J. Exp. Med.*, 72, 49, 1940.

111. Stanley, N. F., Leak, P. J., Waiters, M. N., Joske, R. A., Murine infection with reovirus. II. The chronic disease following reovirus type 3 infection, *Br. J. Exp. Pathol.*, 45, 142, 1964.

112. Walters, M. N., Joske, R. A., Leak, P. J., Stanley, N. F., Murine infection with reovirus. III. Pathology of infections with reoviruses types I and II. *Br. J. Exp. Pathol.*, 46, 200, 1965.

113. Stanley, N. F., Joske, R. A., Animal model: chronic murine hepatitis induced by reovirus type 3, *Am. J. Pathol.*, 80, 181, 1975.

114. Brennan, P. C., Fritz, T. E., Flynn, R. J., Poole, C. M., Citrobacter freundii associated with diarrhea in laboratory mice, *Lab. Anim. Care*, 15, 266, 1965.

115. Ediger, R. D., Kovatch, R. M., Rabstein, M. M., Colitis in mice with a high incidence of rectal prolapse, *Lab. Anim. Sci.*, 24, 488, 1974.

116. Barthold, S. W., Osbaldiston, G. W., Jonas, A. M., Dietary, bacterial and host genetic interactions in the pathogenesis of transmissible murine colonic hyperplasia, *Lab. Anim. Sci.*, 27, 938, 1977.

117. Fujiwara, K., Yamada, A., Ogawa, H., Oshima, Y., Comparative studies on the Tyzzer's organisms from rats and mice, *Jpn. J. Exp. Med.*, 41(2), 125, 1971.

118. Fujiwara, K., Kurashina, H., Magaribuchi, T., Takenaka, S., Yokoiyama, S., Further observations on the difference between Tyzzer's organisms from mice and those from rats, *Jpn.. J. Exp. Med.*, 43(4), 307, 1973.

119. Hansen, A. K., The use of mongolian gerbils as sentinels for infection with Bacillus piliformis in laboratory rats, in *Proc. 4th FELASA Symp.*, 449, FELASA, L'Arbresle Cédex, 1992.

120. Percy, D. H., Bond, S. J., Paturzo, F. X., Bhatt, P. N., Duration of protection from reinfection following exposure to sialodacryoadenitis virus in Wistar rats, *Lab. Anim. Sci.*, 40(2), 144, 1990.

121. Charles River Breeding Laboratories Inc., *Charles River Technical Bulletin,* Vol. 2, No. 2, 1983.

122. Besch-Williford, C., Wagner, J. E., Eradication of enzootic Sendai virus infection from a production colony of Sprague-Dawley rats, *Lab. Anim. Sci.*, 33(5), 502, 1983.

123. Oldstone, M. B. A., Dixon, F. J., Lymphocytic choriomeningitis: production of antibody by "tolerant" infected mice, *Science*, 158, 1193, 1967.

124. Trahan, C. J., Stephenson, E. H., Ezzell, J. W., Mitchell, W. C., Airborne-induced experimental Bordetella bronchiseptica pneumonia in Strain 13 guinea pigs, *Lab. Anim.*, 21, 226, 1987.

125. Allen, A. M., Nomura, T., *Manual of Microbiologic Monitoring of Laboratory Animals*, U.S. Department of Health and Human Services, Bethesda, 1986.

126. Waller, T., Eradication of encephalitozoonosis in rabbit breeding colonies by carbon immunoassay, in *New developments in biosciences: their implications for laboratory animal science,* Beynen, A. C., Solleveld, H. A., Eds., Martin Nijhoff Publishers, Dordrecht, 385, 1988.

127. Arison, R. N., Cassaro, J. A., Pruss, M. P., Studies on murine ascites-producing agent and its effect on tumor development, *Cancer Res.*, 26, 1915, 1966.

128. Kunstyr, I., Ed., A list of pathogens for specification in SPF laboratory animals, GV-SOLAS, Bibberach an der Riss, 1988.

129. Kunstyr, I., Ed., Mikrobiologische Diagnostik bei Laboratoriumstieren, GV-SOLAS, Bibberach an der Riss, 1989.

130. Bhatt, P. N., Jacoby, R. O., Morse, H. C., III, New, A. E., Eds., *Viral and Mycoplasmal Infections of Laboratory Rodents, Effects on biomedical research*, Academic Press Inc., Orlando, 1986.

131. Lussier, G., Potential detrimental effects of rodent viral infections on long-term experiments, *Vet. Res. Commun.*, 12, 199, 1988.

132. Owen, D. G., *Parasites of laboratory animals*, Royal Society of Medicine Services Ltd., London, 1992.

133. Vavra, J., Kučera, K., Pneumocystis carinii Delanoë, its ultrastructure and ultrastructural affinities, *J. Protozool.*, 17, 463, 1970.

134. Long, E. G., Smith, J. S., Meier, J. L., Attachment of Pneumocystis carinii to rat pneumocytes, *Lab. Invest.*, 54, 609, 1986.

135. FELASA Working Group on Animal Health (Blanchet, H. M., Boot, R., Deeny, A, Hansen, A. K., Hem, A., Van herck, H., Kraft, V., Kunstyr, I. Milite, G., Needham, J. R., Nicklas, W., Perrot, A., Rehbinder, C., Richard, Y., De vroy, G.), *Draft to recommendations for health monitoring of mouse, rat, hamster, guinea pig and rabbit breeding colonies*, Hannover, 1992.

136. Mutters, R., Ihm, P., Pohl, S., Frederiksen, W., Mannheim, W., Reclassification of the genus Pasteurella Trevisan 1887 on the basis of DNA homology with proposals for the new species Pasteurella dagmatis, Pasteurella canis, Pasteurella stomatis and Pasteurella langaa, *Int. J. System. Bacteriol.*, 35, 309, 1985.

137. Cole, B. C., Miller, M. L., Ward, J. R., The role of mycoplasma in rat arthritis induced by 6-sulfanilamidoindazole (6-SAE), *Proc. Soc. Exp. Biol. Med.*, 130, 994, 1969.

138. Jasmin, G., Experimental polyarthritis in rats injected with a tumor exudate, *Ann. Rheum. Dis.*, 16, 365, 1957.

139. Pearson, C., Development of arthritis in the rat following injection with adjuvant. In *Mechanisms of hypersensitivity*, Shafer, J. H., LoGrippo, G. A., Chase, M. W. Eds., Little Brown, Boston, 647, 1959.

140. Turnbull, G. J., The needs of the toxicologist, In *Microbiological Standardisation of Laboratory Animals*, Roe, F. J. C., Ed., Ellis Horwood Ltd., Chicester, 1983, chap. 1.

141. Huldt, S., Gard, S., Olovson, S. G., Effect of Toxoplasma gondii on the thymus, *Nature*, 244, 301, 1973.

142. Strickland, G. T., Ahmed, A., Sells, K. W., Blastogenic response of Toxoplasma-infected mouse spleen cells to T- and B-cell mitogens, *Clin. Exp. Immunol.*, 22, 167, 1975.

143. Swartzberg, J. E., Krahenbuhl, J. L., Remington J. S., Dichotomy between macrophage activation and degree of protection against Listeria monocytogenes and Toxoplasma gondii in mice stimulated with Corynebacterium parvum, *Infect. Immun.*, 12, 1037, 1975.

144. Mahmoud, A. A., Warren, K. D., Strickland, G. T., Acquired resistance to infection with Schistosoma mansoni induced by Toxoplasma gondii, *Nature*, 263, 56, 1976.

145. Ruskin, J., Remington, J. S., A role for the macrophage for the acquired immunity to phylogenetically unrelated intracellular organisms, *Antimicrob. Agents Chemother.*, 474, 1969.

146. Ruskin, J., Remington, J. S., Immunity and intracellular infection: resistance to bacteria in mice infected with a protozoan, *Science*, 160, 72, 1968.

147. Remington, J. S., Merigan, T. C., Resistance to virus challenge in mice infected with protozoa or bacteria, *Proc. Soc. Exp. Biol. Med.*, 131, 1184, 1969.

148. Gentry, L.O., Remington, G. S., Resistance against Cryptococcus conferred by intracellular bacteria and protozoa, *J. Infect. Dis.*, 123, 22, 1971.

149. Mims, C., Virus-Related Immunomodulation, in *Viral and Mycoplasmal Infections of Laboratory Rodents, Effects on biomedical research*, Bhatt, P. N., Jacoby, R. O., Morse, H. C., III, New, A. E., Eds., Academic Press, Orlando, 1986, chap. 28.

150. Rowe, W. P., Capps, W. I., A new mouse virus causing necrosis of the thymus in newborn mice, *J. Exp. Med.*, 113, 831, 1961.

151. Hamilton, J. D., Fitzwilliam, J. F., Cheung, K. S., Lang, D. J., Effect of murine cytomegalovirus infection on the immune response to a tumor allograft, *Rev. Infect. Dis.*, 1, 976, 1979.

152. Loh, L., Hudson, J. B., Immunosuppressive effect of murine cytomegalovirus, *Infect. Immun.*, 27, 54, 1979.

153. Loh, L., Hudson, J. B., Murine cytomegalovirus infection in the spleen and its relationship to immunosuppression, *Infect. Immun.*, 32, 1067, 1980.

154. Loh, L., Hudson, J. B., Murine cytomegalovirus-induced immunosuppression, *Infect. Immun.*, 36, 89, 1982.

155. Shanley, J. D., Pesanti, E. L., Effects of antiviral agents on murine cytomegalovirus-induced macrophage dysfunction, *Infect. Immun.*, 36, 918, 1982.

156. Shanley, J. D., Pesanti, E. L., Replication of murine cytomegalovirus in lung macrophages: effect on phagocytosis of bacteria, *Infect. Immun.*, 29, 1152, 1980.

157. Bixler, G. S., Booss, J., Establishment of immunologic memory concurrent with suppression of the primary immune response during cytomegalovirus infection of mice, *J. Immunol.*, 125, 893, 1980.

158. Bixler, G. S., Booss, J., Adherent spleen cells from mice acutely infected with cytomegalovirus suppress the primary antibody response in vitro, *J. Immunol.*, 127, 1294, 1981.

159. Griffith, B. P., Askenase, P. W., Hsiung, G. D., Serum and cell-mediated viral-specific delayed cutaneous basophil reactions during cytomegalovirus infection of guinea pigs, *Cell. Immunol.*, 69, 138, 1982.

160. Griffith, B. P., Lavallee, J. T., Booss, J., Hsiung, G. D., Asynchronous depression of responses to T- and B-cell mitogens during acute infection with cytomegalovirus in the guinea pig, *Cell. Immunol.*, 87, 727, 1984.

161. Stevenson, M., Rees, J. C., Meltzer, M. S., Macrophage function in tumor-bearing mice: evidence for lactic dehydrogenase-elevating virus-associated changes, *J. Immunol.*, 124, 2892, 1980.

162. Isakov, N., Feldman, M., Segal, S., Acute infections of mice with lactic dehydrogenase virus (LDV) impairs the antigen-presenting capacity of their macrophages, *Cell. Immunol.*, 66, 317, 1982.

163. Garlinghouse, L., van Hoosier, G., Studies on adjuvant-induced arthritis, tumor transplantability, and serologic response to bovine serum albumin in Sendai virus-infected rats, *Am. J. Vet. Res.*, 39, 297, 1978.

164. Tattersall, P., Cotmore, S. F., The rodent parvoviruses, in *Viral and Mycoplasmal Infections of Laboratory Rodents, Effects on biomedical research*, Bhatt, P. N., Jacoby, R. O., Morse, H. C., III, New, A. E., Eds., Academic Press Inc., Orlando, 1986, chap. 16.

165. Guignard, R., Potworowski, E. F., Lussier, G., Mouse thymic-virus-mediated immunosuppression; association with decreased helper T cells and increased suppressor T cells, *Viral Immunol.*, 2(3), 215, 1989.

166. Cole, B. C., Lombardi, P. S., Overall, J. C., Jr., Glascow, L. A., Inhibition of interferon induction in mice by mycoplasmas, *Proc. Soc. Exp. Biol. Med.*, 157, 83, 1978.

167. Thomsen, A. C., Heron, I., Effect of mycoplasmas on phagocytosis and immunocompetence in rats, *Acta Pathol. Scand., Sect. C*, 87, 67, 1979.

168. Kaklamanis, E., Pavlatos, M., The immunosuppressive effect of mycoplasma infection. I. Effect on the humoral and cellular response, *Immunology,* 22, 695, 1972.

169. Simberkoff, M. S., Thorbecke, G. J., Thomas, L., Studies on PPLO infection. Inhibition of lymphocyte mitosis and antibody formation by mycoplasmal extracts, *J. Exp. Med.*, 129, 1163, 1969.

170. Specter, S. C., Bendinelli, M., Ceglowski, W. S., Friedman, H., Macrophage-induced reversal of immunosuppression by leukemia viruses, *Fed. Proc.*, 37, 97, 1978.

171. Berquist, L. M., Lav, B. H. S., Winter, C. E., Mycoplasma-associated immuno-suppression: effect on hemagglutinin response to common antigens in rabbits, *Infect. Immun.*, 9, 410, 1974.

172. Westerberg, S. C., Smith, C. B., Wiley, B. B., Jensen, C., Mycoplasma-virus interrelationships in mouse tracheal organ cultures, *Infect. Immun.*, 5, 840, 1972.

173. Irvani, J., van As, A., Mucous transport in the tracheobronchial tree of normal and bronchitic rats, *J. Pathol.*, 106, 81, 1972.

174. Korotzer, T. L., Weiss, H. S., Hamparian, V. V., Somerson, N. L., Oxygen uptake and lung function in mice infected with Streptococcus pneumoniae, influenza virus, or Mycoplasma pulmonis, *J. Lab. Clin. Med.*, 91, 280, 1978.

150

175. Pollack, J. D., Weiss, H. S., Somerson, N. L., Lecitin changes in murine Mycoplasma pulmonis respiratory infection, *Infect. Immun.*, 24, 94, 1979.

176. Laubach, H. E., Kocan, A. A., Sartain, K. E., Lung lysophospholidase activity in specific-pathogen-free rats infected with Pasteurella pneumotropica or Mycoplasma pulmonis, *Infect. Immun.*, 22, 295, 1978.

177. Wells, A. B., The kinetics of cell proliferation in the tracheobronchial epithelia of rats with and without chronic respiratory disease, *Cell. Tissue Kinet.*, 3, 185, 1970.

178. Ventura, J., Domaradzki, M., Role of mycoplasma infection in the development of experimental bronchiectasis in the rat, *J. Pathol. Bacteriol.*, 93, 342, 1967.

179. Green, G. M., The Burns Amberson Lecture — In defense of the lung, *Am. Rev. Respir. Dis.*, 102, 691, 1970.

180. Hunneyball, I. M., The needs of the immunologist, in *Microbiological Standardisation of Laboratory Animals*, Roe, F. J. C., Ed., Ellis Horwood Ltd., Chicester, 1983, chap. 5.

181. Hsu, C.K., Parasitic diseases: how to monitor them and their effects on research, *Lab. Anim.*, 9, 48, 1980.

182. Anderson, M., Innate cytotoxicity of CBA mouse spleen cells to Sendai virus-infected L. cells, *Infect. Immun.*, 20, 608, 1978.

183. Anderson, M., Pattison, J., Heath, R., The nature of the effector cells of cell-mediated immune responses to Sendai and Kunz virus infections in mice, *Br. J. Exp. Pathol.*, 60, 314, 1979.

184. Ziesenis A., Röllinger B., Franz, B., Hart, S., Hadam, M., Leibold, M., Changes in rat leukocyte populations in peripheral blood, spleen, lymph nodes, and synovia during Erysipelas bacteria-induced polyarthritis, *J. Exp. Anim. Sci.*, 35, 2, 1992.

185. Blandford, G., Studies on the immune response and pathogenesis of Sendai virus infection of mice. III. The effects of cyclophosphamide, *Immunology*, 28, 871, 1975.

186. Blandford, G., Charlton, D., Studies of pulmonary and renal immunopathology after nonlethal primary Sendai viral infection in normal and cyclophosphamide-treated hamsters, *Am. Rev. Resp. Dis.*, 115, 305, 1977.

187. Cassell, G. H., Davis, J. K., Simecka, J. W., Lindsey, J. R., Cox, N. R., Ross, S., Fallon, M., Mycoplasmal infections: disease pathogenesis, implications for biomedical research, and control, In *Viral and Mycoplasmal Infections of Laboratory Rodents, Effects on biomedical research*, Bhatt, P. N., Jacoby, R. O., Morse, H. C., III, New, A. E., Eds., Academic Press, Orlando, 1986, chap. 8.

188. Notkins, A. L., Mergenhagen, S. E., Rizzo, A. A., Scheele, C., Waldmann, T. A., Elevated gamma-globulin and increased antibody production in mice infected with lactic dehydrogenase virus, *J. Exp. Med.*, 123, 347, 1966.

189. Taurog, J. D., Leary, S. L., Cremer, M. A., Mahowald, M. L., Sandberg, G. P., Manning, P. J., Infection with Mycoplasma pulmonis modulates adjuvant- and collagen-induced arthritis in Lewis rats, *Arthritis Rheum.*, 27, 943, 1984.

190. Garlinghouse, L., van Hoosier, G., Studies on adjuvant-induced arthritis, tumor transplantability, and serologic response to bovine serum albumin in Sendai virus-infected rats, *Am. J. Vet. Res.*, 39, 297, 1978.

191. Thomsen, A. C., Rosendal, S., Mycoplasmosis — experimental pyelonephritis in rats, *Acta Pathol. Microbiol. Scand.*, 82, 94, 1974.

192. Kloeting, I., Sadewasser, S., Lucke, S., Vogt, L., Hahn, H. J., Development of BB rat diabetes is delayed or prevented by infections or applications of immunogens. In *Frontiers in diabetes research*, Shafrir, E., Renolds, A. E., Eds., John Libbey, London, 190, 1988.

193. Wilberz, S., Partke, H. J., Dagnæs-Hansen, F., Herberg, L., Persistent MHV (mouse hepatitis virus) infection reduces the incidence of diabetes mellitus in non-obese diabetic mice, *Diabetologia*, 34, 2, 1991.

194. Howard, R. J., Notkins, A. L., Mergenhagen, S. E., Inhibition of cellular immune reactions in mice infected with lactic dehydrogenase virus, *Nature*, 221, 874, 1969.

195. Michaelides, M. C., Schlesinger, S., Effect of acute or chronic infection with lactic dehydrogenase virus (LDV) on the susceptibility of mice to plasmacytoma MOPC-315, *J. Immunol.*, 112, 1560, 1974.

196. Lai, W. C., Pakes, S. P., Owusu, I., Wang, S., Mycoplasma pulmonis depresses humoral and cell-mediated responses in mice, *Lab. Anim. Sci.*, 39(1), 11, 1989.

197. Weir, E., Green, D., Brownstein, D., Influence of Sendai virus infection on regulation of the *in vitro* immune response in C57Bl/6J mice, *Lab. Anim. Sci.*, 34, 514, 1984.

198. Brownstein, D. G., Sendai virus, in *Viral and Mycoplasmal Infections of Laboratory Rodents, Effects on biomedical research*, Bhatt, P. N., Jacoby, R. O., Morse, H. C., III, New, A. E., Eds., Academic Press, Orlando, 1986, chap. 6.

199. Notkins, A. L., Enzymatic and immunologic alterations in mice infected with lactic dehydrogenase virus, *Am. J. Pathol.*, 64, 733, 1971.

200. Brinton, M. A., Lactate dehydrogenase-elevating virus, in *The Mouse in Biomedical Research*, Foster, H. L., Small, J. D., Fox, J. G., Eds., Academic Press, New York, 1982, chap. 10.

201. Ruebner, B. H., Hirano, T., Viral hepatitis in mice. Changes in oxidative enzymes and phosphatases after murine hepatis virus (MHV-3) infection, *Lab. Invest.*, 14, 157, 1965.

202. Tiensiwakul, P., Husain, S. S., Effect of mouse hepatitis virus infection on iron retention in the mouse liver, *Br. J. Exp. Pathol.*, 60, 161, 1979.

203. Friis, A.S., Ladefoged, O., The influence of Bacillus piliformis (Tyzzer) infections on the reliability of pharmacokinetic experiments in mice, *Lab. Anim.*, 13, 257, 1979.

204. Osborn, J. E., Cytomegalovirus and other herpesviruses of mice and rats, in *Viral and Mycoplasmal Infections of Laboratory Rodents, Effects on biomedical research*, Bhatt, P. N., Jacoby, R. O., Morse, H. C., III, New, A. E., Eds., Academic Press, Orlando, 1986, chap. 19.

205. Makino, S., Seko, S., Nakao, H., Midazuki, K., An epizootic of Sendai virus infection in a rat colony, *Exp. Anim.*, 22, 275, 1972.

206. Coid, C. R., Wradman, G., The effect of maternal respiratory disease induced by parainfluenza type 1 (Sendai) virus on foetal development and neonatal mortality in the rat, *Med. Microbiol. Immunol.*, 157, 181, 1972.

207. Utsumi, K., Ishikawa, T., Maeda, T., Shimizy, S., Tasumi, H., Fujiwara, K., Infectious sialoadenitis and rat breeding, *Lab. Anim.*, 14, 303, 1980.

208. Fujiwara, K., Takenaka, S., Shuyima, S., Carrier state of antibody and viruses in a mouse breeding colony persistently infected with Sendai and Mouse Hepatitis viruses, *Lab. Anim. Sci.*, 26, 153, 1976.

209. Cheever, F. S., Mueller, J. H., Epidemic diarrheal disease of suckling mice. I. Manifestations, epidemiology, and attempts to transmit the disease, *J. Exp. Med.*, 85, 405, 1947.

210. Vonderfecht, S. L., Huber, A. C., Eiden, J., Mader, L. C., Yolken, R. H., Infectious diarrhea of infant rats produced by a rotavirus-like agent, *J. Virol.*, 52, 94, 1984.

211. Moody, K. D., Brownstein, D. G., Johnson, E. A., Cryptosporidiosis in suckling laboratory rats, *Lab. Anim. Sci.*, 41(6), 625, 1991.

212. Parker, J. C., Igel, H. J., Reynolds, R. K., Lewis, A. M., Rowe, W. P., Lymphocytic choriomeningitis virus infection in fetal, newborn and young adult Syrian hamsters (Mesocricetus auratus), *Infect. Immun.*, 13, 967, 1976.

213. Kilham, L., Margolis, G., Transplacental infection of rats and hamsters induced by oral and parenteral inoculations of H1 and Rat Viruses (RV), *Teratology*, 2, 111, 1969.

214. Schwanzer, V., Deerberg, F., Frost, J., Liess, B., Schwanzerova, I., Pittermann, W., Zur intrauterinen Infektion der Maus mit Ektromelie-virus, *Z.Versuchstierkd.*, 17, 110, 1975.

215. Friis, A. S., Demonstration of antibodies to Bacillus piliformis in SPF colonies and experimental transplacental infection by Bacillus piliformis in mice, *Lab. Anim.*, 12, 23, 1978.

216. Friis, A. S., Studies on Tyzzer's disease: transplacental transmission by Bacillus piliformis in rats, *Lab. Anim.*, 12, 23, 1978.

217. Okewole, P. A., Uche, E. M., Oyetunde, I. L., Odeyemi, P. S., Dawaul, P. B., Uterine involvement in guinea pig salmonellosis, *Lab. Anim.*, 23, 275, 1989.

218. Blackmore, D. K., Cassillo, S., Experimental investigation of uterine infections of mice due to Pasteurella pneumotropica, *J. Comp. Pathol.*, 82, 471, 1972.

219. Cassell, G. H., Wilborn, W. H., Silvers, S. H., Minion, F. C., Adherence and colonization of Mycoplasma pulmonis to genital epithelium and spermatozoa in rats, *Isr. J. Med. Sci.*, 17, 593, 1982.

220. Cassell, G. H., Lindsey, J. R., Baker, H. J., Davis, J. K., Mycoplasmal and rickettsial diseases, in *The Laboratory Rat*, Baker, H. J., Lindsey, J. R., Weisbroth, S. H., Eds., Academic Press, New York, Vol. 1, 243, 1979.

221. Cassell, G. H., The pathogenic potential of mycoplasmas: Mycoplasma pulmonis as a model, *Rev. Infect. Dis.*, 4, 18, 1982.

222. Cassell, G. H., Lindsey J. R., Davis, J.K., Respiratory and genital mycoplasmosis of laboratory rodents: Implications for biomedical research, *Isr. J. Med. Sci.*, 17, 548, 1981.

223. Hill, A. C., Stalley, G. C., Mycoplasma pulmonis infection with regard to embryo freezing and hysterectomy derivation, *Lab. Anim. Sci.*, 41(6), 563, 1991.

224. Juhr, N. C., Ratsch, H., Modifikation der Teratogenese von Actinomycin-D und Cyclophosphamid durch eine Mycoplasma pulmonis-Infektion bei der Ratte, *Z.Versuchstierkd.*, 33, 265, 1990.

225. Uchiyama, Y., Fukuyasu, T., Ashida, K., Effect of the infection of non-pathogenic bacteria in the uterus on the successful implantation of blastocysts in rats, *Jpn. J. Fertil. Steril.*, 33(2), 425, 1988.

226. Bia, F. J., Thornton, G. F., Main, A. J., Fong, C. K. Y., Hsiung, G. D., Western equine encephalitis mimicking herpes simplex encephalitis, *JAMA*, 244, 367, 1980.

227. Barthold, S. W., Brownstein, D. G., The effect of selected viruses on Corynebacterium kutscheri, *Lab. Anim. Sci.*, 38, 50, 1988.

228. Kaspareit-Rittinghausen, J., Deerberg, F., Rapp, K., Wislo, A., Mortality and tumour incidence of Han:SPRD rats, *Z.Versuchstierkd.*, 33, 23, 1990.

229. Kimbrough, R., Gaines, T. B., Toxicity of hexylmethylphosphoramide in rats, *Nature*, 211, 146, 1966.

230. Barthold, S., Research complications and state of knowledge of rodent coronaviruses, in *Complications of Viral and Mycoplasma Infections in Rodents to Toxicology Research*, Hamm, T. E., Jr., Ed., Hemisphere Press, Washington, D.C., 1985, chap. 4.

231. Nettesheim, P. H., Schreiber, H., Cresia, D. A., Richter, C. B., Respiratory infections in the pathogenesis of lung cancer, *Recent Results Cancer Res.*, 44, 138, 1974.

232. Barthold, S. W., Jonas, A. M., Morphogenesis of early 1,2-dimethylhydrazine-induced lesions and latent period reduction of colon carcinogenesis in mice by a variant of Citrobacter freundii, *Cancer Res.*, 37, 4352, 1977.

233. Zurcher, C., Nooteboom, A. L., van Zwieten, M. J., Solleveld, H. A., Hollander, C. F., Influence of severe lung disease following a Sendai virus infection on survival and tumor incidence in two inbred rat strains and their F1 hybrid, in *Animal Quality and Models in Biomedical Research. Proc. 7th ICLAS Symp.*, Utrecht 1979. Spiegel, A., Erichsen, S., Solleveld, H. A., Eds., Gustav Fischer Verlag, Stuttgart/New York, 133, 1980.

234. Koten, P., Wisely, D. Y., Production of lung cancer in mice by inhalation exposure to influenza virus and aerosols of hydrocarbons, *Prog. Exp. Tumor Res.*, 3, 186, 1963.

235. Nettescheim, P., Schrieber, H., Creasia, D. A., Richter, C. B., Respiratory infection and the pathogenesis of lung cancer, *Recent Results Cancer Res.*, 44, 138, 1974.

236. Theiss, J. C., Shimkin, M. B., Stoner, G. D., Kniazeff, A. J., Effect of reovirus infection on pulmonary tumor response to urethan in strain A mice, *J. Natl. Cancer Inst.*, 61, 131, 1978.

237. Ashley, M. P., Neoh, S. H., Kotlarski, I., Hardy, D., Local and systemic effects in the non-specific tumor resistance induced by attenuated Salmonella enteritidis 11RX in mice, *Aust. J. Exp. Biol. Med. Sci.*, 54, 157, 1976.

238. Toolan, H. W., Lack of oncogenic effect of the H-viruses, *Nature*, 214, 1036, 1967.

239. Toolan, H. W., Ledinko, N., Inhibition by H1 virus of the incidence of tumors produced by adenovirus 12 in hamsters, *Virology*, 35, 475, 1968.

240. Toolan, H. W., Rhode, S. L., III, Gierthy, J. F., Inhibition of 7,12-dimethylbenz(a)anthracene-induced tumors in Syrian hamsters by prior infection with H1 parvovirus, *Cancer Res.*, 142, 2552, 1982.

241. Riley, V., Spontaneous mammary tumors: decrease of incidence in mice infected with an enzyme-elevating virus, *Science*, 153, 1657, 1966.

242. Öbrink, K. J., Rehbinder, C., The defined animal, *Scand. J. Lab. Anim. Sci.*, 20(1), 5, 1993.

243. Ganaway, J. R., Allen, A. M., McPherson, C. W., Prevention of acute Bordetella bronchiseptica pneumonia in a guinea pig colony, *Lab. Anim. Care*, 15(2), 156, 1965.

244. Stephenson, E. H., Trahan, C. J., Ezzell, J. W., Mitchell, W. C., Abshire, T. G., Oland, D. D., Nelson, G. O., Efficacy of a commercial bacterin in protecting Strain 13 guinea pigs against Bordetella bronchiseptica pneumonia, *Lab. Anim.*, 23, 261, 1989.

245. Kimura, Y., Aoki, H., Shimokata, K., Protection of mice against virulent virus infection by a temperature-sensitive mutant derived from an HVJ (Sendai virus) carrier culture, *Virology*, 61, 297, 1979.

246. Cassell, G. H., Davis, J. K., Lindsey, J. R., Control of Mycoplasma pulmonis infection in rats and mice: detection and elimination by vaccination, *Isr. J. Med. Sci.*, 17, 674, 1981.

247. Tolpin, M. D., Starr, S. E., Arbeter, A. M., Plotkin, S. A., Inactivated mouse cytomegalovirus vaccine: preparation, immunogenecity and protective effect, *J. Infect. Dis.*, 142, 569, 1980.

248. Howard, R. J., Balfour, H. H., Jr., Protection of morbidity and mortality of wild murine cytomegalovirus by vaccination with attenuated cytomegalovirus, *Proc. Soc. Biol. Med.*, 186, 365, 1977.

249. Tonari, Y., Minashima, Y., Pathogenecity and immunogenecity of temperature-sensitive mutants of murine cytomegalovirus, *J. Gen. Virol.*, 64, 1983, 1983.

250. Jordan, M. C., Adverse effects of cytomegalovirus vaccination in mice, *J. Clin. Invest.*, 65, 798, 1980.

251. van Hoosier, G. L., Answer on a question concerning Sendai virus vaccination, in *Viral and Mycoplasmal Infections of Laboratory Rodents, Effects on biomedical research*, Bhatt, P. N., Jacoby, R. O., Morse, H.C., III, New, A. E., Eds., Academic Press, Orlando, 61, 1986.

252. Bywater, J. E. C., Kellett, B. S., Waller, T., Encephalitozoon cuniculi antibodies in commercially-available rabbit antisera and serum reagents, *Lab. Anim.*, 14, 87, 1980.

Chapter 12

Health Monitoring

Claes Rehbinder

CONTENTS

INTRODUCTION

There is good evidence that infections in laboratory animals, whether producing clinical disease or not, can influence experimental data and thereby the outcome of many experiments.[1-6] The health of laboratory animals is at permanent risk, owing to microbial and other exogenous factors. The effects of these factors may remain clinically inapparent or be clinically apparent when the animal is challenged, e.g., exposed to stress, chemicals, etc. Depending on the specific infection, a variety of biological parameters may be affected, including behavior, growth rate, relative organ weights, immune responses, tumor development, enzyme levels, etc.[1-3,6-16]

Latent or overt infections may, in addition, lead to contamination of organ or cell transplants, tissue cultures, tumors, or biological products. More importantly, with respect to human health, some laboratory animal infections are zoonotic.[1-3,9-12,17-19]

A health monitoring program is of vital importance as research data obtained from defined, health-monitored animals are more reliable and reproducible. In addition, the risk of zoonotic infection of personnel handling laboratory animals or products derived from such animals is considerably decreased. It should be emphasized that in many kinds of experiments certain infections are of secondary importance and do not disqualify animals or results derived from their use.

The main purpose of health monitoring is to achieve "calibrated", defined animals, thereby avoiding the detrimental effects of experimental results which may be caused by various microorganisms and pathological conditions affecting the animal stock. Health monitoring thus creates possibilities to avoid misinterpretations.

OBJECTIVES OF HEALTH MONITORING

Health monitoring (or health surveillance) is used to determine, or define, by employing systematic laboratory investigations, the general health status of the animal population and to state whether investigated animals have pathological lesions or are carriers of pathogens and other microbiological agents that could interfere with the outcome of scientific investigations. The laboratory investigations generally included in health monitoring programs are pathology, bacteriology, mycoplasmology, serology (viral, bacterial, and parasitological infections), and parasitology.[8,17-20]

Even though it is generally accepted that health monitoring is necessary, there are great variations in the services offered by different laboratories. Some of them carry out very comprehensive programs while others are more limited in scope. For practical and economical reasons most health monitoring programs comprise tests only for the most common pathogens, for zoonotic agents, and for agents that may significantly interfere with research. Efforts are being made to achieve an international agreement on a generally accepted program which would comprise testing for the most important and common micro-biological agents, and recommended methods for carrying out the testing. A harmonization of procedures will provide reliable and comparable information on the health and microbiological status of laboratory animals for both suppliers and users. Specific research programs, however, may require animals that have been subject to extensive and specific laboratory checks.

With the development of research models using immunocompromised animals such as nude and SCID mice, the need to protect the animals is most important. Therefore, it can also be necessary to monitor the environment (breeding facility, water, air, feed, etc.) for the presence of bacteria, chemicals, endot-oxins, fungi, mycotoxins, gases, etc.[21]

The use of appropriate health monitoring and well-defined animals will:

- produce more reliable and repeatable research data
- considerably decrease the risk for personnel of all categories handling laboratory animals or their products of being infected with zoonotic diseases
- reduce the risk of spreading infectious agents by means of biological products
- reduce the number of animals used
- prevent unnecessary harm to the animals used

Disease control at both clinical and subclinical levels is probably the most important contribution that can be made to animal welfare.

TROUBLE SHOOTING

Health monitoring is also a valuable tool for solving cases of clinical disease and for the evaluation of the effects of infectious agents that do not cause apparent disease but interfere with research results, so-called "trouble shooting". Hence diagnostic services, in the hands of professionals, and based on necropsies and samples, ought to be used when disease outbreaks occur and also when experimental results seem improbable or inconsistent.

SAMPLING STRATEGIES

The number of animals to be tested and the intervals between tests are of great importance. Two main strategies are applied. Either groups of animals or sentinels are regularly submitted for testing. For large breeding colonies or units, groups of animals are usually submitted for monitoring purposes at regular intervals. For the surveillance of small-scale breeding units and for specially bred strains and animals in experiments, sentinels are regularly used. This is done to avoid using valuable and sometimes rare animals for the sole purpose of health monitoring.

The number of animals required for ascertainment of freedom from infection in any specific unit of laboratory animals is dependent on the nature of the infections monitored. In case of diseases with a low spread from animal to animal, e.g., lymphocytic choriomeningitis,[22] the use of a considerable number of animals is required, whereas the detection of a highly infectious disease like Sendai, often with a morbidity rate close to 100%, demands only few animals.[23-25] Among the considerations involved in choosing the appropriate number of animals for testing are the size of the colony or breeding unit, the importance of random sampling, the sensitivity and selectivity of the test, and the desired degree of reliability of results.

Practical and economical reasons, however, have created the need for a standardized sample size and composition. The recommendation of the Federation of European Laboratory Animal Science Associa-tion (FELASA) working group on animal health[17] is a sample of 10 animals from mouse, rat, hamster, and guinea pig units, and of 8 animals from rabbit breeding units per test (Table 1A and B).

The sample should be composed of different age classes in order to yield relevant results from different tests. Hence, as weanlings have usually not seroconverted they should not be used for serological tests, but, being more prone to harbor parasites than adults, they are suited for parasitological examination. The sampling frequency should agree with reproductive periodicity intervals between generations.

Table 1. Health Monitoring Sampling Frequency and Sample Size

A. Mouse, rat, hamster, and guinea pig breeding units

Sampling frequency	Sample size		Testing/animal			
	Age	No. animals	Ser.	Bact.	Par.	Path.
Every 3 months	Weanling	≥2	-	+	+	+
	10–14 weeks (young adults)	≥4	+	+	+	+
	> 6 months (retired breeders)	≥4	+	+	+	+

B. Rabbit breeding units

Sampling frequency	Sample size		Testing/animal			
	Age	No. animals	Ser.	Bact.	Par.	Path.
Every 6 months	12-14 weeks (young adults)	≥4	+	+	+	+
	> 6 months (retired breeders)	≥4	+	+	+	+

Key: Ser. = serology; Bact. = bacteriology; Par. = parasitology; Path. = pathology.
Source: FELASA Health Monitoring Recommendations.

The FELASA recommendation, however, is a practical and economical compromise. It contains only minimal requirements for health monitoring and constitutes a common baseline for breeders. If an explicit certainty of freedom from or prevalence of certain infections is desired, the sample size and sampling frequency and extent of tests must be adequately statistically calculated.[26,27] Important to remember is that results of health monitoring reflect the status of the colony at the time of sampling and thus are purely retrospective.

It is advantageous if the various investigations are carried out on each animal submitted for screening. This gives the opportunity to correlate microbiological findings with possible morphological changes. Hence the sampled animals are preferably subjected to histopathological investigations (not included in the FELASA recommendations), which in addition may reveal conditions not observed by means of microbiological investigation methods, such as nutritional disorders, lesions caused by mycotoxins in feed and bedding material or by other environmental factors, infections for which tests are not available,[14,28,29] parasitic disorders, e.g., *Klossiella* sp., etc.

Usually animals are well defined when initially obtained. It might, however, especially in long-term experiments, be useful to recheck their microbiological status during and at the end of experiments in order to ascertain that they have remained the same "calibrated measuring instruments" throughout the experiment.

SENTINEL ANIMALS

Sentinel animals are animals that are introduced into a laboratory animal population for health surveillance purposes. Thus, they replace samples of animals otherwise taken from the principal population. Sentinels are put into open cages which are placed either systematically or randomly throughout the unit or in places where exposure to infectious agents is thought or known to be at its maximum. Transmission of infectious agents from the principal population to the sentinels may be furthered by placing the sentinels in cages used by the principal population and containing used, dirty bedding. Sentinels may also in exceptional cases be mixed, in the same cage, with the principal population. Sentinels could be of the same stock as the principal population or of a second strain which is microbiologically well defined and preferably isolator-bred. If a second stock is used, it is an advantage if the animals have a known susceptibility to infectious agents against which the experimental animals ought to be primarily protected.

Immunosuppressed or immunodeficient animals (e.g., nude mice) may not produce sufficient amounts of antibodies to allow reliable test results and may not be suitable as sentinels for serological testing. Instead, immunocompetent animals (e.g., heterozygous litter mates) should be used. Immunodeficient animals are well suited for bacteriological and parasitological investigations. The principal population as well as the sentinel strain should be thoroughly tested prior to being used. The tests performed should be the same as used for health monitoring.

The number of sentinels used on each occasion should be related to the kind of experiment, the risk of microbiological contamination, the housing size, and the frequency of sampling. The more frequent the sampling, the less sentinels are needed per sample. The total number of sentinels used depends on the duration of the experiment but ought not to fall below the number of animals used for ordinary health monitoring of breeding colonies during the same time.[17] Hence, a regular sample of 3 to 4 animals per month and unit would be satisfactory. Sentinels ought to be 6 to 8 weeks old when introduced, and preferably examined 6 to 8 weeks later.

TRANSPORT

Animals for health monitoring should always be delivered alive to the diagnostic laboratory. Barrier-bred animals or animals of higher quality should be transported in carefully sealed crates or cages with special ventilation filters protecting the animals from ambient microbiological contamination (Figure 1).

EUTHANASIA

It is of prime concern that methods for killing animals fulfill the definition of euthanasia — induction of unconsciousness and death with a minimum of distress and pain. Animal welfare, safety of personnel, and scientific aspects must be considered when selecting the adequate method. In general, blood samples for serology are obtained when the animals are unconscious.

Different euthanasia methods produce different macroscopic and microscopic alterations which are generally connected with effects on the circulatory system. However, different species of animals may respond differently when exposed to identical or similar methods. Hence, it is important, especially for the gross and microscopical interpretations by the pathologist, always to use the same standardized species-adapted method of euthanasia.

Stunning of animals should not be used in connection with health monitoring due to the obvious risk of microbiological contamination by fodder aspiration.[30] Using carbon dioxide, an induction with a mixture of carbon dioxide (CO_2) and oxygen (O_2) (80/20) for 1 minute is recommended, followed by pure CO_2 until death has occurred. However, this method produces lung edema and marked extravasation of blood, especially so in guinea pigs. In this species the lesions produced may easily reach an extent where they conceal other lesions.[30]

COLLECTION OF BLOOD

Collection of blood can be performed on the anesthetized animal during the procedure of euthanasia. Cardiac puncture is a convenient method to collect a large quantity of blood from rodents. The needle is inserted through the ventral abdominal wall just behind the xiphoid process (Figure 2). For animals larger than mice, the needle may also be inserted through the lateral thoracic wall in the region of maximum pulsation of the heart.

Large quantities of blood can be obtained by severing large vessels, i.e., the brachial vessels or the abdominal aorta, or by aspirating with a needle and syringe from the abdominal aorta. These latter methods, however, may negatively influence the post-mortem examination and the sterile collection of samples for bacteriology. Decapitation results in blood contaminated with tracheal and salivary secretions.

In the rabbit, blood is easily collected from the auricular artery or the marginal ear veins. Blood samples are preferably obtained by means of a needle and syringe.

SEROLOGY

Viral infections, as well as some bacterial, mycoplasmal, and parasitic infections, are usually screened for by means of serology. Sampling is recommended from a minimum of 8 individuals (4 young adults

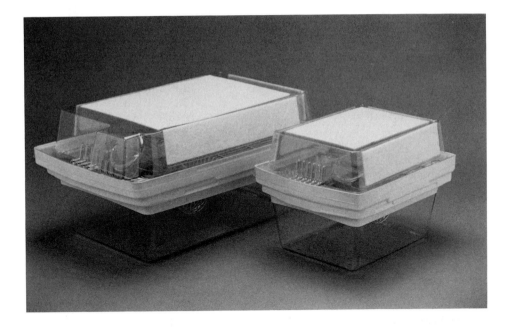

Figure 1. Filter top equipped cages suitable for transport of laboratory rodents (courtesy of SCANBUR a/s).

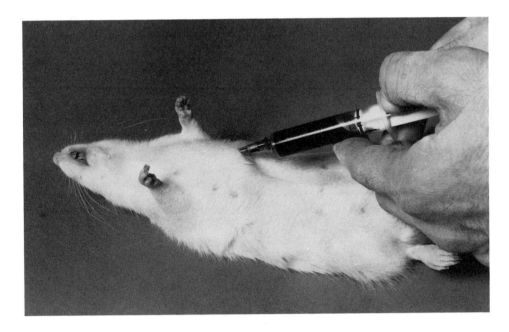

Figure 2. Blood sampling on anesthetized rat performed during the procedure of euthanasia (photo B. Ekberg).

[10 to 14 weeks old], and 4 retired breeders).[17] Equivocal or unexpected positive serological test results should be confirmed by an alternative test method and/or repeated investigation.[17]

Lists of viral infections to be monitored for and suitable test methods for the monitoring of rodent and rabbit breeding units are found in Tables 2 to 6. A list of bacterial, mycoplasmal, and parasitic infections suitable for detection by means of serology is found in Table 7.

Table 2. Viral Infections to be Serologically Monitored in Mouse Breeding Units

No. antigens	Suitable test methods*
1. Minute virus of mice (MVM)	ELISA, HI, IFA
2. Mouse hepatitis virus (MHV)	ELISA, IFA
3. Pneumonia virus of mice (PVM)	ELISA, HI, IFA
4. Reovirus type 3 (Reo3)	ELISA, IFA
5. Sendai virus	CF, ELISA, HI, IFA
6. Theiler's encephalomyelitis virus (TMEV)	ELISA, HI, IFA
7. **Ectromelia virus	ELISA, IFA
8. **Hantaviruses	ELISA, HI, IFA
9. **Lactic dehydrogenase virus (LDV)	LDH plasma test
10. **Lymphocytic choriomeningitis virus (LCM)	ELISA, IFA
11. **Mouse adenovirus (MAd)	ELISA, IFA
12. **Mouse rotavirus (EDIM)	ELISA, IFA
13. **Mouse K virus (K)	ELISA, HI
14. **Mouse polyoma virus	ELISA, HI, IFA
15. **Mouse thymic virus (MTV)	ELISA, IFA
16. **Mouse Cytomegalovirus (MCMV)	ELISA, IFA

* Abbreviations used for test: CF = complement fixation, ELISA = enzyme-linked immunosorbent assay, HAI = hemagglutination inhibition, IFA = indirect immunofluorescence assay, NT = neutralization test.

** Viruses for which evidence exists of rare infections in European mouse colonies. However, they should be tested in rederived or restocked colonies and in animals prior to use in mouse antibody production (MAP) testing.

Sampling frequency: every three months, antigen numbers 1 to 6; once a year, antigen numbers 7 to 12.
Source: FELASA Health Monitoring Recommendations.

Table 3. Viral Infections to be Monitored Serologically in Rat Breeding Units

No. antigens	Suitable test methods*
1. Hantaan Virus	ELISA, HI, IFA
2. Kilham rat virus (KRV)	HI, (ELISA, IFA)**
3. Pneumonia virus of mice (PVM)	ELISA, HI, IFA
4. Reovirus type 3 (Reo3)	ELISA, IFA
5. Sendai virus	CF, ELISA, HI, IFA
6. Sialodacryoadenitis (SDA)/Rat corona virus (RCV)	ELISA, HI, IFA
7. Theiler's encephalomyelitis virus (TMEV)	ELISA, HI, IFA
8. Toolan (H-1)	HI, (ELISA, IFA)**

* Abbreviations used for tests, see Table 2.

** In the case of rat parvoviruses (KRV, H-1) antibodies to these viruses cross-react with the antigens in IFA and ELISA. However, these infections can be differentiated by, e.g., HI tests.

Sampling frequency: every three months, antigen numbers 1 to 8.
Source: FELASA Health Monitoring Recommendations.

Table 4. Viral Infections to be Monitored Serologically in Hamster Breeding Units

No. antigens	Suitable test methods*
1. Lymphocytic choriomeningitis virus (LCM)	ELISA, IFA
2. Pneumonia virus of mice (PVM)	ELISA, HI, IFA
3. Reovirus type 3 (Reo3)	ELISA, IFA
4. Sendai virus	CF, ELISA, HI, IFA
5. Simian virus 5 (SV5)	ELISA, IFA

* Abbreviations used for tests, see Table 2.
Sampling frequency: every three months, antigen numbers 1 to 5.
Source: FELASA Health Monitoring Recommendations.

Table 5. Viral Infections to be Monitored Serologically in Guinea Pig Breeding Units

No. antigens	Suitable test methods*
1. Guinea pig adenovirus (GpAd)	IFA
2. Lymphocytic choriomeningitis virus (LCM)	ELISA, IFA
3. Pneumonia virus of mice (PVM)	ELISA, HI, IFA
4. Reovirus type 3 (Reo3)	ELISA, IFA
5. Sendai virus	CF, ELISA, HI, IFA
6. Simian virus 5 (SV5)	ELISA, IFA

* Abbreviations used for tests, see Table 2.
Sampling frequency: every three months, antigens numbers 1 to 6.
Source: FELASA Health Monitoring Recommendations.

NECROPSY PROCEDURES

The necropsy procedure involves not only a gross pathological investigation, but also sampling for bacteriology, parasitology, and histopathology. It may also include, if necessary, sampling for virology and mycoplasmology. It is thus essential to take all precautions not to contaminate sample material. Hence, a strict protocol of measurements, standard operating procedures (SOPs), must always be followed in order to maintain sterility of instruments and organs.[31]

It is important that surfaces and cut surfaces of all organs are examined *in situ* and in the case of visceral organs, also when removed. It should be remembered that pathological lesions may not only appear as a result of infectious agents, but may also be of genetic, nutritional, toxic, or other origin.

The post-mortem examination should be carried out by a pathologist or an otherwise trained, competent person. The necropsy procedure must never decline to being a mere sampling routine. The following organs ought to be examined for changes or lesions at necropsy: skin, oral cavity, salivary glands (rat only), Harderian glands (rat only), respiratory system, aorta (rabbit only), heart, liver, spleen, gastrointestinal tract, kidneys, adrenals, urogenital tract (including testes), body lymph nodes, muscles, joints, and the vertebral column. Selected organs ought to be regularly examined by histopathology, i.e., lungs and trachea (CAR-bacillosis), kidneys (*Klossiella* spp.), prostate, and uterus. All organs with macroscopical lesions should also be examined by histopathology.

Sick or dead animals, although not submitted for health monitoring, are valuable sources of information and should be investigated by necropsy and appropriate laboratory methods, including histopathology, as an aid in health maintenance.

It is to be expected that, in the future, the use of immunohistochemistry, polymerase chain reaction (PCR), and related techniques will play an important role in direct and rapid demonstration of infectious agents, especially in the case of immunodeficient animals.

Table 6. Viral Infections to be Monitored Serologically in Rabbit Breeding Units

No. antigens	Suitable test methods*
1. Pneumonia virus of mice (PVM)	ELISA, HI, FA
2. Rabbit hemorrhagic disease virus (RHDV)	ELISA, IFA
3. Rabbit pox virus (myxomatosis)	ELISA, IFA
4. Rabbit rotavirus	ELISA, IFA
5. Sendai virus	CF, ELISA, HI, IFA
6. Simian virus 5 (SV5)	ELISA, IFA

* Abbreviations used for tests, see Table 2.

Sampling frequency: every six months, antigen numbers 1 to 6.

Sample size: a minimum of 8 individual animal sera (not pooled) from rabbits randomly sampled from each breeding unit:

Age	No. of animals
12–14 weeks (young adults)	≥4
>6 months (retired breeders)	≥4

Source: FELASA Health Monitoring Recommendations.

Table 7. Examples of Bacterial, Mycoplasmal and Parasitic Infections Suitable for Detection by Means of Serology

Antigen	Mouse	Rat	Hamster	Guinea pig	Rabbit
Bacillus piliformis	x	x	x	x	x
Leptospira spp	x	x	x	x	x
CAR-bacillus		x			
Treponema cuniculi					x
Mycoplasma pulmonis	x	x			
Mycoplasma arthritidis	x	x			
Encephalitozoon cuniculi	(x)	(x)	(x)	x	x
Toxoplasma gondii	(x)	(x)	(x)	x	x

BACTERIAL, MYCOPLASMAL, AND FUNGAL INFECTIONS

The best sampling method for bacteriology may be to plate the material directly onto appropriate agar plates or to transfer it into growth media by means of a sterile loop or swab. If transport to the laboratory is short, organs may be placed in Petri dishes or soaked swabs may be used. If transports of a long duration are needed, the choice is swabs or organ pieces kept in appropriate transport media.

Bacteriological investigations must always include nonselective media, e.g., blood agar. If the bacteriological investigations are limited to a direct use of only selective media the growth of other pathogenic or otherwise important bacteria may be partly or totally suppressed and thereby overlooked, or not growing and thus not reported. Aerobic culture conditions are sufficient for most bacteria. Where possible, identification of microorganisms should be pursued to the specific name, e.g., *Pasteurella pneumotropica* or *Mycoplasma pulmonis*. Samples from the following organs ought to be cultured: nasopharynx, trachea, prepuce/vagina, and cecum.[17,27]

Samples for *Mycoplasma pulmonis* may be obtained by means of a swab or by lung wash technique. When a swab is used it should preferably be soaked in culture medium or in a solution of phosphate-buffered saline (PBS) + serum + antibiotics (Ampicillin) at a pH of around 7.5. When lung wash technique is used, mycoplasma basal broth is introduced by means of a needle and syringe into the trachea and the lower airways and recovered for culture.[32,33] Culture of multiple sites within the respiratory and

Table 8. FEASA-Approved Health Monitoring Report

Name and address of the breeder:

Date of issue:	Unit No.:	Latest test date:	Rederivations:

Species: Rats	Strains:		

	Historical results	Latest Test results	Laboratory	Method
VIRAL INFECTIONS	_____	_____	_____	_____
Hantaan virus	_____	_____	_____	_____
Kilham rat virus	_____	_____	_____	_____
Pneumonia virus of mice	_____	_____	_____	_____
Reovirus type 3	_____	_____	_____	_____
Sendai virus	_____	_____	_____	_____
Sialodacryadenitis/Rat corona virus	_____	_____	_____	_____
Theilers encephalomyelitis virus	_____	_____	_____	_____
Toolans HI virus	_____	_____	_____	_____
BACTERIAL AND FUNGAL INFECTIONS				
Bacillus piliformis	_____	_____	_____	_____
Bordetella bronchiseptica	_____	_____	_____	_____
Citrobacter freundii (4280)	_____	_____	_____	_____
Corynebacterium kutscheri	_____	_____	_____	_____
Leptospira sp.	_____	_____	_____	_____
Serotype: _____	_____	_____	_____	_____
Serotype: _____	_____	_____	_____	_____
Mycoplasma sp.	_____	_____	_____	_____
Biotype: _____	_____	_____	_____	_____
Biotype: _____	_____	_____	_____	_____
Pasteurella sp.	_____	_____	_____	_____
Biotype: _____	_____	_____	_____	_____
Biotype: _____	_____	_____	_____	_____
Salmonellae	_____	_____	_____	_____
Serotype: _____	_____	_____	_____	_____
Seortype: _____	_____	_____	_____	_____
Streptobacillus moniliformis	_____	_____	_____	_____
β–hemolytic streptococci	_____	_____	_____	_____
Lancefield group: _____	_____	_____	_____	_____
Lancefield group: _____	_____	_____	_____	_____
Lancefield group: _____	_____	_____	_____	_____
Lancefield group: _____	_____	_____	_____	_____
Spreptococcus pneumonias	_____	_____	_____	_____
Other species associated with lesions:	_____	_____	_____	_____
_____	_____	_____	_____	_____
_____	_____	_____	_____	_____
_____	_____	_____	_____	_____
_____	_____	_____	_____	_____
PARASITOLOGICAL INFECTIONS				
Arthropods				
_____	_____	_____	_____	_____
_____	_____	_____	_____	_____

Table 8. FEASA-Approved Health Monitoring Report (continued)

Name and address of the breeder:

Date of issue: Unit No.:   Latest test date: Rederivations:

Species: Rats   Strains:

	Historical results	Latest Test results	Laboratory	Method
Helminths				
	_____	_____	_____	_____
	_____	_____	_____	_____
Eimeria sp.				
	_____	_____	_____	_____
Entamoeba muris	_____	_____	_____	_____
Giardia sp.				
	_____	_____	_____	_____
	_____	_____	_____	_____
Spironucleus sp.				
	_____	_____	_____	_____
	_____	_____	_____	_____
Other flagellates	_____	_____	_____	_____
Klossiella sp.				
	_____	_____	_____	_____
Encephalitozoon cuniculi	_____	_____	_____	_____
Toxoplasma gondii	_____	_____	_____	_____
Trichosomoides crassicauda	_____	_____	_____	_____

PATHOLOGICAL LESIONS OBSERVED

Strain: _____ Lesions: _____
Strain: _____ Lesions: _____
Strain: _____ Lesions: _____
Strain: _____ Lesions: _____
Strain: _____ Lesions: _____
Strain: _____ Lesions: _____
Strain: _____ Lesions: _____

ABBREVIATIONS FOR LABORATORIES

_____   _____
_____   _____
_____

genital tracts is required for optimal recovery.[33] Temperature is important for the survival of mycoplasms and samples should, if not directly cultivated, be kept cool (+4°C) or deep-frozen.

Samples for fungal investigation are taken according to the localization of the lesions. For dermatophytes affecting epidermis and hair the material should consist of scrapings, flakes, and hair plucked from the rim of the lesion. Contamination of samples with blood should be avoided as it has a toxic effect on dermatophytes. Before collecting the material, the lesion is preferably disinfected with 70% alcohol, which is allowed to evaporate before sampling. The material should be kept clean until cultured. It can be cultured or mounted on slides in 10% potassium hydroxide for visualization of hyphae and arthrospores. From subcutaneous or deep mycotic lesions, material is taken from the actual lesions for direct microscopy as well as for culture and histology. The non-fixed material should be kept so as to avoid drying before being cultured or examined by microscopy. Scrapings from mouth, throat, nose, ears, etc., that are not cultured or investigated directly should be kept in transport medium.[34]

PARASITIC INFECTIONS

Weanlings (Table 1A) are often most suited for sampling as they may carry a heavier parasitic burden than adult animals[17] owing to their less developed immunity against parasites. They should, however, not be used for serology. Pooled samples may be used when convenient, if the methods used (not serology) eliminate a dilution effect.

Ectoparasites are detected *in situ* in the pelage by aid of a dissecting or stereoscopic microscope.[27] For the detection of *Sarcoptes* (rabbit) and *Demodex* (hamster) mites living in the skin, pieces of the skin or deep scrapings are transferred to a 10% potassium hydroxide solution in order to dissolve organic matter before the microscopic investigation.

Endoparasites are detected by means of microscopic examination of fecal flotations, of fresh wet mounts of cecal contents, and of the inner lining of the ileum. In addition stomach, small intestine, and large colon may be submitted.[27] This protocol eliminates the earlier commonly used, but more unreliable, method for demonstration of *Syphacia* eggs, namely that of pressing a cellophane tape first to the perianal area and then to a glass slide to be examined by microscopy. For *Encephalitozoon cuniculi* and *Toxoplasma gondii* serology is preferably used.

Rarely reported parasites in laboratory rat, mouse, and guinea pig are *Klosiella* spp. and in rat *Trichosomoides crassicauda*. *Klosiella* spp. are detected by means of histopathology and *T. crassicauda* by means of urine sedimentation or histopathology. Tests for these organisms should be performed on request. When reported, all arthropods, all helminths, and all protozooans should be identified as far as possible, preferably by species. The following organisms ought to be included in the laboratory report stated as present or not, or not tested: all arthropods, all helminths, all flagellates, and all coccidia. Special interest may be devoted to *Giardia* spp., *Spironucleus* spp., *Klosiella* spp. (mouse, rat, guinea pig), *Encephalitozoon cuniculi* (important in rabbit and guinea pig), *Toxoplasma gondii* (important in rabbit and guinea pig), and *Trichosomoides crassicauda* (rat only).[17]

THE HEALTH MONITORING REPORT

The report should always contain general statements as to the name of the diagnostic laboratory performing screening, date of the report, date of screening, identification of all strains/stocks within the investigated unit, number of animals screened, breeder's code for the unit, date when the colony was established, year when it was last rederived or restocked, and a description of the strain/stock screened (International Council for Laboratory Animal Science [ICLAS] designation).[17,18,21-25,35] The microorganisms monitored, viruses, bacteria, mycoplasma, fungi, endoparasites, and ectoparasites; the methods used in serological testing; the name of the laboratory carrying out the test (if other than the laboratory issuing the report) should all be listed.

An agent, whether virus, bacterium, mycoplasma, fungus, or parasite, must be stated as present in the unit if antibodies to it are detected in one or more animals examined. For breeding units the results should then continue to be reported as positive (historical results) at successive screenings until the agent has been eradicated by means of, e.g., rederivation or restocking. Agents known to be present in a colony need not be monitored at subsequent screenings provided they are declared present in the health report.

The pathological lesions found should be listed separately and the list should comprise a full description of gross and microscopical lesions. An example of a health monitoring report is given in Table 8.

It is important to keep in mind that negative results only mean that the microorganisms monitored have not been found present in the animals screened by the tests used. The results are not necessarily a reflection of the status of all the animals in the breeding unit.

DIAGNOSTIC LABORATORIES

Diagnostic laboratories specialized in health monitoring programs are valuable assets in the production and maintenance of animals for high-quality research. The laboratories usually also carry out diagnostic necropsies, as diseased or dead animals can be valuable sources of information and should be examined by necropsy and appropriate laboratory methods, including histopathology. Diagnostic necropsies, however, differ from those performed in health monitoring. Diagnostic necropsies are used to determine the cause of disease or death, while the necropsies performed in connection with health monitoring are intended to determine whether there are pathological lesions or not.

The reliability of the tests performed is of crucial importance. As mentioned earlier, there are great variations in the services offered by different laboratories. The demands of the individual research program must guide the choice of laboratory services. It is important that the laboratories performing health monitoring follow the code of good laboratory practice (GLP). This implies that the work follows a written plan and that the work is documented in such a way that it is possible to reconstruct it from stored data. In addition, the investigations should be performed by trained workers with facilities adequately equipped for the work at their disposal.

For the majority of laboratories using animals in research, routine quality controls should be part of good laboratory practice. Whereas GLP and protocols dictate which tests should be made, detailed written procedures, standard operating procedures (SOPs), dictate how they should be made. The SOPs must be sufficiently detailed to allow a trained person to perform each procedure in the same manner on each occasion. SOPs are supposed to be approved by the laboratory manager, signed, dated, and kept available for inspection on request. The purpose of the GLP code and SOPs is to ensure that the results obtained are true reflections of the sampled animals. Preferably, diagnostic laboratories should participate in quality assurance programs.

REFERENCES

1. Animal quality and models, in *Biomedical Research;* 7th ICLAS Symposium, Utrecht, 1979, Spiegel, A., Erichsen, S. and Solleveld, H. A., Eds., Gustav Fischer Verlag, Stuttgart, 1980.
2. Hamm, T. E., Jr., *Complications of Viral and Mycoplasmal Infection in Rodents to Toxicology Research and Testing,* McGraw-Hill, London, 1985.
3. Detection methods for the identification of rodent viral and mycoplasmal infections prepared by the subcommittee on rodent viral and mycoplasmal infections of the American Committee on Laboratory Animal Disease (ACLAD), Lussier, G., Ed., *Lab. Anim. Sci., 41 (3), 199, 1991.*
4. Dresser, R., Developing standards in animal research review, *J. Am. Vet. Med. Assoc., 194 (9), 1184, 1989.*
5. Gledhill, A. W., Bilbey, B. L. J. and Niven, J. S. F., Effect of certain murine pathogens on phagocytic activity, *Br. J. Exp. Pathol., 46, 433, 1965.*
6. Lussier, G., Potential detrimental effects of rodent viral infections on long-term experiments, *Vet. Res. Commun., 12, 199, 1988.*
7. Allen, A. M. and Nomura, U. S., Eds., *Manual of Microbiologic Monitoring of Laboratory Animals,* Department of Health and Human Service. National Institutes of Health. NIH Publ. No. 86-2499, 1986.
8. *Infectious Diseases of Mice and Rats.* Committee on Infectious Diseases of Mice and Rats. Institute of Laboratory Animal Resources, Commission on Life Sciences, National Research Council, National Academy Press, Washington, D.C., 1988.
9. Murtagh, A., The importance of quality control with reference to laboratory animals, *Anim. Technol., 39(1), 69, 1988.*
10. O'Donoghue, P. N., The establishment of Laboratory Animal Science in the United Kingdom. In *Lab. Anim. Sci. Assoc. Silver Jubilee 1988,* Seamer, J. H., Ed., Published by Royal Society of Medicine Services for Laboratory Animals Ltd., on behalf of the Laboratory Animals Science Association, 1988, p. 2.
11. Rehbinder, C., Advantages of health monitoring, *Scand. J. Lab. Anim. Sci., 13(3), 89, 1986.*
12. Bhatt, P. N., Jacoby, R. O., Morse, H. C., III, and New, A. E., Eds., *Viral and Mycoplasmal Infections of Laboratory Rodents. Effects on Biomedical Research,* Academic Press, New York, 1986.
13. Gärtner, K., Ed., *Qualitätskriterien der Versuchstierforschung,* VCH Verlagsgesellschaft, Weinheim, Bundesrepublik Deutschland, 1991.
14. Feinstein, R. E. and Rehbinder, C., Health monitoring of purpose bred laboratory rabbits in Sweden: major findings, *Scand. J. Lab. Anim. Sci., 15, 49, 1988.*

15. Roe, F. J. and Beeny, A.A., Ed., *Microbiological Standardization of Laboratory Animals,* Ellis Horwood Ltd., Chichester, 1983.

16. Davai, C., Ed., *Virus Diseases in Laboratory and Captive Animals,* Martinus Nijhoff Publishing, Boston, 1988.

17. *Recommendations for Health Monitoring of Mouse, Rat, Hamster, Guinea Pig and Rabbit Breeding Colonies,* Federation of European Laboratory Animal Science Associations (FELASA), FELASA Working Group on Animal Health, in press.

18. Wagner, J. E., Besch-Williford, C. L. and Steffen, E. K., Health surveillance of laboratory rodents, *Lab. Anim., 20(5), 40, 1991.*

19. Whittaker, D., The importance of and difficulties encountered with diagnosis of disease in laboratory animals, *Anim. Technol., 40(1), 23, 1989.*

20. Bantin, G. C. and Smith, M. W., The Laboratory Animal Breeders' Association accreditation scheme for commercially bred laboratory animals within the United Kingdom, *Anim. Technol., 36(1), 1, 1985.*

21. Heine, W., Laboratory animal quality determining factors, *Scand. J. Lab. Anim. Sci., 12(4), 99, 1985.*

22. Jacoby, R. O. and Fox, J. G., Biology and disease of mice, in *Laboratory Animal Medicine,* Fox, J. G., Cohen, B. J. and Loew, F. M., Eds., Academic Press Inc., New York, 1984, 59.

23. ILAR (Institute of Laboratory Animal Resources). Long-term holding of laboratory rodents, a report of the Committee on Long-term Holding of Laboratory Rodents, *ILAR News, 19, L1, 1976.*

24. Hsu, C. K., New, A. E. and Mayo, J. G., Quality assurance of rodent models, in *Proc. 7th ICLAS Symp.,* Spiegel, A., Erichsen, S. and Solleveld, H.A., Eds., Gustav Fischer Verlag, Stuttgart, 17, 1980.

25. Dubin, S. and Zietz, S., Samples for animal health surveillance, *Lab. Anim., 20(3), 29, 1991.*

26. Kornerup Hansen, A., Statistical aspect of health monitoring of laboratory animal colonies, *Scand. J. Lab. Anim. Sci.,* in press.

27. *Mikrobiologishe Diagnostik bei Laboratoriumstieren.* Society for Laboratory Animal Science. GV-SOLAS, Biberqach a. d. Riss, 1989.

28. Feinstein, R. E., Uzal, F. A. and Rehbinder, C., Chronic inflammatory lung lesions in rabbits free of known respiratory pathogenes, *Scand. J. Lab. Anim. Sci., 16, 74, 1989.*

29. Uzal, F. A., Feinstein, R. E., Rehbinder, C. and Nikkilä, T., An ultrastructural study of spontaneous chronic lung lesions in asymptomatic rabbits, *J. Vet. Med. A, 36, 721, 1989.*

30. Iwarsson, K. and Rehbinder, C., A study of different euthanasia techniques in guinea pigs, rats and mice. Animal response and post mortem findings, *Scand. J. Lab. Anim. Sci.,* in press.

31. Feinstein, R. E., Post-mortem procedures, Chapter 23, this volume.

32. Needham, J. R., *Handbook of Microbiological Investigations for Laboratory Animal Health,* Academic Press, London, 1979.

33. Tully, J. G. and Raxin, S., *Methods in Mycoplasmology Vol. I. Diagnostic Mycoplasmology,* Academic Press, New York, 1983.

34. Rippon, J. W., *Medical Mycology: The Pathogenic Fungi and the Pathogenic Actinomycetes,* 2nd edition. W. B. Saunders, New York, 1982.

35. Guidelines for specification of animals and husbandry methods when reporting the results of animal experiments. Working Committee for the Biological Characterization of Laboratory Animals GV-SOLAS, *Lab. Anim., 19, 106, 1985.*

Chapter 13

Nutrition and the Importance of Nutrients in Animal Experiments

Andre Chwalibog

CONTENTS

INTRODUCTION

The nutritional status of laboratory animals is gaining increasing importance in biomedical research. Nutrition may influence growth, reproductive performance, and health status of animals and, subsequently, animal responses to a variety of toxicological and pharmacological treatments. The response, which is measured by number parameters such as growth, litter size, body composition, blood constituents, and pathological changes, is the combined result of the treatment and the external and internal factors, as demonstrated in Figure 1.

The essential external factors are food composition, quantity and quality, while the internal factors are related to the animal's ability to transform nutrients into products. Both groups of factors interact with each other, concomitantly influencing animal response to experimental treatments.

In general, the nutritional requirements of farm animals and laboratory animals are similar. All require energy, protein, carbohydrate, lipid, minerals, and vitamins supplied in diets, which should be palatable and free from chemical and biological contamination. Therefore, much information regarding farm animal nutrition may be applied to laboratory animals. However, we have to keep in mind that the aim of laboratory animal nutrition is not the highest production, but optimum performance and nutritionally unbiased response to biomedical treatments.

A diet deficient in composition or quantity may influence not only animal growth or reproductive performance but also immune response and resistance to diseases. Furthermore, prior to changes in animal performance, a number of physiological and anatomical changes caused by a deficiency or an excess of nutrients may interact with the action of medical treatments. This chapter will outline some of the important effects of nutrition on the performance of laboratory animals, concomitantly emphasizing possible interactions between nutrition and experimental results.

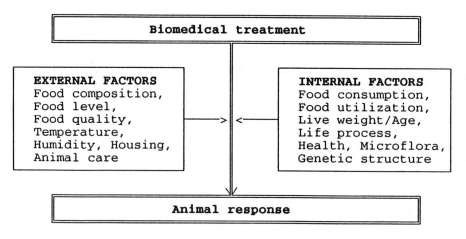

Figure 1. The relation between biomedical treatments and animal response.

FOOD INTAKE AND DIGESTION

VOLUNTARY FOOD INTAKE

Most laboratory animals are given food mixtures *ad libitum*. It is generally accepted that the voluntary food intake is related to the energy requirement of the animal. The classical experiments of Adolph in 1947 demonstrated that when rat diets were diluted with inert materials to produce a wide range of energy concentration, the animals were able to adjust the amount of food eaten so that their energy intake remained constant.[1] However, the concept that "animals eat for energy" has several aspects. In case of extensive dilution of the diet with materials of low digestibility, the ability to adjust the intake may be overcome by the gastrointestinal capacity being a limiting factor. In this case food intake may be insufficient to cover energy and often also nutrient requirements. On the other hand, when the dietary energy density is high enough to cover the energy requirements, increase in energy density by supplementing the diet with extra fat or carbohydrate may result in nutrient deficiencies. This occurs because the animal usually stops eating when its energy requirement has been met. Furthermore, not only the energy density of a diet and the capacity of the gastrointestinal tract influence food intake, but reduced intake is commonly observed in deficiency states, especially with diets low in protein or with an imbalance in amino acids,[2] or in the case of deficiency or excess of some trace minerals and vitamins. The physiological state of the animal also plays an essential role in food intake; several reports show increased intake with the onset of pregnancy, but other reports suggest little or no changes. Lactation is usually associated with a marked increase in food intake, which may, in a rat at peak lactation, be nearly three times that of a non-lactating rat. Considering that the voluntary food intake may be subjected to marked variation depending on nutritional and physiological factors, it is difficult to specify an expected daily consumption; consequently Table 1 demonstrates the approximate voluntary daily food intake in the most common laboratory animals when fed commercial pelleted diets.

For growing animals the wide range of daily food intake is directly related to the age and live weight (LW), increasing during the growth period. For example, the voluntary food intake of growing rats, reported by Thorbek et al.,[3] was 15 g/day at the age of 5 weeks and a LW of 100 g, while from the 7th to 8th week (200 g LW) up to the 18th week of age (400 g LW), it was remarkably constant, about 25 g/day. With a dietary energy concentration of 16.5 MJ/kg food, the values correspond to about 1400 kJ/LW per kilogram metabolic live weight (LW, $kg^{0.75}$) at 100 and 200 g LW, but only to 820 kJ/LW, $kg^{0.75}$ at 400 g LW. Comparable values can be calculated from the experiments of Pullar and Webster[4] with "lean" rats, indicating a pattern of decreasing energy consumption and thereby food consumption in relation to metabolic body weight. Kleiber[5] has suggested that the maximum food intake, for all species, is proportionally related to basal metabolic rate (BMR) with the ratio 4:1. Assuming a constant BMR of 320 kJ/LW, $kg^{0.75}$ the maximum intake in growing laboratory animals should be 1280 kJ/LW, $kg^{0.75}$. In correspondence with Kleiber's principle, Clarke et al.[6] presented general equations for growth, pregnancy, and lactation in all laboratory animals, suggesting constant proportions between energy supply for different life processes and metabolic live weight. Despite the fact that such approaches may give some indication of the level of voluntary food intake, the accuracy of the predicted values is

Table 1. Average Food Intake, g/day

Species	Growing	Adult	Pregnant	Lactating
Mouse	3–5	5–7	6–8	7–15
Rat	8–25	25–30	25–35	35–65
Hamster	6–12	10–12	12–15	20–25
Guinea pig	35–45	45–70	70–80	100–130
Rabbit	120–200	200–300	300	300–400

doubtful since, at least in rats, energy intake in relation to metabolic live weight is not constant either at maintenance level[7] or during growth.[3]

DIGESTION

The supply of nutrients required for the body functions depends on the transformation of the dietary constituents into simpler elements (amino acids, glucose, fatty acids) before they can pass through the mucous membrane of the gastrointestinal tract into the blood and lymph. The process of digestion results from muscular contraction of the alimentary canal, microbial fermentation, and action of digestive enzymes secreted in digestive juices. In monogastric animals like rats and mice microbial activity in the large intestine is low; these animals mainly process food compounds by means of the digestive enzymes and acids.

In suckling rats or mice the action of the digestive system and the secretion of enzymes are restricted to hydrolysis of the components of maternal milk. The serous glands of the tongue produce a lingual lipase which is important for the digestion of milk triglycerides.[8] In contrast to the serous glands, the salivary glands of neonatal rats and mice are functionally immature, and amylase activity is negligible during the first 2 postnatal weeks. In the pancreas, amylase activity does not begin to increase until 2 weeks after birth.[9] The gastric secretion of HCl, pepsinogen and pepsin is minimal, thus allowing intact protein to pass into the small intestine where it is absorbed as intact macromolecules by the process of pinocytosis.[8] Weaning of rats and mice, which normally begins at 17 days of age and is completed by day 26, constitutes a significant change in dietary composition from milk with a high content of lipids (9%) and a low content of carbohydrate (4%) to a diet low in fat and high in carbohydrate, as demonstrated in Table 2.

The change in dietary composition necessitates changes in digestive function. The intestinal hydrolases (maltase, sucrase, isomaltase, trehalase) which are involved in digestion of carbohydrate from solid food cannot be detected in the intestines of rats during the first 2 postnatal weeks, but their activities rise rapidly later on.[10] The activities of amylase, chymotrypsin, trypsinogen, and lipase change little before weaning but increase dramatically at the time of weaning.[11] The gastric secretion of acids and pepsinogen rises to adult levels during the 3rd and 4th postnatal weeks coincident with the transition to solid food.[8] Although the enzymatic changes that occur in the gastrointestinal tract about weaning time seem to be directly related to the change of diet from milk to solid food, there is evidence that the primary cause of the enzymatic development is not a change of diet. Henning[12] described similar changes occurring during the 3rd postnatal week in animals which were prevented from weaning. Among other regulatory factors that have been suggested, glucocorticoids, thyroxine, glucagon, gastrin, cholecystokinin, prostaglandins and insulin may play an important role as potential regulators of postnatal development of the gastrointestinal tract.[8] There is no doubt that the changes in digestive capacity occurring during the first 4 weeks of life should be considered in order to attain optimum utilization of food. In older rats, the digestive capacity is stabilized and almost constant under normal feeding conditions.

The presence of food in the stomach may have a significant influence on the bioavailability and pharmacokinetics of certain drugs.[13] Rats are night eaters, and usually they are fasted overnight prior to dosing with different drugs, assuming that overnight fasting will result in the postabsorptive state.[14] However, there is substantial evidence that the rate of gastric emptying, e.g., the rate of passage in the alimentary tract, depends on diet composition. In balance experiments with rats at about 140 g LW, using glass beads as a marker, Raczynski et al.[15] demonstrated that the highest amount of marker was recovered in feces about 30 hours after the beginning of eating, and only marginal amounts could be detected in the digestive tract at 72 hours after feeding. Protein and fat levels in the diet did not affect the rate of passage. However, crude fiber strongly increased the rate of passage, with the highest recovery of the marker about 20 hours from feeding. It was also demonstrated that reduced level of microbial activity in the hind-gut

172

decreased the rate of passage time by about 15 hours. It is interesting to note that in these experiments the level of microbial activity was regulated by the administration of the antibiotic Nebacitin, thereby indicating that compounds which alter microbial metabolism might affect the rate of food passage in the alimentary tract and subsequently the digestibility of nutrients.

SUPPLY OF NUTRIENTS AND ENERGY

The principle for estimation of nutrient and energy supply

Table 2. Composition of Rat Milk and a Diet for Weaned Rats

Components	Milk g/kg	Diet[a] g/kg
Protien	87	219
Fat	93	35
Carbohydrate	37	559
Energy, MJ/kg	6.3	16.4

[a]"Rostock diet"[11] as analyzed by Thorbek at al.[3]

is generally the same for different nutrients and for different life processes. It is based on the knowledge of the amount of nutrients and energy retained in the body during growth or deposited in fetal and maternal tissues during pregnancy, or in the body and milk during lactation, as well as the animal's ability to digest, absorb, and utilize nutrients and energy. However, several other nutritional factors have to be elucidated in order to supply animals with an optimal diet. Therefore, each nutrient has to be evaluated regarding its chemical structure, its action in the body, and its possible interaction with other nutrients. Because of the diversity of aspects associated with the supply of nutrients and energy for laboratory animals, it is impossible to debate all effects of nutrition on experimental results, so only some of the major nutritional characteristics will be discussed in the following sections.

OUTLINE OF NUTRIENT METABOLISM

The starting point of metabolism is the substances produced by the digestion of food. Digested carbohydrate (DCHO), protein (DP), and fat (DF) are the main groups of nutrients involved in a variety of catabolic and anabolic processes in the body. The general relations between the intake of digested nutrients and the end products of their metabolism in the body are demonstrated in Figure 2.

The soluble part of DCHO is mainly absorbed as glucose, of which the major part is oxidized and used as a source of energy, while a smaller part is utilized in the lipogenesis of body fat. The insoluble carbohydrates (fibers) are fermented and transformed into volatile fatty acids (VFA), which finally are sources of energy and precursors in the synthesis of body fat. Although VFA are a significant source of energy for herbivorous animals (in the guinea pig and the rabbit approximately 30% of the energy is supplied from VFA metabolism), the microbial capacity for VFA production in the rat and the mouse is limited. Amino acids from DP are synthesized and retained in the body or milk and partly degraded and oxidized with concomitant transfer of their carbon skeletons in lipogenesis. An efficient use of dietary protein requires an adequate level of energy-yielding substrates and of all essential fatty acids, minerals, and vitamins. The free fatty acids and triglycerides from DF are transformed into body fat, and they can be oxidized, becoming an efficient energy source. In case of inadequate energy supply from a diet, body fat can be mobilized as an additional energy source.

There have hitherto been no quantitative measurements of nutrient distribution in laboratory animals. However, recent data for growing pigs may be descriptive also for rats and mice because, generally, the same dietary ingredients are used for these species, and the biochemical pathways of nutrient metabolism are not different. Chwalibog et al.[16] demonstrated for growing pigs that at sufficient daily energy supply (metabolizable energy >1.2 MJ/LW, $kg^{0.75}$) as the result of the oxidation of nutrients depends on the amount and quality of DP and the amount of DCHO, but not on the amount of DF. Hence, independent of dietary fat level there was no fat oxidation in these experiments. Thus, the sole source of energy was oxidation of DCHO and DP. Generally, 85% of the total oxidation was caused by DCHO, the remaining part being caused by DP. When, with sufficient energy supply, animals received more DP than needed for maintenance and growth, the surplus was deaminated, causing a higher oxidation (20 to 25% of the total oxidation) and a higher lipogenesis from protein sources. In contrast, when the energy supply was too low to cover the requirements, the pattern of oxidation was quite different. At this stage a marked oxidation of DF occurred, supported by oxidation of fat mobilized from body reserves (40 to 45% of the total oxidation). At the same time, the oxidation of DP was markedly reduced to about 10% of the total oxidation in order to save protein for retention, indicating the animal's ability to regulate protein and fat metabolism in relation to the dietary supply. Therefore, generally, nutrient oxidation and use for retention can be placed in the following order of preference:

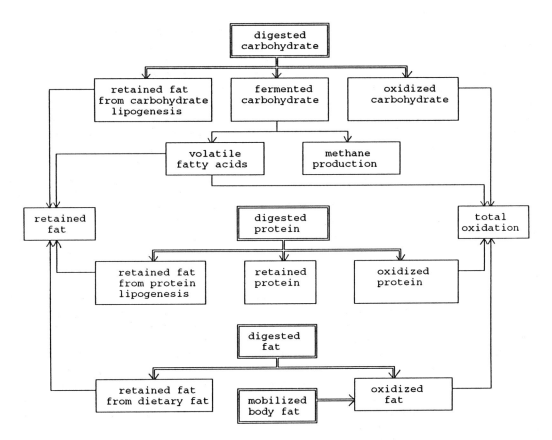

Figure 2. Nutrient oxidation and retention, input-output relations.

1. Protein retention
2. Protein oxidation and use for lipogenesis
3. Carbohydrate oxidation and use for lipogenesis
4. Fat retention from dietary lipids
5. Fat oxidation

CARBOHYDRATE

Carbohydrates (CHO) constitute the largest proportion of food consumed by laboratory animals, except carnivores. They are the most important components of plants, constituting up to 75% of the dry matter present in feeds of plant origin. Dietary CHO, consisting of α-monosaccharide units (soluble CHO), are readily digested by endogenous enzymes and constitute the major energy source for laboratory animals. A number of CHO can be used by the rat, and as reviewed by the National Research Council,[17] glucose, sucrose, maltose, fructose, and starch support similar levels of performance. However, too high contents of lactose or galactose in the diet may cause diarrhea and poor performance. Diets for rats and mice are mainly based on starch, which is a relatively inexpensive energy source, yielding 17.6 kJ/g. There is a direct relation between CHO intake and the degree of fatness of the animals, because CHO, exceeding the amount needed to meet the energy requirement, will be stored as body fat. Although rats and mice are able to regulate food intake, depending on the energy density of the diet, an extensive supply of soluble CHO may result in obesity, especially in animals with genetic predispositions to obesity like Zucker "fatty" rats.[18] Obesity is also more likely to occur when the diet is high in sugar, since sugar is utilized more efficiently than starch.[19] All rodents exhibiting obesity or obesity-related diabetes syndrome are characterized by diminished glucose tolerance, which may result in hyperinsulinemia and inappropriate hyperglycemia,[20] and thereby in reduced longevity.

The CHO composed of ß-monosaccharide units are called insoluble CHO, collectively referred to as "dietary fiber". They resist the action of digestive enzymes but can be utilized by micro-organisms in the large intestine. Plant cell wall material, which is the major source of dietary fiber, is composed chiefly of cellulose, hemicellulose, and pectins. Microbial metabolism is severely limited in rats and mice compared with herbivorous animals, and fiber digestion is almost entirely confined to microbial activity in the hind-gut.[21] However, a small amount of dietary fiber (2 to 5% of the diet) can be processed by micro-organisms and ought to be included in the diets. It is important because of the water-holding capacity of the fiber and its influence on the peristaltic mobility of the intestines by which food components are driven forward through the alimentary tract. Furthermore, dietary fiber components influence the composition and function of the intestinal microflora and activate the microbial synthesis of several vitamins (Table 6). It has been demonstrated that pectin stimulates the microbial synthesis of thiamin, riboflavin, and niacin.[22] Pectin can absorb various antimetabolites and thus reduce their degree of absorption.[23] There are also indications that fiber increases peripheral sensitivity to insulin, perhaps by increasing the number of insulin receptors.[24] On the other hand, an excess of dietary fiber has a negative influence on nutrient and energy digestibility, since it increases the rate of passage of food components in the digestive tract and subsequently reduces the time of action of digestive enzymes. Total glucose, lipid, and protein absorption is decreased when high levels of dietary fiber are consumed.[25] Furthermore, an association between dietary fiber and periodontitis and oro-nasal fistulation in rats has been reported in several investigations,[26] and is presumed to relate to the presence of long sharp fibers of oats or barley.[27]

FAT

Dietary fat is required as a source of essential fatty acids (EFA), for the absorption of the fat-soluble vitamins, and to enhance the palatability of the food. Lipids are an excellent source of energy, providing 2.5 times more energy (39.8 kJ/g) than carbohydrate (17.6 kJ/g) and protein (18.4 kJ/g). However, if a diet contains adequate CHO and protein, fat is not used as a source of energy, but is transformed to body lipids. Both the amount and composition of dietary fat are important in laboratory animal nutrition. A high fat level in the diet increases cholesterol synthesis. Especially high inputs of saturated fat furnish acetyl-CoA in excess of that required for energy production and body fat synthesis, and the excess acetyl-CoA is used for cholesterol formation. The type of fat in the diet influences the fatty acid profile of body lipids.[28] The fatty acid composition of the dietary fat affects antioxidant mechanisms in the colon mucosa, presumably because the composition of cell membranes reflects the fatty acid composition of the diet.[29]

There is evidence that high-fat diets elevate the toxic effects of nuclear-damaging agents and carcinogens.[30] It has been demonstrated that increase in fat level may alter the acute genotoxic effects of carcinogens, a phenomenon associated with the initiation of colon cancer.[31] Furthermore, mammary tumor incidence is related to the fatty acid composition of the diet, with a greater incidence of tumors in rats fed diets containing polyunsaturated fatty acids (PUFA) when compared to diets with saturated fat. In the rat increasing levels of linoleic acid were correlated with increasing chemically induced mammary tumor incidence up to maximum at 4.5% of dietary linoleic acid.[32,33] The same effect was observed in the mouse, but at a higher level of linoleic acid (8.4%).[34] Feeding high levels of fat, particularly PUFA, may depress immune responsiveness,[35] which may lead to an increased susceptibility to infections.

The early works of Burr and Burr[36,37] first established that the rat does not thrive on diets rigidly devoid of fat, but develops a number of deficiency syndromes. The linoleic acid family of PUFA was shown to reverse the effects of fat-free diets. The linoleic, linolenic, and arachidonic acids are usually referred to as essential fatty acids (EFA). Mammals lack the enzymes which introduce double bonds at carbon atoms beyond C-6 in the fatty acid chain. This makes the double bond at the 12th carbon atom of linoleic acid "essential". After absorption, linoleic acid can be oxidized, accumulated in the adipose tissue, and/or converted to PUFA and incorporated into structural lipids.[38] The list of symptoms ascribed to EFA deficiency ranges from classical signs such as reduced growth rate, dermal lesions, increased water permeability of the skin, increased susceptibility to bacteria, decreased prostaglandin synthesis and reproductive failure, reduced myocardial contractility, abnormal thrombocyte aggregation, swelling of rat liver mitochondria, and increased heat production. Dietary requirements of EFA are usually stated in terms of linolate. An amount equivalent to 1 to 1.5% of the metabolizable energy (ME) of the diet has been found adequate for most monogastric animals.[6] However, studies on growing pigs indicate an even lower requirement of 0.26% of the ME.[39] This level is likely to be present in all natural food compounds used for laboratory animals, but not in highly refined or purified diets, which must be fortified with EFA-rich sources like soybean oil. Also diets containing a high level of saturated fatty acids (>5%) may require a greater supply of EFA, since EFA enhance the utilization of saturated fatty acids.[40]

PROTEIN

The nutritive effects of a protein depend on the amino acids which are released from the protein by digestive processes. For nutritional purposes amino acids are classified into two groups: non-essential (NEAA) and essential (EAA) amino acids. The NEAA are not necessary as dietary components, since they can be synthesized in the body via intermediates of carbohydrate metabolism or by transformation of some EAA into certain NEAA. EAA, however, cannot be synthesized in the body, at least not at a rate adequate to meet physiological requirements, and they must therefore be supplied with the diet. Table 3 shows the classification of amino acids for growing rats.

Despite the fact that arginine can be synthesized by mammals from ornithine, it is considered to be an essential amino acid, since, in the urea cycle, nearly all arginine is converted to ornithine and urea. Cystine and tyrosine, included in the NEAA group, are often called semi-essential, hence their synthesis in the animal cells requires EAA as precursor substances. Cystine is formed from methionine + serine and tyrosine from phenylalanine.

Protein synthesis can only take place when all the amino acids required to form a certain protein are present together; thus, a relative inadequacy of one amino acid impairs utilization of the rest. The amino acid in lowest concentration in relation to the requirement will therefore determine the rate at which protein can be synthesized in the body. Subsequently, amino acids present in excess of the requirement for protein synthesis will not be used for synthesis, but their nitrogen-free components (keto acids) will be oxidized and used in lipogenesis, while the nitrogenous component (ammonia) is converted by the liver to urea and excreted by the kidneys. Animals can synthesize EAA from their respective keto acids, but this is only of theoretical interest because these specific keto acids are not present in natural feeds.[41] Therefore, it is evident that EAA must be present in the diet in correct quantities and proportions in order to be synthesized into animal protein. However, the animal must also receive a sufficient amount of NEAA. They are beneficial because they have a sparing effect on the oxidation of EAA.[42] If an inadequate amount of NEAA is absorbed (and produced from body protein turnover), they will be resynthesized from dietary EAA.

Inadequate amino acid supply is the most common of all nutrient deficiencies. Signs of protein deficiency include reduced protein concentration in the blood, reduced protein synthesis rate in the tissues and synthesis of certain enzymes and hormones, decreased food intake, reduced growth rate, and infertility. On the other hand, an excess supply of one or more amino acids may cause amino acid imbalance and consequently decreased protein utilization. The classical experiments with growing rats fed a rice diet with lysine and threonine as limiting amino acids demonstrated that if the lysine content of the diet was held constant and the threonine content was increased stepwise, a point was reached at which the growth of rats fed on a threonine-supplemented diet was retarded unless the lysine content of the diet was also increased.[43] The same phenomenon was seen in the reverse situation with threonine being held constant and lysine increased. Furthermore, the sites in the brain that regulate food intake are sensitive to an alteration in the proportion of amino acids in the blood plasma, and imbalance of amino acids may cause a reduced food intake.[44] There is also evidence that a surplus of arginine and histidine may depress protein utilization, while the ingestion of a large amount of methionine or tyrosine (20 to 50 g/kg food) is followed by serious metabolic and histopathological changes apart from depressed food intake and retarded growth of the rat.[45] Excess methionine inhibits ATP synthesis, causing irregularities in energy metabolism, and excess tyrosine causes a specific toxic syndrome with histopathological changes in skin, pancreas, liver, and testes, and severe eye lesions. For some amino acids, the negative effects of an excess supply may only be prevented by addition of other amino acids which are structurally similar. Growth depression in rats caused by surplus isoleucine and valine can be prevented by addition of their "antagonistic" amino acid leucine. It is also interesting to note that a high-quality protein is much less affected by an excess of a single amino acid than is a protein source of poorer quality, as demonstrated for egg protein versus barley and potato protein.[46] Too high protein consumption may accelerate amyloid deposits in the kidney, being indicative of future renal disease, as demonstrated in adult mice.[47] However, more recent studies showed no significant indication of amyloidosis in growing mice fed 21% protein in the diet.[48] Also the source of protein affects the animal's health. Pronounced nephrocalcinosis was found in rats fed a Na-caseinate semisynthetic diet, but not when Na-caseinate had been replaced by lactoalbumin, which in turn reduced kidney weight.[49]

The other important aspect of protein nutrition is its significance in oncological research. Recent results indicate that supplementation of methionine to soybean protein isolates increased mammary tumor progression in the rat.[50] It was also suggested that a decreased level of dietary methionine may decrease tumor cell proliferation.

When discussing the role of dietary protein in laboratory animal nutrition, it has to be emphasized that the utilization of protein for different life processes is dependent on energy supply. The relationship between protein balance and both protein and energy intake has been recognized for years and was recently discussed by Young.[42] In summary, the available data indicate that the level of energy intake determines the changes in protein turnover and retention, and the level of protein intake determines the magnitude of the effect of energy intake on protein retention. These interrelationships between energy and protein are outlined in Figure 3.

Table 3. Essential and Non-essential Amino Acids for Growing Rats

Essential	Non-essential
Histidine	Alanine
Isoleucine	Aspartic acid
Leucine	Cystine
Lysine	Glutamic acid
Methionine	Glycine
Phenylalanine	Hydroxyproline
Threonine	Proline
Tryptophan	Serine
Valine	Tyrosine
Arginine	

For a low-protein diet, an increase of energy intake to point A will increase protein retention, while the extended energy supply from A to B will not have any effect on protein retention. For a high-protein diet, the pattern is the same; however, because of higher protein supply, protein retention is elevated. For this diet, the increase from A to B will stimulate protein retention until the limit is reached at point B. The relationship presented between energy and protein is, of course, a simplification, and other factors should also be considered, such as the extent to which energy is supplied from carbohydrate or fat,[51,52] the supply of other nutrients,[53] amino acid profile in the diet,[42,52] and endocrinological regulation of anabolic and catabolic processes.[42]

ENERGY

All functions of the body require energy, which is supplied from carbohydrate, fat, and protein. The results of inadequate energy supply are obvious, but too high energy intake can be harmful as well. Excess energy intake produces obesity, several obesity-associated diseases, and reproductive failure, and reduces longevity.[54,55] There is evidence that rapid growth rates and obesity are associated with an increased occurrence of spontaneous and induced tumors in laboratory animals.[56,57]

The total energy, gross energy (GE), available in food can be determined by complete combustion in the calorimetric bomb. As shown in Figure 4 the animals cannot use all GE, as some energy is lost in feces, urine, and methane. The remaining energy, called metabolizable energy, is the energy available in the animal for maintenance, growth, reproduction, lactation, and work.

The ME value of a food varies according to the species of animal to which it is given. For rats and mice ME values are almost similar as these animals digest foods to much the same extent and losses in the form of methane are negligible (Figure 5). However, for herbivorous animals like guinea pigs and rabbits the same foods are digested to a lower extent and, due to the fermentation processes, more methane is lost, consequently reducing the ME value.

Because of energetic expenses of the digestion and absorption of nutrients and due to energetic inefficiency of the reactions by which absorbed nutrients are metabolized, part of the ME is lost as heat increment (also referred to as specific dynamic action, diet-induced thermogenesis, or thermal energy). The deduction of the heat increment of a food from its ME gives the net energy (NE) value of the food. The NE is the remaining part of food energy which is used for different life processes, and is therefore the unique measure of the energetic value of the food. Theoretically, energy systems based on NE would be the most accurate systems to evaluate energetic values of foods, but from a practical point of view it is a question whether ME should not be preferred for evaluation of foods for laboratory animals. Relatively few types of feedstuffs are used for laboratory animals, primarily grain and oilseed cakes, where the utilization of ME does not vary much. Extensive studies on different animals have shown that ME can be calculated with reasonable certainty on the basis of the digested quantities of nutrients, as follows:[58]

		Rats	Rabbits	
ME, kJ	=	18.4	18.2	× digest. crude protein, g
	+	39.4	39.5	× digest. fat, g
	+	15.2	18.8	× digest. crude fiber, g
	+	17.5	17.1	× digest. nitrogen-free extract, g

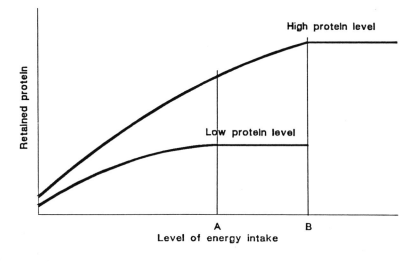

Figure 3. Relationship between protein retention and energy intake.

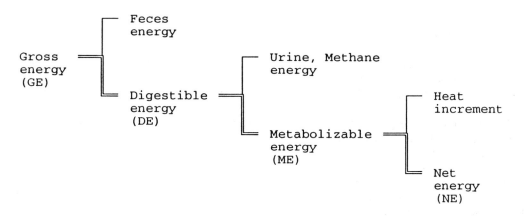

Figure 4. The partition of food energy in the animal.

The calculation of ME will always be subject to some uncertainty concerning the energy constants for the respective nutrients. In practice the same accuracy can be obtained by using only the content of organic matter (OM) as a basis. From 147 measurements on growing rabbits, Thorbek and Chwalibog[59] found the following relation between ME and digestible OM: ME, kJ = 18.7 × digested OM, g. The factor 18.7 corresponds to the factors of 17.0, 18.4, and 20.6 found for calves, pigs, and poultry, respectively. Since the digestibility of organic matter is generally about 65%, ME in feed for rabbits (guinea pig) could be calculated as: ME, kJ = OM, g × 0.65 × 18.7. For rats (mice and hamsters), a factor between 18 and 20 can probably be used. On the assumption that the digestibility of organic matter is 85%, the following calculation could be used: ME, kJ = OM, g × 0.85 × 19.[60]

If the energy value of foods is expressed in ME units, the requirements must be expressed in the same units, thus we need to know the animal's maintenance requirement for metabolizable energy (MEm) as well as the efficiency of ME utilization for growth, pregnancy, and lactation. Theoretically, the maintenance requirement is defined as the amount of energy necessary to balance anabolism and catabolism, giving an energy retention around zero. There are different methods to assess MEm and to estimate the efficiency of ME utilization for different body functions, as recently discussed for farm animals.[61] However, for laboratory animals, there are few empirical results about MEm.[17,62] In summary, MEm values for rats and mice are usually suggested to be around 100 kcal (420 kJ) per LW, kg[0.75]. Although

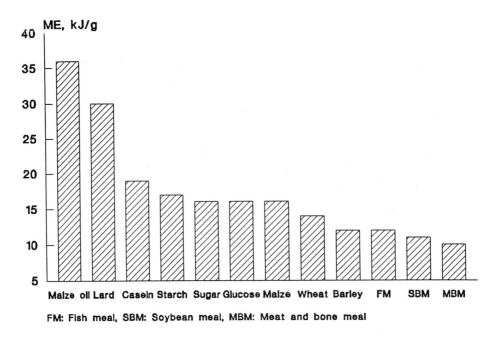

FM: Fish meal, SBM: Soybean meal, MBM: Meat and bone meal

Figure 5. Metabolizable energy (ME) in different feedstuffs for rats and mice.

this value has been extensively used as the measure of MEm in laboratory animals, it has to be emphasized that it is debatable whether there is any constant value of MEm independent of nutritional, genetic, and environmental conditions.[7,61,63] There is substantial information about ME utilization for growth, pregnancy, and lactation,[63,64] but surprisingly, these values are not used for laboratory animals.

The standards for energy requirements of laboratory animals are based either on the measurements of the voluntary food intake at different physiological states[17] or on equations produced by Clarke et al.[6] According to these equations the maintenance requirement of rats is 450 kJ/LW, $kg^{0.75}$ and requirements for the other body functions (inclusive of maintenance) are calculated as: growth = 1200 kJ/LW, $kg^{0.75}$, pregnancy = 600 kJ/LW, $kg^{0.75}$, lactation = 1300 kJ/LW, $kg^{0.75}$. The values are presumed to be in terms of ME, although this is not stated. Major discrepancies between the energy requirements derived from these equations and the values proposed by the National Research Council[17] were demonstrated by Eggum and Beames[62] for growing rats above 200 g LW. There is no doubt that another approach has to be applied in order to estimate requirements for energy in a more precise way. Possibly, a factorial method based on the separation of the metabolic processes contributing to the energy requirement, as demonstrated later in this chapter, would provide less erroneous values.

MINERALS

Minerals are nutritionally divided into two groups: macrominerals and microminerals. The macrominerals (calcium, phosphorus, potassium, sodium, and magnesium) maintain the following functions:

1. Structural integrity
2. Transmembrane potentials needed for a variety of cellular functions
3. Osmotic pressure regulations needed for body fluid balances
4. Acid-base balances

Microminerals (zinc, copper, manganese, and selenium) are needed as components of metalloenzymes, which are employed in a broad variety of metabolic processes. Iodine is a necessary constituent of thyroid hormone, iron of hemoglobin and myoglobin, and cobalt of vitamin B_{12}. The function of minerals, deficiency signs, and occurrence in feeds are outlined in Table 4.

Two major concepts related to the mineral supply must be emphasized. First, it is the balanced amount of all minerals in the diet that is important. A deficient supply of one mineral may affect absorption and metabolism of other minerals; also an excess supply of one or several minerals may often be more harmful than beneficial. Second, it is the biological availability of the minerals that is important. It is generally

Table 4. Mineral Fuctions, Deficiency Symptoms and Content in Feeds

	Function	Deficiency symptom	Content in feed	
			High	Low
Ca	Bone formation, muscle function, blood coagulation	Increased muscle tonus, rickets, osteomalacia	Animal origin (bone meal)	Grain, oilseed meal/cakes
P	Bone formation, enzymes, ATP, phosphoproteins, phospholipids	Rickets, osteomalacia, disturbances in energy metabolism	Animal origin, rye, barley, wheat, oats	Tapioca, oilseed meal/cakes
Na	Fluid balance, nerve function, osmotic pressure, acid-base balance, enzyme activator	Reduced utilization of protein and energy, reduced growth, polyuria, eye lesions, reproductive disturbances	Animal origin (milk and fish products)	Vegetables, grass
K	Osmotic pressure, acid-base balance, heart/muscle function, enzyme activator	Anorexia, lethargy, muscular weakness	Grass, oilseed meal/cakes, fish products	Grain
Mg	Enzyme activator, nerve function	Convulsions, heart arrhythmia	Oilseed meal/cakes, wheat bran	Potato, blood meal
Mn	Bone formation, enzyme activator	Reduced growth and fertility, embryonic morality	Oilseed meal/cakes, wheat bran	Animal origin, grain
Cu	Red blood cells, iron absorption, (enzyme activator)	Anemia, reduced growth, depigmentation of hair	Oilseed meal/cakes	Milk, maize
Fe	Hemoglobin, transferrin, cytochromes	Anemia	Blood, meat, fish products	Milk
Zn	Insulin, enzymes, Ca-P turnover	Parakeratosis, diarrhea, anorexia	Widely distributed	Soy meal
Se	Mitochondrial enzymes, vitamin E absorption	"White muscle disease", infertility	Oilseed meal/cakes, fish products	Grain

recognized that the total content of a mineral element in a particular dietary compound or in a complete diet has little significance unless it is qualified by its biological availability to the animal.

Mineral deficiencies or excess supplies are characterized by a number of animal responses, which can be divided into primary and secondary responses. The primary, or the most immediate, responses are changes in body levels and circulation levels of the elements. Theoretically, these are the best indications of a suboptimal supply, but they are difficult to assess. Contrary to changes in body pools, the secondary responses can be quantified from different clinical and performance signs. Although there are numerous typical deficiency symptoms for particular minerals, the variety of interactions between minerals and other nutrients often makes it very difficult to judge which specific mineral might be responsible for the clinical or performance symptoms. Another problem regarding reliance on clinical and performance signs is that their appearance may be a consequence of reduced food intake caused by housing conditions, temperature, humidity, etc., and not necessarily due to nutritional factors.

Concerning the problem of the biological availability of minerals, there are several factors which may influence mineral utilization. Absorption and utilization of minerals depend on the chemical and physical form of the minerals in the diet, ratios between specific minerals, the supply of other nutrients and energy, and several other factors, like age and sex of animals, disease, parasites, microbial activity in the alimentary tract, and hormonal regulation. The availability of calcium is known to vary according to the presence of phosphorus, magnesium, and vitamin D. The availability of calcium (and some other

Table 5. Total Phosphorus (%), Phytic Acid (%), and Phytase Activity (μg Released Phosphorus/min per g dry matter) in Different Feeds

Feed	Total P	Phytic acid-P	Phytase activity
Barley	0.35	0.27	24
Wheat	0.32	0.24	53
Oats	0.32	0.24	0
Wheat bran	0.99	0.84	150
Rapeseed meal	1.53	1.09	0

minerals) appears to be lower in older than in younger animals.[65] The availability of phosphorus is known to depend on the chemical form of phosphorus in the diet; of particular importance is the availability of phytate phosphorus. Phosphorus bound to phytic acid is not readily available for monogastric animals, unless the enzyme phytase is present in the food. Because foods vary in content of phytic acid and phytase activity, the amount of available phosphorus is seldom coincident with the total amount of phosphorus in the natural foods (Table 5).

Apart from the fact that phytic acid phosphorus is not a reliable source of phosphorus, phytic acid has a negative effect on the absorption of other minerals, because acid-phosphorus groups of phytic acid link with other metals in the gastrointestinal tract into unavailable components. High concentrations of calcium can also reduce the amount of phosphorus absorbed.[66] Contrary to phosphorus deficiency problems (Table 4), too-high levels of phosphorus in the diet may induce nephrocalcinosis. This common finding, particular in female rats, has been extensively studied in the recent years. Schoenmakers et al.[67] and Marsman et al.[68] showed that 0.4% phosphorus in semipurified rat diets produces nephrocalcinosis, while a restriction to 0.2%, or a calcium:phosphorus ratio above 1,[69] or high levels of manganese and protein[70] prevent calcification of the kidney. Absorption of iron can be reduced by high intakes of calcium and manganese, but is increased by the presence of zinc. It is now well established that an interaction occurs between copper and zinc so that high levels of dietary zinc reduce liver copper levels. On the other hand, an increase in the concentrations of calcium, copper, phytic acid, and vitamin D reduces the availability of zinc. Also the dietary protein level can affect zinc utilization. Pedersen and Eggum[71] reported that absorption and retention of zinc in growing rats apparently increase with increasing protein intake. These findings were recently confirmed by Hunt and Johnson,[72] who demonstrated that high-protein diets rich in sulfur-containing amino acids increased bone zinc deposition. However, they suggested that this effect was not a consequence of improved zinc availability, but altered bone zinc metabolism.

VITAMINS

The primary function of vitamins is to promote and regulate a wide variety of physiological processes. The outline of functions, deficiency symptoms, and the contents in foods is demonstrated in Table 6. As in the case of minerals, not only the amount of a particular vitamin, but also the balance between vitamins and other nutrients, must be considered. The well-established interrelationship between vitamin D, calcium, and phosphorus indicates that the requirement for vitamin D declines with increasing concentrations of calcium and phosphorus.

Requirements for vitamin E always refer to α-tocopherol; however, the contents of different tocopherols vary from food to food, and consequently different biological potencies of tocopherols (Table 7) should be considered in the formulation of the diet. The action of tocopherols in animals is influenced by a number of dietary factors. Antioxidants and selenium complement vitamin E in some functions by reducing the vitamin oxidative function in the diet and the digestive tract. For diets with a high level of unsaturated fatty acids and without an adequate supplementation with chemical antioxidants higher levels of vitamin E are required to prevent lipid peroxidation.[73]

Dietary factors may also influence the requirements of water-soluble vitamins. An increase in fat level may reduce the thiamin requirement, but increase the requirements for riboflavin and pantothenic acid, and animals fed high-protein levels may also require an extended supply of riboflavin.

Normally it has been considered that there is no need to supply biotin, folic acid, vitamin K, and vitamin B_{12}, since these are available by microbial synthesis in the intestine, and via coprophagy. However, in germ-free and associated animals, or in case of reduced microbial activity, for example during antibiotic treatment, supplementation with these vitamins may be necessary. In the case of choline, which is synthesized in the body from methionine, the requirements are influenced by the amount of methionine in the diet. There is also evidence that rats fed a choline-free diet have decreased lipid content in the liver and may develop liver cancer.[74]

Table 6. Vitamin Functions, Deficiency Symptoms and Contents in Feeds

	Function	Deficiency symptom	Content, high
A	Bone formation, reproduction, mucous membranes, vision	Impaired fertility, abortion, small litters, blindness, lowered resistance to infections, disturbances in bone development	Cod liver oil, green plants, yellow maize
D	Ca and P metabolism, protein transport	Rickets, osteomalacia	Animal origin (milk, fish)
E	Antioxidant, resistance to infections, reproduction	Muscle dystophy, infertility, abortion, small litters, liver necrosis	Green plants, grain
K	Coagulation of blood	Gastrointestinal hemorrhages, increase in blood-clotting time	Microbially synthesized, supply via coprophagy, green plants, fish meal
B_1	Carbohydrate metabolism, nerve and muscular function	Anorexia, vomiting, muscular fatigue, cardiac disorders, reduced ferility	Supply via coprophagy, grain, oilseed meal, milk products
B_2	Protein and fat metabolism	Enteritis, cataract, reduced fertility	Supply via coprophagy, milk and fish products
Niacin	As B_2, function of skin and digestive organs	Eczema, damaged mucous membranes, nervous systems	Synthesized from tryptophane, cod liver oil, sunflower meal
B_6	Transport-absorption of amino acids, lipids and carbohydrates	Reduced growth, anemia, nervous symptoms, skin inflammation	Cod liver oil, milk, grain
Panto-thenic acid	Nutrient metabolism, function of skin and mucous, resistance to infections	Skin changes, gastrointestinal disorders, anorexia	Milk and fish products
Biotin	Fatty acid synthesis, energy metabolism	Loss of hair, eczema	Microbially synthesized, cod liver oil, milk
Choline	Transport and metabolism of lipids, neural impulses	Disturbed fat metabolism, reduced growth	Synthesized from methionine, all feeds
Folic acid	Protein and nucleic acids metabolism, formation of hemo-immunoglobulin	Hematological disorders, anemia	Soybean meal, fish meal
B_{12}	Coenzyme, growth factor — necessary for protein metabolism	Reduced growth, anemia, skin inflammations	Microbially synthesized, animal origin (milk, meat)
C	Coagulation, resistance to infections and to stress, function of collagenous tissues	Internal hemorrhagia, increased susceptibilty to infections	Synthesized except in primates, Dalmatian dogs, and guinea pig

Table 7. Content of Tocopherols in Different Feeds and Relative Biological Activity of Tocopherols

Tocopherol: mg/kg	α-	β-	γ-	δ-	Compound	Relative activity, %
Barley	4	3	0.5	0.5	d-α-tocopherol	100
Wheat	10	9			d-β-tocopherol	50
Rye	8	4	6		d-γ-tocopherol	10
Maize	6		38		d-δ-tocopherol	3
Maize oil	112	50	602	18	d-α-tocotrienol	30
Soy oil	101		593	264	d-β-tocotrienol	5

Finally, it has to be mentioned that processing and storage of foods decreases the active vitamin content. Pasteurization or autoclaving may cause losses in the order of 90% of vitamin C and thiamin, 45% of pantothenic acid, 35% of pyridoxine, and 10% of riboflavin. Gassing may cause considerable losses of niacin and pyridoxine, and gamma radiation may destroy vitamin A.[60]

Although there are many aspects concerning vitamin deficiencies in laboratory animals, cases of "true" dietary vitamin deficiency are rare, primarily because commercial diets are usually fortified with vitamins. This means that the content of natural vitamins is essentially ignored, albeit they provide additional activity. However, this concept is often a reason for hypervitaminosis, which is probably more common than are vitamin deficiencies. Therefore, a careful estimation of vitamin content available from the natural feedstuffs should be included in the calculations of dietary vitamin supply.

WATER

Water is a very important, but often overlooked, nutritional component. An animal can survive after losing almost all of its glycogen and storage fat and half of its protein, but 10% loss of total body water causes serious illness, and a 15% loss results in death.[75] Animals have two basic sources of water: metabolic water and drinking water. Metabolic water results from the oxidative reactions of carbohydrate, fat, and protein. Approximately 5 to 8 g of water is produced for each 100 kJ of energy released from oxidized nutrients. The amount of consumed water is closely related to food intake; in small rodents the ratio of water to food eaten is about 2.5 to 3:1 under normal dietary and climatic conditions. The average daily consumption of water by some laboratory animals is demonstrated in Table 8.

Water quality standards for laboratory animals do not exist. However, the water quality recommendations for human consumption can also be applied to laboratory animals (Table 9).

Bacterial contamination of drinking water may be a most important vector of infections, and in order to prevent bacterial growth, it is suggested that water should be acidified and drinking bottles regularly autoclaved.[76,77] Apart from palatability and toxicity problems other aspects of water composition ought to be considered in particular investigations. For example, in experiments involving feeding mineral-deficient diets, the animals might cover their copper requirement from the drinking water, or obtain substantial amounts of zinc, chromium, and iron leaching from rubber stoppers used to cork water bottles. Especially the acidification of water can increase leaching of these minerals.[78]

NUTRITIONAL REQUIREMENTS AND ALLOWANCES

REQUIREMENTS

Knowledge of the quantitative relations between catabolic and anabolic processes in the body (see previous section) is essential in predicting the effect of a diet on the metabolic response, and is consequently necessary for the estimation of nutrient and energy requirements for growth, pregnancy, and lactation. However, the primary element in the evaluation of nutritional requirements is knowledge of the ability of animals to transform nutrients and energy obtained from a diet into body components and products. In spite of much information available on different aspects of laboratory animal nutrition, there are no reports on methodical investigations

Table 8. Average Water Intake, ml/d

Species	Growing	Adult
Mouse	3–10	5–10
Rat	5–80	25–35
Hamster	8–10	5–15
Guinea pig	100–250	200–300
Rabbit	100–400	300–400

concerning nutrient and energy balances during pregnancy or lactation, and only a few exist on growth.

A series of methodical studies concerning protein and energy metabolism in growing rats during 5 months after weaning was carried out by Thorbek et al.[3] The results of these studies furnish valuable data concerning nutrient and energy utilization and accretion during growth, providing the necessary basis for calculation of the requirements. The experiments were performed with male *Rattus norvegicus albinus* fed *ad libitum* on non-purified commercial diets. The average nitrogen balance (corresponding to protein balance; $N \times 6.25$) for the growth period between 5 and 18 weeks of age is demonstrated in Figure 6.

Table 9. Quality Requirements for Drinking Water

Substance	Max. content mg/l	Remarks
Aluminum	0.2	Water gets cloudy
Ammonium	0.5	Promotes corrosion of pipes and bacterial growth
Calcium	200	Precipitation of calcium
Fluoride	1.5	Affects health
Phosphorus	0.15	Indicates pollution
Iron	0.2	Precipitation of ochre
Potassium	10	Indicates pollution
Nitrogen	1	Indicates pollution with organic N compounds
Chloride	300	Off-flavor
Magnesium	50	Off-flavor
Sodium	175	Off-flavor
Nitrate	50	Methemoglobinemia
Sulfate	250	Off-flavor

In relation to the nitrogen intake, 56% was excreted in urine and 18% in feces, while 26% was retained in the body. During the same period energy excreted in urine constituted only 2% of dietary energy, and 18% of the energy intake was excreted in feces, but the major part, 53%, was measured as the total heat energy, and subsequently the remaining 27% was retained in the body protein and fat (Figure 7). These relations clearly indicate that only about 20 to 30% of the consumed protein or energy is finally retained in the growing laboratory rat kept under ordinary dietary and housing conditions.

From the same experimental data we have also recalculated daily protein and fat retention, as demonstrated in Figure 8. Protein retention followed the same pattern as described for growing farm animals,[61,79] showing increasing protein retention (RP) to about 1.7 g/day at the age between 7 and 8 weeks and then decreasing to a constant plateau of 0.5 g/day at 16 to 18 weeks of age. Daily fat retention (RF) gradually increased above 2 g/day until 10 to 14 weeks of age, after which a slow decrease was observed. The amount of retained energy (RE), which is a function of energy retained in protein and fat, reached the highest level of 125 kJ/day at the age of 8 to 10 weeks; then it gradually decreased to about 80 kJ because of decreasing protein and fat retention.

Based on the values presented, the requirements for protein and energy in the growing rat are calculated by the factorial approach, as demonstrated in Tables 10 and 11. The calculations are performed for weeks 5, 8 (about maximum RP), 10 (about maximum RF), and 18 (mature animals). Concerning the protein requirement, it was assumed that protein digestibility in commercial standard diets for rats is 80%, and the biological value averages 75%.[52] The requirement of digestible protein for maintenance (DPm) is calculated from the following function: DPm, g/day = $(0.15 \times LW, kg^{0.75} \times 2 \times 6.25)/0.75$, where $0.15 \times LW, kg^{0.75}$ is endogenous nitrogen excreted in urine multiplied by 2, assuming that the same amount of metabolic nitrogen is excreted with the feces, 6.25 is the factor to recalculate nitrogen to protein, and 0.75 is the biological value of protein.[80]

Metabolizable energy required for maintenance (MEm) is calculated from the function: MEm, kJ/day = $32.5 + 251 \times LW, kg^{0.75}$, while the amount of ME required for energy retention in protein (RPE) and in fat (RFE), i.e., for growth, is calculated with the efficiencies of ME utilization as 0.50 and 0.77 for RPE and RFE, respectively.[7,61]

The pattern of protein retention showed that the highest requirement for digestible protein was at 8 weeks of age; with relatively low fat retention at 5 weeks of age, the total requirement for ME was markedly lower than in the later part of the growth period. The values presented demonstrate the pattern of requirement during growth, but for practical diet formulation it is interesting to note the changes in the required concentration of DP per 100 kJ ME. It decreased linearly from 1.2 g/100 kJ at 5 weeks to 0.7 g/100 kJ at 18 weeks of age, thus indicating the necessity to provide diets with different concentrations of protein during the growth period.

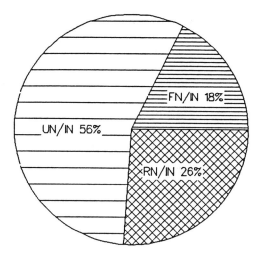

Figure 6. Nitrogen excretion in feces (FN), and urine (UN) and retained nitrogen (RN) in relation to nitrogen intake (IN). Average percentage in male Wistar rats in the growth period from 5 to 18 weeks of age.

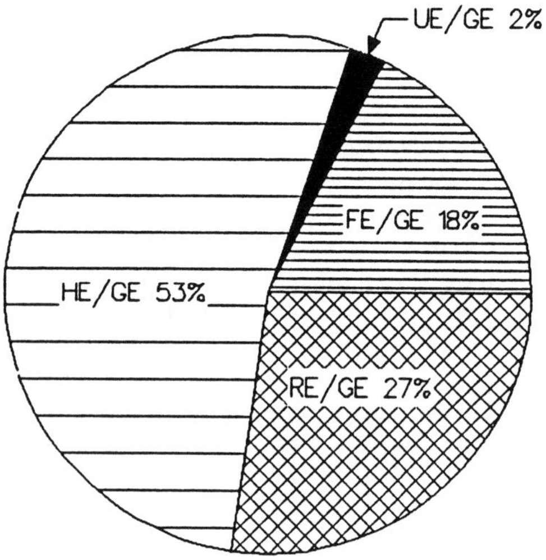

Figure 7. Energy excreted in feces (FE), and urine (UE), heat loss (HE) and retained energy (RE) in relation to energy intake (GE). Average percentage in male Wistar rats in the growth period from 5 to 18 weeks of age.

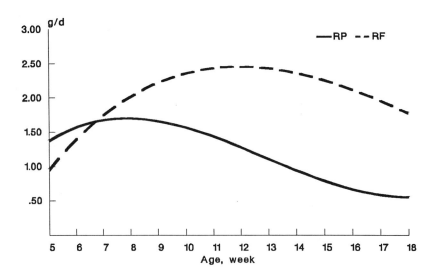

Figure 8. Retained protein (RP) and fat (RF) in male Wistar rats during the growth period from 5 to 18 weeks of age. Extrapolated polynomial functions.

Table 10. Requirement of Digestible Protein for Growing Rats in Relation to Live Weight (LW) and Retained Protein (RP)

Age week	LW g	RP g/d	Requirement, g/d		
			Maintenance	Growth	Total
5	100	1.3	0.4	1.7	2.1
8	220	1.7	0.8	2.3	3.1
10	290	1.3	1.0	1.7	2.7
18	400	0.5	1.3	0.7	2.0

Mean values based on the data from Thorbek et al.[3]

Table 11. Requirement of Metabolizable Energy for Growing Rats in Relation to Live Weight (LW), Retained Energy in Protein (RPE) and Retained Energy in Fat (RFE)

Age week	LW g	RPE kJ/d	RFE kJ/d	Requirement, kJ/d		
				Maintenace	Growth	Total
5	100	30	20	80	90	170
8	220	40	80	110	180	290
10	290	30	95	130	180	310
18	400	12	70	160	120	280

Mean values based on the data from Thorbek et al.3

ALLOWANCES

Knowledge of the amount of nutrients and energy required by animals is necessary to establish nutritional allowances for laboratory animals. There is a clear distinction between the term requirement and allowance. The requirement is a statement of what animals on average require for a particular function, but the allowance is greater than this amount by a safety margin designed principally to allow for variations in requirements between individual animals, and to account for possible variations of nutrient content in the same foods or diets. Unfortunately, this distinction between the two terms is not strictly defined for laboratory animals, and in many publications it is not clear whether the "requirements" or so-called nutritional standards refer to requirements or to allowances. This is one of the main reasons for many of the discrepancies between different recommendations. Keeping in mind the possible confusion caused by the use of inconsistent terminology, the tables in this section present only a general outline of nutritional allowances recommended for common laboratory animals. For detailed descriptions of nutritional standards the publications by Coates,[81] Clarke et al.,[6] the National Research Council,[17] and Eggum and Beames[62] are suggested.

Nutrient and energy allowances for laboratory animals are rarely expressed in terms of quantity per day, but, because the animals are usually fed *ad libitum*, by means of the concentrations of nutrients and energy in the diet. In practice most laboratories use only two different diets within each animal species, one for adult, non-producing animals, and the other for growing, pregnant, or lactating animals.

Knowledge of the requirements for the individual amino acids for different laboratory animals and different life processes is limited. The most abundant information exists for laboratory rats, although, depending on the source of information, there is a considerably broad range of recommended values, as demonstrated in Table 12.

The recommendations for protein, fat, fiber, and metabolizable energy allowances are demonstrated in Table 13. Concerning protein supply generally, the adult mouse, rat, and hamster require 70 to 120 g crude protein per kilogram of diet with 90% of dry matter. Depending on protein digestibility and biological value, this is equivalent, in the natural diets, to a supply of about 50 to 70 g digestible protein per kilogram of food. For the other body functions a supply of 200 to 240 g crude protein per kilogram of food may be recommended, corresponding to 120 to 140 g digestible protein for both maintenance and productive functions.

The level of crude fat in the diet for adult animals is recommended at about 20 g/kg diet, but for productive animals at about 50 g/kg. For mouse, rat, and hamster the crude fiber in the diet should preferably not exceed 80 g/kg. On the other hand in guinea pigs and rabbits, considerable amounts of

Table 12. The Range of Recommended Levels of Essential Amino Acids for Laboratory Rats as g/100 g Protein, as mg/kg.[75] per d, and as g/MJ, ME per d

Amino acid	g/100g protein[a]	mg/kg$^{0.75}$ [b]	g/MJ[c]
Arginine	5.0 – 6.0	0 – 10	0.39
Histidine	2.5 – 3.0	0 – 17	0.19
Isoleucine	5.0 – 6.0	30 – 49	0.32
Leucine	7.5 – 8.0	16 – 64	0.49
Lysine	6.0 – 9.0	10 – 33	0.45
Methionine+cystine	5.0 –10.0	20 – 43	0.30
Phenylalanine+tyrosine	6.0 –10.0	16 – 52	0.52
Threonine	4.0 – 4.5	20 – 54	0.32
Tryptophan	1.2 – 1.5	5 – 10	0.10
Valine	5.0 – 6.0	18 – 47	0.39

[a]Data from References 54 and 60.
[b]Data from References 82 and 83.
[c]Data from Reference 62.

Table 13. Recommended Supply of Nutrient, g/kg Food and Energy, MJ/kg Food[a]

Species	Crude protein	Crude fat	Crude fiber	Metabolizable energy
Adult				
Mouse, rat	70 - 120	20	40 - 60	12
Hamster	70 - 120	20	50 - 80	12
Guinea pig	140 - 180	20	150 - 200	11
Rabbit	140 - 180	25	150 - 200	11
Growing, pregnant, lactating				
Mouse, rat	200 - 240	30 - 50	30 - 50	12 - 14
Hamster	200 - 240	20 - 80	30 - 50	12 - 14
Guinea pig	180 - 230	50	100 - 150	12
Rabbit	180 - 230	50	100 - 150	12

[a]Based on calculations on approximate *ad libitum* food intake, containing 90% dry matter.

Table 14. Recommendations for Mineral and Vitamin Supply

Mineral	g/kg Food	Mineral	mg/kg Food
Ca	5	Fe	35
P	4	Cu	5
Mg	2	Mn	50
Na	0.5	Se	0.1
K	3.6	Zn	12
S	0.3	J	75

Vitamin per kg food			
Retinol	10000 i.u.	Thiamin	4 mg
Cholecalciferol	1000 i.u.	Riboflavin	3 mg
α-Tocopherol	30 mg	Pyridoxine	6 mg
Phylloquinone	50 mcg	Pantothenic acid	8 mg
Ascorbic acid[a]	1000 mg	Niacin	10 mg
		Folic acid	1 mg
		Cyanocobalamin	50 mcg

[a]For guinea pig.

cellulose, hemicellulose and pectin are broken down in the large intestine (50 to 75% of the digestion capacity of ruminants). For these animals, a content of 100 to 200 g crude fiber per kilogram is recommended.

There is a wide range of recommended supply of minerals and vitamins, and the values presented in Table 14 are on the minimum side of the recommendations. However, these refer to the supply of minerals and vitamins in excess of their content in the feedstuffs.

The standards given for fat-soluble vitamins predominantly apply to the small rodents. As vitamin C cannot be synthesized by guinea pigs, a minimum of 1000 mg L-ascorbic acid per kilogram of food or added to the drinking water is recommended.

As mentioned before, the nutritional standards for laboratory animals are not comprehensive and much work will be required to establish nutrient and energy requirements and consequently nutritional allowances for different species and life processes, as well as for animals kept under different conditions, and used for different research purposes. Therefore, the values for nutritional allowances presented can only be considered as general recommendations.

REFERENCES

1. McDonald, P., Edwards, R. A., and Greenhalgh, J. F. D., *Animal Nutrition*, Longman, London, 1981, chap. 16.
2. Balch, C. C., and Campling, R. C., Voluntary intake of food, in *Handbuch der Tierernährung*, Lenkeit, W., Breirem, K., and Crasemann, E., Eds., Verlag Paul Parey, Hamburg, 1969, chap. 17.
3. Thorbek, G., Chwalibog, A., Eggum, B. O., and Christensen, K., Studies on growth, nitrogen and energy metabolism in rats, *Arch. Tierernähr.*, 32, 827, 1982.
4. Pullar, J. D., and Webster, A. J. F., Heat loss and energy retention during growth in congenitally obese and lean rats, *Br. J. Nutr.*, 31, 377, 1974.
5. Kleiber, M., *The Fire of Life*, John Wiley & Sons, New York, 1961, chap. 18.
6. Clarke, H. E., Coates, M. W., Eva, J. K., Ford, D. J., Milner, C. K., O'Donoghue, P. N., Scott, P. O., and Ward, R. J., Dietary standards for laboratory animals: Report of the Laboratory Animal Centre Diets Advisory Committee, *Lab. Anim.*, 11, 1, 1977.
7. Eggum, B. O., and Chwalibog, A., A study on requirement for maintenance and growth in rats with normal or reduced gut flora, *Z. Tierphysiol. Tierernähr. Futtermittelkd.*, 49, 104, 1983.
8. Henning, S. J., Functional development of the gastrointestinal tract, in *Physiology of the Gastrointestinal Tract*, Johnson, R., Ed., Raven Press, New York, 1987, chap. 9.
9. Prochazka, P., Hahn, P., Koldovsky, O., Noh Ynek, M., and Rokos, J., The activity of alpha-amylase in homogenates of the pancreas of rats during early post-natal development, *Physiol. Bohemoslov.*, 13, 288, 1964.
10. Rubino, A., Zimbalatti, F., and Auricchio, S., Intestinal disaccharidase activities in adult and suckling rats, *Biochem. Biophys. Acta*, 92, 305, 1964.
11. Descholdt-Lanckman, M., Robberecht, P., Camus, J., Baya, C., and Christophe, J., Hormonal and dietary adaptation of rat pancreatic hydrolases before and after weaning, *Am. J. Physiol.*, 226, 39, 1974.
12. Henning, S. J., Postnatal development: coordination of feeding, digestion and metabolism, *Am. J. Physiol.*, 241, G199, 1981.
13. Melander, A., Influence of food on the bioavailability of drugs, *Clin. Pharmacokinet.*, 3, 337, 1978.
14. Jefery, P., Burrows, M., and Bye, A., Does the rat have an empty stomach after an overnight fast? *Lab. Anim.*, 21, 330, 1987.
15. Raczynski, G., Eggum, B. O., and Chwalibog, A., The effect of dietary composition on transit time in rats, *Z. Tierphysiol. Tierernähr. Futtermittelkd.*, 47, 160, 1982.
16. Chwalibog, A., Jakobsen, K., Henckel, S., and Thorbek, G., Oxidation and fat retention from carbohydrate, protein and fat in growing pigs, *Z. Tierphysiol. Tierernähr. Futtermittelkd.*, in press.
17. National Research Council, *Nutrient Requirements of Laboratory Animals*, National Academy of Sciences, Washington, D.C., No. 10, 1978.
18. Rafecas, I., Esteve, M., Remesar, X., and Alemany, M., Plasma amino acids of lean and obese Zucker rats subjected to a cafeteria diet after weaning, *Biochem. Int.*, 25, 797, 1991.
19. Glick, Z., Bray, A., and Teague, R. J., Effect of prandial glucose on brown fat thermogenesis in rats: Possible implications for dietary obesity, *J. Nutr.*, 114, 1934, 1984.

20. Herberg, L., Interrelationships between obesity and diabetes, *Proc. Nutr. Soc.*, 50, 605, 1991.
21. Eggum, B. O., Andersen, J. O., and Rotenberg, S., The effect of dietary fibre level and microbial activity in the digestive tract on fat metabolism in rats and pigs, *Acta Agric. Scand.*, 32, 145, 1982.
22. Rotenberg, S., and Andersen, J. O., The effect of antibiotica on some lipid parameters in rats receiving cornstarch, potato flour or pectin in the diet, *Acta Agric. Scand.*, 32, 151, 1982.
23. Rotenberg, S., Eggum, B. O., Hegedüs, M., and Jacobsen, I., The effect of pectin and microbial activity in the digestive tract on faecal excretion of amino acids, fatty acids, thiamin, riboflavin and niacin in young rats, *Acta Agric. Scand.*, 32, 310, 1982.
24. Anderson, J. W., Physiological and metabolic effects of dietary fiber, *Fed. Proc.*, 44, 2902, 1985.
25. Cummings, J. H., Nutritional implications of dietary fiber, *Am J. Clin. Nutr.*, 31, 521, 1978.
26. Robinson, M., Hart, D., and Pigott, G. H., The effects of diet on the incidence of periodontitis in rats, *Lab. Anim.*, 25, 247, 1991.
27. Madsen, C., Squamous-cell carcinoma and oral, pharyngeal and nasal lesions caused by foreign bodies in feed. Cases from a long-term study in rats, *Lab. Anim.*, 23, 241, 1989.
28. Widdowson, E. M., Dauncey, M. J., Gairdner, D. M. T., Jonxis, J. H. P., and Pelikan-Filipkova, M., Body fat of British and Dutch infants, *Br. Med. J.*, i, 653, 1975.
29. Kuratko, C., and Pence, B., Rat colonic antioxidant status: Interaction of dietary fats with 1,2-dimethylhydrazine challenge, *J. Nutr.*, 122, 278, 1992.
30. Bird, R., and Bruce, R., Effect of dietary fat levels on the susceptibility of colonic cells to nuclear-damaging agents, *Nutr. Cancer*, 8, 93, 1986.
31. Bull, A., Bronstein, J., and Nigro, N., The essential fatty acid requirement for azoxymethane-induced intestinal carcinogenesis in rats, *Lipids*, 24, 340, 1989.
32. Ip, C., Carter, C. A., and Ip, M. M., Requirement of essential fatty acid for mammary tumorgenesis in the rat, *Cancer Res.*, 45, 155, 1985.
33. Ip, C., Fat and essential fatty acid in mammary carcinogenesis, *Am. J. Clin. Nutr.*, 45, 218, 1987.
34. Fisher, M. S., Claudio, J. C., Locniskar, M., Belury, M. A., Maldve, R. E., Lee, M. L., Leyton, J., Slaga, T. J., and Bechtel, D. H., The effect of dietary fat on the rapid development of mammary tumors induced by 7,12-dimethylbenz(a)anthracene in SENCAR mice, *Cancer Res.*, 52, 662, 1992.
35. Crevel, R. W. R., Friend, J. V., Goodwin, B. F., and Parish, W. E., High-fat diets and the immune response of C57 B1 mice, *Br. J. Nutr.*, 67, 17, 1992.
36. Burr, G. O., and Burr, M. M., A new deficiency disease produced by the rigid exclusion of fat from the diet, *J. Biol. Chem.*, 82, 345, 1929.
37. Burr, G. O., and Burr, M. M., On the nature and role of the fatty acids essential in nutrition, *J. Biol. Chem.*, 86, 587, 1930.
38. Innis, S. M., Essential fatty acids in growth and development, *Prog. Lipid Res.*, 30, 39, 1991.
39. Christensen, K., Determination of linoleic acid requirements in slaughter pigs, *Nat. Inst. Anim. Sci., Rep.*, 577, 1, 1985.
40. Holman, R. T., Essential fatty acid deficiency, in *Progress in the Chemistry of Fats and Other Lipids*, Vol. 9, Pergamon Press, Elmsford, New York, 1968, 619.
41. Eggum, B. O., Biochemical and methodological principles, in *Protein Metabolism in Farm Animals*, Bock, H. D., Eggum, B. O., Low, A. G., Simon, O., and Zebrowska, T., Eds., Oxford Scientific Publications, Deutscher Landwirtschaftsverlag, Berlin, 1989, chap. 1.
42. Young, V. R., Nutrient interactions with reference to amino acid and protein metabolism in non-ruminants — particular emphasis on protein-energy relations in man, *Z. Ernährungswiss.*, 30, 239, 1991.
43. Harper, A. E., and Rogers, Q. R., Amino acid imbalance, *Proc. Nutr. Soc.*, 24, 173, 1965.
44. Rogers, Q. R., and Leung, P. M. B., The influence of amino acids on the neuroregulation of food intake, *Fed. Proc. Fed. Am. Soc. Exp. Biol.*, 32, 1709, 1973.
45. Harper, A. E., Benevenga, N. J., and Wohlhueter, R. M., Effects of ingestion of disproportionate amounts of amino acids, *Physiol. Rev.*, 50, 428, 1970.
46. Eggum, B. O., Bach Knudsen, K. E., and Jacobsen, I., The effect of amino acid imbalance on nitrogen retention (biological value) in rats, *Br. J. Nutr.*, 45, 175, 1981.
47. Dunn, T. B., Relationship of amyloid infiltration and renal disease in mice, *J. Nat. Cancer Inst.*, 5, 17, 1944.
48. Conell, D. I., Street, W., Pendry, R. A., Yeboah, J., and Godfrey, A., Comparative feeding trials of 2 maintenance diets containing different crude protein levels, *Lab. Anim.*, 15, 13, 1981.

49. Meyer, O. A., Kristiansen, E., and Würtzen, G., Effects of dietary protein and butylated hydroxytoluene on the kidneys of rats, *Lab. Anim.*, 23, 175, 1989.

50. Hawrylewicz, E. J., Huang, H. H., and Blair, W. H., Dietary soybean isolate and methionine supplementation affect mammary tumor progression in rats, *J. Nutr.*, 121, 1693, 1991.

51. Yoshida, A., Harper, A. E., and Elvehjem, C. A., Effects of protein per calorie ratio and dietary level of fat on calorie and protein utilization, *J. Nutr.*, 63, 555, 1957.

52. Eggum, B. O., A study of certain factors influencing protein utilization in rats and pigs, *Natl. Inst. Anim. Sci. Rep.*, 406, 1, 1973.

53. Szelényi-Galàntai, M., Jacobsen, I., and Eggum, B. O., The influence of dietary energy density on protein utilization in rats, *Acta Agric. Scand.*, 31, 204, 1981.

54. Solleveld, H. A., McAnulty, P., Ford, J., Peters, P. W. J., and Tesh, J., Breeding, housing and care for laboratory animals, in *Laboratory Animals.*, Ruitenberg, E. J., and Peters, P. W. J., Eds., Elsevier Science Publishers B.V., Amsterdam, 1986, chap. 1.

55. Suzuki, T., Tana-Ami, S., Fujiwara, H., and Ishibashi, T., Effect of the energy density of non-purified diets on reproduction, obesity, alopecia and aging in mice, *Exp. Anim.*, 40, 499, 1991.

56. Ross, M. H., and Brass, G., Influence of protein under- and overnutrition on spontaneous tumour prevalence in the rat, *J. Nutr.*, 103, 944, 1965.

57. Roe, F. J. C., Testing for carcinogenicity and the problems of pseudo-carcinogenicity, *Nature*, 303, 657, 1983.

58. Schiemann, R., Nehring, K., Hoffmann, L., Jentsch, W., and Chudy, A., *Energetische Futterbewertung und Energinormen*, VEB Deutsch. Landwirtschaftsverlag, Berlin, 1971.

59. Thorbek, G., and Chwalibog, A., Tilvækst, fordøjelighed, kvælstof- og energiomsætning hos voksende kaniner målt ved forskellige foderkombinationer, *Nat. Inst. Anim. Sci. Rep.*, 510, 1, 1981.

60. Chwalibog, A., *Ernæring af laboratoriedyr*, DSR Forlag, The Royal Veterinary and Agricultural University, Copenhagen, 1989.

61. Chwalibog, A., Energetics of animal production, *Acta Agric. Scand.*, 41, 147, 1991a.

62. Eggum, B. O., and Beames, R. M., Use of laboratory animals as models for studies on nutrition of domestic animals, in *Laboratory Animals*, Ruitenberg, E. J., and Peters, P. W. J., Eds., Elsevier Science Publishers B.V., Amsterdam, 1986, chap. 9.

63. Blaxter, K., *Energy Metabolism in Farm Animals*, Cambridge University Press, Cambridge, 1989, chap. 8.

64. Klein, M., and Hoffmann, L., Bioenergetics of protein retention, in *Protein Metabolism in Farm Animals*, Bock, H. D., Eggum, B. O., Low, A. G., Simon, O., and Zebrowska, T., Eds., Oxford Scientific Publications, Deutscher Landwirtschaftsverlag, Berlin, 1989, chap. 11.

65. Wiseman, J., and Cole, D. J. A., *Feedstuff Evaluation*, Butterworths, London, 1990.

66. Peeler, H. T., Biological availability of nutrients in feeds: availability of major mineral ions, *J. Anim. Sci.*, 35, 695, 1972.

67. Schoenmakers, A. C. M., Ritskes-Hoitinga, J., Lemmens, A. G., and Beynen, A. C., Influence of dietary phosphorus restriction on calcium and phosphorus metabolism in rats, *Int. J. Vitam. Nutr. Res.*, 59, 200, 1989.

68. Marsman, G., Pastoor, F. J. H., Mathot, J. N. J. J., Theuns, H. M., and Beynen, A. C., Vitamin D, within its range of fluctuation in commercial diets, does not influence nephrocalcinosis in female rats, *Lab. Anim.*, 25, 330, 1991.

69. Ritskes-Hoitinga, J., Mathot, J. N. J. J., Danse, L. H. J. C., and Beynen, A. C., Commercial rodent diets and nephrocalcinosis in weanling female rats, *Lab. Anim.*, 25, 126, 1991.

70. Van Camp, I., Ritskes-Hoitinga, J., Lemmens, A. G., and Beynen, A. C., Diet-induced nephrocalcinosis and urinary excretion of albumin in female rats, *Lab. Anim.*, 24, 137, 1990.

71. Pedersen, B., and Eggum, B. O., Interrelations between protein and zinc utilization in rats, *Nutr. Rep. Int.*, 27, 441, 1983.

72. Hunt, J. R., and Johnson, L. K., Dietary protein, as egg albumen: effects on bone composition, zinc bioavailability and zinc requirements of rats, assessed by a modified broken-line model, *J. Nutr.*, 122, 161, 1992.

73. Verschuren, P. M., Houtsmuller, U. M. T., and Zevenbergen, J. L., Evaluation of vitamin E requirement and food palatability in rabbits fed purified diet with a high fish oil content, *Lab. Anim.*, 24, 164, 1990.

74. Kapoor, R., Ghoshal, A. K., and Farber, E., Changes in fatty acid composition of phospholipids from liver microsomes and nuclei in rats fed a choline-free diet, *Lipids*, 27, 1, 1992.

75. Lewis, L. D., Morris, M. L., and Hand, M. S., *Small Animal Clinical Nutritiom*, Mark Morris Associates, Topeka, Kansas, 1987, chap. 1.

76. Tober-Meyer, B. K., and Bieniek, H. J., Studies on the hygiene of drinking water for laboratory animals. 1. The effect of various treatments on bacterial contamination, *Lab. Anim.*, 15, 107, 1981.

77. Tober-Meyer, B. K., Bieniek, H. J., and Kupke, I. R., Studies on the hygiene of drinking water for laboratory animals. 2. Clinical and biochemical studies in rats and rabbits during long-term provision of acidified drinking water, *Lab. Anim.*, 15, 111, 1981.

78. Kennedy, B. W., and Beal, T. S., Minerals leached into drinking water from rubber stoppers, *Lab. Anim. Sci.*, 41, 233, 1991.

79. Thorbek, G., Chwalibog, A., and Henckel, S., Energetics of growth in pigs from 20 to 120 kg live weight, *Z. Tierphysiol. Tierernähr. Futtermittelkd.*, 49, 238, 1983.

80. Chwalibog, A., *Husdyrernæring*, DSR Forlag, The Royal Veterinary and Agricultural University, Copenhagen, 1991, chap. 4.

81. Coates, M. E., The nutrition of laboratory animals, in *The UFAW Handbook on the Care and Management of Laboratory Animals*, Hume, C.W., Ed., UFAW, Churchill Livingstone, Edinburgh, 1976, chap. 3.

82. Owens, F. N., and Pettigrew, J. E., Subdividing amino acid requirements into portions for maintenance and growth, in *Absorption and Utilization of Amino Acids*, Friedman, M., Ed., CRC Press, Boca Raton, Florida, 1989, chap. 2.

83. Shin, I.-S., *Subdividing amino acid requirements for maintenance from requirements for growth*, Thesis, Oklahoma State University, 1990.

Chapter 14

ENVIRONMENTAL IMPACT ON ANIMAL EXPERIMENTS

Per Svendsen

CONTENTS

INTRODUCTION

In the wild, animals may survive in a changing environment because of the genetic variance within the population. Those individuals which adapt best to the new conditions will reproduce more efficiently than the rest and become dominant in the population.

When animals are kept in captivity, their environment is altered dramatically. As in nature, this leads to selection of individuals with a greater tolerance of the new conditions. This is known as domestication. In general the most successful domestic animals originate from wild species with a high degree of environmental adaptability.

The species used as laboratory animals are no different from other domestic animals in this respect. Wild mice and rats can survive almost all climatic conditions on Earth, whereas their laboratory relatives have lost the genetic background for this remarkable adaptability. The more inbred the animals are, the more vulnerable they become to changing environmental conditions.

When breeding animals for experimental use, the major concern is to produce individuals or populations in which the genetic variance is as small as possible. The price for this is an animal that reacts in various ways to even small changes in the environment. For some types of experiment these reactions are of little or no significance, whereas other types of experiment may be severely affected.

THE ANIMAL ROOM ENVIRONMENT

Most laboratory animals, in particular the small rodents, live all their lives in a closed plastic box, in the bottom of which is a mixture of bedding, feces, and urine. The temperature inside the cage will certainly differ from that of the animal room, and depend on the number of animals kept in the cage and the efficiency of the ventilation in the room. The composition of the air in the cage will also differ from that of the animal room, again depending on the efficiency of the ventilation system, and even more on the animal husbandry, e.g., on how frequently the bedding is changed and the cage washed.

Noise in the animal room may originate from many sources, e.g., slamming of doors, telephone bells, movement of equipment, etc. Most animals will react to loud noise, and some species may also react to high-frequency sounds that are outside the range of human hearing. These sounds may come from vibrations in water pipes or from electrical equipment.

In nature, animals are strongly affected by the intensity and duration of daylight. Their reproductive cycles and daily behavior are regulated by light. The laboratory animal may also be affected by changing light intensity if the animal room is constructed with windows to the outside or if the artificial lighting is not properly regulated.

Laboratory animals may be affected by chemicals via their feed and bedding, and by airborne pollutants. The composition of the feed in relation to nutrients is of great importance for enzymatic reactions and the metabolism of bioactive compounds. The feed may be contaminated by pesticides used on the original crop, or by micro-organisms during storage. Similarly, the bedding may be contaminated by chemicals or contain natural substances that can affect the animals.

The social environment of laboratory animals is affected by other animals of the same or a different species, and by the people caring for the animals or using them. Keeping male animals of the same species together in a cage often leads to fighting and mutilation. Besides the welfare aspect this may also lead to stress and changes in metabolism, and hence changes in response to experimental conditions. Similar stress-induced metabolic changes can be provoked by animals of another species, especially in the case of prey and predator. Handling of animals, even the moving of a cage from one room to another, may cause stress reactions and changes in homeostasis.

Sick animals and animals suffering from subclinical disease have been shown to metabolize drugs abnormally because certain bacterial and viral infections affect hepatic microsomal drug-metabolizing enzymes directly, leading to decreased liver enzyme function.[1]

PHYSICAL FACTORS AFFECTING LABORATORY ANIMALS

The physical factors that most often affect laboratory animals are changes in ambient temperature and humidity, changes in the light-dark cycle, and changes in the level of noise.

SURROUNDING TEMPERATURE

The homeotherm animal can maintain a constant body temperature when subjected to external temperatures within a range specific to each species. This is known as the homeotherm zone. Within this temperature range there is a smaller range, known as the thermoneutral zone, where body temperature is regulated exclusively by variations in the flow of heat between the core of the body and the body surface, known as conduction and convection of heat. Above the thermoneutral zone body temperature is maintained by evaporative heat loss, i.e., by sweating or panting.

If the surrounding temperature falls below the thermoneutral zone, the body temperature is regulated by behavioral changes, and, if this is not sufficient, by increased metabolic rate and consequent heat production. This phenomenon is illustrated in Figure 1, showing an experiment involving three groups of mice, caged singly, in pairs, or five together. The animals are kept at -4, 4, and 20°C, and the daily feed consumption is recorded. The animals in the cold environment eat significantly more than those in the warm environment, and furthermore animals kept alone in the cage in the cold environment eat more than animals caged two or five together. The experiment demonstrates both behavioral thermoregulation — when there are several animals in a cage, they will nest close together and thus keep each other warm, and metabolic thermoregulation — the animals will eat more feed and thus increase metabolism and produce more heat.[2]

Laboratory animals are usually kept under conditions where room temperature lies between 16 and 26°C. This temperature interval, however, is well below the thermoneutral zone, and consequently changes in the surrounding temperature cause changes in the metabolic rates of the animals.

Figure 2 illustrates how enzyme activity is influenced by a temporary fall in the surrounding temperature. The activity of the liver enzymes anilin p-hydroxylase and cytochrome P-450 was measured in mice following a 9-hour cold stress (2°C). A significant increase in activity was recorded for both enzymes lasting up to one week. Considering the importance of cytochrome P-450 in the metabolism of drugs and other foreign compounds, toxicity testing using these animals during the adjustment period would be meaningless.[3]

An example (Figure 3) may illustrate the importance of this phenomenon. If the acute toxicities of chlorpromazine, amphetamine, and caffeine are examined in mice at different room temperatures, great variations are found.[4]

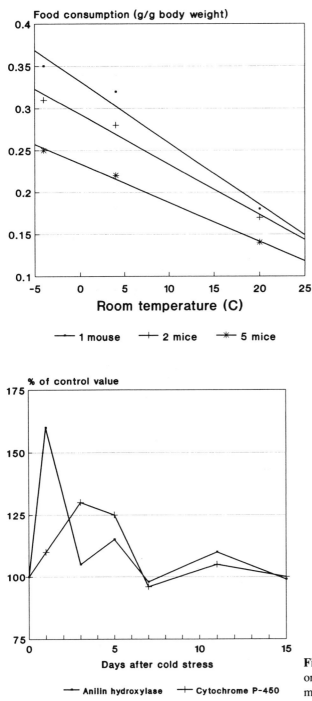

Figure 1. Feed consumption in mice kept at different room temperatures and at different cage densities.[2]

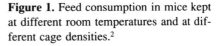

Figure 2. The effect of cold stress (9 hours at 2°C) on the level of drug-metabolizing enzymes in mice.[3]

LIGHT-DARK CYCLE

Rhythmical patterns of behavior are frequently observed in animals with periods ranging from seconds to a whole year. The shortest rhythms (less than 24 hours) are known as ultradian rhythms, examples of which are the cyclic contractions of the ruminant stomach and the heart beat. Biorhythms of about 24 hours' duration are called circadian rhythms. Alterations in body temperature, defecation, metabolic rate, and alertness are examples of circadian rhythms.[5,6] Infradian rhythms are longer than 24 hours: weekly, seasonally, or even yearly cycles. An example of an infradian rhythm is the estrous cycle.

194

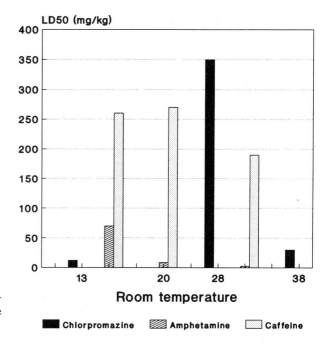

Figure 3. The acute toxicity of chlorpromazine, amphetamine and caffeine in mice kept at different room temperatures.[4]

Biorhythms are dictated by the suprachiasmatic nucleus of the anterior hypothalamus. Specialized cells of the retina feed information about day length and light intensity to the suprachiasmatic nucleus, which in response produces antidiuretic hormone and vasoactive intestinal peptide. These compounds indirectly stimulate the pineal body to produce melatonin and other hormones, which pass to the part of the hypothalamus that produces the various releasing hormones that stimulate the adenohypophysis to release ACTH, gonadotropins, growth hormone, prolactin and thyrothropin.

The estrous cycle is affected by the light-dark ratio. In rats, for example, the cycle lasts 4 days with a light-dark ratio of 12:12 hours. Changing the ratio to 16:8 hours results in an estrous cycle of 5 days, and at 22:2 hours the cycle becomes irregular, and the animals will not reproduce.

Changes in light intensity may also affect the enzyme activity of the liver, and alter the metabolism of drugs and toxic compounds. Figure 4 shows an example of this: given a fixed dose of hexobarbital at different times of the day, rats will react by sleeping different lengths of time in relation to the light-dark ratio and in relation to the activity of the oxidizing enzyme. The longest sleeping time is recorded during the light period, when enzyme activity is lowest. The highest enzyme activity is recorded in the dark period, when sleeping time is reduced by 25%. In the wild, rodents are nocturnally active animals. This observation demonstrates the importance of organizing animal experiments in such a way that compounds are given and samples taken at the same time every day.[7]

NOISE

The human ear will register sound waves of a frequency between 20 and 16,000 Hertz. Most animals, however, can hear sounds of a higher frequency: dogs will react to sound waves of 30,000 Hertz, and rats have their optimum hearing capacity at 40,000 Hertz. The noise level in animal houses may vary between <30 to 102 dB throughout the day.[8,9] Exposure to noise induces stress reactions that include neural and endocrine activation, resulting in increases in blood pressure, blood glucose, serum corticosteroids, and changes in the adrenal glands.

If rats are exposed to sound waves of 220 Hertz and 130 dB for 1 hour, the corticosterone content of the adrenals increases to three times the normal value.[10] Other experiments have demonstrated changes in white blood cell counts, increased Na^+ and K^+ excretion from the kidneys, and irregularities of the estrous cycle.[11-14]

Metabolism may also be affected by intense noise in the animal room. Figure 5 shows an experiment where rabbits were fed a fat-rich diet, and the plasma level of cholesterol was measured over a period of several months. One group of animals, exposed to a constant noise level of 102 dB, showed significantly

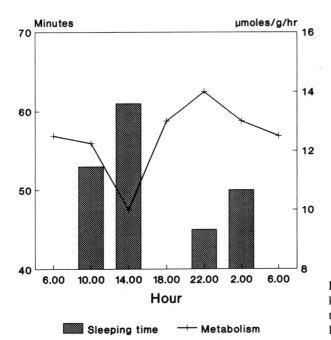

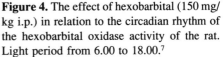

Figure 4. The effect of hexobarbital (150 mg/kg i.p.) in relation to the circadian rhythm of the hexobarbital oxidase activity of the rat. Light period from 6.00 to 18.00.[7]

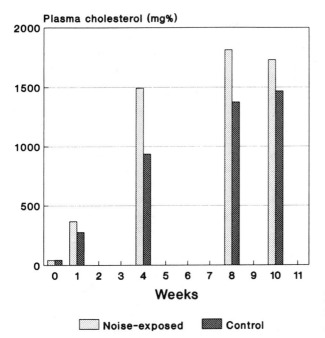

Figure 5. Plasma cholesterol levels of rabbits fed a fat-rich diet. One group was exposed to a constant noise level of 102 dB.[15]

higher cholesterol levels than control animals living in a silent environment. This example demonstrates the importance of efficient sound protection in the animal department.[15]

CHEMICAL FACTORS AFFECTING LABORATORY ANIMALS

Laboratory animals can, unintentionally or because of negligence, be exposed to chemical compounds. These may affect the health of the animals or cause changes in their metabolism. The most important sources of chemical contamination are animal excretions, bedding, feed, insecticides, and household chemicals.

196

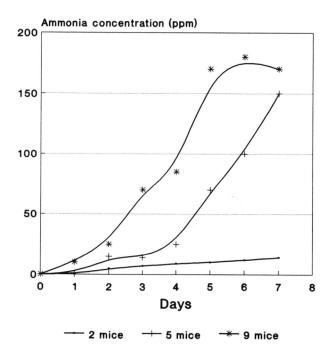

Figure 6. The daily increase in ammonia concentration in cages (26 ¥ 20 ¥ 14 cm) housing 2, 5, or 9 mice respectively.[16]

AMMONIA

Figure 6 shows the relationship between animal density and ammonia concentration in the cage. With only two mice in the cage, ammonia production is very low, whereas a density of nine animals causes the ammonia concentration to rise to toxic levels in 2 to 3 days. Frequent changing of the bedding is thus necessary to avoid pathological changes.[16] The use of filters or cage covers exerts a major influence on the composition of the air in the cages. They cause the accumulation of ammonia, carbon dioxide, and probably other gases to levels considerably higher than in cages with open covers.[17]

The threshold limit value for ammonia is 25 ppm. This level is reached after 3 to 4 days at recommended stocking density. Pathological changes are especially seen in the respiratory tract[16] and in the cornea.[18]

Reduction of the activity of drug-metabolizing liver enzymes has been reported in rats kept in cages where urine and feces were allowed to accumulate for 1 week, compared to rats kept in cages that were changed twice daily (Figure 7). The inhibition of drug metabolism in rats kept under these dirty conditions may arise from hepatic toxicity caused by increased ammonia concentration in the cages. A similar decrease in liver enzyme activity due to ammonia build-up is likely to occur in cages with protective filter tops (Figure 8).[19]

VOLATILE COMPOUNDS IN THE BEDDING

Small laboratory animals are usually kept in cages with bedding made from wood shavings. Certain types of wood contain volatile compounds that may induce enzyme systems in the liver. Alpha-pinene is a volatile compound found in spruce and pine, and cedrene and cedrol are present in red cedar wood. These compounds are strong enzyme inducers, and animals kept in cages with bedding produced from these types of soft wood have a significantly higher cytochrome P-450 activity compared to animals kept on bedding produced from hard wood such as beech and aspen or chippings made from corn cob, resulting in an increased metabolism of some foreign compounds by the liver (Figure 9).[20,21] The influence of this compound on toxicological testing is evident.[22]

INSECTICIDES

A number of insecticides may affect laboratory animals. In most cases they will increase enzyme activity and thus reduce the toxicity of test substances. In some cases, however, the reverse reaction is observed. This occurs when the metabolite rather than the compound itself is toxic. The oral threshold doses for rats for insecticides like chlordane, DDT, aldrin, and dieldrin are probably less than 10 ppm and may be as

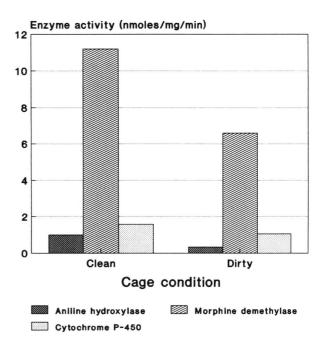

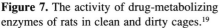

Figure 7. The activity of drug-metabolizing enzymes of rats in clean and dirty cages.[19]

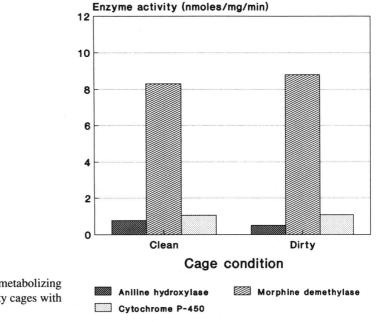

Figure 8. The activity of drug-metabolizing enzymes of rats in clean and dirty cages with filter tops.[19]

low as 1 ppm.[23] Stimulation of hepatic microsomal drug metabolism will occur in hypophysectomized or adrenalectomized rats, indicating that the effects of these insecticides are not merely via a pituitary-adrenal stress reaction, but rather associated with a proliferation of the smooth endoplasmic reticulum of the liver.[24]

SOCIAL FACTORS AFFECTING LABORATORY ANIMALS

Different types of social stress, like handling, presence of other species in the animal room, or animal density in the cage may affect the animals and consequently their response to experimental exposures.

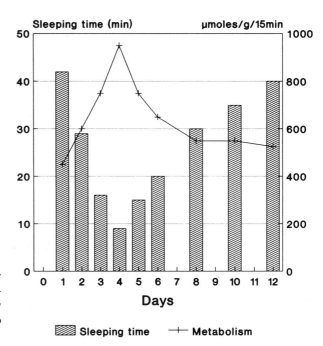

Figure 9. Hexobarbital-metabolizing activity and hexobarbital sleeping time in mice exposed to red cedar bedding from day 1 to day 3, and on hard wood bedding from day 4 to day 12.[22]

HUMAN CONTACT

The importance of a standardized handling of laboratory animals is illustrated by experiments performed by Weininger.[25] It was demonstrated that rats gentled for 10 minutes a day for 21 days following weaning had a significantly higher body weight than comparable non-gentled rats (Figure 10). This difference appeared to be due to better utilization of the feed rather than increased feed intake. Exposure to severe immobilization stress was better tolerated by the gentled animals than by the control animals. The gentled rats showed less heart muscle damage and less gastrointestinal bleeding, and their adrenal glands were smaller. This indicates that the pituitary-adrenal response to physical and non-physical stress was triggered at a higher threshold for the gentled animals, i.e., the ACTH output was smaller in these animals, thereby causing less organic change in the cardiovascular and gastrointestinal systems.

The stressor effect of handling and experimental procedures was examined by Gärtner et al.[26] The presence of a familiar attendant working in the room without touching the cages did not affect the homeostasis of the animals, while moving rats in their cages from the racks to the floor or to a table increased the serum concentrations of prolactin, corticosterone, thyroid-stimulating hormone, follicle-stimulating hormone (FSH), luteinizing hormone (LH), and thyroxine 150 to 500% compared to control animals which were decapitated within 100 seconds of entering the room. Heart rate, hematocrit, hemoglobin, and plasma protein were elevated 10 to 20% following cage movement, indicating microcirculatory shock reactions.

In the rabbit exposure to a new environment for 10 minutes resulted in a 2 to 3-fold increase in plasma corticosterone, indicating a similar susceptibility to handling stress in this species.[27] If rabbits have to be moved prior to an experiment, at least 2 hours should pass before the experimental procedure begins, to allow stress-induced reactions to normalize.[28]

Handling and immobilization of rats leads to activation of adrenal-medullary excretion of epinephrine and sympathetic neuronal release of norepinephrine. In immobilized rats plasma levels of epinephrine reach peak levels about 40-fold higher than in undisturbed animals in about 20 minutes, and then decline to about one third of the peak levels (Figure 11). The plasma level of corticosterone is similarly elevated (Figure 12).[29]

CAGE DESIGN

The acute toxicity of drugs or chemicals is affected by the type of cage in which the animals are kept. The mortality in different strains of rats after s.c. injection of morphine and anileridine was found significantly higher in sheet metal cages than in open-mesh cages due to respiratory failure, because severely depressed animals placed their noses against the metal surface of the closed cage. A more than

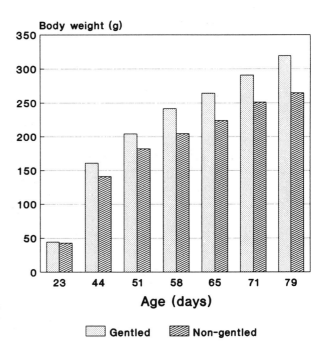

Figure 10. Mean body weights of rats. One group was gentled for 10 minutes daily for 3 weeks following weaning.[25]

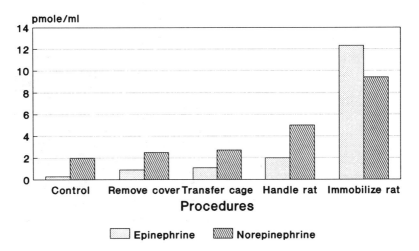

Figure 11. Plasma catecholamine levels of rats exposed to various procedures.[29]

10-fold increase in LD50 could be obtained by placing the animals in cages made entirely from wire mesh compared to animals placed in sheet metal cages.[30]

ANIMAL INTERACTIONS

The effect of animal density on behavior, physiological responses to stress, food consumption, body weight, pathological changes and drug metabolism has been thoroughly investigated. If mice are housed in groups of one, two, four, or eight per cage ($27 \times 21 \times 14$ cm) for 18 months, the more densely housed groups show markedly reduced food consumption, decreased body weight, and increased frequence of gastritis.[31] The adrenal response in mice, i.e., the plasma corticosterone concentration, increases with increased animal density. When housed in pairs, the subordinate animal has a higher adrenal weight and plasma corticosterone level than the dominant partner (Figure 13).[32]

Isolation of rats also appears to cause a stress reaction. The hepatic microsomal enzyme activity of rats isolated for 3 weeks was found to be significantly higher than for group-caged rats, and consequently hexobarbital sleep time was reduced (Figure 14). The individually caged rats can, however, adapt to their

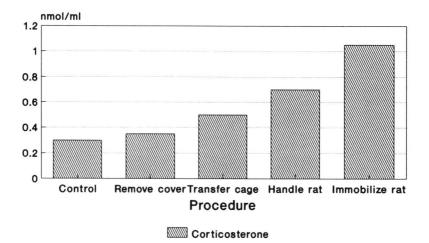

Figure 12. Plasma corticosterone levels of rats exposed to various procedures.[29]

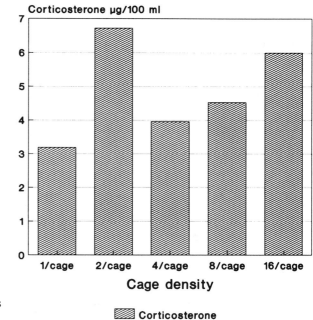

Figure 13. The plasma corticosterone levels of mice kept at different densities.[32]

environment, and after 6 weeks of isolation there was no longer any difference between individually and grouped caged animals with respect to barbiturate metabolism.[33]

The toxicity of certain compounds, e.g., amphetamine, in mice is related to the density of the animals in the cages. As the floor area per animal decreases, the acute toxicity increases. This reaction is probably due to the increased catecholamine release in the stressed animals, since it can be reduced or prevented by administration of neuroleptics or by adrenalectomy.[34]

As it appears from the above-mentioned investigations, the effect of social stress on laboratory animals is considerable and well documented, and should be taken into account in many types of experiments, especially such that involve endocrinology and metabolism of foreign compounds. Animals should always be housed in equally sized groups in standardized cages. Experimental procedures and daily care should be carried out by the same person using the same routine every day, and the animals should not be moved from the animal room — not even from the rack, unless absolutely necessary.

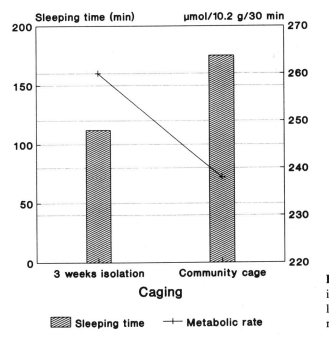

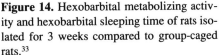

Figure 14. Hexobarbital metabolizing activity and hexobarbital sleeping time of rats isolated for 3 weeks compared to group-caged rats.[33]

CONCLUSION

These few examples of environmental impact on animal experiments indicate the magnitude of the problem. The standard of animal facilities has improved considerably over the last decades, and scientists and animal technicians are better trained in procedures and care. Most experimenters rely on animal technicians for the care of their animals, and sometimes they also rely on laboratory technicians for dosing the animals and for the collection of samples. The experienced technician is well aware of the problems of environmental impact on animal experiments, but if he or she is not informed about the type of experiment being performed, he may not consider it relevant. Therefore, it is important to inform the animal technician about the project, and together with the technician analyze all possible environmental factors that could influence the animals and have an impact on the experiment.

REFERENCES

1. Fouts, J.R., Overview of the Field: Environmental Factors Affecting Chemical or Drug Effects in Animals, *Fed. Proc.*, 35, 1162, 1976.
2. Prydchodko, H., Effect of Aggregation of Laboratory Mice (Mus musculus) on Food Intake at Different Temperatures, *Ecology*, 39, 500, 1958.
3. Shysh, A. and Noujaim, A.A., Alterations in Hepatic Microsomal Drug Metabolizing Systems in Cold Stressed Mice, *Can. J. Pharm. Sci.*, 7, 23, 1972.
4. Benti, T. and Cima, L., Einfluss der Temperatur auf die pharmakologische Wirkung des Chlorpromazins, *Arzneimittel-Forschung*, 5, 73, 1955.
5. Jilge, B., The Phase Relation Between a Circadian Rhythm of the Rabbit and Different Light:Dark Ratios, *Z. Versuchstierk.*, 26, 111, 1984.
6. Davis, W.M., Day-Night Periodicity in Pentobarbital Response of Mice and the Influence of Socio-Psychological Conditions, *Experientia*, 18, 235, 1962.
7. Nair, V. and Casper, R., The Influence of Light on Daily Rhythm in Hepatic Drug Metabolizing Enzymes in Rat, *Life Sci.*, 8, 1291, 1969.
8. Peterson, E.A., Noise and Laboratory Animals, *Lab. Anim. Sci.*, 30, 422, 1980.
9. Pfaff, J., Noise as an Environmental Problem in the Animal House, *Lab. Anim.*, 8, 347, 1974.
10. Henkin, R.I. and Knigge, K.M., Effect of Sound on the Hypothalamic-Pituitary-Adrenal Axis, *Am. J. Physiol.*, 204, 710, 1963.

11. Zondek, B. and Tamari, I., Effect of Audiogenic Stimulation on Genital Function and Reproduction, *Acta Endocrinol.*, 45, 227, 1964.

12. Stephens, D.B. and Adams, C.E., Observations on the Effects of Vibration Stress and Sound on Pregnancy, Parturition and Respiration in the Rabbit, *Lab. Anim.*, 16, 341, 1982.

13. Geber, W.F., Anderson, T.A. and van Dyne, B., Physiologic Responses of the Albino Rat to Chronic Noise Stress, *Arch. Environ. Health*, 12, 751, 1966.

14. Ogle, C.W. and Lockett, M.F., The Release of Neurohypophysal Hormone by Sound, *J. Endocrinol.*, 36, 281, 1966.

15. Friedman, M., Byers, S.O. and Brown, A.E., Plasma Lipid Responses of Rats and Rabbits to an Auditory Stimulus, *Am. J. Physiol.*, 212, 1174, 1967.

16. Gamble, M.R. and Clough, G., Ammonia Build-up in Animal Boxes and its Effect on Rat Tracheal Epithelium, *Lab. Anim.*, 10, 93, 1976.

17. Serrano, L.J., Carbon Dioxide and Ammonia in Mouse Cages: Effect of Cage Covers, Population, and Activity, *Lab. Anim. Sci.*, 21, 75, 1971.

18. Van Winkle, T.J. and Balk, M.W., Spontaneous Corneal Opacities in Laboratory Mice, *Lab. Anim. Sci.*, 36, 248, 1986.

19. Vesell, E.S., Lang, C.M., Passananti, G.T. and Tripp, S.L., Hepatic Drug Metabolism in Rats: Impairment in a Dirty Environment, *Science*, 179, 896, 1973.

20. Cunliffe-Beamer, T.L., Freeman, L.C. and Myers, D.D., Barbiturate Sleeptime in Mice Exposed to Autoclaved or Unautoclaved Wood Beddings, *Lab. Anim. Sci.*, 31, 672, 1981.

21. Nielsen, J.B., Andersen, O. and Svendsen, P., Effekt af strøelse på leverens Cytochrom P-450 system i mus, *Scand. J. Lab. Anim. Sci.*, 11, 7, 1992.

22. Vesell, E.S., Lang, C.M., White, W.J., Passananti, G.T., Hill, R.N., Clemens, T.L., Liu, D.K. and Johnson, W.D., Environmental and Genetic Factors Affecting the Response of Laboratory Animals to Drugs, *Fed. Proc.*, 35, 1125, 1976.

23. Fouts, J.R., Some Effects of Insecticides on Hepatic Microsomal Enzymes in Various Animal Species, *Rev. Can. Biol.*, 29, 377, 1970.

24. Hart, L.G. and Fouts, J.R., Studies of the Possible Mechanisms by which Chlordane Stimulates Hepatic Microsomal Drug Metabolism in the Rat, *Biochem. Pharmacol.*, 14, 263, 1965.

25. Weininger, O., The Effects of Early Experiences on Behavior and Growth Characteristics, *J. Comp. Physiol. Psychol.*, 49, 1, 1956.

26. Gärtner, K., Bütner, D., Döhler, K., Friedel, R., Lindena, J. and Trautschold, I., Stress Response of Rats to Handling and Experimental Procedures, *Lab. Anim.*, 14, 267, 1980.

27. Fenske, M., Fuchs, E. and Probst, B., Corticosteroid and Catecholamine Plasma Levels in Rabbits Stressed Repeatedly by Exposure to a Novel Environment or by Injection of (1-24) ACTH or Insulin, *Acta Endocrinol.*, 99 (suppl.246), 110, 1982.

28. Knudtzon, J., Plasma Levels of Glucagon, Insulin, Glucose and Free Fatty Acids in Rabbits During Laboratory Handling Procedures, *Z. Versuchstierk.*, 26, 123, 1984.

29. Kvetnansky, R., Sun, C.L., Lake, C.R., Thoa, N., Torda, T. and Kopin, I.J., Effect of Handling and Forced Immobilization on Rat Plasma Levels of Epinephrine, Norepinephrine, and Dopamine-beta-Hydroxylase, *Endocrinology*, 103, 1868, 1978.

30. Winter, C.A. and Flataker, L., Cage Design as a Factor Influencing Acute Toxicity of Respiratory Depressant Drugs in Rats, *Toxicol. Appl. Pharmacol.*, 4, 650, 1962.

31. Chvédoff, M., Clarke, M.R., Irisarri, E., Faccini, J.M. and Monro, A.M., Effects of Housing Conditions on Food Intake, Body Weight and Spontaneous Lesions in Mice. A Review of the Literature and Results of an 18-Month Study, *Food. Cosmet. Toxicol.*, 18, 517, 1980.

32. Brain, P.F. and Nowell, N.W., The Effects of Differential Grouping on Endocrine Function of Mature Male Albino Mice, *Physiol. Behav.*, 5, 907, 1970.

33. Dairman, W. and Balazt, T., Comparison of Liver Microsome Enzyme Systems and Barbiturate Sleep Times in Rats Caged Individually or Communally, *Biochem. Pharmacol.*, 19, 951, 1970.

34. Doggett, N.S., Reno, H. and Spencer, P.S.J., A Comparison of the Acute Toxicity of Some Centrally Acting Drugs Measured under Crowded and Uncrowded Conditions, *Toxicol. Appl. Pharmacol.*, 39, 141, 1977.

Chapter 15

Experimental Design and Statistical Evaluation

Aage Vølund

CONTENTS

INTRODUCTION

The general desire to reduce the number of animals in biological experimentation can be fulfilled in a rational way by means of statistical methods for design and analysis. With a specifically formulated experimental objective and utilization of prior knowledge, it is possible to determine the optimal number of animals in each experimental group, in the sense that using more animals would be an inefficient waste, while fewer animals would make the experiment inconclusive. More advanced methods for design of experiments and statistical data analysis offer additional possibilities for reducing the number of animals and/or obtaining more information from an experiment of a given size. These include sequential methods, multifactorial designs, block designs and regression methods to reduce the effect of the inherent biological variation.

It is not possible in a short text to give a complete coverage of the statistical methods which are useful for design and analysis of animal experiments. Some general knowledge of basic statistical methods[1,2] will be assumed or briefly described, but the main focus will be on explaining when and how it is possible to improve the efficiency of experimental work through the use of suitable statistical methods. This will be supported by examples and references to more detailed descriptions of the methods. A large number of packages of statistical computer programs are available for data analysis and — to a lesser extent — for design of experiments. However, it is important to realize that once the design has been determined, the method of analysis cannot be chosen freely. Thus, a correct interpretation of the results requires an understanding of the interplay between possibilities and limitations of the design and the statistical analysis.

DESCRIPTIVE METHODS

A fundamental characteristic of a set of data is its size, i.e., the number of observations, and counting may be regarded as the primary statistical task. Next comes classification into groups and ordering of the data, whereas calculations of means, proportions, standard deviations, coefficients of variation, etc., represent fairly advanced arithmetic operations, which were laborious to carry out on large data sets before the advent of the computer. These methods imply a data reduction where a (large) number of observations such as a collection of numerical measurements are summarized as a few characteristic values such as a mean and range.

The idea of describing a large number (or just a handful) of observations by means of a few numbers, for example their mean value, is presumably motivated by a genuine desire to communicate some essential information in a more simple, practical and efficient manner than by presenting all the individual values. In addition there may also be the notion involved that the mean is a more representative value than any single observation one might choose from the data set. The latter is linked to the experience that a

0-8493-4378-X/94/$0.00+$.50
© 1994 by CRC Press Inc.

mean value will exhibit less variability than individual values. However, in addition to describing a set of data by its mean value it is equally important to characterize the variability of the observations. To this end one may quote the range, i.e., the minimum and the maximum, or the standard deviation. Thus, we may distinguish between statistics that describe the systematic (non-random) properties of the data and those that describe the random variability. From a practical point of view one is inclined to focus on the non-random measures and regard the presence of random variation as a nuisance. However, from a statistical point of view both are important for extracting useful information and necessary for drawing reliable conclusions.

With large data sets, say 50 to 100 observations or more, which are not often obtained in animal experimentation, the standard way to describe the variability is to group the observations into successive intervals of equal length, count the number in each group, and calculate the frequency distribution. Its graphical representation is the histogram, which characterizes the distribution of the observations. By adding the frequencies successively from the lowest to the highest interval the sum distribution is obtained. This allows determination of percentiles, e.g., the 10% percentile is the value for which 10% of the observations fall below and consequently, 90% above. The 50% percentile (the median) is a useful measure of the midpoint of the distribution. The so-called interquartile range, being the difference between the 75% and the 25% percentiles, is a useful simple measure of the variability of the data. Figure 1 shows an example of a descriptive analysis of the body weight of 80 rabbits.

These classical descriptive methods have in recent years been supplemented by a number of useful primarily graphical methods known as exploratory data analysis.[3] The methods are included in some statistical computer packages and are being increasingly used. Figure 2 illustrates some of these methods applied to the same data set as in Figure 1.

The stem and leaf plot makes it easy to determine the values of the median, quartiles and other percentiles. The methods described in Figure 2 are also useful for comparative description of several data sets. Another objective of descriptive methods besides data reduction is detection of relations or structures in data, e.g., deviations from homogeneity or purely random variation. A plot of the observations versus the order in which they were obtained, e.g., a time series plot, may be very useful to reveal interesting patterns or anomalous behavior. It may also indicate the presence of errors in the data, which should be checked and possibly corrected before any further analysis. Thus, descriptive methods are also useful for quality control of the data. The scatter plot of paired observations is undoubtedly the most widely used method for exploring relations between variables. This plot should precede calculation of any numerical measure of the association such as the correlation coefficient.

TESTS OF HYPOTHESES

Reading scientific journals may give the impression that statistical tests of significance are the most important and widespread class of statistical methods in use. The results of such tests are usually communicated in terms of P-values, like $P<0.05$ or $P = 0.003$. A typical statement may be: The difference in mean value between the control and treated group (of animals) was statistically significant, $P<0.05$. What does this mean? First it does not mean that the probability of no difference is less than 0.05. A correct and complete description may run as follows: a so-called null hypothesis H_0 has been set up, stating that the means of two groups are equal: $\mu_1 = \mu_2$. Under this and certain other assumptions the probability of observing a difference equal to or larger than the actual difference can then be calculated. This probability is the P-value. If it is relatively small, either a correspondingly rare event has been observed, or the null hypothesis may be regarded as false. If the P-value is sufficiently small, the investigator (and other scientists) rejects the null hypothesis and concludes that there is a real (true) difference between the means, i.e., the alternative hypothesis H_1: $\mu_1 \neq \mu_2$ is accepted. Apparently most researchers begin to agree about this conclusion when $P<0.05$. This is, however, an empirical limit which cannot be justified otherwise. With this decision rule there is a risk of being wrong in 5% of the cases, i.e., of committing an error of the first kind. The probability of this error is called the significance level α of the test. Other significance levels typically used in statistical tables are $\alpha = 0.01$ and 0.001. There is, however, a tendency to report the actual P-value rather than the standard significance levels, which gives the reader a better background for judging the significance of the test result.

Tables 1 and 2 list a number of frequently used statistical tests for hypotheses about means (μ and variances (σ^2) associated with one or two samples. The sample mean $\bar{x}$ and variance s^2 are defined in Table 1. The corresponding values for two samples $\bar{x}_1$ and $\bar{x}_2$ and s_1^2 and s_2^2 are defined in complete

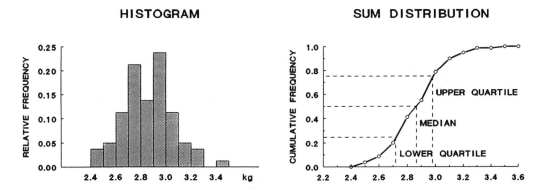

Figure 1. Distribution of body weight of 80 rabbits.

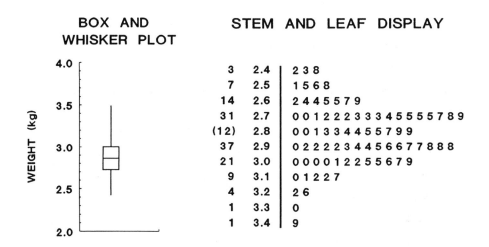

Figure 2. The box shows the median and quartiles and the whiskers the range of the body weight of the 80 rabbits. The stem gives the first 2 digits of the weight and the leaves show the third — one digit per rabbit. The numbers to the left of the stem give the number of rabbits cumulated from below and above while the number in the mid-class is shown in brackets.

analogy, and it is shown how the two sample variances are combined to a single estimate. These tests are all derived for observations that are statistically independent and follow a Gaussian (or normal) distribution. Independence means, generally speaking, that the random variation associated with any single observation has no relation to the random variation of any other observation. Fulfillment of this requirement may be achieved in experimental studies by adherence to the principle of randomization (see the section on experimental design). In non-experimental studies independence can be achieved by random sampling from the population in question. Tables of the percentiles corresponding to standard α-values for the u- (standard Gaussian), the t- (Student's), the χ^2- and the F-distribution can be found in almost any textbook on statistical methods. The P-values may be obtained from sufficiently detailed tables of the standard distributions or provided by computer program packages.

An error of the second kind is when the null hypothesis is incorrectly accepted. The probability of committing such an error obviously depends on the size of the true difference between the two means: $\Delta=|\mu_1-\mu_2|$. The larger Δ is, the smaller is the error probability. Figure 3 shows schematically the 4 possibilities in the test situation. Figure 3 also illustrates the probability of making the correct decision as a function of the difference between the means. This is the so-called power function of the test, which is 1 minus the probability of a type 2 error. Note that when the difference approaches zero, the power approaches the significance level. Apart from its dependence on the true difference the power will for a given difference increase with increasing significance level and sample sizes. Examples of this dependence are also shown in Figure 3. This forms the basis for determination of sample sizes that are optimal

Table 1: One and two sample u- and t-tests for means based on the normal distribution

Assumptions	H_0	Test Statistic	Reject H_0 ,if
σ known	$\mu = \mu_0$	$u = \dfrac{\bar{x} - \mu_0}{\sigma/\sqrt{n}}, \quad \bar{x} = \Sigma x_i / n$	$\|u\| > u_{1-\alpha/2}$
σ unknown	$\mu = \mu_0$	$t = \dfrac{\bar{x} - \mu_0}{s/\sqrt{n}}, \quad s^2 = \dfrac{\Sigma(x_i - \bar{x})^2}{n-1}$	$\|t\| > t_{1-\alpha/2}(n-1)$
(σ_1, σ_2) known	$\mu_1 = \mu_2$	$u = \dfrac{\bar{x}_1 - \bar{x}_2}{\sqrt{(\sigma_1^2/n_1) + (\sigma_2^2/n_2)}}$	$\|u\| > u_{1-\alpha/2}$
$\sigma_1 = \sigma_2 = \sigma$ unknown	$\mu_1 = \mu_2$	$t = \dfrac{\bar{x}_1 - \bar{x}_2}{s\sqrt{(1/n_1) + (1/n_2)}}$ $s^2 = \dfrac{s_1^2(n_1 - 1) + s_2^2(n_2 - 1)}{n_1 + n_2 - 2}$	$\|t\| > t_{1-\alpha/2}(n_1 + n_2 - 2)$

Table 2: One and two sample χ^2- and F-tests for variances based on the normal distribution

Assumptions	H_0	Test Statistic	Reject H_0 ,if
μ known	$\sigma^2 = \sigma_0^2$	$\chi^2 = \dfrac{\Sigma(x_i - \mu)^2}{\sigma_0^2}$	$\chi^2 < \chi^2_{\alpha/2}(n)$ or $\chi^2 > \chi^2_{1-\alpha/2}(n)$
μ unknown	$\sigma^2 = \sigma_0^2$	$\chi^2 = \dfrac{\Sigma(x_i - \bar{x})^2}{\sigma_0^2}$	$\chi^2 < \chi^2_{\alpha/2}(n-1)$ or $\chi^2 > \chi^2_{1-\alpha/2}(n-1)$
(μ_1, μ_2) known	$\sigma_1^2 = \sigma_2^2$	$F = \dfrac{\Sigma(x_{1i} - \mu_1)^2/n_1}{\Sigma(x_{2i} - \mu_2)^2/n_2}$	$F < F_{\alpha/2}(n_1, n_2)$ or $F > F_{1-\alpha/2}(n_1, n_2)$
(μ_1, μ_2) unknown	$\sigma_1^2 = \sigma_2^2$	$F = \dfrac{\Sigma(x_{1i} - \bar{x}_1)^2/(n_1 - 1)}{\Sigma(x_{2i} - \bar{x}_2)^2/(n_2 - 1)}$	$F < F_{\alpha/2}(n_1 - 1, n_2 - 1)$ or $F > F_{1-\alpha/2}(n_1 - 1, n_2 - 1)$

in the sense that with a given (high) probability they will lead to rejection of the null hypothesis if the true difference is equal to or larger than the value specified. This method for calculation of sample sizes applies to other types of statistical tests, and the reader is referred to standard textbooks on statistical methods and design of experiments, which give details and tables for determination of sample sizes based on power specifications.[4,5]

It follows that the power is a measure of the sensitivity of the test, and if there is a choice among several tests for testing the same hypothesis the most powerful test is normally preferred. For a given significance level and a given power at a specified difference Δ, expressed relative to the (known) standard deviation σ, i.e., Δ/s, is specified, it is possible to calculate the corresponding sample sizes. These are necessary and sufficient to achieve the desired protection against errors of the first and second kind. Furthermore, it can be shown that it is optimal to have the same number of observations in both groups.

In practice it is difficult to ensure that observations are distributed normally, especially with small group sizes, say below 50. There exist a variety of statistical tests for assessment of normality, but the power of these tests becomes very low for the sample sizes usually encountered. The descriptive methods mentioned in the preceding section may, however, indicate whether there are deviations from normality, such as skew distributions or mixtures of distributions. It is sometimes possible by means of a suitable transformation of the observations to obtain normality. Nevertheless, there may be situations where it is not possible to justify normality of the raw or transformed data. In such cases it is advisable to apply a

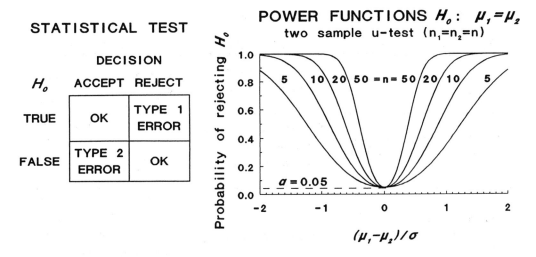

Figure 3. Statistical test and power function.

so-called non-parametric or distribution free test. There exist a number of such tests which supplement the tests listed in Table 1. However, it is important to remember that the assumption of independence must still be fulfilled. Table 3 lists some of the most widely used non-parametric tests based on the ranking of the observations. Many more can be found in the special literature.[6]

The significance of the sign test can be evaluated by means of a table of the binomial distribution. $SR_a(n)$ refers to the special table for the Wilcoxon signed rank test, and $MW_a(n_1, n_2)$ refers to the table value for the Mann Whitney Wilcoxon rank test. The approximative u-test can, however, often be used with sufficient approximation.

Since non-parametric tests are valid under more general assumptions than those based on the Gaussian distribution, it might be preferable only to use non-parametric methods. There are at least three reasons for not adopting this apparently safe approach to statistics in general. First, it is well known that the non-parametric tests have less power than the standard tests when the assumptions for both types of tests are fulfilled. In fact, for very small sample sizes the standard non-parametric tests may have zero power, which means that they cannot reject the null hypothesis at all. Second, studies have shown that the standard tests are quite robust against deviations from normality. The robustness usually means that the significance levels are not changed severely, while the power sometimes falls considerably. Hence, the standard tests may be regarded as conservative. Third, the null hypothesis and especially the alternative hypotheses are more difficult to specify for the non-parametric tests. For example, in a two-sample test the null hypothesis may be formulated as equality of the corresponding distributions, but it may be very difficult or arbitrary to define alternatives for assessment of the power of the non-parametric test, and it may be difficult to understand and describe what caused a rejection of the null hypothesis.

Table 4 shows two examples of application of the standard two-sample t-test (Student's test) and the corresponding rank sum test (Mann Whitney Wilcoxon's test) to the same data. The purpose in both examples was to compare the results from groups 1 and 2. The x_{ji}-values represent measurements of antibody binding (expressed in percent) in sera from groups of 10 rabbits immunized with different antigens. Note that identical (tied) observations are assigned the average rank. In the first case both tests can be used with similar results, but the t-test should be preferred due to its higher power. In the second case the assumption of Gaussian distributions with the same variance is apparently not fulfilled, due to a single "outlier", which of course cannot be discarded for that reason only. The t-test is therefore not applicable, while the assumptions for applying the rank sum test are still fulfilled. It is seen that the (unreliable) t-test would not have led to the same conclusion in this case as the rank sum test.

Statistical tests appear to be used for two different purposes in data analysis. In the first place tests are used for making decisions about the appropriate statistical model, primarily to check its validity or to see whether it can be simplified. Ideally the situation would then be that the assumptions for the subsequent statistical test(s) corresponding to the scientific objective of the investigation can be regarded as fulfilled. Thus, the second use of statistical tests is to provide an objective basis for drawing conclusions with regard to the objective of the study. As an example one may, as in Table 4, test the assumption of equal variances for two samples before applying the t-test to test the equality of the means according to the

Table 3: One and two sample non-parametric tests

Type of Test	H_0	Test Statistic	Reject H_0 ,if
Sign test	*median*$=\theta_0$	$x=$*number of obs.*$<\theta_0$ $n=$*number of obs.*$\neq\theta_0$	$\sum_0^x \binom{n}{i}0.5^i <\alpha/2 \ or \ >1-\alpha/2$ *(binomial distribution)*
Wilcoxon signed rank sum test	*position (mean)*$=\mu_0$	$S_-=\Sigma rank\lvert x_i-\mu_0\rvert; \ x_i<\mu_0$ $S_+=\Sigma rank\lvert x_i-\mu_0\rvert; \ x_i>\mu_0$ $n=$*number of obs.*$\neq\mu_0$	$S=\min(S_-,S_+)<SR_{\alpha/2}(n)$ *or approx. for* $n\geq 10$ $\dfrac{\lvert S-n(n+1)/4\rvert}{\sqrt{n(n+1)(2n+1)}}>u_{1-\alpha/2}$
Mann Whitney Wilcoxon rank sum test	*equal position* $\mu_1=\mu_2$	$x_{1j}, \ j=1,...,n_1 \quad x_{2j}, \ j=1,...,n_2$ $S_1=\sum_{j=1}^{n_1} rank(x_{ij}); \ n_1\leq n_2$ *(rank all obs. as one group)*	$S_1<MW_{\alpha/2}(n_1,n_2) \ or$ $S_1>MW_{1-\alpha/2}(n_1,n_2)$ *or approx. for* $n_1\geq 5$ $\dfrac{\lvert S_1-n_1(n_1+n_2+1)/2\rvert}{\sqrt{n_1n_2(n_1+n_2+1)/12}}>u_{1-\alpha/2}$

objective of the study. From a theoretical point of view it can of course be argued that both tests are concerned with inference about the model. The distinction is therefore dependent upon the scientific objective(s) of the experiment or the data analysis which can be translated to statistical tests of specific hypotheses. It follows that in the reporting of results the primary focus is on the outcome of these tests, while the tests of the model assumptions are usually not or only very briefly mentioned.

ESTIMATION AND MODELS

In the previous section we have already described tests of means and variances without any explicit definition of these terms. The cumulative distribution function $F(x)$ of a random variable X describes the probability of observing a value of X less than or equal to x, i.e., $P(X\leq x) = F(x)$. The density function is the derivative: $f(x) = dF(x)/dx$. The mean of X is defined as: $E(X) = \int xf(x)dx$, and its variance: $V(X) = \int(x-E(X))^2f(x)dx$. The integration is over the domain of x. The square root of the variance is the standard deviation $s(X)$. A distribution function is determined by certain parameters. For example, the density of the normal or Gaussian distribution $f(x) = (\sigma\sqrt{2\pi})^{-1} exp(-[(x-\mu)/\sigma]^2/2)$ depends on two parameters μ and s. The mean and variance of a distribution will therefore depend on the parameters. This dependence is very simple in the case of the normal distribution, where $E(X) = \mu$ and $V(X) = s^2$.

A fundamental task of statistical analysis is to estimate the parameters from a sample of observations from a distribution whose parameter values are unknown. In the case of the normal distribution the sample mean would intuitively be used as an estimate of μ and the sample variance s^2 as an estimate of σ^2. There is, however, a well-developed statistical theory of estimation, the method of maximum likelihood, which leads to estimates of parameters that have desirable optimal properties, e.g., minimum variance. This theory states that the sample mean and variance are the "best" estimates that can be found for the parameters of the normal distribution. Note that such estimates are also subject to random variation, i.e., random variables with certain distributions. For example, in the case of the normal distribution the sample mean $\bar{x}$ corresponds to a random variable $\bar{x} = \Sigma x_i/n$, which is also normally distributed with mean μ, but with a smaller variance σ^2/n.

In addition to finding the "best" possible value for a parameter it may also be desirable to determine the set or range of values that in some sense is in agreement with the (raw) data. This has been formalized as determination of confidence sets or intervals. The underlying principle for defining a confidence set is the testing of a statistical null hypothesis, say $H_0: \mu = \mu_0$, the $(1-\alpha)$-confidence set is then the set of

Table 4: Examples of F-test, t-test and rank sum test

Number	Example 1 Group 1 x_{1i}	Rank	Group 2 x_{2i}	Rank	Example 2 Group 1 x_{1i}	Rank	Group 2 x_{2i}	Rank
1	30	3	32	4.5	18	19	3	9
2	45	11.5	37	9	5	10	1	3
3	35	8	27	1	2	6.5	1	3
4	49	14	72	19	59	20	13	18
5	34	6.5	47	13	10	16	2	6.5
6	60	17	65	18	10	16	2	6.5
7	57	15.5	57	15.5	9	13.5	1	3
8	28	2	32	4.5	9	13.5	10	16
9	39	10	75	20	7	11.5	2	6.5
10	34	6.5	45	11.5	7	11.5	0	1
$\bar{x}$	41.10		48.90		13.60		3.50	
s	11.18		17.48		16.48		4.35	
rank sum		94		116		137.5		72.5
F-test $H_0: \sigma_1^2 = \sigma_2^2$	$F = 11.18^2/17.48^2 = 0.41$, $F_{0.025}(9,9) = 0.25$ $F_{0.975}(9,9) = 4.03$, Accept H_0 $s^2 = (9 \cdot 11.18^2 + 9 \cdot 17.48^2)/18 = 14.34^2$				$F = 16.48^2/4.35^2 = 14.34$, $F_{0.025}(9,9) = 0.25$ $F_{0.975}(9,9) = 4.03$, Reject H_0 Don't calculate s^2 ($= 12.05^2$)			
t-test $H_0: \mu_1 = \mu_2$	$t = |41.10 - 48.90|/[14.34/\sqrt{(2/10)}] = 1.19$ $t_{0.975}(18) = 2.10$, Accept H_0				Assumptions for calculation of t-test are not fulfilled ($t = 1.87$)			
rank sum test $H_0: \mu_1 = \mu_2$	$MW_{0.025}(10,10) = 78$, $MW_{0.975}(10,10) = 132$ Accept H_0, (approx. u-test: $u = 0.83$)				$MW_{0.025}(10,10) = 78$, $MW_{0.975}(10,10) = 132$ reject H_0, (approx. u-test: $u = 2.46$)			

values that leads to acceptance of H_0 at significance level α. Table 5 gives formulas for calculation of confidence intervals in some common one- or two-sample situations. Figure 4 shows some examples of calculation of confidence intervals from real data.

Since point and interval estimation represents statistical inference about parameters or functions of parameters, it is obvious that non-parametric statistical methods cannot contribute much to these activities. It should, however, be mentioned that it is possible to determine a confidence interval for the median (and other percentiles) of an unspecified distribution using the sign test (and modifications thereof). It is also possible to determine confidence intervals for some unspecified "position parameter" based on the signed one-sample rank sum test or for the shift in position by means of the corresponding two-sample test.[6] It may, however, be difficult to interpret what such non-parametric confidence intervals represent from a practical point of view.

It is common practice to report mean values with some ± error estimate. This error may be the estimated standard deviation s which is often denoted SD (see Table 1). This value estimates the magnitude of the variation of the (individual) observations and describes the variability of the population from which the observations are sampled. The coefficient of variation CV, which is defined as $CV = s/\bar{x}$, is also frequently reported, usually expressed in percent. Although these error estimates become more precise as the number of observations is increased, they are in principle independent of the sample size and therefore do not reflect the precision of the estimated mean.

The standard deviation of the mean of n observations is $s/\sqrt{n}$ and to avoid confusion with SD it is preferably referred to as the standard error (of the mean), i.e., SE or SEM. Because the ± notation does not tell whether the estimates reported are SD or SEM, it should be avoided unless special efforts are made to define its meaning. It is preferable to report the mean with SD or SEM plus, of course, the number of observations. The choice between SD or SEM depends on whether it is the variability of the individual observations (the population distribution) or the variability of the mean (the parameter estimate) which is most relevant to emphasize. In the first case SD is given, and in the second SEM or SE is given. Even though values for SEM or SE describe the precision of the associated means, they are nevertheless

Table 5: Confidence intervals for means based on the normal distribution

Assumptions	$(1-\alpha)$-confidence interval
Interval: μ σ known	$[\bar{x}-u_{1-\alpha/2}\,\sigma/\sqrt{n}\,;\,\bar{x}+u_{1-\alpha/2}\,\sigma/\sqrt{n}]\,;\,\bar{x}=\Sigma x_i/n$
Interval: μ σ unknown	$[\bar{x}-t_{1-\alpha/2}(n-1)s/\sqrt{n}\,;\,\bar{x}+t_{1-\alpha/2}(n-1)/\sqrt{n}]\,;\,s^2=\Sigma(x_i-\bar{x})^2/(n-1)$
Interval: $\mu_1-\mu_2$ (σ_1,σ_2) known	$[\bar{x_1}-\bar{x_2}-u_{1-\alpha/2}\sqrt{\dfrac{\sigma_1^2}{n_1}+\dfrac{\sigma_2^2}{n_2}}\,;\,\bar{x_1}-\bar{x_2}+u_{1-\alpha/2}\sqrt{\dfrac{\sigma_1^2}{n_1}+\dfrac{\sigma_2^2}{n_2}}]$
Interval: $\mu_1-\mu_2$ $\sigma_1=\sigma_2=\sigma$ unknown	$[\bar{x_1}-\bar{x_2}-t_{1-\alpha/2}(n_1+n_2-2)s\sqrt{\dfrac{n_1+n_2}{n_1n_2}}\,;\,\bar{x_1}-\bar{x_2}+t_{1-\alpha/2}(n_1+n_2-2)s\sqrt{\dfrac{n_1+n_2}{n_1n_2}}]$ $s^2=\dfrac{s_1^2(n-1)+s_2^2(n-2)}{n_1+n_2-1}$

insufficient to allow a precise probability statement about the precision of the parameter in question. To achieve this the precision of the SE itself must be included in the assessment. This is exactly what is done by calculation of confidence intervals as described in Table 5. Moreover, confidence intervals are very useful to supplement tests of significance, especially when no significant difference is found, because in that case the confidence interval will provide a measure of how large the difference could have been without reaching statistical significance. The size of the confidence interval is also useful to judge the scientific or practical "significance" of a statistically significant difference, since a small and unimportant difference associated with an even smaller confidence interval may be highly significant only from statistical point of view.

So far we have only considered very simple statistical models for observed data, for example that the observations grouped as two samples have the same or different means and/or variances. Data may be analyzed according to models with a more complicated mean value structure as well as a structure in the variances. In this way we are again focusing on a description of the systematic variation in the data (mean value structure) and the random variation as separate entities. In the following section such statistical models will be presented in connection with statistically designed experiments.

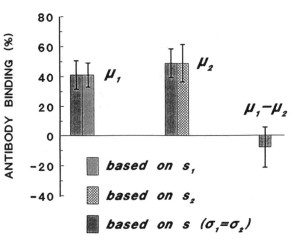

95% CONFIDENCE INTERVALS
Data from Table 4, Example 1

Figure 4. The confidence intervals are calculated according to the equations in Table 5. The intervals based on the common standard deviation are preferable in this example.

Table 6: Death rates from pneumonia in 1849

Treatment	Number of patients	Number of deaths	Percent deaths
Blood-letting	85	17	20.0%
Emetic powder	106	22	20.7%
Placebo	189	14	7.4%

DESIGN OF EXPERIMENTS

It has already been mentioned that statistical methods make it possible to determine sample sizes based on power specifications. This makes it possible to design experiments of optimal size in the same way. A more fundamental aim is to ensure that the experiment is valid in the sense that it is possible to draw a valid conclusion with respect to its objective. It is, for example, well known that in order to determine whether a given treatment has an effect in an animal experiment one must compare the results from a group of animals receiving the actual treatment with the results from a control group treated in the same way except for the specific treatment, e.g., by using a placebo. It is, however, apparently not so widely recognized that the principle of randomization is essential for drawing a valid conclusion about a causal relation between the treatment and the observed effect. This principle guarantees that effects of all other factors conceivably able to cause a difference between the treatment group and the control group can only be due to random variation, whose probability of occurrence or interference (i.e., a type 1 error) is controlled by the significance level of the statistical test. The following example may serve to clarify the importance of randomization.

In 1849 the Polish-Austrian physician Joseph Dietl reported results of treating three groups of pneumonia patients with either the standard treatments of that time, which were blood-letting and emetic powder, or with a (placebo) treatment consisting of confinement to bed and a light diet.[7] The results are shown in Table 6. They can be analyzed formally by statistical methods described later on, but it is quite obvious that the patients in the placebo group did much better than those given the intervention treatments, and these results contributed to the abandoning of the old-fashioned and ineffective treatments. The point is, however, that the conclusion about the relative efficacy of the treatments is strictly dependent on the (implicit) assumption that the patients in the three groups are comparable. Only a formal randomization could have ensured that the patients in the three groups would have reacted identically — apart from random variation — if they had received the same treatment. If, for example, the placebo treatment was preferably given to the less ill patients, it would not be possible to draw any valid conclusion from this study.

In addition to the randomization principle and the optimization of size there are two other important advantages to be gained with designed experiments. These are the reduction of the effects of experimental variability and the possibility to analyze effects of several experimental factors in the same experiment. In order to give an introduction to these methods it is useful to introduce some general notational concepts. First of all it is assumed that the purpose of an experiment is to compare and assess the effects of two or more treatments on a response variable. The simplest experiment will thus have two treatments, say a test (or active) treatment and a control (or placebo) treatment. We may also say that this experiment has a single experimental factor with two levels, while the example in Table 6 had a single factor with three levels. The levels of a factor may be qualitative, such as in the medical example, or they may be quantitative, for example representing different doses of the same drug.

An experimental design is thus conceptually defined as the combination of the experimental treatments and the experimental units. For example, two treatments may each be applied to 10 experimental units to give a design with a total of 20 unit experiments. A unit experiment — not to be confused with an experimental unit — consists of the combination of a single treatment with a single experimental unit. The principle of randomization should of course be used for assigning the treatments to the experimental units. While the concept of an experimental treatment has a clear intuitive meaning, it is less apparent what constitutes an experimental unit. It might be thought to correspond to the experimental animal or the physical material which is used for carrying out a unit experiment; however, the experimental unit includes everything that can affect the response of the experiment apart from the treatment itself. Thus,

212

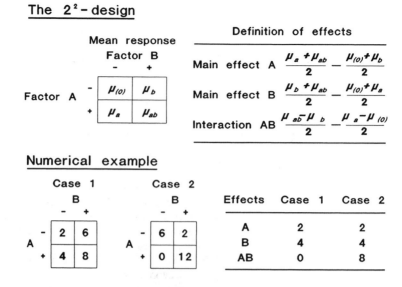

The 2^2 – design

Mean response

Factor B

Factor A		B −	B +
	−	$\mu_{(0)}$	μ_b
	+	μ_a	μ_{ab}

Definition of effects

Main effect A $\dfrac{\mu_a + \mu_{ab}}{2} - \dfrac{\mu_{(0)} + \mu_b}{2}$

Main effect B $\dfrac{\mu_b + \mu_{ab}}{2} - \dfrac{\mu_{(0)} + \mu_a}{2}$

Interaction AB $\dfrac{\mu_{ab} - \mu_b}{2} - \dfrac{\mu_a - \mu_{(0)}}{2}$

Numerical example

Case 1

B

A		−	+
	−	2	6
	+	4	8

Case 2

B

A		−	+
	−	6	2
	+	0	12

Effects	Case 1	Case 2
A	2	2
B	4	4
AB	0	8

Figure 5. The 2^2-factorial design. Definition of main effects and interaction. The numerical example shows no interaction in case 1 and large interaction in case 2.

the experimental unit comprises all experimental conditions, all steps in the performance and measuring method, the apparatus and measuring instruments, influences from the operator, effects of the environment, as well as the physical and biological materials involved in the experiment.

It is straightforward to extend the structure of the treatments to multifactorial designs. Suppose two drugs are to be tested at three and four dose levels, respectively. This could be carried out in a complete factorial design comprising all 12 combinations of the factor levels or in some incomplete design. The so-called "one-factor-at-a-time" design is an incomplete design often seen used in practice. This design allows only determination of separate effects of the factors, whereas the combined effects of two or more factors cannot be predicted. The use of a complete factorial design, however, enables estimation and testing of interaction (or non-additive) effects of combinations of the factors. Consider for example the design with two factors A and B each with two levels, say a low (-) and a high (+) level. Figure 5 gives the definitions of the main effects and the interaction effect as well how these effects are estimated in this 2×2 or 2^2-design. In the next section it will briefly be explained how analysis of variance is used for systematic testing of the various effects.

Suppose a simple experiment is to be carried out with only one factor at two levels. To achieve sufficient power for the test of (no effect of) the factor it may, for example, have been calculated that 8 replicates, i.e., a total of 16 observations, are required. In such a situation it may be considered "good experimental practice" to study the effect of additional factors rather than performing the 8 identical unit experiments at each level of the single factor. A second factor could be introduced at two levels and each treatment of the 2×2 design is then repeated four times. A third factor might also be introduced and each treatment is still repeated twice. In this way it becomes possible to test and estimate the effects of several factors in a single experiment of the same size as required for studying only a single factor. Moreover, the power for the tests of the various factors is not reduced appreciably, and finally the multifactorial design enables assessment of interactions between two or more factors. Thus, it can be concluded that multifactorial designs are more efficient and provide more information than the traditional "one-factor-at-a-time" approach.

It should be mentioned — with some support from theoretical considerations as well as practical experience — that interactions of a high order are unlikely. This may be utilized in the design to introduce more factors. If a fourth factor is introduced into the example just mentioned, there are no longer any replicates for estimation of the variance, but if it can be assumed that interaction terms between three or four factors only represent random variation, a complete analysis of all (4) main effects and (6) interactions between two factors can still be carried out. This process may even be extended to include more factors than can be estimated separately. Such designs are termed fractional factorial designs. Although these designs may not be able to identify the effects of all interesting main effects and interactions, the analysis can show that certain groups of effects are present or absent, and it is possible to add on additional fractional designs to identify the individual significant effects. It is, however, not possible here to give a more detailed description of this sequential use of fractional factorial designs to screen for effects of many factors with a limited experimental effort. The reader is advised to consult textbooks on experimental design, which also provide details on multifactorial designs with more than two factor levels.[4,5]

Until now we have only been concerned with the (factorial) structure of the experimental treatments, while the experimental units have been regarded as homogeneous or indistinguishable. Therefore, a completely random allocation of treatments to experimental units is performed. In practice, however, there is often some heterogeneity or structure present in the experimental units. Although a completely randomized design may still be used, and can lead to valid analysis and conclusions, there may be considerable advantages to be gained by exploiting the heterogeneity of the experimental units. This of course requires that the heterogeneous structure can be identified at the planning stage before the experiment is carried out. Suppose that the response to be measured in an animal experiment is genetically dependent or dependent on environmental effects early in life. In such cases animals from the same litter would be expected to be more alike than animals from different litter groups. Such structured heterogeneity of the experimental units can be utilized for the design of a so-called block experiment. In its basic form a block design is constructed by allocating the different treatments to a number (n) of litter groups (blocks) of the same size (t) as the number of treatments. The treatments are randomized independently to the experimental units within each block, and the structure of the design has one treatment factor at t levels and one block "factor" at n levels. The t treatments may themselves have a multifactorial structure.

Animals may be matched in pairs or larger groups which are similar with respect to certain characteristics that might influence the response. This defines a block structure in the design which must be taken into account in the analysis of the results. The essential advantage of a block design is that the (undesirable) effect of the (large) variation between blocks (litters) is eliminated, and the effect of the treatments will be evaluated relative to the smaller variation within blocks. Another frequently occurring cause of heterogeneity is the "time" factor. Animals or, more generally, the experimental units may undergo changes during the period over which the experiment is performed, since all the unit experiments usually cannot be carried out in parallel. The number of experimental units that can be handled in parallel or during a reasonably short period are thus taken as a block, and the treatments are randomly allocated to the units within each block. More complex block designs with two or more block factors may also be designed. There exist classes of ingenious block designs known as Latin squares or Graeco-Latin squares, which enable reduction of the heterogeneity due to more than one block factor. Figure 6 shows some examples of various block designs.

In addition to the complete block designs, where the block size is equal to the number of treatments, there exists a large literature on so-called incomplete block designs in which the number of treatments exceeds the block size. With multifactorial designs incomplete block designs may be constructed in such a way that certain (high order) interaction effects become confounded with the block variation while the (interesting) main effects and low order interactions can still be assessed with optimal precision. When there is no structure in the treatments (t levels of a single factor) there are balanced incomplete or partially balanced incomplete block designs, which are characterized by a high degree of efficiency compared to corresponding complete block designs. More designs and detailed descriptions can be found in textbooks on experimental design.[4,5]

Two other types of experimental design should also briefly be mentioned. These are the so-called split plot designs and the cross-over designs. Split plot designs may be described as designs in which some experimental treatments (factors) are randomized to different blocks while others are randomized to experimental units within blocks. For example, if certain treatments (levels of a factor A) are randomized to pregnant females while others (levels of factor B) are randomized to the litter groups, this would constitute a split plot design, where the effect of factor A on the offspring has to be evaluated relative to the inter-block variation, whereas B as well as the interaction between A and B can be measured relative to the (smaller) intra-block (within litter) variation.

In the cross-over design (Figure 6) two or more treatments are applied successively to the "same" experimental unit. Since the unit may change with time, the basic idea is to change the order of the treatments to balance out or reduce the influence of this source of variation. The simplest cross-over design with two treatments consists of two groups of experimental units where one gets treatment 1 followed by 2 and the other gets treatment 2 followed by 1. The advantage of the cross-over design is

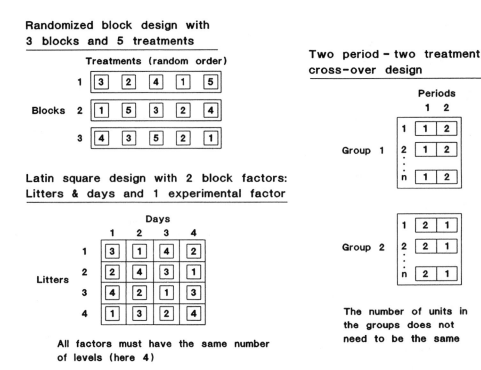

Figure 6. Examples of a randomized block design, a Latin square design and a cross-over design. Note that both treatments are tested on each experimental unit in the cross-over design.

primarily that in theory the effect of heterogeneity between experimental units (animals) is reduced to a minimum, i.e., treatment effects are evaluated relative to intra-individual variation. The main problem with cross-over designs is that they may become invalidated if the treatments have long-term effects, or if more complex so-called carry-over effects are present.

In repeated measures designs there are, as the name implies, two or more measurements or observations of the same response variable after applying a given treatment. The measurements are usually taken at successive time intervals, but they may also be taken simultaneously, e.g., at different locations of the body. The timing or positioning of the repeated measurements appears to be determined more by practical considerations and general experience than by statistical principles. It would also be difficult to develop generally applicable methods for the design of such experiments. Consequently most effort has been devoted to improving the methods of analysis of repeated measures experiments. One approach is to carry out a two-step analysis, where the first step consists of modeling the repeated measurements within the unit experiments in order to obtain (a few) characteristic measures (summary statistics) that describe the important aspects of the response, e.g., a peak value and when or where it occurs. These characteristic values are then analyzed separately or simultaneously with univariate or multivariate methods according to the objective of the experiment. Another approach aims at a more general modeling of the data, which allows a one-step simultaneous analysis without the need for making more or less arbitrary intermediate decisions. However, this leads to a rather complex analysis, which may be difficult to interpret relative to the objective of the experiment.

Finally, before leaving the subject of experimental design it should be mentioned how randomization can be performed in practice. What is required is a random permutation of the number of treatments. Special tables of random permutations have been published and tables of random numbers may also be used. Randomization may also be carried out as a random physical procedure such as throwing dice or setting up a specific lottery drawing. It is also possible and becoming more common to use computer-generated random permutations. In any case the randomization procedure should be well defined and controlled in detail. It is not sufficient to assume that consecutive animals, e.g., as they are picked from a cage, are coming along as if they were randomized (by nature), and then apply one treatment to the first animal, a second to the next, and so on. Groups of animals defined in this way might respond differently if they were given the same treatment.

In some types of experiments, where the observers or other individuals involved may influence the results, it is customary to use some unbreakable coding of the treatments. This "blinding" of the treatments may conveniently be combined with randomization and it is used extensively in clinical investigations. It is arguable that such measures should be used more widely even in situations where one would not expect any observer bias. For example, it would seem unlikely that animals would respond differently depending on whether the treatments are coded or not, but the persons handling the animals may unwittingly handle them slightly differently, perhaps enough to bias the responses and invalidate the experiment. Needless to say coding will also protect against deliberate fraud or suspicions of fraud.

ANALYSIS OF VARIANCE

This statistical method is used extensively for analysis of designed experiments, and there is a close connection between the design and the subsequent analysis of variance of the experimental results.[4,5] The primary objective of the analysis is to estimate and test the effects of the experimental factors. In the simplest case, analysis of variance may be regarded as a generalization of the two-sample t-test to a test of the hypothesis: $H_0 : \mu_1 = \mu_2 = ... = \mu_t$ against non-homogeneity of the means of the t groups. This analysis is often referred to as one-way analysis of variance. Two-way analysis of variance is used when there are two experimental factors or a block factor and a single experimental factor. This implies that there exist k-way analyses of variance for experiments with k factors. Table 7 shows the analysis of variance tables for one-way and two-way designs. Analysis of variance methods for the other types of experimental designs mentioned in the preceding section are described in textbooks on experimental design.[4,5]

The total sum of squared deviations (SSD_T) is partitioned into components corresponding to the design factors and an error term that measures the random variation between replicates or the residual variation that cannot be attributed to the factors. By dividing the sum of squared deviations with the associated degrees of freedom one gets the so-called mean square, which will represent independent estimates of the variance between replicates or residuals under the assumption that the null hypothesis is true, i.e., the factor in question has no effect. The ratio between the mean squares will therefore provide an F-test of the null hypothesis for no effect of the design factor. The simplest one-way analysis of variance leads to an F-test which is equivalent to the two-sample t-test in Table 4, as $F(1, f_0) = t^2(f_0)$; $f_0 = n_1 + n_2 - 2$. Similarly, the paired t-test, which corresponds to the one-sample t-test in Table 4 with the paired differences $(x_{1i} - x_{2i})$; $i = 1, ..., n$ substituted for x_i, is equivalent to the test of treatment effect (F_t) in the two-way analysis of variance with n blocks of size two and two treatments.

If the null hypothesis is rejected it can be concluded that the means at the different levels of the factor in question are not all identical. To help evaluate how they may differ, it is recommended to calculate confidence intervals for the means or for differences between pairs of means using the formulas given in Table 5. As an estimate of the standard deviation $S_o = \sqrt{S_o^2}$ should be used along with a table value for $t_{1-\alpha/2}(F_o)$. In block experiments it is of interest to see whether the mean square for the block factor exceeds the residual mean square. The larger the difference or the corresponding F-statistic is, the more has been gained in efficiency by using the blocking principle to reduce the effect of the heterogeneity of the experimental units. However, it is usually not of any particular interest to carry out a formal test of the statistical significance of the block factor. After having found a significant treatment effect by the analysis of variance it is often of interest to make further tests to determine which means are significantly different. A number of methods have been developed for this purpose. They are known as the least significant difference method (LSD), Dunnett's method, Duncan's method, Student-Newman-Keul's method, and Scheffe's method. It is not possible to describe these methods here, but it should be mentioned that a main objective is to control the overall significance level α of the test procedure. Standard t-tests of differences between pairs of treatment means should not be carried out, since the value of α increases with the number of t-tests. The so-called Bonferroni adjustment may be used. It guarantees an overall significance level $\leq \alpha$, if k t-tests are carried out with a significance level α/k. However, one of the above-mentioned special methods may provide a more powerful test.

When there is more than one experimental factor, the first step should be to test the interaction effect of the highest order (among all factors). Only if higher order interaction effects are insignificant, is it meaningful to test lower order interaction effects between the factors involved and eventually their main effects. For example, in the two-way analysis of variance with factors A and B in Table 7 the interaction effect AB should be tested first. Only if the null hypothesis for this effect can be accepted, will it be

Table 7: One-way and two-way analysis of variance

One-way ANOVA of completely randomized experiment with t treatments (index i) and n_i replicates (index j)

Variation	Sum of squares	Degrees of freedom	Mean square	F-statistic
Treatments	$SSD_t=\Sigma n_i(\overline{x_{i\cdot}}-\overline{x_{\cdot\cdot}})^2$	$f_t=t-1$	$s_t^2=SSD_t/f_t$	$F_t=s_t^2/s_0^2$
Replicates	$SSD_0=\Sigma\Sigma(x_{ij}-\overline{x_{i\cdot}})^2$	$f_0=\Sigma(n_i-1)$	$s_0^2=SSD_0/f_0$	
Total	$SSD_T=\Sigma\Sigma(x_{ij}-\overline{x_{\cdot\cdot}})^2$	$f_T=\Sigma n_i-1$		

Two-way ANOVA of randomized block experiment with t treatments (index i) and n blocks (index j)

Variation	Sum of squares	Degrees of freedom	Mean square	F-statistic
Treatments	$SSD_t=\Sigma n(\overline{x_{i\cdot}}-\overline{x_{\cdot\cdot}})^2$	$f_t=t-1$	$s_t^2=SSD_t/f_t$	$F_t=s_t^2/s_0^2$
Blocks	$SSD_b=\Sigma t(\overline{x_{\cdot j}}-\overline{x_{\cdot\cdot}})^2$	$f_b=n-1$	$s_b^2=SSD_b/f_b$	$F_b=s_b^2/s_0^2$
Residuals	$SSD_0=\Sigma\Sigma(x_{ij}-\overline{x_{i\cdot}}-\overline{x_{\cdot j}}+\overline{x_{\cdot\cdot}})^2$	$f_0=(n-1)(t-1)$	$s_0^2=SSD_0/f_0$	
Total	$SSD_T=\Sigma\Sigma(x_{ij}-\overline{x_{\cdot\cdot}})^2$	$f_T=nt-1$		

Two-way ANOVA of completely randomized experiment with two factors A (n_A levels, index i) and B (n_B levels, index j) and n replicates of each treatment (index k)

Variation	Sum of squares	Degrees of freedom	Mean square	F-statistic
A	$SSD_A=\Sigma n_B n(\overline{x_{i\cdot\cdot}}-\overline{x_{\cdot\cdot\cdot}})^2$	$f_A=n_A-1$	$s_A^2=SSD_A/f_A$	$F_A=s_A^2/s_0^2$
B	$SSD_B=\Sigma n_A n(\overline{x_{\cdot j\cdot}}-\overline{x_{\cdot\cdot\cdot}})^2$	$f_B=n_B-1$	$s_B^2=SSD_B/f_B$	$F_B=s_B^2/s_0^2$
AB	$SSD_{AB}=\Sigma\Sigma n(\overline{x_{ij\cdot}}-\overline{x_{i\cdot\cdot}}-\overline{x_{\cdot j\cdot}}+\overline{x_{\cdot\cdot\cdot}})^2$	$f_{AB}=(n_A-1)(n_B-1)$	$s_{AB}^2=SSD_{AB}/f_{AB}$	$F_{AB}=s_{AB}^2/s_0^2$
Replicates	$SSD_0=\Sigma\Sigma\Sigma(x_{ijk}-\overline{x_{ij\cdot}})^2$	$f_0=n_A n_B(n-1)$	$s_0^2=SSD_0/f_0$	
Total	$SSD_T=\Sigma\Sigma\Sigma(x_{ijk}-\overline{x_{\cdot\cdot\cdot}})^2$	$f_T=n_A n_B n-1$		

The dot notation indicates that a mean value has been calculated over the index being replaced by the dot, e.g. $\overline{x_{i\cdot}}=\Sigma x_{ij}/n$. The null hypothesis of no treatment or factor effect is rejected if $F>F_{1-\alpha}(f,f_0)$, where f is the degrees of freedom associated with the mean square for the effect in question.

meaningful to proceed by testing the main effects of factors A and B. In this case an improved estimate s^2 for the error variance is obtained by pooling s_0^2 and s_{AB}^2, i.e., $s^2 = (SSD_0 + SSD_{AB})/(f_0 + f_{AB})$. The pooled estimate has $f = f_0 + f_{AB}$ degrees of freedom and leads to more powerful F-tests of the main effects of A and B, and it should also be used for calculation of confidence intervals. If a significant interaction effect between two or more experimental factors has been found, it is usually not possible to describe the results of the experiment otherwise than by reporting the means at all combinations of the levels of the factors involved, preferably supplemented by confidence limits. In analogy with the rank sum tests for the means given in Table 3 there are non-parametric tests corresponding to one-way and two-way analysis of

Table 8: Analysis of variance of 2^2-factorial experiment

	Factor												Mean	SD
Antigen	Adjuvant	Antibody binding (%) in individual rabbits											Mean	SD
I (−)	no (−)	0	2	1	3	0	3	2	3	2	4	2.00	1.33
II (+)	no (-)	5	3	0	3	3	6	5	1	3	6	3.50	2.01
I (−)	yes (+)	1	2	3	-1	1	3	5	2	5	2	2.30	1.83
II (+)	yes (+)	7	4	6	5	9	2	1	4	9	7	5.40	2.72

Variation	Sum of squares	Degrees of freedom	Mean square	F-statistic
A (Antigen)	52.90	1	52.90	12.78 (12.59)
B (Adjuvant)	12.10	1	12.10	2.92 (2.88)
AB (interaction)	6.40	1	6.40	1.55
Replicates	149.00	36 (37)	4.14 (4.20)	
Total	220.40	39		

Estimates of means and 95% confidence intervals

Antigen I ($\mu_{(0)}$)	2.15	(1.22; 3.08)
Antigen II (μ_a)	4.45	(3.52; 5.38)
Adjuvant effect ($\mu_b - \mu_{(0)}$)	1.10	(-0.21; 2.41)

variance. The former is known as Kruskall Wallis' test and the latter as Friedman's test. The reader is referred to standard statistical textbooks for details about these tests.[1,2,4]

The following example shows how the two-way analysis of variance of a completely randomized experiment with a 2^2-factorial design may be analyzed. Four groups of 10 rabbits were immunized with two different antigens (factor A) which were administered with or without adjuvant (factor B). The data are similar to those analyzed in Table 4 and are listed in Table 8, which also shows the analysis of variance and the subsequent calculation of confidence intervals. According to the testing strategy outlined above, the F-value for the interaction effect (AB) would first be compared with the values from the table of the F-distribution. Because $F_{0.95}(1,36) = 4.11$ it is concluded that there is no significant interaction.

The numbers shown within brackets in the analysis of variance scheme have been obtained after pooling the sum of squared deviations and the degrees of freedom for the non-significant interaction term (AB) with the residual *SSD* and degrees of freedom. In this way an improved mean square is calculated and used as denominator to provide (in this case only slightly) more powerful tests for the main effects of factors A and B. The results of these tests are, however, practically unchanged, and the conclusion is that factor A has a significant effect, while the effect of factor B does not reach statistical significance. The pooled mean square estimate is also used in the calculation of the confidence intervals. The confidence intervals for the means at each level of factor A correspond to the same precision as if 20 replicates had been used for each antigen. For factor B a 95% confidence interval for its effect in terms of the difference between the means at its two levels has been calculated. This interval includes 0 since the effect was not significant at the 5% level. The interval endpoints give the maximal sizes of the effects that would not have been found significant, and the size of the interval in this way constitutes a measure of the sensitivity of the experiment.

REGRESSION ANALYSIS

It is important in connection with the analysis of designed experiments to make a clear distinction between two different applications of regression analysis. In the present context regression analysis will be used in a restricted sense where the purpose is to analyze the relation between a response variable and one or more quantitative experimental factors. In another frequently used terminology the response is denoted the dependent variable, which is described as a function of some independent variables. When the data are obtained in a correctly designed and performed experiment, it is possible to draw conclusions regarding a causal relation between variation in the levels of the experimental factors and the response. Regression analysis methods are, however, also used for analyzing correlations between uncontrolled variables arising in observational studies. In such cases it is, in principle, not possible to assess causal relationships. In fact, it may be difficult to determine which variable should be regarded as dependent and which as independent. Moreover, it cannot usually be excluded that other unobserved variables or factors are to some extent or even completely responsible for the observed correlation. Such applications of regression analysis are nevertheless very important and may, when due care is taken, contribute valuable information, e.g., lead to new scientific hypotheses, which eventually may be confirmed by means of designed experiments.

Regression analysis may be described as a method for making statistical inference, i.e., estimation and tests of hypotheses, about a mathematical model for the mean value of the response variable Y and the levels of k experimental factors, i.e., $E(Y) = f(x_1, ..., x_k)$. The linear models have been the most extensively studied and applied. The linear model in k independent variables is: $E(Y) = \alpha + \Sigma B_i x_i; i = 1, ..., K$. From a statistical point of view a linear model is defined as a model where the mean is a linear function of the (unknown) coefficients or parameters. For example, the polynomial model of degree p for a single factor, i.e., $E(Y) = \alpha + \Sigma B_j x^j; j=1, ...p$, is also regarded as a linear model.

A priori it is frequently not possible or advisable to assume that a specific mathematical model will fit the data. Thus, the first objective of a regression analysis is to determine a minimal model that will fit the data sufficiently well. Since polynomial models of increasing degree should in principle be able to approximate any "well-behaved" mathematical function, it is not surprising that such models have found widespread use, especially in applications where models based on theoretical considerations are not available or are very complicated. The dual goal of the modeling phase of the regression analysis, i.e., to determine which factors affect the response as well as the appropriate mathematical model to describe the effects of these factors, is conveniently accomplished in analogy with the analysis of variance of experiments with qualitative factors.

Table 9 illustrates schematically how the regression analysis of an experiment with two quantitative factors may be carried out. The technique is fairly complex and the remainder of this section may be skipped at the first reading. The following polynomial model with terms for main effects of up to the second degree and the corresponding interaction terms is used:

$$E(Y) = a + \beta_{11}x_1 + \beta_{12}x_1^2 + \beta_{21}x_2 + \beta_{22}x_2^2 + \gamma_{11}x_1x_2 + \gamma_{21}x_1^2x_2 + \gamma_{12}x_1x_2^2 + \gamma_{22}x_1^2x_2^2$$

The terms with the β coefficients correspond to the so-called linear and quadratic main effects, while the γ coefficients represent the interaction terms between the two factors. In the simplest case with equidistant levels of the factors it is possible by means of so-called orthogonal polynomials to calculate all terms in Table 9 directly. In more general cases with non-equidistant levels and/or unbalanced designs where n may vary between combinations of factor levels, it is possible to calculate the various terms in the table by means of the general method for multivariate regression analysis. Without going into details about how these calculations are made it will suffice to realize that with a given regression model such as the polynomial model stated above one obtains a residual sum of squares:

$$SSD_{min} \, Min \sum_{i=1}^{n_A} \sum_{j=1}^{n_B} \sum_{l=1}^{n} \left(y_{ijl} - E(Y) \right)^2$$

where y_{ijl} is the observed response at replicate l of the i-th level of factor A and the j-th level of factor B, $E(Y)$ is the polynomial defined above, and the minimization is performed over all values of the α, β, and γ parameters. This is the well-known least squares estimation method, which for normally distributed data is equivalent to the maximum likelihood method.

In the present case SSD_{min} will be equal to $SSD_{rep} + SSD_{res}$. If there are no replicates, i.e., $n = 1$, it is not possible to calculate SSD_{rep} and to carry out the F-test of the full model. This test is based on the ratio: $F = s_{res}^2 / s_{rep}^2$, which will lead to rejection of the model if $F > F_{1-\alpha}(n_A n_B.9, n_A n_B n-1)$. In that case a model of higher order or perhaps another type of model than a polynomial should be tried. When there are

Table 9: *Analysis of variance for a polynomial regression model of second degree with two factors A and B at $n_A \geq 3$ and $n_B \geq 3$ levels and n replicates at each combination of factor levels.*

Variation	Sum of squares	Degrees of freedom	Mean square	F-statistic
Linear A	$SSD_{lin.A}$	1	$s^2_{lin.A}$	$s^2_{lin.A}/s^2_p$
Linear B	$SSD_{lin.B}$	1	$s^2_{lin.B}$	$s^2_{lin.B}/s^2_p$
Quadratic A	$SSD_{qua.A}$	1	$s^2_{qua.A}$	$s^2_{qua.A}/s^2_p$
Quadratic B	$SSD_{qua.B}$	1	$s^2_{qua.B}$	$s^2_{qua.B}/s^2_p$
Lin.A × Lin.B	$SSD_{lin.A \times lin.B}$	1	$s^2_{lin.A \times lin.B}$	$s^2_{lin.A \times lin.B}/s^2_p$
Lin.A × Qua.B	$SSD_{lin.A \times qua.B}$	1	$s^2_{lin.A \times qua.B}$	$s^2_{lin.A \times qua.B}/s^2_p$
Qua.B × Lin.B	$SSD_{qua.A \times lin.B}$	1	$s^2_{qua.A \times lin.B}$	$s^2_{qua.A \times lin.B}/s^2_p$
Qua.A × Qua.B	$SSD_{qua.A \times qua.B}$	1	$s^2_{qua.A \times qua.B}$	$s^2_{qua.A \times qua.B}/s^2_p$
Residuals	SSD_{res}	$n_A n_B - 9$	s^2_{res}	s^2_{res}/s^2_{rep}
Replicates	SSD_{rep}	$n_A n_B(n-1)$	s^2_{rep}	
Total	SSD_{tot}	$n_A n_B n - 1$		

replicates it is possible to calculate SSD_{rep} by means of a one-way analysis of variance with $n_A n_B$ groups, as shown in Table 7.

If the full model is accepted the analysis proceeds by calculating the pooled variance estimate: $s_p^2 = (SSD_{rep} + SSD_{res})/(n_A n_B n - 9)$ which is that used for the F-tests of the individual mean squares corresponding to the various polynomial terms as shown in Table 9. The sum of squared deviations for these terms can be found as the differences between the residual sum of squares from multiple regression analyses without and with the term in question included, i.e., for example, $SSD_{qua.Axqua.B} = SSD_{min}$(model without $_{\gamma 22}$)$-SSD_{min}$(full model). In analogy with the analysis of factorial experiments the first step is to test interaction terms and polynomial terms of the highest order in this way, and if the null hypothesis can be accepted, the model is gradually simplified. In this connection it should be pointed out that it is usually not meaningful to test and possibly omit an interaction or polynomial term if a term of higher order with the same variable(s) is statistically significant.

When this testing strategy, which aims at finding the simplest regression model that can adequately describe the relation between the dependent and independent variables, has been completed, the estimates of the regression coefficients (α, β, γ) and their standard errors may be reported. These values are normally provided by the multiple regression program. Estimated values with SEs or confidence limits can also be calculated for the model at given values of the independent variables, and two- or three-dimensional graphical presentations of the fitted curve or surface can be prepared.

While multiple regression analysis based on linear models could only be carried out in the simplest cases before the advent of computers, it was even more laborious to use non-linear regression models. Again, it is not possible to give a detailed description of how such models are analyzed, and the reader is referred to textbooks that describe such methods.[8,9] There are, however, many similarities to the analysis of linear models. The most distinct differences are that the least squares estimation requires iterative calculations and that various tests of the model are of an approximate character, because the parameter estimates usually have very complicated, intractable, non-normal distributions. However, it has been found that under certain general assumptions the estimates will approach Gaussian distributions as the number of observations increases or their variance decreases.

It is possible to analyze a general non-linear model according to the same strategy as in the case of the multivariate linear model, although this is only an approximation, assuming the sample size is large. For example, in pharmacokinetics one may want to analyze the disappearance of a drug according to a non-linear model consisting of a sum of k exponential terms:

$$E(Y) = \sum_{j=1}^{k} \alpha_j exp(-\beta_j t),$$

where Y represents the amount or concentration of the drug at time t after injection. With observations of Y at different times (y_i, t_i), $i = 1, ..., n$, the best model fit is usually determined by minimizing the sum of squared deviations with respect to (a_j, β_j), $j = 1, ..., k$:

$$SSD_k = Min \sum_{i=1}^{n} [y_i - \sum_{j=1}^{k} \alpha_j exp(-\beta_j t_i)]^2$$

It is then possible to test whether a model with k-1 exponential terms gives an equally good fit to the observations by means of the following approximate F-statistic with 2 and n-2k degrees of freedom:

$$F \cong [(SSD_{k-1} - SSD_k)/2] / [SSD_k/(n-2k)]$$

This process may be continued until it is not possible to reduce the model further. Before leaving this example it may be noted that the experiment has a repeated measures design, which may lead to complications in the analysis, since successive observations may not be statistically independent.

Another regression example with repeated measurements is the so-called growth curve model. The purpose is to describe measurements of a growth variable, such as the weight of an animal, as a function of time. This may be accomplished by means of a linear model, e.g., a polynomial in time, or a non-linear regression model. After having found the simplest type of model that fits the data for individual animals according to the methods described above, the next step may consist of comparisons of the growth curves themselves or perhaps the growth rate curves, which are determined by differentiating the growth model functions. The analyses may be carried out as comparisons of the estimated regression parameters or simply as comparisons of estimated (interpolated) values at given time points. It should be pointed out that tests of different parameters or tests of estimated values at different times are not independent, and that the distribution of the test statistics is usually only approximate. There are also other methods for analysis of data from repeated measurement designs, which are described in the special literature on these subjects.

DOSE RESPONSE ANALYSIS AND BIOASSAY

In toxicology and pharmacology, as well as in many basic biological research studies, it is of interest to analyze the relation between a response variable and the dose of the biologically active material.[10,11] Dose response analysis is primarily an application of regression methods. Depending on the specific purpose of the study there is, however, often a need for certain extensions of the standard linear or non-linear regression analysis. In toxicology the purpose may be to determine the dose that causes a specific reaction in a given proportion of the animals being tested, for example assessment of ED_{50}, i.e., the dose that provokes the response in 50% of the animals. The experiment consists of testing groups of animals with different doses and observing the number of responders in each group. With a properly randomized design this response variable follows a binomial distribution, and the expected or mean proportion of responders may be described as a function of the dose variable. Thus we have a regression model of the type: $E(Y)=F(z)$, where Y is the response variable corresponding to the fraction of positive responders at the dose level $z \geq 0$. Over relatively narrow response and dose ranges it may be possible to use a linear model in dose or in the logarithm of dose, but it is often preferred to test a wide range of doses to obtain responses over the whole range from 0 to 1. This calls for non-linear dose response models which for low doses approach 0 and for large doses approach 1. Thus, cumulative distribution functions with $F(0)=0$ and $F(\infty)=1$ may be used as dose response models.

Two of the most widely used dose response models are the lognormal and the logistic distribution functions. They are referred to as the probit and logit models, respectively. These models allow a special interpretation of the dose response relation, i.e., as the distribution of tolerances for the population of the biological individuals. The probit model thus corresponds to a lognormal distribution of tolerances. A randomly selected individual will respond to a dose z if its tolerance is less than z and the probability of a positive response is $P(Z \leq z)=\phi((logz-\mu)/\sigma)$, where $\phi(\bullet)$ is the standardized normal distribution function. Likewise the logit model corresponds to a logistic tolerance distribution, which may be written as $F(z)=z^\lambda/(z^\lambda+\xi^\lambda)$; $\lambda>0$, $\xi>0$. Both models exhibit a symmetrical sigmoid-shaped dose response curve when $F(z)$ is plotted versus **logz** (see Figure 7). The parameter ξ of the logit model corresponds to ED_{50} as **exp(μ)** does in the case of the probit model. The parameter λ is proportional to the slope of the linear part of the dose

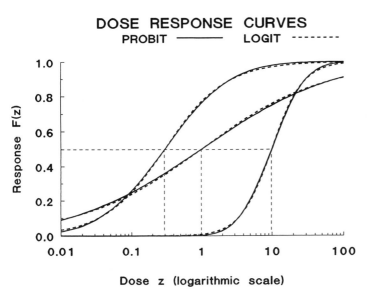

DOSE RESPONSE CURVES
PROBIT ———— LOGIT ‑‑‑‑‑‑‑‑

Figure 7. Similarity of logit and probit dose response curves plotted for $(\lambda,\xi)=(0.5,1), (1,0.3), (2,10)$ and intersecting at $ED_{10}, ED_{50}, ED_{90}$, i.e. the pairs of logit and probit curves are equal at these three dose levels.

response curve around ED_{50}, whereas σ is inversely proportional to this slope. Figure 7 illustrates that the two models are nearly identical. In practice positive responses may be observed with the zero dose, or some individuals may be resistant and unable to respond at all. The dose response models based on distribution functions can be modified to account for this by inclusion of two extra parameters to give the following generalized model: $\theta_1+\theta_2F(z)$, where $0\leq\theta_1\leq1$ is the probability of response at zero dose or the fraction of the population that will always respond, and $0^-1-\theta_1 + q_2^-1$ is the fraction that cannot respond.

Figure 8 shows a dose response analysis of results from an experimental study of the teratological effect of thiourea.[12] Groups of rats were treated with different doses and the number of fetuses with anomalies out of the total number was analyzed as a binomially distributed response according to the logistic model. The maximum likelihood estimates of the ξ and the λ parameters were 29.08 and 4.404, respectively. The fitted curve is shown together with the observed response rates, and the actual number of positive responses out of the total number is shown next to the dot representing the observed response rate. It should be mentioned that a control group of 167 tested with a zero dose of thiourea showed zero positive responses. The statistical analysis includes inverse estimation of doses corresponding to given response rates such as ED_{50} with a 95% confidence interval. The example also includes a calculation of the so-called virtually safe dose, which corresponds to a very low response rate, e.g., 10^{-6}. Considerable care should, however, be taken with such calculations, since it has been observed that different dose response models, which can describe the data equally well, may yield very different estimates of the virtually safe dose. For example, if the probit model is fitted to the data in Figure 8, a virtually safe dose (risk=10^{-6}) of 4.2 mg/kg is found. This is considerably higher than the corresponding dose obtained with the logistic because the lognormal approaches zero more rapidly for small doses than the logistic.

So far dose response analysis has been presented for experiments with a single population of individuals and a single drug. Obviously, one could compare dose response relations for two populations, e.g., compare toxicity of a drug in two animal species. If the two dose response curves can be regarded as parallel, shifted along the logarithmic dose axis, the difference in sensitivity to the drug may be described by the size of the shift. This constitutes a convenient and sufficient measure of the relative toxicity of the drug. In complete analogy dose response curves for two drugs tested on individuals from the same population may also be compared. If the curves are parallel the drugs are said to be similar, and the shift measures the relative potency of the two drugs. One of the drugs is usually regarded as a standard or reference, and the estimation of the relative potency of the other is thus a measurement of its biological activity or a bioassay. The experimental determination of the dose response relation for a single drug in a single population as in Figure 8 is, however, also referred to as a bioassay.

The bioassay of insulin according to the mouse convulsion method has been used extensively to assess the biological activity of production batches of the protein hormone before they are approved for treatment of diabetic patients. The experimental procedure for the assay as well as the statistical analysis of the results is described in detail in various pharmacopoeia.[13] Briefly, in its simplest version the experiment consists of injecting two groups of mice with a low and a high dose of the test preparation

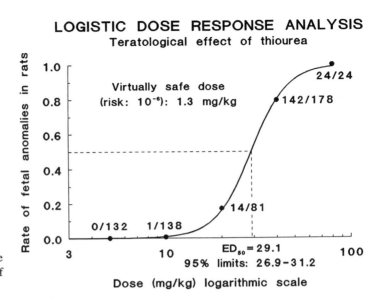

Figure 8. Logistic dose response analysis of teratological effect of thiourea on rat fetuses.

and two other groups with low and high doses of the standard preparation. The doses are chosen from experience so that about 20% of the mice will show a characteristic convulsion response to the low dose and about 80% to the high dose, if the test preparation, as expected, has a relative potency of 1. Figure 9 shows the results of such a bioassay carried out with four groups of 24 mice. The doses of the insulin standard preparation were 6 and 10 mU per mouse. Since the new production batch was expected to have the same potency as the standard, the same nominal doses of the test preparation were administered, and the purpose of the assay was to check that the relative potency of the new batch was sufficiently close to 1. In fact, the pharmacopoeias give limits for the potency estimate as well as the size of the 95% confidence interval.

The dose response analysis is based on the probit model using the middle part of the dose response relation. First the similarity or parallelism of the two lines is tested by means of an approximate χ^2-test. If this hypothesis is acceptable, the relative potency is estimated with an approximative 95% confidence interval, which serves as a measure of the precision of the potency estimate. Figure 9 shows the best-fitting parallel probit dose response curves, and the similarity hypothesis is clearly acceptable. This example is typical of the precision that is obtained in such assays with a qualitative binary response. If a higher precision is required, the group sizes could be increased, but for practical reasons it is preferable to repeat the assay with other animals, and calculate a combined estimate with as narrow confidence limits as desired.

Although the methods and examples presented so far have been based on binary responses, it should be emphasized that dose response analysis and bioassay methods also apply to responses measured on a continuous scale. As in other applications of regression analysis, linear models play a leading role. In bioassay such dose response models are known as parallel line models and slope ratio models. They may be regarded as approximations to more complex non-linear models. The modified dose response model based on a suitable distribution function, for example the logistic: $F(z)=\theta_1+\theta_2 z^\lambda/(z^\lambda+\xi^\lambda)$ can also be used to describe the sigmoid-shaped dose response relations that are often obtained when a continuous response variable is plotted against the logarithm of the dose. This so-called four-parameter logistic dose response model has been used extensively in bioassays and immunoassays.[14]

Figure 10 shows an example of a bioassay of insulin analyzed according to the four-parameter logistic model.[14] In this bioassay suspensions of free fat cells from mice are incubated with different concentrations (doses) of insulin and tritiated tracer glucose. The response is the amount of tritium incorporated into the lipid fraction of the cells. Parallel sigmoid-shaped dose response curves could be fitted to the data (mean and SEM of triplicate measurements), and the horizontal distance between the curves measures (the logarithm of) the relative potency. The precision of the potency estimate will increase with an increasing slope of the middle part of the dose response curves and with decreasing error variance. Thus, it is predominantly the middle near-linear part of the dose response relation that determines the potency, and it is therefore preferable to place as many dose levels as possible in that range. On the other hand,

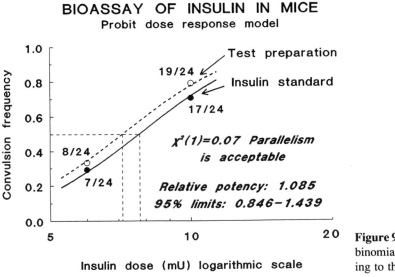

Figure 9. Example of bioassay with a binomial response analyzed according to the parallel line probit model.

in such assays it is of importance to determine the whole sigmoid curve in order to check that the same minimal and maximal response levels are achieved with both preparations.

CATEGORICAL DATA AND SURVIVAL ANALYSIS

Categorical data may be divided into three types. The first is the binomial or multinomial type, where the observations fall into a given number of $q \geq 2$ classes, which do not have a natural ordering. The second type is when the q classes can be ordered or ranked, but it is not possible to assign meaningful numerical values to the classes. The third is the Poisson type of observations, where a number of events are observed. As an example of the first type, animals in a toxicology study may be classified according to cause of death, and as an example of the ordinal scale data, responses in a study of allergic reactions may be classified as: severe, strong, moderate, doubtful, and absent. An example of the third type of categorical

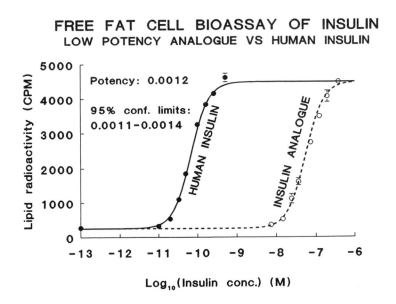

Figure 10. Example of bioassay analyzed according to the four-parameter logistic model. Although the count of radioactivity in principle is a discrete response variable it can in this case be approximated very well by a continuous normal distributed variable.

Table 10: *The χ^2-test of homogeneity for a q by r table*

		Classes					
		1	...	*i*	...	*q*	*Sum*
	1	O_{11}	...	O_{i1}	...	O_{q1}	$S_{\bullet 1}$
	:	:		:		:	:
Groups	*j*	O_{1j}	...	O_{ij}	...	O_{qj}	$S_{\bullet j}$
	:	:		:		:	:
	r	O_{1r}	...	O_{ir}	...	O_{qr}	$S_{\bullet r}$
	Sum	$S_{1\bullet}$	...	$S_{i\bullet}$	...	$S_{q\bullet}$	$S_{\bullet\bullet}$

The expected number in cell no. ij is:

$$E_{ij} = \frac{S_{i\bullet} S_{\bullet j}}{S_{\bullet\bullet}}$$

The test statistic is:

$$\chi^2((q-1)\cdot(r-1)) = \sum_{i=1}^{q} \sum_{j=1}^{r} \frac{(O_{ij} - E_{ij})^2}{E_{ij}}$$

data could be the number of transformed cells in a blood sample. In many situations it is possible to analyze the categorical data by methods that are analogous to the analysis of variance and regression analysis, which have been developed for continuous observations.

The idea behind the general method of analysis of such data is to describe the structure of the underlying parameters (such as class probabilities or count rates) by means of a linear model. The primary task of the analysis is to test the goodness of fit of the model. If it is acceptable an attempt can be made to simplify the model as much as possible in analogy with the testing strategy presented for analysis of variance and regression models. These general methods for categorical data are known as generalized linear models (GLIM),[15,16] and they have been implemented in computer program packages. There are, however, some classical methods that are useful and fairly easy to apply.

The data reported in Table 6 (death rates from pneumonia, 1849) may be analyzed by means of the χ^2-test of homogeneity, i.e., a test of the hypothesis of equal death rates with the three treatments. The general version of this test applies to *r* groups and *q* classes, and the test statistic is defined in Table 10. The expected number of deaths in the three treatment groups in Table 6 are in the order given: 11.86, 14.78, 26.36, and the expected number of survivors is the total minus the expected number of deaths. The test statistic is then readily calculated as: $\chi^2(2)=13.42$, which corresponds to a P-value of about 0.002, and the null hypothesis is rejected. The test-statistic defined in Table 10 is only approximately χ^2-distributed, and it is usually recommended not to rely on the approximation if the expected number in some classes falls below 5.

For two-by-two tables with small numbers it is preferable to use an exact test such as Fisher's test based on the hypergeometric sampling distribution. It can be applied to test different hypotheses depending on how the two-by-two table was obtained. We may for example want to test whether two symptoms, such as the presence or absence of two different types of tumors, occurs independently in a given group of animals. This problem is clearly different from a situation where we want to compare the frequency of tumors in two groups of given size that have received different treatments. Fisher's test or the χ^2-test may, however, be used in both cases. There are classification tables, also called contingency tables, with more than two cross-classification criteria. Although they apparently have a simple structure, it quickly becomes very complicated to define and test relevant hypotheses as the dimension of the table increases. This also stems from the difficulties associated with making clear distinctions between dependent (response) variables and independent or explanatory variables and specification of relevant hypotheses.

With data from designed experiments there is no problem in identifying the classification criteria corresponding to the experimental factors. If, furthermore, the response can be identified as a single classification criterion, for example a positive or negative response, it follows that the situation is similar to that considered with the dose response models. Logistic models or generalizations thereof to more than two response classes have consequently found widespread use for analysis of the relation between a response variable and variables corresponding to the experimental factors. These multivariate logistic methods can also be applied for analysis of data from non-experimental sampling studies.

Data classified on an ordinal scale may also be analyzed according to the methods described above, but the information contained in the ordering is not utilized. On the other hand it is clearly not warranted to analyze the data after assignment of arbitrary numerical values to the ordered classes. It may, though, be acceptable to analyze the ordering as if it represents a ranking, i.e., by applying non-parametric rank-based statistical methods. However, these methods only allow for analysis according to rather simple models. Recently logistic models for ordinal observations have been developed.[16] They rely on certain assumptions that link the ordering to the logistic model, and experience with these methods is rather limited.

In long-term toxicology and in studies of diseases in animals it is of importance to analyze the time until some characteristic response or symptom occurs, because the adverse effect may often be an earlier appearance rather than an increased rate of the toxic response. The most fundamental response is the death of the individual, and this has given name to the statistical methods for survival analysis which have undergone an impressive development in recent years.[17] These methods are not limited to studies of risk of death as a function of time. They can be applied to analyze any specific change of state whose time of occurrence can be observed, such as appearance of disease or aging symptoms, failure to function, etc. The methods are also useful for analyzing reliability of physical components and systems.

A primary task in survival analysis is to estimate the survival function, i.e., the probability of being alive or, more generally, in the same state as a function of time. From an experimental point of view this may seem like a very simple problem. A group of individuals are followed until they have all changed state, e.g., have died, and the individual times of death are recorded. From these data it would be easy to calculate the survival function as 1 minus the cumulative distribution of the times of death. The situation, however, quickly becomes more complicated if so-called censoring occurs. In a pure survival study censoring means that information about death is missing for some individuals. It is only known that they were alive up to a certain time. This may be regarded as a lack of control of the experiment, which should normally be avoidable, but consider instead of death the occurrence of some other specific change of state, e.g., development of a disease. When rats who are likely to develop diabetes are followed from birth, some may die before development of diabetes, and this kind of censoring should be taken into account in the estimation of the survival function (without diabetes) as a function of time. This is what the Kaplan Meier method for estimation of the survival function actually does.

The principle behind the Kaplan Meier estimator is best described by considering a simple example. Suppose that a group of ten animals are observed from birth. After a certain period, say 67 days, one develops diabetes. The survival (without diabetes) is thus 100% until 67 days, and it drops to 9/10 (90%) immediately thereafter. After 92 days one animal (without diabetes) is found dead. This censoring does not change the survival estimate, but the number of animals at risk is now eight. When the next case of diabetes is observed say on day 107 the survival changes from 90% to 90·(7/8) = 78.75%. If then on day 113 one animal (without diabetes) dies and another develops diabetes the survival changes to 78.75·(6/7) = 67.5%, since seven were at risk. Finally, if two animals develop diabetes on day 120 the survival drops to 67.5·(3/5) = 41.5%. Figure 11 shows a realistic example of calculation of survival curves for two groups of animals.

It is possible to calculate the approximative variance of the survival function estimated according to the Kaplan Meier method and compare survival rates from two or more groups at a given time by means of an approximate test based on this variance. However, it is usually preferable to carry out a test of the equality of the survival curves as such. The so-called logrank test is widely used for this purpose. It is not possible here to give a detailed description of how this test-statistic is calculated.[17] It leads to an approximate χ^2-distributed statistic with k-1 degrees of freedom for a comparison of k survival curves. This test was carried out for the two groups of rats in Figure 11, and the test showed clearly that survival without diabetes (or the rate of development of diabetes) was significantly different in the two groups.

Survival analysis has been extended to enable incorporation of explanatory variables (risk factors) for the individuals into a rather general model, the so-called proportional hazards model or the Cox model.[17] This analysis may give new information about the importance of the risk factors and lead to less biased and more powerful tests of differences in survival between treatment groups. For a continuous survival function $S(t)$ the hazard function is defined as:

$$\lambda(t) = -\frac{dS(t)}{dt} \cdot \frac{1}{S(t)}$$

226

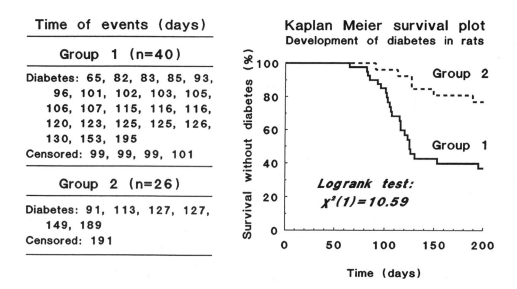

Time of events (days)	Kaplan Meier survival plot

Development of diabetes in rats

Group 1 (n=40)

Diabetes: 65, 82, 83, 85, 93,
96, 101, 102, 103, 105,
106, 107, 115, 116, 116,
120, 123, 125, 125, 126,
130, 153, 195
Censored: 99, 99, 99, 101

Group 2 (n=26)

Diabetes: 91, 113, 127, 127,
149, 189
Censored: 191

Figure 11. Survival analysis of development of diabetes in two groups of rats. Group 1 was untreated, while Group 2 received an antidiabetic treatment. The times when individual animals developed diabetes or were censored (died without diabetes) are given in the left panel. The right panel shows the survival curves and the result of the logrank test.

The negative value of the derivative of $S(t)$ is the density of the life-time distribution: $F(t) = 1-S(t) = P(T \le t)$, where $P(T \le t)$ is the probability of death at time t or earlier. The hazard $\lambda(t)$ can be interpreted as a measure of the risk of dying during a short interval after time t, given that the individual has survived until time t.

The proportional hazards model describes the hazard for an individual characterized by a set of explanatory variables (risk factors) $z_1,...,z_k$ as:

$$\lambda\left(t, z_1, \cdots, Z_k\right) = \lambda_0(t) exp\left(\sum_{i=1}^{k} \beta_i z_i\right)$$

where $\lambda_0(t)$ is an underlying unspecified hazard function and $\beta_1, ..., \beta_k$ are regression coefficients. In standard applications it is usually assumed that $\lambda_0(t)$ is the same for all individuals, and that differences between groups, e.g., due to experimental factors, can be modeled by means of suitable explanatory variables. In analogy with the testing strategy presented in connection with analysis of variance and regression analysis it is then possible by means of approximative tests to determine which of the explanatory variables have statistically significant effects on survival. These effects can be estimated and expressed quantitatively with approximative confidence intervals.

REFERENCES

1. Daniel W.W. *Biostatistics: A Foundation for Analysis in the Health Sciences*. 5th Ed. John Wiley, New York, 1991.
2. Snedecor G.W. and Cochran W.G. *Statistical Methods*. 7th Ed. Iowa State University Press, Ames, 1980.
3. Tukey J.W. *Exploratory Data Analysis*. Addison-Wesley, Reading, MA, 1977.
4. Cochran W.G. and Cox G.M. *Experimental Designs*. John Wiley, New York, 1957.
5. Cox D.R. *Planning of Experiments*. John Wiley, New York, 1958.
6. Conover W.J. *Practical Non-Parametric Statistics*. 2nd Ed. John Wiley, New York, 1980.
7. Dietl J. *Der Aderlass in der Lungenenzündung*, 1849.
8. Draper N.R. and Smith H. *Applied Regression Analysis*. 2nd Ed. John Wiley, New York, 1981.
9. Daniel C. and Wood F.S. *Fitting Equations to Data*. 2nd Ed. John Wiley, New York, 1980.
10. Finney D.J. *Probit Analysis*. 3rd Ed. The University Press, Cambridge, 1971.

11. Finney D.J. *Statistical Method in Biological Assay*. 3rd Ed. Ch. Griffin, London, 1978.
12. Scientific Committee, Food Safety Council. Proposed system for food safety assessment. *Food Cosmet. Toxicol.* 1978; 16 (Suppl.): 109.
13. British Pharmacopoeia 1980, Her Majesty's Stationery Office, London, 1980.
14. Vølund A. Application of the four-parameter logistic model to bioassay: Comparison with slope ratio and parallel line models. *Biometrics* 1978; 36: 225.
15. McCullagh P. and Nelder J.A. *Generalized Linear Models*. 2nd Ed. Chapman & Hall, London, 1989.
16. Agresti A. *Categorical Data Analysis*. John Wiley, New York, 1990.
17. Kalbfleisch J.D. and Prentice R.L. *The Statistical Analysis of Failure Time Data*. John Wiley, New York, 1980.

Chapter 16

Common Non-Surgical Techniques and Procedures

Krister Iwarsson, Lennart Lindberg, and Tage Waller

CONTENTS

0-8493-4378-X/94/$0.00+$.50
© 1994 by CRC Press Inc.

INTRODUCTION

Laboratory animals should be subjected to laboratory routines based on species-specific, well-documented, and humane techniques of handling, restraint, sampling, and dosing. This is best achieved with experienced staff, and with proper adaptation of the animals to the laboratory environment and routines.[1]

New techniques should be practiced on anesthetized animals before being used in experiments to reduce failure and prevent unnecessary suffering. Certain procedures require the use of sedatives, analgesics, or anesthetics to reduce the awareness, apprehension, distress, or pain of the animals.[2]

This chapter presents basic techniques in handling, restraining, and performing common non-surgical procedures in the most commonly used laboratory animal species. The procedures are recommended because they are easy to carry out and gentle to the animals. For topics and techniques not dealt with in this chapter or for more detailed discussions the reader is referred to specific textbooks.[3-14]

The metric system is used for measurements. Needle sizes and catheter diameters in relation to gauge systems are shown in Table 1 and Table 2, respectively. Dosing volumes in various species and needle sizes for different injection routes are summarized in Table 3.

PRE-EXPERIMENTAL ROUTINES AND CLINICAL EXAMINATION

Before an animal is used in an experiment, it is necessary to ensure that it is in good condition and accustomed to the different procedures in the experiment. "Poor animals lead to poor experiments" and misleading results. Laboratory animals should, as far as possible, be obtained from recognized breeders, capable of producing reliable genetic and health certificates.

All newly arrived animals should be clinically examined, and animals with signs of disease should not be allowed into the animal department. Sick animals must be kept in isolation until diagnostic procedures have been completed. Guinea pigs and rabbits should be tested for encephalitozoonosis if they are not certified free from this disease. Dogs and cats must be free from internal and external parasites, and it must be ascertained that the relevant vaccinations have been performed. If possible pigs should originate from a specific pathogen-free herd, and animals designated for surgical experiments should be tested for porcine stress syndrome (malignant hyperthermia) by the halothane test.

It is very important to accustom the animals to the new environment before they are used in experiments. Transport to and arriving at a new place is stressful for all animals. To overcome this stress they need time for acclimatization (quarantine). The length of this acclimatization period has been estimated by measuring the stress hormone levels and the immune response, and is reported to be a minimum of 48 hours for rats.[15] It has also been shown that changes in the external environment, staff, and the laboratory routines, as well as the experiment itself, can induce a stress response.[16,17] The following quarantine periods are recommended: rodents and guinea pigs, 5 days; rabbits, 2 weeks; cats, 3 weeks; dogs, 4 weeks; pigs and chickens, 1 week. Depending on the time and kind of transportation, the recommended periods can be adjusted up or down. In-house transports can also induce stress.[18]

On arrival from the breeder, after the end of the quarantine period, and before starting an experiment, the health and physical condition of the animals must be checked. The check list should contain the following items: behavior and movements, respiration, appearance of fur, skin, eyes, ears, nose, mouth, anal and genital openings, urine and feces, water and feed intake.

The Good Laboratory Practice (GLP) regulations[19] and national laws[20] require scientific procedures, detailed research protocols, and record-keeping. Written standard operating procedures (SOPs) for animal caretaking and handling and for research routines as well as detailed recording forms for documentation are important for meeting these requirements.

HANDLING AND PHYSICAL RESTRAINT

HANDLING

It is important to avoid stressing the animals before and during the experiment. As a general rule all animals should be handled in a safe, firm, and gentle way and kept in an environment which fulfils their ethological needs. If possible the same person should take care of feeding and watering, cleaning and cage changing, and perform minor procedures. If the animals are handled by different persons, the same routines must be used by all. Training of animals to accept new situations and procedures should be carried out before the experiment starts.[1]

Moving of animals should be reduced to a minimum.[18] Minor procedures can be performed in the animal room, as long as stress to other animals in the same room can be avoided.[21]

Rat — The best way to lift a rat is shown in Figure 1. The adult rat must not be lifted by its tail, as this may cause a circular disruption of the skin of the tail. Young rats (<3 weeks) can be lifted by the base of the tail. Rats can become very cooperative if handled and trained properly.

Mouse — The mouse is picked up from a cage by the tail as seen in Figure 2 and handled as shown in Figures 7A, B, and C. Mice are more difficult to train than rats.

Hamster — The hamster is picked up by lifting the animal with both hands. Aggressive hamsters can be removed safely from a cage if they are first allowed to hide in a small tube (plastic or paper) placed in the cage. Once they are inside the tube, the openings can be covered with both hands and the tube lifted out of the cage.

Guinea pig — Guinea pigs are handled like rats, except that larger animals must be held with two hands (Figure 3). Guinea pigs are easily frightened; in particular, they dislike sudden movements in their immediate surroundings. Panic reactions due to events outside the cage may result in severe injury to the animals.

Rabbit — Figure 4 shows how to move a rabbit to and from a cage. Figure 5A shows how to hold a rabbit and Figure 5B how to carry it. The rabbit should be placed on a table with a rough surface. Slippery surfaces are not accepted well by the rabbit. Both hands should be used when lifting and holding a rabbit. If only one hand is

Table 1. Needle Sizes in Relation to Standard Wire Gauge

External diameter	
Metric gauge (mm)	Standard wire gauge
0.25	30
0.35	28
0.40	27
0.45	26
0.50	25
0.55	24
0.65	23
0.70	22
0.80	21
0.90	20
1.10	19
1.25	18
1.45	17
1.65	16
1.80	15
2.10	14
2.40	13
2.80	12
3.00	11
3.25	10
3.65	9
4.06	8

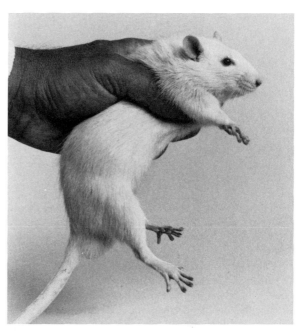

Figure 1. The correct way to lift a rat. The rat is firmly held behind the front legs.

Table 2. Catheter Dimensions in Relation to French Size

External diameter	
Metric gauge (mm)	**French gauge/*Charrière* no.**
0.33	1
0.67	2
1.00	3
1.33	4
1.67	5
2.00	6
2.33	7
2.67	8
3.00	9
3.33	10
3.67	11
4.00	12
4.33	13
4.67	14
5.00	15
5.33	16
5.67	17
6.00	18
6.33	19
6.67	20
7.00	21
7.33	22
7.67	23
8.00	24
8.33	25
8.67	26
9.00	27
9.33	28
9.67	29
10.00	30
10.33	31
10.67	32
11.00	33
11.33	34
11.67	35
12.00	36
12.33	37
12.67	38
13.00	39
13.33	40

used the rabbit may perform an escape movement involving a forceful extension of the back, which may lead to a fracture of the vertebral column. The major symptom of this fracture is complete paralysis of the hind legs. The condition is incurable, and the affected animal should be euthanized immediately. Vertebral fracture is best prevented by supporting the hind quarters when lifting the animal.

Cat — Cats bred for experimental purposes are usually docile but may react against a new situation or person and become intractable. When lifting a cat from the floor, one hand should be placed under the chest with one or two fingers between the front legs and the other hand under the belly. Kittens can be lifted with a one-hand grip of the body. Figures 6A and B show two examples of how to hold a cat. Most cats can easily be trained to accept minor experimental procedures without restraint.

Table 3. Recommended needle outer diameters and maximum injected volumes for different routes of injection route.

Species	s.c.		i.m.		i.p.		i.v.	
	Needle outer diameter, mm	Maximum volume, ml	Needle outer diameter, mm	Maximum volume, ml	Needle outer diameter, mm	Maximum volume, ml	Needle outer diameter, mm	Maximum volume, ml
Rat, 200 g	0,5-0,6	2	0,5	0,1	0,6	4-5	0,4-0,5	0,5
Mouse, 25g	≤0,5	0,5	0,4-0,5	0,05	≤0,6	2	≤0,5	0,3
Hamster, 100 g	0,5	1	≤0,5	0,1	≤0,6	2-3	≤0,5	0,3
Guinea pig, 200 g	≤0,9	2-3	0,5	0,1	0,6	4-5	≤0,4	0,5
Rabbit, 4 kg	0,9	20-30	0,6	0,5	0,8	50	0,8-0,9	10
Cat, 3 kg	0,8	20	0,8	0,5	0,8	30	0,6-0,8	5
Dog, 10 kg	0,9	50	0,8	1,0	0,8	100	0,6-0,9	10
Pig, 25 kg	0,8-1,0	10	0,9	2,0	0,9	250	0,6-0,8	20
Chicken, 1 kg	0,6	0,5-1,0	0,6-0,8	0,5	0,8	10	0,6	1

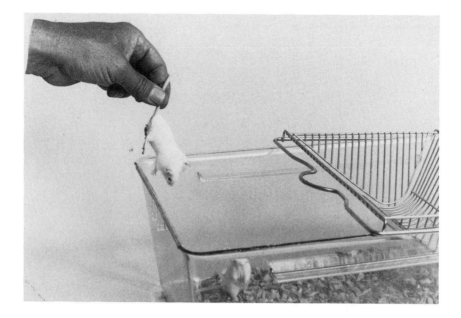

Figure 2. The mouse is picked up from a cage by the base of the tail. See also Figure 7.

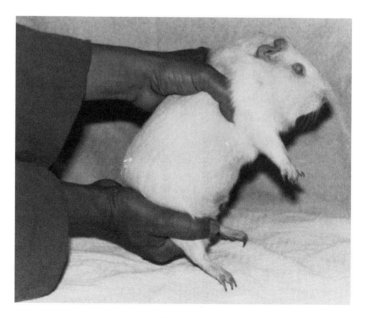

Figure 3. The correct way to hold an adult guinea pig by supporting the hind quarters.

Dog — Dogs should be lifted with one arm behind the thighs and the other in front of the chest. They should always be placed on a rough surface to prevent the paws from slipping.

Pig — Young pigs (<25 kg) can be handled without difficulty. They can be lifted and carried like dogs for short distances. Heavier pigs require special equipment, for instance trolleys.

Chicken — Chickens are lifted and held as shown in Figure 37A. Chickens are easily frightened and sudden movements should be avoided.

PHYSICAL RESTRAINT

Animals can be restrained manually or by using special restrainers. The keywords for physical restraint of animals are safety, firmness and gentleness.

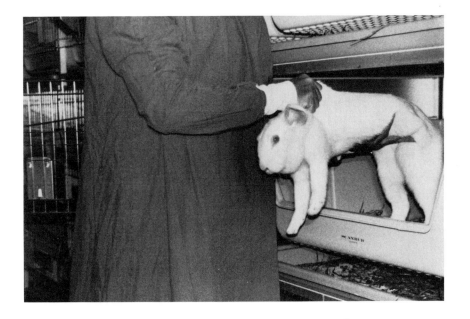

Figure 4. The correct way to remove a rabbit from its cage.

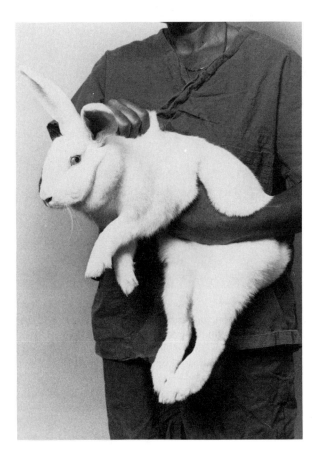

Figure 5(A). Holding a rabbit close to the body by grasping the scruff with one hand and placing the other hand under the abdomen.

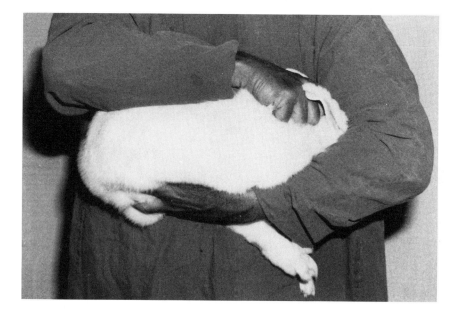

Figure 5B. The correct way to carry a rabbit with its head hidden under the arm and the body supported by arm and hand.

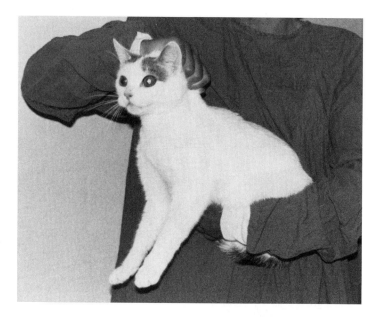

Figure 6. Correct ways to hold a cat. The cat is supported on one arm and hand close to the body: (A) with the other hand grasping the scruff.

Rat — For simple procedures rats can be held with one hand round the neck and shoulders and the other hand holding the hind legs as shown in Figures 15A and B. For procedures on the tail, like intravenous injections and blood sampling, a restrainer such as shown in Figure 17A can be used. However, increased heart rate has been demonstrated in rats kept in restraining tubes, indicating that this is a stressful experience for the animals.[22]

Mouse — The mouse is restrained with one hand for simple procedures, as shown in Figures 7A, B, and C. For procedures on the tail, like blood sampling and intravenous injections, various restrainers are in use. Figure 8 shows three different mouse restrainers.

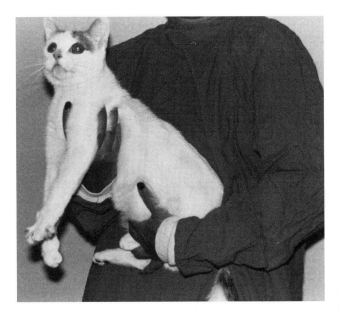

Figure 6B. With the other hand holding the front legs.

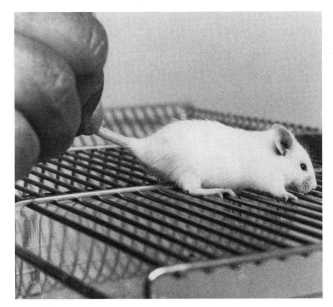

Figure 7. Holding a mouse for simple procedures. (A) The mouse is placed on the lid of the cage and held by the tail.

Hamster — Hamsters are restrained as shown in Figure 9. The loose skin on the neck and back is suitable for gripping, and if gently pressed against the table the animal will be immobilized for simple procedures.

Guinea pig — Simple procedures on guinea pigs can be performed with the animal placed on a table. It is an advantage to let an assistant restrain the animal by holding it gently over the shoulders and the back. For some procedures the guinea pig is lifted with one hand round the thorax and the other hand supporting the hind legs. Pregnant females should be handled with special care to prevent abortion.

Rabbit — Rabbits can be trained to sit in open restraining boxes for simple procedures like subcutaneous injections (Figure 10) or intravenous injections (Figure 24B) and blood sampling from the ear (Figure 35). Another method is to roll a towel round the rabbit and fasten the towel with safety pins. Restrainers of the pillory type may cause vertebral fracture, and should be avoided.

Cat — Cats can be trained to accept simple procedures without restraint. For some procedures, like intravenous injections on the legs, the cat must be held firmly by an assistant, who grasps the skin of the

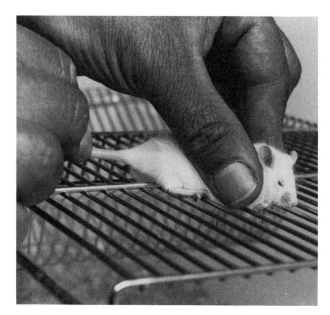

Figure 7B. When the mouse is clinging to the bars, it can be grasped by the scruff with the free hand and lifted up.

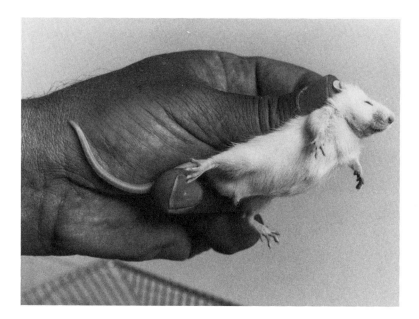

Figure 7C. The tail is fixed between the ring finger and the palm.

scruff with one hand, and the skin over the back or the hind legs above the hock joint with the other hand. For control of a difficult animal, sedatives are recommended.

Dog — Dogs are restrained as shown in Figures 11A and B for simple procedures performed on unanesthetized animals. Dogs can also easily be trained to cooperate with the researcher for simple procedures like injections and blood sampling.

Pig — Small pigs (<30 kg) are easy to restrain.[23] One way is to place them in dorsal recumbency on a specially constructed V-shaped restrainer. Large pigs may cause problems. They can be restrained in the standing position using a loop twitch as illustrated in Figure 12. With this technique, however, some apprehension and stress is unavoidable. Alternatively the pig is sedated.

Chicken — Chickens are restrained as shown in Figures 37A and B.

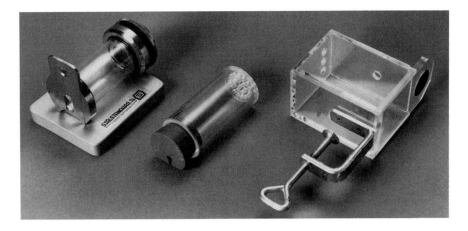

Figure 8. Equipment for restraint of mice. The left restrainer is made by B&K Stålstandard A/S, Nittedal, Norway. The other two are purpose-made.

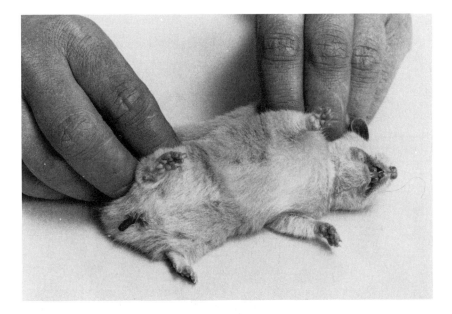

Figure 9. Restraining a hamster by grasping the loose skin of the scruff and back and pressing it against the table.

IDENTIFICATION METHODS

The GLP regulations are very strict regarding identification of animals, and animals, cages, cage-racks as well as rooms should be marked so that they can be easily identified. Various methods to identify laboratory animals have been reviewed.[6,24]

TATTOOING

Tattooing is a reliable and widely used identification method in laboratories working according to GLP. Rats and mice are mainly tattooed on the dorsal side of the tail, without damage to the blood vessels commonly used for injections or blood sampling. Rats may also be tattooed on the ears as well. Guinea pigs, rabbits, cats, dogs, and pigs are tattooed on the ears. Two types of equipment are available: tongs and tattooing pencils (Figure 13A). Tongs are suitable only for tattooing the ears. In most situations where

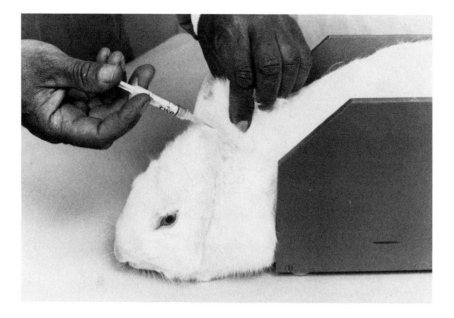

Figure 10. A rabbit in a restraining box being given a subcutaneous injection.

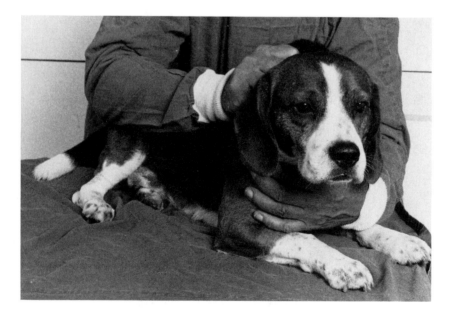

Figure 11. Two correct ways to restrain a dog for simple procedures. (A) The dog is restrained on a table in sternal recumbency by an assistant holding the scruff with one hand and supporting the chest with the other.

animals are tattooed it is recommended to have an assistant hold the animals. Tattooed figures will stay permanently and are recommended for acute as well as long-term experiments (Figure 13B). A method for tattooing the palms of the paws of newborn rats using a syringe and a needle with an external diameter of 0.8 mm has been described.[25]

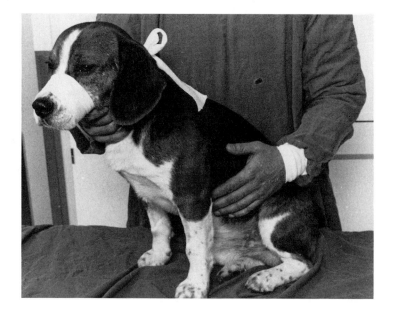

Figure 11B. To avoid bites a tape muzzle is applied with a clove hitch round the jaws and the ends tied in a bow behind the ears.

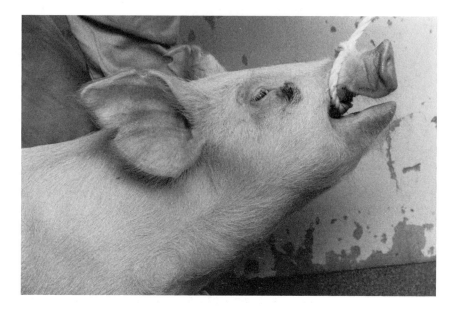

Figure 12. Restraint of a large pig with a loop twitch.

EAR TAGS

Numbered metal ear tags are commercially available. They are applied to the ear using a special instrument. Ear tags are of limited use for rodents, guinea pigs, and rabbits, as they frequently cause inflammation in the adjacent tissues and the animals often scratch them off. Possible disturbing effects on animal behavior must also be considered.

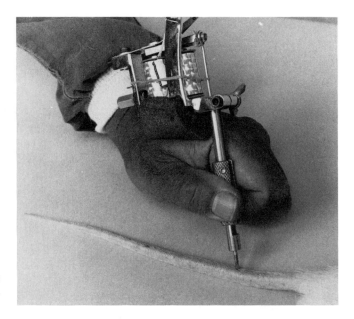

Figure 13. Identification of rodents. (A) Tattooing a rat tail with a tattooing pencil (AIMS Inc., Piscataway, NJ).

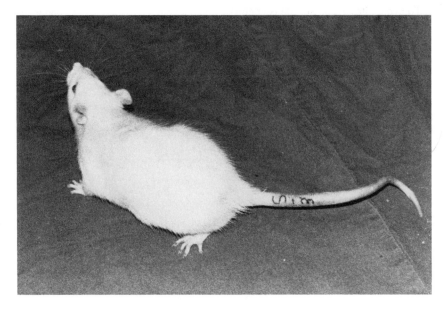

Figure 13B. Tattooed rat.

EAR PUNCHING

Ear punching is frequently used for identification of laboratory animals. Various code systems are used.[6,24] A purpose-made ear punch for rodents is shown in Figure 13C. The effect of ear punching on normal behavior is not known.

IMPLANTABLE MICROCHIPS

Biocompatible, glass-encased microchips encoded with identification numbers are now available (Bio Medic Data Systems, Inc., Maywood, NJ). The chips are injected subcutaneously using a needle with an external diameter of 3 mm. Special equipment must be used to read the numbers. Microchips can stay in the tissues of rats for up to one year without any problems.[26] The cost of microchips is relatively high.

RINGS

Numbered or variously colored plastic or metal rings applied to the legs are often used to identify chickens (Figures 37A and B).

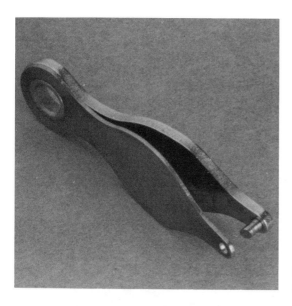

Figure 13C. Purpose-made ear punch for small rodents.

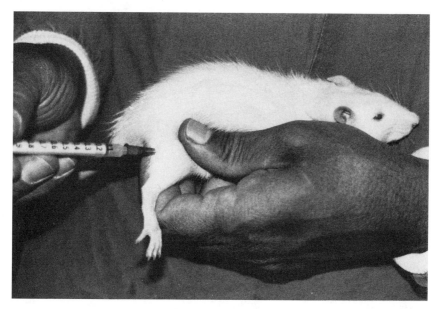

Figure 14. Intramuscular injection in the back of the thigh of a rat.

OTHER METHODS

Other methods for identification are also in use, e.g., toe clipping, fur coloring, collars, etc., but for various reasons, e.g., animal welfare and marking reliability, these methods are not generally recommended.

ADMINISTRATION OF DRUGS

INJECTIONS

Injections may be given into the skin (intracutaneous, i.c.); under the skin (subcutaneous, s.c.); into the muscles (intramuscular, i.m.); into the peritoneal cavity (intraperitoneal, i.p.); into the brain (intracerebral); and into the venous blood (intravenous, i.v.). It is important that fluids for i.c., s.c., and i.m. injections have a pH of about 7.4, are isotonic, and are injected slowly in moderate volumes to prevent pain and unnecessary tissue damage.[27] Nonisotonic fluids must be injected i.p. or i.v. The normal daily requirement of water is about 50 ml/kg body weight and larger amounts of fluid should not be injected

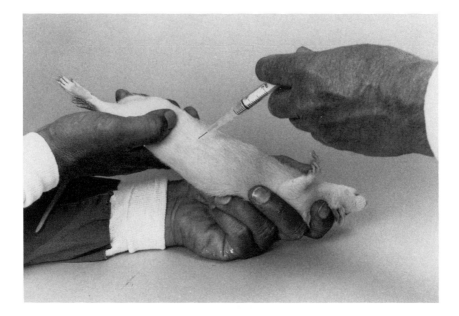

Figure 15. Intraperitoneal injection in a rat held with the hind legs stretched backwards to expose the abdomen. (A) The plastic needle case is cut about 10–15 mm from the top and the needle is passed through. The cut case will function as a stopper and prevent the needle from being inserted too deeply into the abdomen.

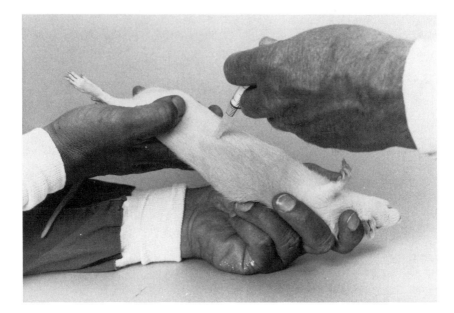

Figure 15B. The injection is performed in the lower half of the abdomen on the right or left side of the midline.

at one time. Large isotonic fluid volumes can be injected subcutaneously at several sites instead of intravenously.

Warming part of an animal or the whole body will cause vasodilatation and make the blood vessels more visible. For intravenous injections in small rodents and rabbits it is recommended to use indwelling plastic catheters[28] or butterflies. A useful method is to cut a standard hypodermic needle into two pieces

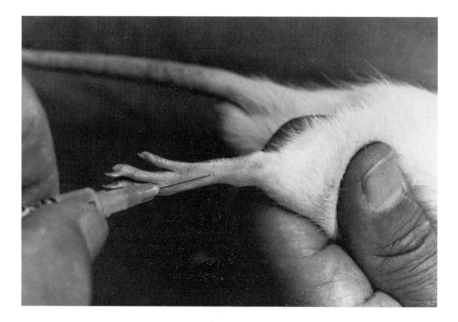

Figure 16. Intravenous injection in the dorsal metatarsal vein on the hind leg above the foot of a rat, using a hypodermic needle with an external diameter of 0.4 mm. Stasis is obtained by gentle pressure of the index finger and thumb.

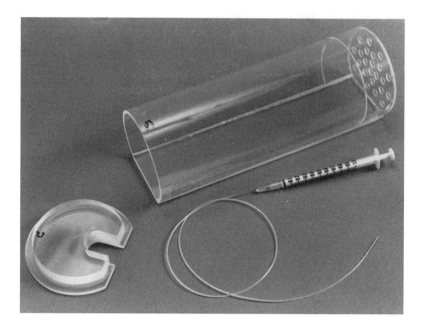

Figure 17. Intravenous injection in the lateral tail vein of a rat. (A) Restrainer and injection needle.

and connect these with a polyethylene tube, as shown in Figures 17A to C, 19, and 24. Recommended dose volumes and needle outer diameters for the different species are presented in Table 3.

Rat
Subcutaneous injection — Subcutaneous injections can best be performed in the scruff or the flank. In young rats (<50 g body weight) the flank is preferable. The maximum volume at each site should be 1 ml per 100 g body weight. Needles with an external diameter of 0.5 to 0.6 mm should be used.

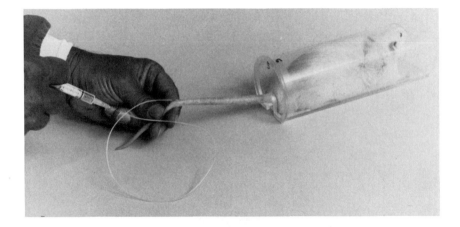

Figure 17B. Injection with a needle, external diameter 0.4 mm, cut into two halves with polyethylene tubing (PE 20) mounted in-between.

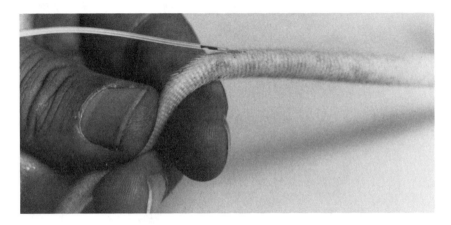

Figure 17 C. Close-up of injection site.

Intracutaneous injection — The animal should be shaved carefully on the site of injection, usually in the shoulder region. The skin is held in a fold between two fingers, and a needle with an external diameter of 0.4 mm is inserted into the cutis without entering into the subcutis, and a maximum volume of 0.1 ml is injected. An anemic bleb will appear after a correct injection.

Intramuscular injection — The best site for an i.m. injection is the back of the thigh, as shown in Figure 14. A maximum of 0.05 ml/100 g body weight can be given. Larger amounts will not stay intramuscularly. A needle with an external diameter of 0.5 mm should be used.

Intraperitoneal injection — Intraperitoneal injection in a rat is illustrated in Figures 15 A and B. The animal is held by an assistant. Needles with external diameters of 0.6 mm should be used. A plastic needle case is used to prevent too deep an injection. The top of the case is shortened to allow the tip of the needle to extrude about 10 mm. The injection is given in the lower half of abdomen on the left or right side at a 90° angle to the skin. A maximum of 5 ml can be injected.

Intravenous injection — A number of veins can be used for i.v. injections in rats. The dorsal metatarsal vein on the hind legs (Figure 16) or the lateral tail veins are used in unanesthetized rats. Young rats are easier to inject than older ones as the tail skin becomes rather thick in old animals. Warming the tail in hot water (45°C) or the whole animal under a heating lamp dilates the tail veins. Needles or indwelling plastic catheters with an external diameter of 0.5 mm are used and a maximum of 0.5 ml can be injected. Equipment for i.v. injections is shown in Figures 17A, B, and C. The sublingual veins can be used for i.v. injections in anesthetized rats. The veins are located on either side of the ventral surface

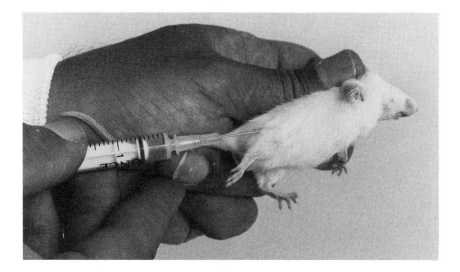

Figure 18. Subcutaneous injection in the flank of a mouse.

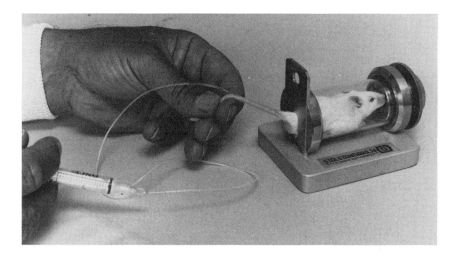

Figure 19. Intravenous injection in the lateral tail vein of a mouse using equipment similar to that shown in Figure 17 for a rat.

of the tongue, which can be pulled out by using a tissue forceps. The dorsal penile vein can also be injected into in anesthetized male rats. Needles with an external diameter of 0.4 mm are used. Repeated intravenous injections of unanesthetized rats are best done after catheterization of the jugular or femoral veins.[29,30]

Mouse

Subcutaneous injection — Subcutaneous injections are given in the scruff or in the flank, as shown in Figure 18, using needles with external diameters of 0.5 mm or less. The recommended maximum volume is 0.5 ml. Leakage from the injection site may occur if larger volumes are injected.

    Intracutaneous injection — The same site and technique are used as described for the rat.

    Intramuscular injection — Intramuscular injections cannot be performed properly in mice due to the limited muscle mass available in this species.

    Intraperitoneal injection — The same protection against injecting too deeply as described for the rat can be used (Figures 15A and B). The needle should have an external diameter of 0.6 mm or less, and

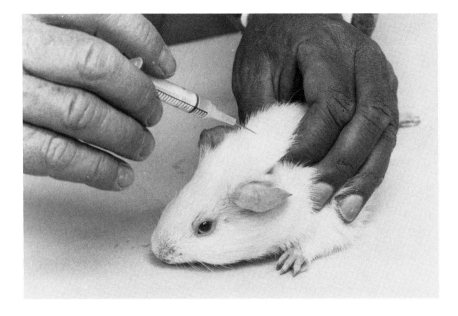

Figure 20. Subcutaneous injection in the scruff of a guinea pig.

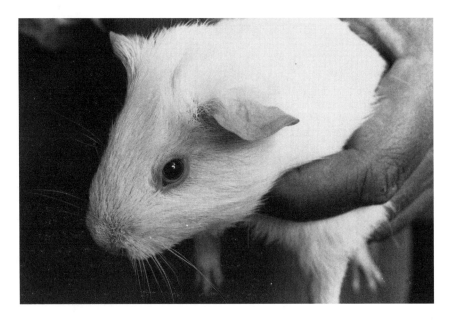

Figure 21. Ear veins of a guinea pig suitable for intravenous injection.

the injection is given in the lower half of the abdomen on either side of the midline. The maximum volume normally tolerated is 2 to 3 ml.

Intravenous injection — The lateral tail veins are preferable for injections in unanesthetized mice (Figure 19). Restraining tubes (Figure 8) or similar devices should be used. Needles should have an external diameter of 0.4 mm or less and the volume of one injection should not exceed 0.5 ml in 20- to 30-g mice. Injection must not be carried out too fast, and all air must be removed from the needle and syringe before injection.

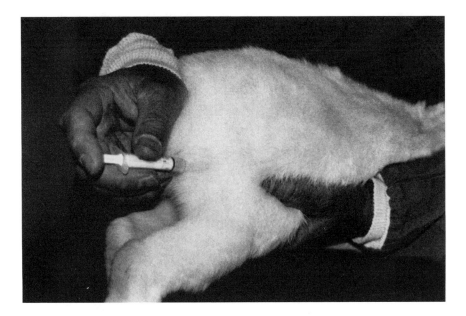

Figure 22. Intramuscular injection in the back of the thigh of a rabbit.

Intracerebral injection — Intracerebral injections should only be performed on anesthetized animals. The needle must be strong enough not to bend when passing through the skull bone. Needles with an external diameter of 0.4 to 0.6 mm are used. The depth of introduction is controlled by a cuff on the needle. The injection site is halfway between the eye and the opposite ear base. Only microliter volumes can be injected.

Hamster
Subcutaneous, intracutaneous, intramuscular, intraperitoneal and intracerebral injections are carried out as described for rats.
   Intravenous injection — The dorsal metatarsal vein on the hind leg above the foot is the best vein for injecting unanesthetized hamsters. In sedated animals the anterior cephalic vein is preferable. The femoral vein is more difficult to find, and other veins, e.g., jugular veins, can be used only after anesthesia and minor surgery.[29] Needles with external diameters of 0.4 to 0.5 mm are used and the maximum volume tolerated is 0.3 ml.

Guinea pig
Intracutaneous, intramuscular, and intraperitoneal injections are performed as described for rats.
   Subcutaneous injection — Any site on the scruff or back is suitable (Figure 20). Needles should have a maximum external diameter of 0.9 mm. Maximum tolerated volumes depend on the body weight, but not more than 5 ml should be injected at one single injection site.
   Intravenous injection — Guinea pigs are not well suited for i.v. injections. Using needles with external diameters of 0.3 to 0.4 mm, i.v. injections into the ear veins of large guinea pigs can be performed (Figure 21). Vasodilatation is obtained by warming the ear or the entire animal with a heating lamp. Other usable veins are the lateral metatarsal vein on the hind leg (Figure 34), the medial saphenous vein,[31] and the dorsal penile vein in males. For these procedures it is necessary to anesthetize the animal. The same needle size as for the ear veins can be used. The recommended maximum volume is 0.25 ml per kg body weight.

Rabbit
   Subcutaneous injection — The scruff and back are suitable sites for subcutaneous injections. In adult animals 20 to 30 ml can be injected at each site; needles with external diameters of 0.9 mm should be used (Figure 10).

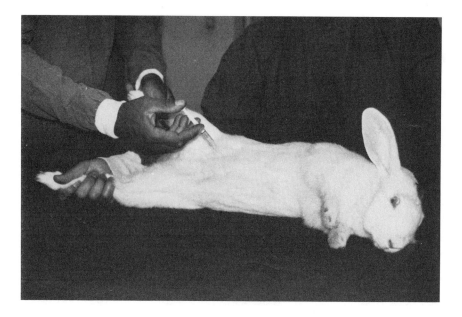

Figure 23. Intraperitoneal injection in a rabbit. The animal is restrained on the table by an assistant holding the scruff firmly with one hand and the hind legs with the other.

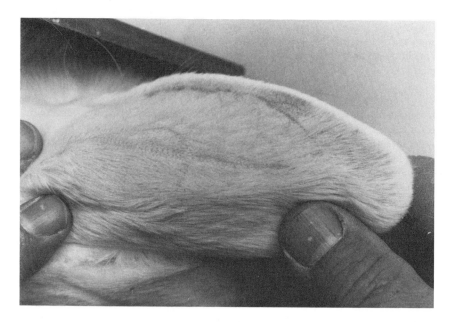

Figure 24. Intravenous injection in a rabbit ear vein. (A) Blood vessels in a rabbit ear with the central artery in the middle and the posterior marginal vein above it.

Intracutaneous injection — Any site of the skin is suitable after shaving. The same volumes, technique, and equipment are used as described for the rat. The rather thin skin on the inner surface of the ear can also be used. This injection site is especially suitable for delayed skin hypersensitivity tests. The advantage is that no shaving is needed and reactions are easy to check.

Intramuscular injection — The back of the thigh is the best site for intramuscular injection in the rabbit (Figure 22). A maximum of 0.5 ml can safely be injected, using a needle with an external diameter of 0.6 mm.

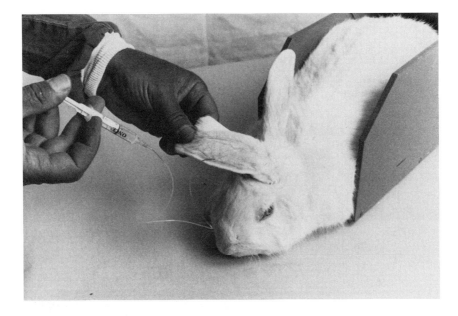

Figure 24B. Injection in the posterior marginal vein with the same type of equipment as described for mice and rats (Figures 17 and 19).

Intraperitoneal injection — The same technique to prevent the needle from being inserted too deeply by using the cut plastic needle case as a stopper, as described for rats, can be employed. Rabbits may be difficult to restrain when injected intraperitoneally and it is recommended to have an assistant hold the rabbit firmly on a table, with one hand grasping the loose skin of the scruff and the other hand holding the hind legs (Figure 23). A rabbit can also be held in dorsal recumbency on the lap of an assistant, restrained between his knees. Needles with external diameters of 0.8 mm are used and injections are given in the lower half of the abdomen on either side of the midline. The volume should not exceed 50 ml in a 3- to 4-kg rabbit.

Intravenous injection — The marginal vein on the rabbit ear is very suitable for intravenous injections (Figure 24). Warming the ear with a heating lamp will dilate the vessels and facilitate injection. Needle catheters or cut needles with external diameters of 0.8 to 0.9 mm with an intermediate polyethylene tubing (PE-60) can be used. A maximum of 10 ml can safely be injected. With infusion pumps for long-time infusions a maximum of 50 ml per kg body weight can be given over a 24-hour period. A method for chronic intravenous infusion via the marginal ear vein by means of vascular access ports has been described.[32]

Intracerebral injection — Intracerebral injection can be performed in anesthetized rabbits on the side of the skull between the eye and the ear base where a sulcus can be felt. Needles with external diameters of 0.9 mm are used and the depth of introduction is controlled by a cuff on the needle.

Cat

Subcutaneous injection — The scruff or the back is the best site for subcutaneous injection, using needles with external diameters of 0.8 mm or more. Not more than 20 ml should be injected at any injection site in adult animals.

Intramuscular injection — Injections can be performed in the muscles on the back of the thigh or the triceps brachii muscle on the back of the front leg above the elbow, using needles with external diameters of 0.8 mm and injecting a maximum of 0.5 ml at each site.

Intraperitoneal injection — Intraperitoneal injection is seldom indicated in the cat. The same injection technique as described for rabbits can be used. Cats can either be restrained by an assistant or be injected without firm restraint, standing on a table while gently grasped by the loose skin of the scruff.

Intravenous injection — The cephalic vein on the front leg is used. The cat is restrained by an assistant firmly gripping the skin of the scruff with one hand and holding the other arm round the body of the animal. Needle catheters, e.g., butterflies (external diameters of 0.6 to 0.8 mm), indwelling

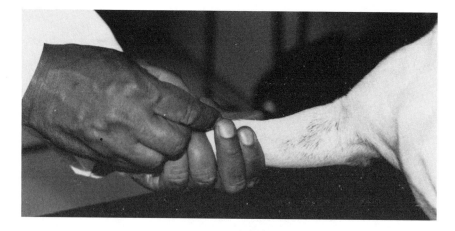

Figure 25. Intravenous injection in the cephalic vein of a dog.

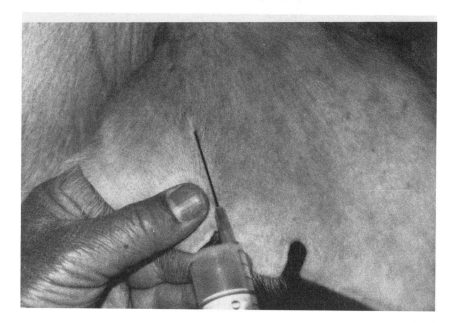

Figure 26. Intravenous injection in the ear vein of a pig.

catheters (external diameters of 0.6 to 1.0 mm) or hypodermic needles with external diameters of 0.6 to 0.8 mm can be used. The injection volumes should not exceed 5 ml.

Dog

Subcutaneous injection — The scruff and the flank are the best sites. Needles with external diameters of 0.9 mm or more are used and injections should be performed slowly, the volume not exceeding 50 ml at each site for a 10- to 15-kg dog.

Intramuscular injection — The muscles on the back of the thigh or the back of the front leg above the elbow are used. Injections should be performed slowly with not more than 0.5 to 1.0 ml at each site, using needles with an external diameter of 0.8 mm.

Intraperitoneal injection — Intraperitoneal injection is seldom indicated in the dog. The injections can be performed in the lower half of the abdomen with an assistant gently restraining the dog on a table. Needles should have an external diameter of 0.8 mm and the maximum volume should not exceed 10 ml per kg body weight.

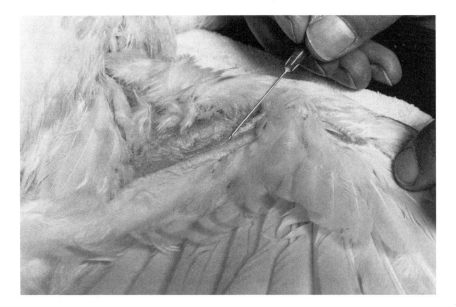

Figure 27. The brachial vein on the wing of a chicken, suitable for intravenous injections and blood sampling.

Intravenous injection — The cephalic vein on the dorsal side of the front leg is the best vein for injections (Figure 25). Needle catheters (e.g., butterflies) with external diameters of 0.5 to 2.1 mm or indwelling-type catheters are recommended. Hypodermic needles with external diameters of 0.6 to 0.9 mm can also be used. Other suitable veins are the femoral vein, the recurrent metatarsal vein on the hind leg, and the jugular vein. The recommended maximum volume for a single injection is 1 ml per kg body weight.

Pig

Subcutaneous injection — The best site for injection is on the side of the neck immediately behind the ears, where the skin and subcutaneous tissues are soft and loose. Needles with external diameters of 0.8 to 1.0 mm are used and the maximum volume at each site is 5 to 10 ml.

Intramuscular injection — Intramuscular injections in the pig are usually given in the neck region or in the thigh. Needles with external diameters of 0.9 mm are used, and the injected volume should not exceed 2 to 5 ml.

Intraperitoneal injection — The injection is given in the lower abdomen to minimize the risk of causing damage to the spleen. Needles with an external diameter of 0.9 mm can be used.

Intravenous injection — Intravenous injection can be performed in the ear veins (Figure 26). However, these veins are rather fragile, and needle catheters (butterflies) with external diameters of 0.6 to 0.8 mm or indwelling-type catheters for pediatric use are recommended rather than hypodermic needles. Large pigs can be restrained with a loop twitch (Figure 12) or tethered in a narrow pen.

Chicken

Subcutaneous injection — Subcutaneous injections are usually performed on the upper dorsal neck using needles with external diameters of 0.6 mm and maximum volumes of 0.5 to 1 ml depending on body weight.

Intracutaneous injection — The skin on the wattles is a suitable place for intracutaneous injections.

Intramuscular injection — The most suitable muscles are the pectoral muscles on either side of the sternum. Needles with an external diameter of 0.6 to 0.8 mm are preferable, and not more than 0.5 ml should be injected at each injection site. It should be ensured that blood vessels have not been perforated.

Intraperitoneal injection — This injection is performed in the midline of the abdomen, halfway between the sternum and the cloaca, using needles with external diameters of 0.8 mm. The maximum volume tolerated is 10 ml.

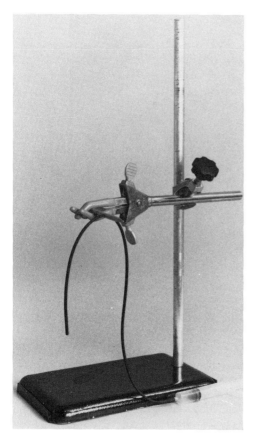

Figure 28. Oral dosing in rats. (A) Equipment consisting of a mouth gag holder, a mouth gag and a rubber tube, external diameter 2 mm, marked with the distance from mouth to stomach and connected to a syringe.

Intravenous injection — The brachial vein on the wing (Figure 27) or the posterior tibial vein (Figure 37 C) on the leg are the best superficial veins for intravenous injections. Feathers over the veins are removed to make the veins visible. Needles with external diameters of 0.6 mm can be used, and the recommended volume is 1 ml. Chronic infusion in unrestrained chickens has been described.[33]

ORAL DOSING

Oral dosing can be performed in different ways: by mixing the test compound or drug in the feed or drinking water, or by gastric intubation. When mixing in the feed or the drinking water it is necessary to control the feed or water intake of each animal and adjust the concentration of the test compound or drug to appropriate values. Animals eating dry feed like pellets drink about 100 ml per kg body weight a day.

Gastric intubation is described for each species below. The recommended maximum volumes are related to the stomach sizes. The stomach should preferably be empty (food withheld), but as small rodents, guinea pigs, and rabbits are coprophaging animals, it is difficult to ensure an empty stomach.

Rubber or PVC stomach tubes should be lubricated with water or an aqueous lubricant to make it easier to pass the esophagus. On reaching the esophagal opening, the insertion of the tube must be stopped to allow the animals to swallow.

Metric and French gauge/*Charriére* numbers are compared in Table 2.

Rat

If properly trained, rats accept repeated oral dosing without struggling or signs of fear. Stomach tubes for intubation of rats are either probe-ended metal tubes with a length of 10 to 12 cm and an external diameter of 2.0 mm, or rubber tubes of the same bore. Before inserting a stomach tube, the distance between the mouth and the stomach (located at the level of the last rib) is marked on the tube. If resistance is noted during introduction of the stomach tube, the tube is withdrawn a few millimeters, and a new attempt made. It is unlikely that the tube will enter the trachea. Figure 28A shows the equipment necessary for oral dosing of a rat and the procedure is shown in Figure 28B. The maximum dose for an adult rat is 5 ml.

Mouse and Hamster

Metal probe-ended tubes are used for gastric intubation of mice and hamsters. Equipment and procedure are shown in Figures 29A, B and C. A maximum of 2 ml may be given each time.

Guinea Pig

Metal probe-ended tubes or rubber tubes with external diameters of 1.6 to 1.8 mm can be used. The distance from mouth to stomach should be marked on the tube. A mouth gag must be used with rubber tubes to prevent damage to the tube. The maximum dose is 5 to 10 ml depending on the size of the animal. Guinea pigs are easily stressed by this procedure and should be sedated.

Rabbit

Figure 30A shows equipment for oral dosing of rabbits and Figure 30B shows how to perform gastric intubation of a rabbit. It is essential to mark the tube with the mouth-stomach distance. The maximum volume accepted by a 3- to 4-kg rabbit is 25 to 30 ml.

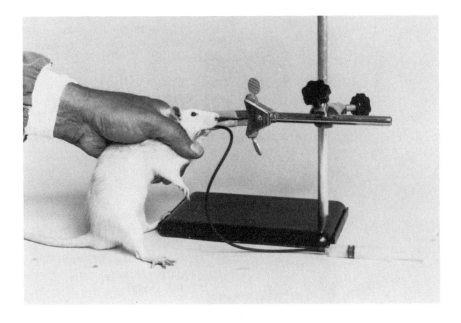

Figure 28B. Oral dosing of a rat using the equipment described.

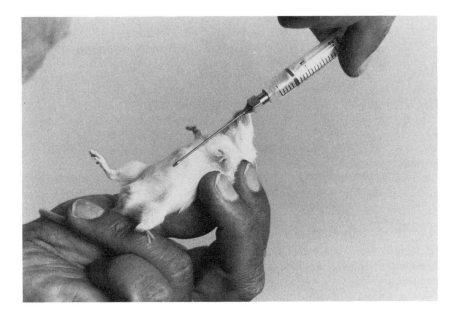

Figure 29. Oral dosing of mouse: (A) probe-ended stainless steel gastric tube measuring the distance to the stomach.

Cat

Fluids can be dosed with a syringe introduced into the corner of the mouth. Small doses (0.5 to 1.0 ml) are given at a time, and the cat is allowed to swallow between each dose. Cats can also be dosed orally using a mouth gag and a rubber stomach tube (external diameter 3 mm). The maximum volume is 15 ml for an adult cat.

Tablets or capsules are pushed to the base of the tongue with the right index finger, while the cat's head is restrained with the left hand and the mouth is opened with the third finger of the right hand by applying pressure to the lower incisors.

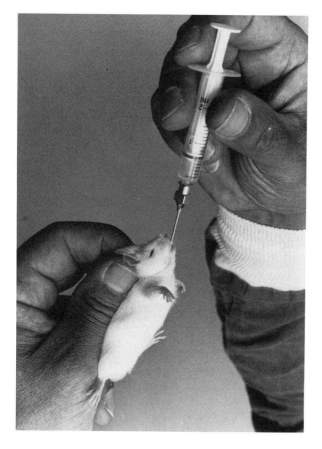

Figure 29B. inserting the tube by extending the head and neck of the animal.

Dog

Fluids can be given via a syringe introduced into the mouth or via a rubber stomach tube, using a technique similar to the one described for rabbits. A mouth gag is necessary to prevent damage to the tube. A maximum of 10 to 20 ml per kg body weight can be given.

Tablets or capsules are given directly into the mouth. Using the left hand, the mouth is forced open by applying pressure to the cheek. The tablet is placed at the base of the tongue, the mouth is closed and the pharynx region massaged until the animal swallows.

Pig

Pigs will usually resist the passing of a stomach tube, and fluids must be given in the mouth with a syringe.

Chicken

A rigid polypropylene catheter connected to a syringe of suitable size is recommended for oral dosing in chickens. The animal should be restrained by an assistant, as shown in Figure 37B. The bill is opened by gently gripping the comb with one hand, while the other hand inserts the tube through the esophagus. It is easy to see the opening of the esophagus and avoid accidental entry into the trachea. Injection should be carried out slowly to prevent vomiting. It may be difficult to pass the crop, so if it is important to deposit a substance directly in the stomach, it may be necessary to choose a bird species with no crop, like the canary.

Tablets and similar substances can be placed far back in the pharynx of the chicken with the fingers or a forceps. The animal will then swallow.

INTRATRACHEAL AND INTRABRONCHIAL INSTALLATION

Intratracheal and intrabronchial installation in anesthetized rats and mice have recently been described in detail.[34,35] Amounts of 50 µl were installed without[34] or with[35] laryngoscopes and illumination equipment. Similar techniques have previously been described in textbooks.[3,6] Gaseous products can also be administered to different animal species using special boxes where the gases are mixed with air and inhaled.

SAMPLING

BLOOD

The total blood volume of the common laboratory animal species is about 80 ml/kg body weight. A maximum of 10 to 15% (8 to 12 ml/kg body weight) of the total blood volume can be drawn without harm to the animal. Larger volumes may be obtained if plasmapheresis (reinjection of red cells) is performed or the animal is anesthetized and euthanized after the bleeding procedure. Plasma-pheresis in rats allows removal of 75% of the total plasma volume or more.[30] It is also possible to stimulate hemopoiesis by taking increasing amounts of blood with subsequent increased blood production. Blood samples are conveniently obtained by using vacuum tube systems. For small animals, 2 to 5 ml vacuum tubes for pediatric use are suitable.[36]

Figure 29C. Tube inserted into the stomach and ready for dosing.

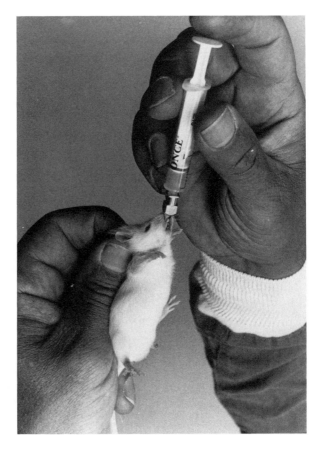

Some of the techniques described below should be used only on anesthetized animals, e.g., blood sampling from the retroorbital plexus of rodents.[37] Warming the animal, or part of it, improves the sampling efficiency. Chronic catheterization of veins or arteries can also be performed to facilitate repeated blood sampling. This needs initial surgery on anesthetized animals.[29]

The effects of blood loss, and recommendations regarding sample volume, have been presented in a review article.[38]

Rat

Ventral tail artery — Relatively large amounts of blood can be obtained from the tail artery of anesthetized rats.[39] The tail is dipped in hot water (45°C) to dilate the artery. The rat is placed in dorsal recumbency and the index finger firmly pressed against the tail about 5 cm from the tip to make the artery more visible. The artery is punctured about 1.5 cm in front of the index finger using a needle with an external diameter of 0.7 mm.

The dorsal metatarsal vein — The dorsal metatarsal vein (Figure 16) is suitable for blood sampling. The rat is held by an assistant, and stasis obtained by compression of the thigh. Puncture is performed with a 0.6 mm diameter needle. Up to 0.5 ml of blood can be obtained in a reasonable time. Warming the animal will increase the blood volume. The use of a dorsal foot vein on anesthetized rats for repeated blood sampling has been described.[40] Methyl salicylate was used for vasodilatation and the vessel was punctured with a needle of an external diameter of 0.9 mm.

Lateral tail veins — The tail should be warmed by dipping in hot water (45°C) to dilate the vessels. The veins can then be punctured using a needle with an external diameter of 0.6 mm, which is cut to a length of about 3 cm. Stasis is obtained by placing a rubber band round the tail base. It is possible to sample up to 5 ml of blood from the tail vein of a rat.[41]

Orbital plexus — The anesthetized rat is placed in lateral recumbency on a table. Stasis is obtained by gently grasping the scruff (Figures 31A and B) while perforating the conjunctiva and underlying tissues of the canthus of the eye with a thin-walled glass tube with an external diameter of about 0.5 to 1.0 mm. Standard hematocrit tubes or pasteur pipettes may be used. The tube ending should be checked for possible damage beforehand. The glass tube is pushed through the tissues while it is gently rotated until the plexus is reached. The stasis should be released before the tube is removed. On each occasion 0.5 ml of blood or more can be obtained. Studies including histological investigation have demonstrated bleeding and inflammatory reaction in the tissues after orbital plexus bleeding.[42] Endocrine stress response has also been observed.[17] The method cannot be recommended, and is discouraged by inspecting authorities in several countries.

Cardiac puncture — Cardiac puncture should only be performed on anesthetized animals followed by euthanasia. The animal is placed on its back and the heart beats are palpated (Figure 32A). A needle with an external diameter of 0.6 mm mounted on a 2- to 5-ml syringe is used. The needle is introduced from the left side where the heart beat is felt most clearly (Figure 32B). Less damage to the heart is done if the needle is cut and a polyethylene tube mounted as shown in Figures 17, 19, and 24. A slight vacuum should be created in the syringe while moving the needle towards the heart, until blood appears. A method for cardiac puncture by using a vacuum tube on CO_2-anesthetized rats has been described.[36]

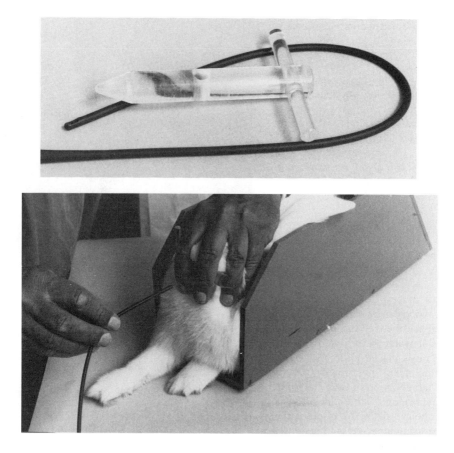

Figure 30. Oral dosing of rabbits. (A) Equipment consisting of mouth gag and rubber tube, external diameter 4 mm, marked with the distance from mouth to stomach. (B) The mouth gag is inserted behind the incisors and held by one hand with the fingers on both sides of the mouth. The tube is then inserted through the hole in the gag as far as the mark on the tube.

Exsanguination — Exsanguination can be performed by heart puncture as described above. Decapitation can be used on unanesthetized animals if special equipment is available. However, the amount of blood obtained is limited and often the blood is contaminated. Exsanguination from the aorta is performed after laparotomy and exposure of the aorta. Hemostats are used to hold the aorta as far back as possible. The aorta is then cut behind the hemostat, dissected from the dorsal surface and placed in a collecting tube.

Mouse

To obtain maximum amounts of blood (>0.5 ml) it is necessary to warm the animal. Care should be taken not to overheat it.

Ventral tail artery — The warmed mouse (Figure 33A) is placed in a restrainer (Figure 33B) and the ventral tail artery is punctured near the base of the tail with a needle with an external diameter of 1.2 mm (Figures 33B and C). A collecting tube is kept ready, as the blood comes quickly and in large drops. Using this method it is possible to obtain 0.5 ml or more from a 25- to 30-g mouse in a very short time.

Lateral tail vein — The warmed animal is placed in a restrainer as described above. Stasis can be obtained by placing a rubber band around the tail base. The vein is punctured with a needle or a small incision. The blood can drop directly into a collecting tube. This method gives smaller amounts and takes longer than blood sampling from the tail artery.

Orbital plexus — Blood sampling from the orbital plexus can be performed on anesthetized mice using the same technique as described for rats. Collection is performed using micro-hematocrit tubes. Although the method appears less traumatic to mice than to rats it is not generally recommended.

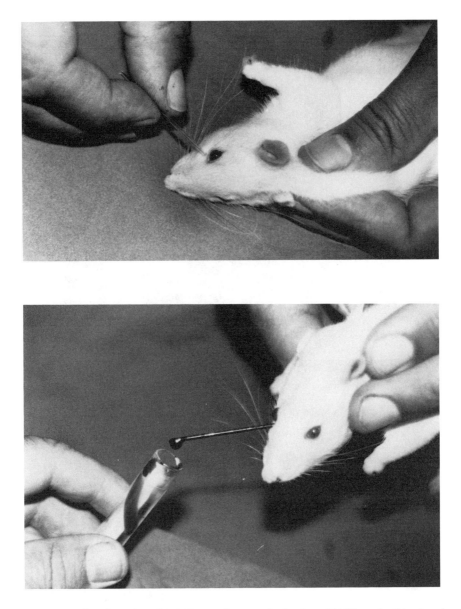

Figure 31. Blood sampling from the orbital plexus of an anesthetized rat. (A) The animal is placed on its side on the table and a fine glass tube, external diameter 1 mm, is introduced in the medial canthus of the orbit into the venous plexus. (B) Blood is collected in a glass tube.

Exsanguination — The same techniques as described for rats can be used on anesthetized mice. Other methods are bleeding from the orbital plexus after removing the eye, or by making an incision in the axillary region including the axillary artery and collecting the blood from the wound with a pasteur pipette.

Hamster
Blood sampling and exsanguination are performed in hamsters using the same procedures as for rats.

Guinea pig
The lateral metatarsal vein — Small amounts of blood (0.5 to 2 ml) can be obtained from the lateral metatarsal vein, which is punctured with a needle (external diameter 0.9 mm) or with a scalpel blade. Stasis is obtained by squeezing the thigh, as shown in Figures 34A and B.

Ear veins — Small amounts (<0.5 ml) can be obtained from the ear veins of a warmed animal.

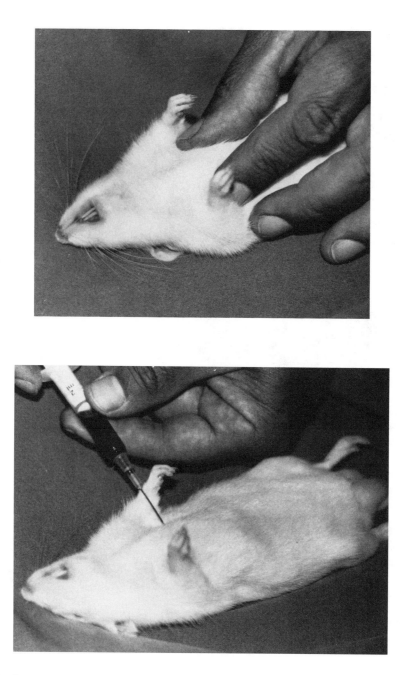

Figure 32. Cardiac puncture in an anesthetized rat; (A) The heart beats are palpated; (B) The needle, external diameter 0.6–0.9 mm, is inserted from the left side.

Cardiac puncture — Heart puncture can be performed on anesthetized animals using the same technique as described for the rat.

Exsanguination — Decapitation and abdominal aorta bleeding as described for rats can be used. Another method is to stun the animal by a blow to the head followed by cutting the carotid arteries. Cardiac puncture on anesthetized animals can also be used for exsanguination.

Rabbit

Central ear artery — Blood can be drawn from the central ear artery of rabbits. The blood flow may be increased by heating the animal or by sedation with fentanyl/fluanisone (Figure 35). A hypodermic

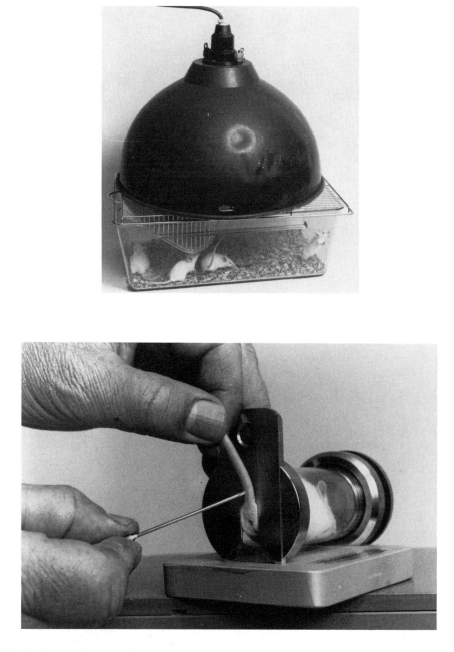

Figure 33. Blood sampling from the ventral artery of the mouse tail. (A) Infrared lamp used for warming the animals in the cage. (B) Mouse placed in a heavy glass/metal restrainer (B&K Stålstandard AS, Nittedal, Norway) with the puncture needle, external diameter 1.2 mm, pointing at the site where the artery is to be punctured

needle with an external diameter of 0.9 mm, cut to about 3 cm, can be used. With a cut needle it takes longer for the blood to coagulate.

Marginal ear veins — The marginal ear veins can be punctured with a needle or a scalpel blade, and blood is collected directly in a tube. The skin over the vein is clipped and the animal is warmed with a heating lamp placed over the ear during collection. Blood flow can also be stimulated by rubbing the ear with gauze moistened with methyl salicylate. If an incision is used, the skin around the incision can be treated with petroleum jelly to facilitate blood collection.

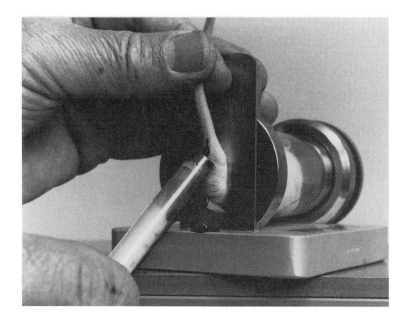

Figure 33C. Blood sampling from the artery.

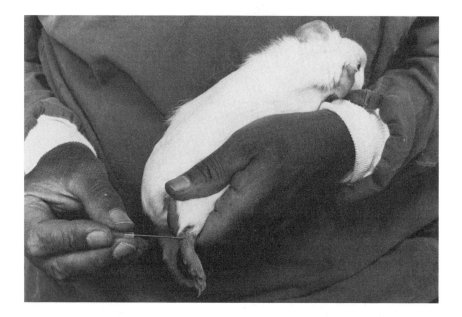

Figure 34. Blood sampling in a guinea pig. (A) The puncture needle, external diameter 1.2 mm, is pointing at the lateral metatarsal vein of the lower hind leg. After performing stasis with the thumb and index finger, the blood vessel is easily seen.

Cardiac puncture — The same technique is applied to rabbits as described for the rat, using a needle with an external diameter of 0.9 mm. The blood is aspirated with a syringe.

Catheterization — Repeated blood sampling from rabbits by catheterization of the ear artery[43] and catheterization of the vena cava via the marginal ear vein[44] has been described. The blood is collected by aspiration with a syringe.

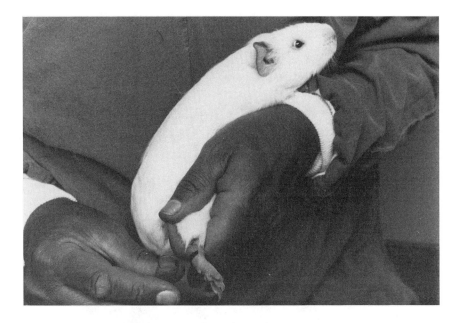

Figure 34B. The vein is punctured and blood collected in a glass tube.

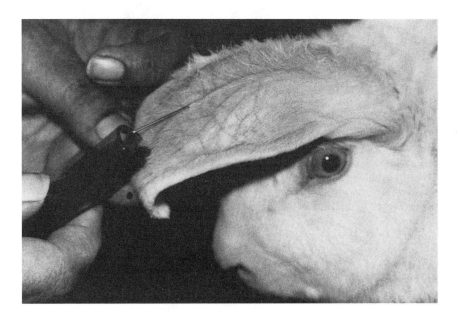

Figure 35. Blood sampling from the central artery of a rabbit ear. The needle, external diameter 0.9 mm, is cut to a length of 25–30 mm.

Exsanguination — Cardiac puncture or catheterization of the carotid artery on anesthetized animals are the best methods. It must be ensured that the animals are dead at the end of the procedure, e.g., by injecting an overdose of an injectable anesthetic.

Cat
Marginal ear vein — The marginal ear vein can be used for collecting small volumes of blood (<0.5 ml). The ear should be shaved over the vein, petroleum jelly applied and the animal placed under a heating

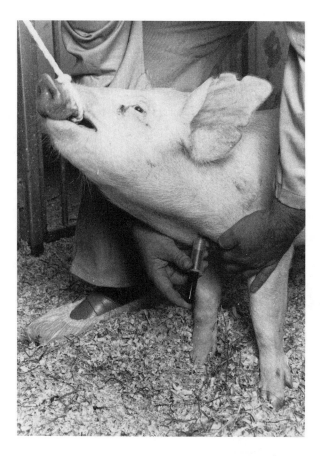

Figure 36. Blood sampling from the anterior vena cava of a pig using a standard vacuum tube set.

lamp. The vein is punctured with a needle or a scalpel, and the blood is allowed to drip into a collecting tube.

Cephalic vein — The cephalic vein puncture is performed with a 0.6 mm-needle cut to a length of about 3 cm. Stasis is obtained by applying compression above the elbow. Two to five ml of blood can be collected by this method.

Jugular vein — The cat is clipped over the vein and sedated or anesthetized. To expose the vein, the head of the cat is turned to the side and upwards. Stasis is obtained by placing a finger on the vein close to the thorax opening. Vein puncture is performed using a needle with an external diameter of 0.8 mm.

Cardiac puncture — The cat must be anesthetized, and the same sampling technique as described for rats is used.

Exsanguination — Exsanguination is performed by cardiac puncture or by catheterization of the carotid artery on anesthetized animals.

Dog

Cephalic vein — The cephalic vein on the dorsal surface of the forelimb is the most commonly used vein for blood sampling in dogs. Stasis is obtained by applying pressure round the elbow with either the hand or a rubber band. The skin over the vein is clipped and a needle with an external diameter of 0.8 to 0.9 mm is introduced into the vein.

Recurrent metatarsal vein — This vein is located on the lateral surface of the hock joint. The skin over the vein is clipped and a needle with an external diameter of 0.8 mm is used.

Jugular vein — Nervous dogs should be sedated or superficially anesthetized. The skin of the jugular groove is clipped and stasis achieved by compression of the vein. Needles with an external diameter of 0.8 to 0.9 mm and vacuum tubes are used to sample up to 10 ml or more.

Exsanguination — Cardiac puncture of anesthetized animals is the best method of exsanguination. The same technique is applied as described for rabbits. A needle with an external diameter of 1.2 mm

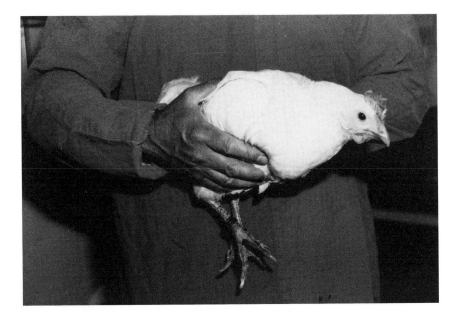

Figure 37. Blood sampling from the posterior tibial vein of a chicken. (A) The chicken is picked up and held by placing both hands over the wings.

connected to a large syringe (20 to 30 ml) is used. An intracardial overdose of an injectable anesthetic may be necessary to ensure that the animal is dead. Exsanguination from jugular veins or carotid arteries after catheterization can also be performed on anesthetized animals.

Pig
Ear vein — Small volumes of blood can be obtained from the ear veins. Stasis is obtained by placing a rubber band round the ear base. The vein can be punctured using a needle with an external diameter of 0.9 mm, or a scalpel.

Anterior vena cava — Large blood samples are obtained from this vein. Small pigs are restrained by placing them in dorsal recumbency on a table or in a V-shaped restrainer; large pigs are restrained in the standing position using a loop twitch (Figure 12). A standard vacuum tube connected to a needle with an external diameter of 1.0 to 1.2 mm and a length of 6 to 10 cm, depending on the size of the pig, should be used. The needle is inserted in a caudo-dorsal direction 20 to 30 mm from the anterior sternum on an imaginary line from the ear base to the Manubrium sterni (Figure 36).

Jugular vein — Catheterization of the jugular vein to enable long-term blood sampling from growing piglets has been described.[45] Using this method it is possible to sample blood without inducing stress reactions such as increased plasma concentrations of cortisol and glucose, increased white blood cell counts and hematocrit values, and changes in rectal temperature and heart rate. A simple technique for jugular catheterization via an ear vein in adult sows without long-term stress responses has also been described.[46]

Chicken
Posterior tibial vein — This vein is located after removal of feathers on the distal part of the thigh where the vein crosses the medial surface (Figure 37C). It is possible to obtain 5 to 10 ml of blood or more from an adult bird. A needle with an external diameter of 0.9 mm cut to a length of about 3 cm is used (Figure 37D).

Brachial vein — The wing vein as shown in Figure 27 is also suitable for blood sampling. The same equipment is used as described for the posterior tibial vein (above). Cannulation of the brachial vein for repeated blood sampling has been described.[47] The tubing is fixed to the inner side of the wing.

Cardiac puncture — The chicken heart is difficult to locate by palpation. Cardiac puncture should be performed on anesthetized animals, using a hypodermic needle with an external diameter of 0.8 mm

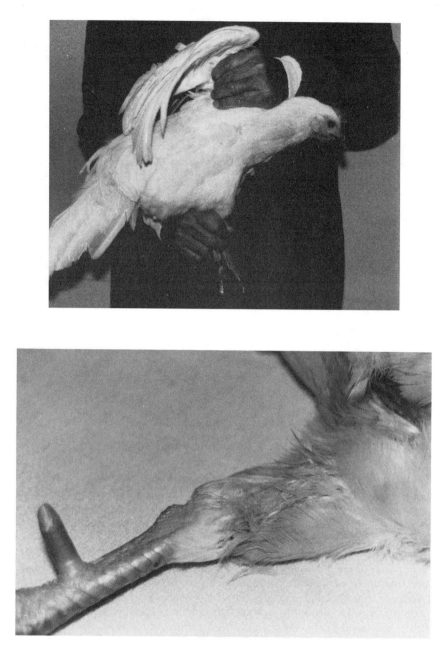

Figure 37. (B) The chicken is restrained by holding the wings together above the body with one hand and holding the legs with the other hand. (C) The vein is made visible by removing the feathers.

and mounted on a syringe. The animal is held in dorsal recumbency by an assistant. The needle can be introduced through the anterior thoracic opening or through the thoracic wall between the two first ribs close to the sternum. A method for vacuum-assisted cardiac puncture has been developed to facilitate the collection of large amounts of blood in a short time.[48]

Exsanguination — Cardiac puncture on anesthetized animals or decapitation are the methods to be used.

URINE AND FECES

Single samples of urine and feces can be collected by sampling when the animals urinate or defecate. Rodents usually urinate and defecate when they are picked up and restrained. This habit differs among

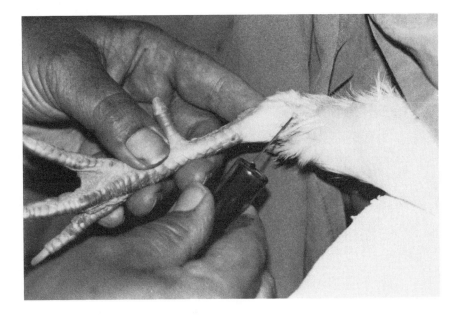

Figure 37(D) The vein is punctured with a needle, external diameter 0.9 mm, cut to a length of about 30 mm.

strains. Manual compression of the lower abdomen may provoke urination. If uncontaminated urine is required, urethral catheterization[6,9,49] or aspiration of the urine through the abdominal wall using a syringe and needle is preferred. When the total amount of urine and feces is required over a period of some time, metabolism cages are used (Figure 38).[8]

CEREBROSPINAL FLUID

Cerebrospinal fluid is obtained in a similar way from all animals. The animals are anesthetized and shaved over the dorsal atlanto-occipital region, the head is flexed, and a needle is introduced in the midline through the atlanto-occipital membrane. Contamination with blood may occur, specially at repeated sampling.

Rat — The Cisterna magna in rats is reached through the atlanto-occipital membrane with a 0.6-mm needle connected to polyethylene tubing.[4] It is possible to obtain 0.1 to 0.15 ml.

Mouse — Collection of cerebrospinal fluid from mice requires a skin incision from a point 4 mm cranial to the external occipital protuberance to a point 1 cm cranial to the shoulder. The membrane is punctured with a 22-gauge needle and 0.025 ml of fluid can be collected.[50]

Guinea pig — Repeated sampling of cerebrospinal fluid can be performed in guinea pigs using a needle with an external diameter of 0.6 mm connected to a syringe.[51] The needle is introduced through the atlanto-occipital membrane with a 20 to 30° angle between the needle and the axis of the head. It is possible to obtain between 0.03 and 0.33 ml on each occasion.

Rabbit — After anesthesia and clipping of the dorsal cervical and occipital areas, the rabbit is placed in lateral recumbency and its head is flexed ventrally. A needle with an external diameter of 0.7 mm is inserted into the 4th ventricle, and 1.5 to 2 ml of cerebrospinal fluid can be collected.[6,52]

Cat — Anesthetized animals should be clipped and disinfected in the atlanto-occipital region. The anesthetized animal is placed in lateral recumbency and the head flexed. A spinal needle with an external diameter of 0.8 mm and a stylet is inserted at a 90° angle to the dorsal neck through the atlanto-occipital membrane. Decreased resistance is noted as the needle enters the Cisterna magna. At this point the stylet is withdrawn and cerebrospinal fluid will appear. A maximum of 0.5 ml can be removed. More details can be found in textbooks of clinical veterinary medicine.[53,54]

Dog — The same technique as described for the cat can be used in dogs. The depth of insertion varies with the size of the animal. A maximum of 1 to 2 ml can be sampled from a 10-kg dog.

Pig — A method for repeated collection of cerebrospinal fluid from conscious pigs and sheep has been described.[55] The method requires initial surgery. Frequent sampling of 0.05 to 0.15 ml of cerebrospinal fluid via polyethylene tubings can be carried out for several weeks.

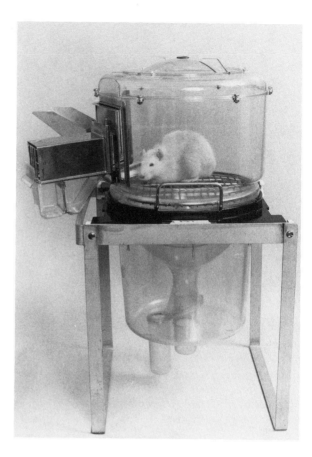

Figure 38. Sampling urine and feces from a rat using a metabolism cage (Techniplast Gazzada S.A.R.L., Italy).

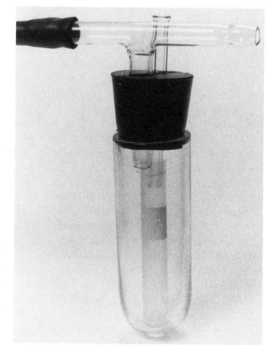

Figure 39. Equipment for sampling milk from rats. The T-shaped glass tube is connected to a vacuum pump via the rubber tubing. The open limb is operated with a finger tip to create intermittent vacuum, simulating sucking. The open straight glass pipe through the stopper ends in a small collecting tube inside the large glass tube and its outer end is applied to the teat.

MILK

A milking machine for small laboratory rodents is shown in Figure 39. A large glass collecting tube with a rubber stopcock, through which two holes have been drilled, is used. One T-shaped glass tubing and one straight glass tubing are inserted in the drilled channels. The straight tubing is connected to a smaller collecting tube inside the large collecting tube and the outer end is applied to the teat. One end of the T-shaped tubing is connected to a vacuum pump or water vacuum. The other end is operated with one finger to obtain an intermittent vacuum resembling sucking. The vacuum level should be between 250 and 300 mm of mercury. The mammary glands are massaged gently towards the teat during the milking process. This device can be used for all laboratory animal species if the size of the equipment is adjusted to the size of the animal.[56] In rats up to 7 ml of milk can be obtained daily.[4]

PERITONEAL FLUID AND PERITONEAL CELLS

Ascitic fluid — Ascitic fluid, for instance from mice innoculated i.p. with hybridoma cells, can be aspirated with a syringe and a needle with the size adjusted to the size of the animal. If the needle becomes obstructed by the intestines or the omentum, fluid is allowed to flow freely through the needle without applying a vacuum. A method for intraperitoneal sampling of ascitic fluid from rats has been described.[57] Silicone rubber tubing is implanted surgically and fluid collected for several hours.

Peritoneal cells — By washing the abdominal cavity with isotonic solutions, e.g., Hank's solution, peritoneal cells can be collected from unanesthetized, anesthetized, or dead animals using a syringe and needle.

BONE MARROW

The proximal part of the tibia is the most common site for collection of bone marrow from anesthetized rodents, guinea pigs, and rabbits. A needle with an external diameter of 1.2 to 1.8 mm is connected to a syringe of a relatively large volume, making it possible to create a sufficient vacuum. Only small samples of bone marrow can be obtained from rodents and guinea pigs. Up to 1 ml can be obtained from rabbits.

Any of the large bones of the legs can be used for collection of bone marrow from dead animals.

BRONCHOALVEOLAR LAVAGE

A semi-automatic method for standardized bronchoalveolar lavage of small laboratory animals has been described.[59] The animals must be anesthetized and then euthanized by cutting the abdominal aorta. The lungs are placed in a purpose-made pressure chamber with valves which make it possible to create and release pressure. Eight ml of lavage buffer solution should be used for a 200-g rat to wash out alveolar macrophages from the lungs.

OTHER TECHNIQUES

BODY TEMPERATURE CONTROL

Small animals with high metabolic rates are sensitive to environmental temperature changes, especially when they are anesthetized. It is important to keep the body temperature at normal values also during short periods of anesthesia. Sensitive experiments are also dependent on a constant body temperature, as even small changes in temperature may result in metabolic changes.

An instrument for control of body temperature (CMA/150) in anesthetized small rodents during experiments is commercially available (CMA Microdialysis AB, Stockholm, Sweden). A picture of this instrument is shown in Figure 40.

NON-INVASIVE BLOOD PRESSURE MEASUREMENT

Arterial systolic blood pressure in rats can be measured by tail cuff methods.[60] A new method using a microphone attached to the tail by a piece of rubber tubing has been described.[61] Tail artery pulsations are transmitted to the microphone via the air inside the tubing and the mean arterial blood pressure is recorded. The values correlate well with the mean femoral artery pressure measured by conventional catheterization of the femoral artery.

Another indirect method of determining mean arterial blood pressure and systolic blood pressure in hypertensive rats is to use a photoelectric oscillometric apparatus (UR-1000, Ueda Electric Works Co.,

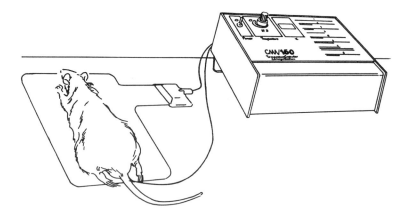

Figure 40. Equipment for temperature control during experiments (CMA/150 Temperature Controller, CMA-Microdialysis AB, Stockholm, Sweden).

Tokyo, Japan).[62] The pressure is measured by inserting the tail into a cuff containing a photoelectric pulse detector connected to an oscillator.

Simple direct blood pressure measurements in conscious dogs can be performed by intra-arterial use of vascular-access-ports (Norfolk Medical Products, Inc., Skokie, IL). The method requires an initial, minor surgical procedure to catheterize the femoral artery.[63]

REFERENCES

1. *Guidelines on the Handling and Training of Animals*, Prepared by The Biological Council, Animal Research and Welfare Panel, Universities Federation for Animal Welfare, Potters Bar, Herts, 1992.
2. *Guidelines on the Care of Laboratory Animals and Their Use for Scientific Purposes, IV, Planning and Design of Experiments*, Laboratory Animal Science Association/Universities Federation for Animal Welfare, Potters Bar, Herts, 1990.
3. Harkness, J. E. and Wagner, J. E., *The Biology and Medicine of Rabbits and Rodents*. Lea & Febiger, Philadelphia, 1977.
4. Waynforth, H. W. and Flecknell, P.A., *Experimental and Surgical Technique in the Rat*. Academic Press Inc., London, 2nd ed., 1992.
5. *Guide to the Care and Use of Experimental Animals*, Vols 1 and 2, Canadian Council on Animal Care, Ontario, 1980, 1984.
6. Bivin, W. S. and Smith, G. D., Techniques of experimentation, in Fox, J. G., Cohen, J. B. and Loew, F. M., Eds., *Laboratory Animal Medicine*, Academic Press, New York, 1984, chap. 19.
7. Poole, T., Ed., *The UFAW Handbook on the Care and Management of Laboratory Animals*, Longmans, London, 1986.
8. Gay, W.J. and Heavner, J.E., *Methods of Animal Experimentation, Vol VII*, Academic Press, New York, 1986.
9. Flecknell, P. A., Non-surgical experimental procedures, in Tuffery, A. A., Ed., *Laboratory Animals. An Introduction for New Experimenters*, John Wiley & Sons, Chichester, 1987, chap. 13.
10. Scobie-Trumper, P., Animal handling and manipulations, in Tuffery, A. A., Ed., *Laboratory Animals. An Introduction for New Experimenters*, John Wiley & Sons, Chichester, 1987, chap. 9.
11. Tuffery, A. A., Ed., *Laboratory Animals. An Introduction for New Experimenters*. John Wiley & Sons, Chichester, 1987.
12. Kesel, M. L., Handling, restraint, and common sampling and administration techniques in laboratory species, in Rollin, B.E. and Kesel, M.L., Eds., *The Experimental Animal in Biomedical Research*, Vol. 1, CRC Press, Boston, 1990, chap. 19.
13. Anderson, R. S. and Edney, A. T. B., *Practical Animal Handling*, Pergamon Press, Oxford, 1991.

14. *Guidelines for the Recognition and Assessment of Pain in Animals.* Prepared by a Working Party of the Association of Veterinary Teachers and Research Workers, Universities Federation for Animal Welfare, Potters Bar, Herts, 1992.

15. Landi, M., Bowman, T. and Campbell, S., Effects of handling and transportation stress on rodents, in Beynen, A. C. and Solleveld, H. A., Eds., *New Developments in Biosciences: Their Implications for Laboratory Animal Science,* Martinus Nijhoff Publishers, Boston, 1988.

16. Gärtner, K., Büttner, D., Dvhler, K., Friedel, R., Lindena, J. and Trautschold, I., Stress response of rats to handling and experimental procedures, *Lab. Anim.,* 14, 267, 1980.

17. Van Herck, H., Baumans, V., De Boer, S. F., Van Der Gugten, J., Van Woerkom, A. B. and Beynen, A. C., Endocrine stress response in rats subjected to singular orbital puncture while under diethyl-ether anaesthesia, *Lab. Anim.,* 25, 325, 1991.

18. Drozdowics, C. K., Bowman, T. A., Webb, M. L. and Lang, C. M., Effect of in-house transport on murine plasma corticosterone concentration and blood lymphocyte populations, *Am. J. Vet. Res.,* 51, 1841, 1990.

19. *Federal Register,* 21 CFR, part 58, Sept. 4, 1987, Food and Drug Administration, Washington, D.C.

20. Wootton, R. and Flecknell, P. A., Record-keeping requirements of the Animals (Scientific Procedures) Act 1986 and how to meet them, *Lab. Anim.,* 21, 267, 1987.

21. Sales, G. D. and Milligan, S. R., Ultrasound and Laboratory animals, *Anim. Technol.,* 43, 89, 1992.

22. Garner, D., McGivern, R., Jagels, G. and Laks M. M., A new method for direct measurement of systolic and diastolic pressures in conscious rats using vascular-access-ports, *Lab. Anim. Sci.,* 38, 205, 1988.

23. Holtz, W., Pigs and minipigs, in Poole, T., Ed., *The UFAW Handbook on the Care and Management of Laboratory Animals,* Longmans, London, 1986, chap. 31.

24. Assal, A. N., Review of the identification methods of laboratory mice, rats, rabbits and guinea pigs, *Scand. J. Lab. Anim.* Sci., 15, 19, 1988.

25. Iwaka, S., Matsuo, A. and Kast, A., Identification of newborn rats by tattooing, *Lab. Anim.,* 23, 361, 1989.

26. Ball, D. J., Argentieri, G., Krause, R., Lipinski, M., Robison, R. L., Stoll, R. E. and Visscher, G. E., Evaluation of a microchip implant system used for animal identification in rats, *Lab. Anim. Sci.,* 41, 195, 1991.

27. Porter, W. P., Bitar, Y. M., Strandberg, J. D. and Charache, P. C., A comparison of subcutaneous and intraperitoneal oxytetracycline injection methods for control of infectious disease in the rat, *Lab. Anim.,* 19, 3, 1985.

28. Nachtman, R. G., Driscoll, T. B., Gibson, L. A. and Johnson, P. C., Jr., Commercial over-the-needle catheters for intravenous injections and blood sampling in rats, *Lab. Anim. Sci.,* 38, 629, 1988.

29. Blouin, A. and Cormier, Y., A technique for repeated I.V. sampling and infusion in small animals, *Lab. Anim.,* 17, 17, 1988.

30. Reding, R., White, D. J. G., Davies, H. S. and Calne, R. Y., Plasma exchange technique in the unheparinized unanaesthetized rat, *Lab. Anim.,* 22, 293, 1988.

31. Carraway, J. H. and Gray, L. D., Blood collection and intravenous injection in the guinea pig via the medial saphenous vein, *Lab. Anim. Sci.,* 39, 623, 1989.

32. Melich, D., A method for chronic intravenous infusion of the rabbit via the marginal ear vein, *Lab. Anim. Sci.,* 40, 327, 1990.

33. Cravener, T. L. and Vasilatos-Younken, R., A method for catheterization, harnessing and chronic infusion of undisturbed chickens, *Lab. Anim.,* 23, 270, 1989.

34. Smith, G., A simple non-surgical method of intrabronchial instillation for the establishment of respiratory infections in the rat, *Lab. Anim.,* 25, 46, 1991.

35. Stacher, B. and Williams, I., A method for intratracheal instillation of endotoxin into the lungs of mice, *Lab. Anim.,* 23, 234, 1989.

36. Sardi, A. and Facundus, E., A simplified aseptic technique to obtain large blood samples in the rat model, *Lab. Anim.,* 20, 51, 1991.

37. Timm, K. I., Orbital venous anatomy of the Mongolian gerbil with comparison to the mouse, hamster and rat, *Lab. Anim. Sci.,* 39, 262, 1989.

38. McGuill, M. W. and Rowan, A. N., Biological effects of blood loss: implications for sampling volumes and techniques, *ILAR NEWS,* 31, 5, 1989.

39. Böber, R., Technical Review: Drawing blood from the tail artery of a rat, *Lab Anim.*, July/Aug. 33, 1988.

40. Snitily, M. U., Bentry, M. J., Mellencamp, M. A. and Preheim, L. C., A simple method for collection of blood from the rat foot, *Lab. Anim. Sci.*, 41, 285, 1991.

41. Omaye, S. T., Skala, J. H., Gretz, M. D., Schaus, E. E. and Wade, C. E., Simple method for bleeding the unanaesthetized rat by tail venipuncture, *Lab. Anim.*, 21, 261, 1987.

42. Van Herck, H., Baumans, V., Van Der Craats, N. R., Hesp, A. P. M., Meijer, G. W., Van Tintelen, G., Walvoort, H. C. and Beynen, A. C., Histological changes in the orbital region of rats after orbital puncture, *Lab. Anim.*, 26, 53, 1992.

43. Smith, P. A., Prieskorn, D. M., Knutsen, C. A. and Ensminger, W. D., A method for frequent blood sampling in rabbits, *Lab. Anim. Sci.*, 38, 623, 1988.

44. Martin, F. R., Alguacil, L. F. and Alamo, C., A method for catheterizing rabbit vena cava via marginal ear vein, *Lab. Anim. Sci.*, 41, 493, 1991.

45. Takahashi, H., Long-term blood-sampling technique in piglets, *Lab. Anim.*, 20, 206, 1986.

46. Zanella, A. J. and Mendl, M. T., A fast and simple technique for jugular catheterization in adult sows, *Lab. Anim.*, 26, 211, 1992.

47. Zhou, C. and Brown, L. A., Intravenous cannulation of chickens for blood sampling, *Lab. Anim. Sci.*, 38, 631, 1988.

48. Foytik, J. E., Satterfield, W. C., Bailey, J. W. and Keeling, M. E., Vacuum-assisted cardiac puncture in chickens, *Lab. Anim. Sci.*, 39, 626, 1989.

49. Wagner, R. W. and Stein, F. J., A new approach to urethral catheterization of female dogs, *Lab. Anim. Sci.*, 37, 111, 1987.

50. Vogelweid, C. M. and Kier, A. B., A technique for the collection of cerebrospinal fluid from mice, *Lab. Anim. Sci.*, 38, 91, 1988.

51. Reiber, H. and Schunk, O., Suboccipital puncture of guinea pigs, *Lab. Anim.*, 17, 25, 1983.

52. Kusumi, R. K. and Plouffe, J. F., A safe and simple technique for obtaining cerebrospinal fluid from rabbits, *Lab. Anim. Sci.*, 29, 681, 1979.

53. Coles, E. H., *Veterinary Clinical Pathology*, 2nd ed., W. B. Saunders Company, Philadelphia, 1974.

54. Oliver, J. E., Jr., Redding, R. W. and Knecht, C. D., Introduction to the central nervous system, in Ettinger, S. J. Ed., *Textbook of Veterinary Internal Medicine*, Vol. 1, W. B. Saunders Company, Philadelphia, 1975, chap. 10.

55. Preluski, D. B. and Hartin, K. E., A technique for serial sampling of cerebrospinal fluid from conscious swine and sheep, *Lab. Anim. Sci.*, 41, 481, 1991.

56. Marcus, E. G., Shum, F. T. F. and Goldman, S. L., A device for collecting milk from rabbits, *Lab. Anim. Sci.*, 40, 219, 1990.

57. Nagel, J. D., Kort, W. J., Varossieau, F. and McVie, J. G., A new method of sampling ascitic fluid from rats, *Lab. Anim.*, 23, 197, 1989.

58. Nashed, N., A technique for the collection of peritoneal cells from laboratory animals, *Lab. Anim. Sci.*, 25, 225, 1975.

59. Van Soolingen, D., Moolenbeek, C. and Van Loveren, H., An improved method of bronchoalveolar lavage of lungs of small laboratory animals: short report, *Lab. Anim.*, 24, 197, 1990.

60. Byron, F. B. and Wilson, C., A plethysmographic method for measurement of systolic blood pressure in the rat, *J. Physiol.*, 93, 301, 1938.

61. Zatz, R., A low cost tail-cuff method for the estimation of mean arterial pressure in conscious rats, *Lab. Anim. Sci.*, 40, 327, 1990.

62. Ikeda, K., Nara, Y. and Yamori, Y., Indirect systolic and mean blood pressure determination by a new tail cuff method in spontaneously hypertensive rats, *Lab. Anim.*, 25, 26, 1991.

63. Mann, W. A., Landi, M. S., Horner, E., Woodward, P., Campbell, S. and Kinter, L. B., A simple procedure for direct blood pressure measurements in conscious dogs, *Lab. Anim. Sci.*, 37, 105, 1987.

Chapter 17

Gnotobiology

Annelise Hem

CONTENTS

INTRODUCTION

Gnotobiology is the science of rearing and keeping animals in a controlled environment, for example in isolators, so that all bacteria, viruses, fungi, and protozoa in or on the animal are known and can be documented. An important use of gnotobionts is as a source of foundation stock to be used in the subsequent production of highly defined barrier-bred animals (SPF-animals). The gnotobiotic animal has also been used in studies of host/microorganism relationships, carcinogenesis, immunology, nutrition, toxicology, and much more. The majority of these studies involve rats and mice, including the mutant

0-8493-4378-X/94/$0.00+$.50
© 1994 by CRC Press Inc.

nude, but many other species and strains have been used: rat,[1-21] nude rat,[22] mouse,[23-41] nude mouse,[42,43] quail,[44] rabbit,[45] chicken,[42-48] pig,[49-52] dog,[53,54] calf,[55,56] cat,[57] lamb,[58] ferret,[59] goat,[60] foal,[60] and guinea pig.[61]

HISTORY

The first steps into the field of gnotobiology were taken over 90 years ago with Pasteur investigating whether higher animals could live without bacteria. Guinea pigs were the first animals to show short-term survival in the absence of microorganisms. In these early years many difficulties resulted from nutritional deficiencies caused by the preparation of sterile diets. In 1914 Küster overcame some of these difficulties and, using specially prepared natural milk, kept goats alive for one month. His procedure involved an early form of isolator. In 1943 Reyniers and Trexler described an isolator which could be used as a surgical and rearing isolator with complete barriers.[62] Reproduction of the germ-free rat was reported in 1946. The first isolators were nonflexible constructions of material such as rigid plastic material or stainless steel, described by Gustafsson in 1948; more recently they were made more flexible, as described by Reynolds and Trexler in 1957.[62]

TECHNOLOGY

The germ-free animal (GF) is born and reared in total isolation from the surrounding environment in an isolator. To achieve the GF state it is essential that GF embryos are delivered into a sterile environment. With small animals hysterectomy is performed, with large animals the technique is cesarian section or hysterotomy. The young have to be reared on an artificial diet if a GF foster mother is not available.

THE ISOLATOR

An isolator is constructed of several components: the body, the air handling system, the entry and exit systems, and the operator access.

Isolator Body

The isolator is an apparatus that creates an enclosed microbiological entity. The isolator body (Figure 1A) can be made of flexible plastic sheets, of rigid plastic material, Plexiglass, stainless steel, or any other suitable material. Any material used must be impervious to liquids, should have a smooth surface, and be able to withstand exposure to disinfectants. In general all isolators are constructed in the same way. The flexible plastic isolator is frequently used with small animals such as rodents and rabbits, and as these animals are most frequently used, this type of isolator will be described in detail.

Flexible plastic isolators are available in many different sizes and forms, which enables the size and specific design to be chosen to fit the purpose of the experiment. The design of an isolator must eliminate any potential health hazards to the technician, such as over-stretching or having to bend down to work. The ergonomy of the procedures involved in maintaining the animals and performing experiments in an isolator should, therefore, be a matter of consideration. When constructing an isolator, consideration must be given to supporting the flexible film body on a framework (Figure 1B). This is to ensure that if the air pressure is lost, the body will not collapse on to the animals inside.

Air Supply System

All air entering the isolator and leaving it must be passed through a high efficiency particulate air (HEPA) filter (Figure 1C and D). This procedure allows the isolator to be supplied with sterile air. The provision of an exhaust filter ensures that there can be no backflush of nonsterile air if the air supply system fails. Air for the isolator may be taken directly from the room where it is situated. The air must be checked to ensure that it has the correct temperature and humidity levels.

If a large number of isolators are situated in a single room, the air supply may need to be adjusted to give a sufficient volume of air for the isolators. Air can be pumped into the isolator in two ways. One method involves each isolator having its own pump (Figure1E). The other pipes air to each isolator from a single large supply (Figure 5A). If this method is used, it is essential to have each isolator fitted with its own filter to prevent problems when servicing or moving the isolators.

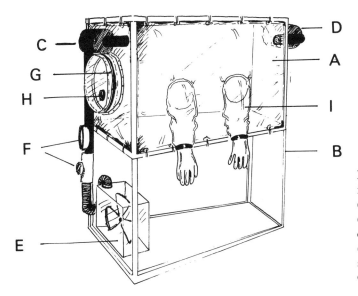

Figure 1. Flexible film isolator: (A) The isolator body, (B) supportive framework, (C) inlet air filter, (D) outlet air filter, (E) air supply pump, (F) air pressure control and manometer, (G) access port, (H) stoppered tube for disinfection, (I) sleeves and gloves. (Courtesy Cecilie Cocozza, Oslo.)

Air Pressure Control

The air flow through the inlet and the outlet is calibrated to keep the air pressure within the isolator slightly above ambient pressure (Figure 1F). This prevents infections from entering the isolator in case of minor accidental perforations and keeps the flexible isolators inflated. The manufacturers of isolators recommend the optimal pressure. It may be easier to work in the flexible isolator if the pressure is reduced during the work phase and then increased to the recommended level when the work is done.

Access Port

Various equipment, all supplies, and livestock can be passed into the isolator and waste materials, samples and livestock can be removed via an access port (Figure 1G). This is a tube through the isolator wall which can be closed at both ends by removable doors. Ideally the outer door should have a means of allowing disinfectant to be sprayed into the access port (Figure 1H). The entry port may be placed on the short or the long end of the isolator. If an access port is very short for practical reasons, it is necessary that some sort of extension to the port is available (Figure 2). This may be another isolator which can be directly coupled to the access port. Isolators may be equipped with a specially designed access port for easy access (Figure 3).

Gloves

To enable manipulation of the animals and materials within the isolator long-sleeved gloves are fixed through the isolator wall (Figure 1I). It is recommended that the material used for the gloves be of sufficient thickness to avoid the possibility of frequent damage. The use of cotton gloves inside the isolator gloves makes it easier to get in and out of the isolator gloves. To prevent bite holes in the isolator gloves a pair of protective gloves may be used over the isolator gloves when working with the animals. Gloves should be placed in such a way that all parts of the isolator can be reached easily. Small isolators may only need one pair of gloves, but large isolators will almost certainly require more than one pair (Figures 4-6). Also, very large isolators may be fitted with a half-suit (Figures 7-8). This is an invaginated plastic sheet which completely covers the worker and allows access to the isolator. The half-suit must be ventilated and cooled for the well-being of the operator (Figures 9-10).

ISOLATOR OPERATION

Starting a New Isolator

The construction of the isolator should follow the instructions supplied by the manufacturer. The cage racking should be introduced and mounted before the isolator is switched on and the air flow monitored for at least 48 hours. During this time the isolator should be thoroughly checked for leakages according to instructions from the manufacturer. By spraying a small amount of gas inside the isolator and checking

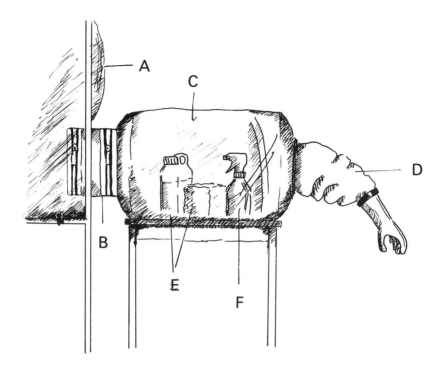

Figure 2. Isolator access port extension: (A) isolator body, (B) access port, (C) isolator port extension, (D) sleeve(s) for manipulation of goods, (E) feed and water, (F) spray bottle. (Courtesy Cecilie Cocozza, Oslo.)

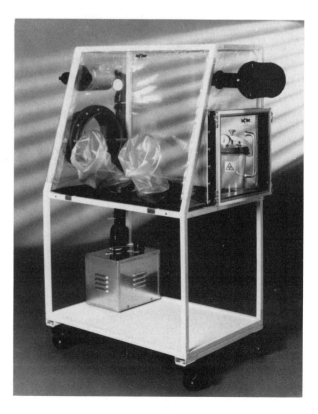

Figure 3. Laboratory isolator with a special access port for easy introduction of large items of equipment. (Courtesy Harlan Olac Ltd.)

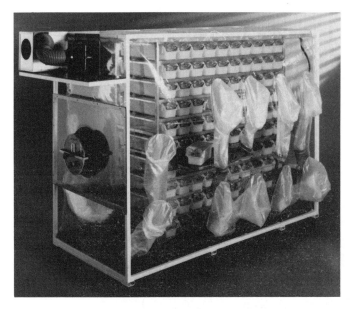

Figure 4. Large isolator fitted with four pairs of gloves, extra storage room with its own gloves, two single gloves for servicing the access port, and a sliding work shelf. (Courtesy Harlan Olac Ltd)

with the detector systematically all over the surface of the isolator, even minute leakages will be detected. During the monitoring phase items to be placed in the isolator should be prepared. At the end of the monitoring period the inside of the isolator and the access port should be cleaned with a disinfectant solution. After the disinfection has been completed, cages, water bottles, disinfectant spray bottle, waste material containers, a scrape for cage cleaning and disinfectant may be introduced into the isolator. When restarting an isolator that has been used, it is necessary to remove all equipment from the isolator for thorough cleaning.

Sterilization — The sterilization of the new isolator is extremely important. Sterilization can be effected by gassing with, e.g., formaldehyde, or by spraying with a liquid disinfectant, e.g., peracetic acid. The air supply and air extract pipes should be plugged in such a way that the filters are exposed to the gas. Equipment should be arranged inside the isolator to allow easy penetration of the gas. After the sterilization procedure has been completed, the air supply should be switched on and the gas removed. It should be remembered that most disinfectants may be toxic, carcinogenic, and/or allergenic and that protection of the operator must be adequate.

Evaluation of sterilization procedure — It is essential that before animals are introduced into a new isolator, it is verified that the isolator is sterile. This may be monitored in two stages. After construction and before disinfection, the inside of the isolator can be swabbed and the swabs cultured for microorganisms. The testing before sterilization should result in various microorganisms growing in the culture media. After sterilization the swabbing procedure is repeated and negative results must be obtained.[63] Also, agar plates should be exposed in the isolator for at least 8 hours and give negative results after culture.

Operation of the Access Port

All nonliving materials that go into the isolator must be sterilized/disinfected. This can be done by packing all goods in a stainless steel cylinder, which is autoclaved and then joined to the entry port. This method has the advantage of allowing the goods to enter the isolator directly from the cylinder without the need for any further treatment. Another procedure involves the surface disinfecting of presterilized items. When starting the isolator sufficient feed, bedding, drinking water, plastic waste bags, and various other utensils are double-bagged and presterilized by autoclaving at 134°C for 4 minutes, or irradiation with 5 Mrad.

A suggested procedure for introducing materials into an isolator is described below: the access port must be thoroughly disinfected and the inner door kept closed. At this stage the bag to be introduced must be immersed in a disinfectant solution. The inner bag is then carefully removed and placed in the access port, while it is being disinfected, and the outer door is closed. When disinfection is complete, the inner door can be opened and the goods introduced into the isolator.

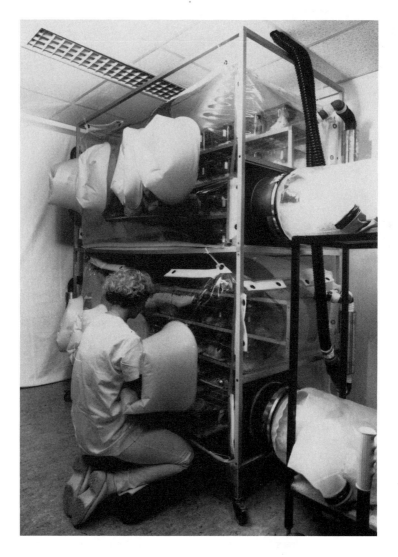

Figure 5. Two separate units placed on top of each other showing a special cushion used when servicing the lower isolator. Pipes from a central air supply are also shown. (Courtesy Helge Vereide, The Norwegian Radiumhospital, Oslo.)

ANIMALS AND THE ISOLATOR

INTRODUCTION OF ANIMALS

The source of animals for entry into an isolator may be another (GF) isolator or a surgical procedure. The donor mother for surgery must be carefully selected. The colony from which she is to be taken should be tested for a wide range of microorganisms and the results obtained interpreted as to the suitability of the mother for surgery. Particular attention must be paid to infections known to be transplacentally transmitted.

Transfer from Another Isolator

When animals are to be transferred from one isolator to another, the procedure is simple if the isolators can be directly connected. If, however, the isolators are housed in separate areas, a transport system must be used. Filter boxes are available commercially that will pass through access ports and can therefore be sterilized and introduced as already described. When the animals are in the box, this box is placed inside a second filtered transport box and this may then be removed from the isolator. After transportation to

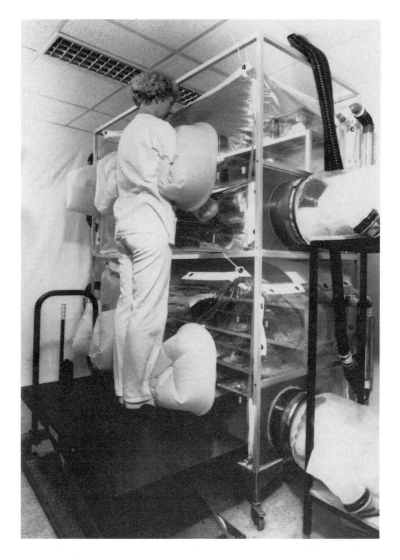

Figure 6. Two separate units placed on top of each other with a platform adjustable to give the right height for servicing the upper isolator. (Courtesy Helge Vereide, The Norwegian Radiumhospital, Oslo.)

the new isolator, the animals must be transferred into the new isolator by a method which ensures complete sterility.

Surgical Methods

Surgical procedures should be carried out before the natural birth process has commenced. There are two surgical methods that can be used: hysterectomy, which involves the removal of the gravid uterus from the mother, and hysterotomy, which involves the removal of the young from the mother. Both these methods can be performed using a filter cabinet (sterile bench) in an open method or a surgical isolator in a closed method. Various surgical isolators are available commercially (Figure 11).

Open method — Many types of filter cabinets are available commercially. The cabinet used must provide a sterile working environment. Before the procedure is started the cabinet must be set up with all materials that will be needed. The donor mother is euthanized, dipped in disinfectant and placed with the abdomen uppermost and the legs secured. The abdomen is shaved or flayed, the exposed surface is disinfected and covered with a sterile drape. The abdomen is opened and the uterus exposed. For hysterectomy the uterus is dissected from the mother's abdomen and the entire uterus is immediately placed in a container with a suitable disinfectant in a physiological solution. For hysterotomy the young

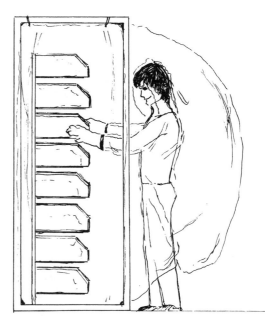

Figure 7. Isolator with one rack fitted with a half-suit in the isolator wall. (Courtesy Cecilie Cocozza, Oslo.)

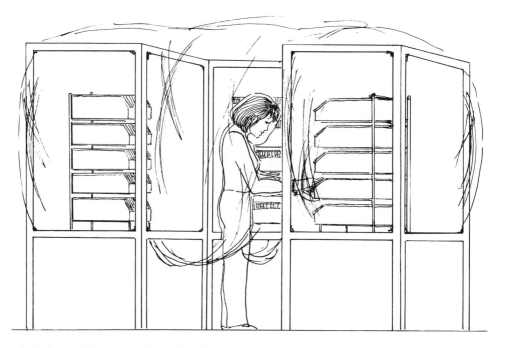

Figure 8. Isolator with racks on three sides fitted with a half-suit from the isolator floor. (Courtesy Cecilie Cocozza, Oslo.)

animals are removed from the uterus in the mother and immediately placed directly in a container as above. This container is then handled as previously described and introduced into the isolator.

Closed method — This method requires the use of a specialized surgical isolator (Figure 11). The isolator must be set up as previously described with all items required. The mother is euthanized. The mother's abdomen is prepared as above, and she is placed on a holder, which is pushed upwards into a specially prepared area of the floor of the isolator. The hysterectomy or hysterotomy is then performed from inside the isolator by cutting through this area of the isolator directly into the abdomen of the mother. The surgical isolator may be directly coupled with the holding isolator. The use of surgical isolators does

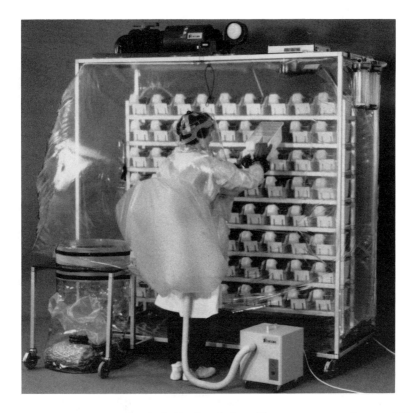

Figure 9. Full rack isolator demonstrating the half-suit technique. The access port can be turned 90 degrees with the port extension functioning as waste basket. The separate air supply system for the operator is shown. (Courtesy B & K Universal Group Ltd.)

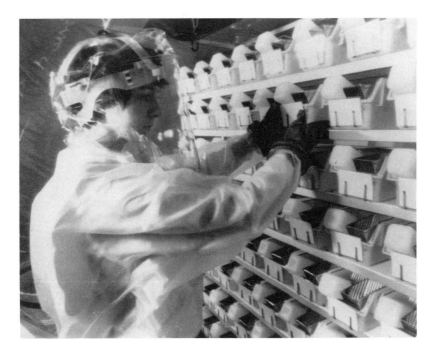

Figure 10. Close-up of a half-suit isolator showing the head gear and the ventilated jacket. These are important to ensure that the working environment is pleasant. (Courtesy B & K Universal Group Ltd.)

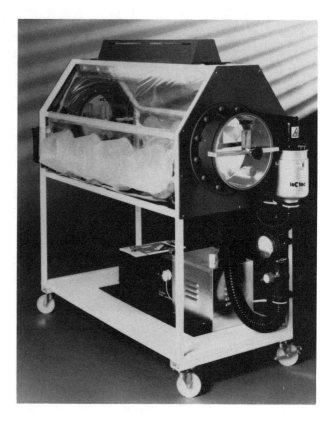

Figure 11. Surgical isolator fitted with two pairs of gloves on both sides, two transfer ports on opposite sides, and an external illuminator. (Courtesy Harlan Olac Ltd.)

not eliminate the necessity of placing either the uterus or the pups in disinfectant solution before introduction into the holding isolator.

Resuscitation and Foster Mothers

It is advisable to use a GF foster mother with the newborn. This eliminates the nutritional problems encountered when using artificial diet for the hand-rearing of the neonate. The foster mother must be selected from stock known to be good mothers and of a contrasting coat color from the donor animal. The foster mother should be mated 1 to 2 days before the donor animal is mated. She is allowed to give birth to her litter. All but two of the foster mother's pups are removed ready for receipt of the newborn. When reviving the newborn pups it is important to keep them warm and to dry them with sterile tissues. Once they have been revived and are judged to be breathing well and have a normal skin color, they are placed with the foster mother.

MAINTENANCE OF ANIMALS IN AN ISOLATOR

In order to maintain the integrity of the isolator the use of the access port should be limited. Therefore, it is advisable to collect together all necessary items and perform the introduction into the isolator in one operation. GF animals generally do not require box changing as frequently as animals with a microflora. The details of the practical, daily work in the isolator will not be discussed, except for a few points. It is advisable to keep equipment in the isolator in a suitable container rather than placing it on the isolator base. Testing the gloves and sleeves for leakages at regular intervals is recommended. A description of the procedure and necessary equipment should be supplied by the manufacturer of the isolator.

ENSURING GERM-FREE QUALITY

GF animals must be demonstrated to be free from contamination with microorganisms. About 10 days after the surgical procedure the foster mother's own pups are removed, necropsied and subjected to a full bacteriological, mycological, and parasitological examination. At weaning the foster mother is removed and she is subjected to the same examination as her pups, but extended to include serological methods for virus infections.[64] The final examination is carried out when the young are about 9 to 10 weeks of age and they are examined in as great a detail as the foster mother. If this series of examinations proves that the isolator contains GF animals, the level of subsequent examinations can be reduced.

It is recommended that samples of feces be collected at two-weekly intervals and examined by aerobic and anaerobic methods. It is suggested that at three-month intervals animals should be sacrificed for full microbiological examination. Because there are still problems of vertical transplacental transmission of organisms to be elucidated, these animals must be examined serologically.[65]

CHARACTERISTICS OF THE GERM-FREE ANIMAL

The GF animal differs from conventional (CV) animals in many ways. The greatest difference is the total lack of intestinal microorganisms. The indigenous microflora of the gastrointestinal tract is involved in a vast number of biochemical processes. The absence of such flora thus influences the animal greatly, accounting for a great many of the characteristics of germ-free animals.

Intestinal Tract

The most notable feature of the intestinal tract of a GF animal is the size of the cecum. In rodents and lagomorphs it is always grossly enlarged and accounts for a large proportion of the animal's body weight. The size of the cecum has been shown to be related to the bulk of the diet. A high fiber content leads to a large cecum.[66] The cecum does not develop its normal musculature and the contents are far more liquid than in CV animals; however, this does not happen in the chicken and the dog.[67] It has been shown that after the introduction of microorganisms into the cecum the volume is reduced, mainly due to muscle contraction.[6] It has been noted in the GF rat that an enlarged cecum reduces cardiac output and oxygen consumption.[62]

The enlarged cecum may rupture. The walls of the intestinal tract of GF animals are always thinner. Szentkuti et al. have shown that in the distal colon of the rat the total gut wall thickness was reduced by 47% compared to the CV rat.[18] The intestinal wall of GF animals is always paler than that of the CV animal, partly due to less connective tissue.[62] The overall mass of the small intestine is decreased, the villi being more slender and uniform, and the crypts shorter, reducing the total surface area of the intestine.[67] Histological examination has shown that the mucin layer of the GF rat colon was thinner than in the CV rat.[18] The GF animal cannot degrade mucin. It cannot convert cholesterol to coprostanol and bilirubin to urobilinogen. The tryptic activity is increased, as is bilirubin deconjugation.[33]

Fecal pellets from GF animals are lighter in color than those of CV animals and are odorless. This is useful when evaluating the isolator, as odor may indicate a contamination of the isolator. It has been demonstrated that the metabolism, uptake, and incorporation by the enterocytes of components of dietary nucleic acid are influenced by the microflora.[41]

Other Organs

In the GF rodent the size of some organs is reduced. There is evidence of smaller livers, lungs, and hearts. Also the blood supply to organs can be 25 to 50% less than in CV animals, most reductions in the blood flow being to the liver and intestines. GF rats also have a smaller blood volume.[68] The levels of lipid peroxide and aniline-hydroxylase activity of the liver and the serum total cholesterol, triglyceride and phospholipid are significantly lower in GF than in CV mice of the same age.[36]

The Immune System

The GF status influences the immune system. A GF pig at 49 days of age has a T cell subset pattern comparable with that of a 5-day-old CV pig.[51] Peripheral lymphoid organs show a reduced development in the GF animal. This is particularly noticeable in the organs associated with the gastrointestinal tract. The immunoglobulin level in the GF animal is reduced because in the absence of intestinal microflora complex proteins in the diet are not broken down and absorbed. The response to antigenic stimulus is delayed in a GF animal, but when it occurs it is more prolonged and results in higher levels of immunoglobulin.[62]

THE FEEDING OF THE GERM-FREE ANIMAL

The lack of intestinal microflora profoundly alters the digestive process in GF animals. If animals are maintained solely as a source of breeding stock, the diet can be of a more general nature than those, for example, destined to be used in immunological experiments. Chemically defined diets to be used in the rearing and keeping of GF animals for immunological studies were described and reviewed by Wostman and Pleasants in 1991.[69] Animals for breeding purposes can be fed a sterilized standard diet, but it must be remembered that if this method is chosen, the animal must be given supplements in some form (vitamins and other substances) to compensate for the lack of production of such substances by the microorganisms of the gut. Such a fortified, autoclavable diet is commercially available.

MICROFLORA AND THE GNOTOBIOTIC ANIMAL

The GF animal can be used to study the effects of microorganisms. This can be carried out by colonizing the GF animal with one or more defined microorganism. In this state the GF animal is termed an associated gnotobiotic animal. When one organism is used, it may be called monoassociated; if two, it is diassociated; if many, it is polyassociated. Associated animals are important models for the study of the possible effects of one or more microorganism on various parameters. The level of association is determined by the intended use of the animal.

When GF animals are maintained as a foundation stock for subsequent breeding in a barrier-maintained colony, they must be polyassociated with a number of microorganisms to ensure that all the expected GF characteristics will be absent.[70] By controlling the number of associating microorganisms specific research projects can be attempted.[33]

Associated gnotobiotic animals must be kept in isolators to maintain their integrity. It is also important to carry out a microbiological evaluation of the isolator to confirm the status of the animals.

COLONIZATION RESISTANCE

Animals that are being associated with microflora, with the intention of releasing the animals from an isolator to a barrier unit where they will be housed in standard rooms, must be given microorganisms that will remove GF characteristics and give rise to colonization resistance. This resistance prepares the animals for the challenge from the wide range of expected organisms outside the controlled isolator environment. Much research effort has been concentrated in the study of colonization resistance and GF animals.[28,31,40,61,71–73] Not only the choice of species of microorganisms, but also nutritional factors may influence the colonization.[45]

HIGHLY DEFINED BARRIER-MAINTAINED ANIMALS

These animals are generally polyassociated and may or may not be maintained in an isolator. In contrast to GF animals these animals are monitored for specific organisms, which may not be a total analysis of their microflora. These animals are referred to as specified pathogen free (SPF). The microbiological quality of these animals is determined by the standard and methods of husbandry used. They must be kept behind some form of barrier to protect them from contamination from the environment, which may come from many sources. The success of detection of the microflora during testing depends on the test methods used, the frequency of testing, the age of the animal when tested, and for a barrier breeding unit recommendations as to how monitoring should be carried out.[64] It is important to remember that the microbiological profile of a unit of highly defined animals is specific for that unit. This difference in microbiological flora can influence various aspects of the animals' biology and thus their reactions to test situations.[29,74,75] Highly defined animals that are removed from barrier units to nonbarrier units will gradually become colonized by new microorganisms. This produces an animal known as a conventional animal.

GNOTOBIOTIC ANIMALS: USE IN RESEARCH

RODENT MODELS
Carcinogenesis/Mutagenesis

The role of the gut flora in the metabolism of various carcinogenic substances has been investigated by a number of researchers. GF rats have been found to excrete less mutagenic metabolites than do CV rats.[1,12] On the other hand it has also been shown in a separate study that intestinal microflora has no influence on the metabolism of some mutagens and that differences cannot be demonstrated between a GF and a CV animal.[9] It has been demonstrated that metabolites derived from *Aspergillus versicolor* in GF rats exposed to this organism resulted in the development of pituitary tumors.[17]

In another study, GF mice infected with a murine leukemia virus were found to be more resistant to the development of disease caused by this virus than CV mice. It was suggested that this is due to the level of the immune system activation, which has an influence on the pathogenicity of the retrovirus tested.[27]

Infections/Immunity

GF animals have been widely used to investigate the relationships between microorganisms, including their pathogenic capabilities. Also, GF mice have been used to investigate strain differences in C*lostridium difficile*, where it was shown that nontoxinogenic strains caused less cecal weight reduction than toxinogenic strains.[32] The same organism was used to produce a vaccine of monoclonal antibodies against *Clostridium difficile* toxin, and this protected GF mice challenged with the organism, as they did not develop pseudomembranous colitis.[25]

Johne's disease, which is caused by *Mycobacterium paratuberculosis*, is an inflammatory bowel disease that affects ruminants and humans. *Mycobacterium paratuberculosis* was inoculated into athymic GF mice in an attempt to investigate the pathogenesis of the organism.[42]

Another human bowel infection involving the protozoan parasite *Entamoeba histolytica* was also investigated in the athymic GF mouse.[43]

It is also interesting that the GF mouse has been used in a study to validate an *in vitro* method of continuous-flow bacterial cell culture. The work compared three genera of bacteria, including *Escherichia coli*, and it was found that the *in vitro* method is likely to be satisfactory to study interaction among bacterial populations in the gastrointestinal tract. If this method proves to be successful it will replace animals for such studies.[28]

GF and CV rats have been used to study septic shock, the method involving cecal ligation and subsequent perforation. Surprisingly the GF status offers no increased protection against septic shock. The results indicate important cardiovascular effects of microflora that need to be considered when developing models for trauma and stress.[76]

Hemorrhagic shock has been studied in GF and CV rats. It was found that if the cecum was removed from a GF rat, the animal was more resistant to hemorrhagic shock than a non-cecectomized GF rat.[76] Resistance to hemorrhagic shock has also been described in the GF rat in a comparative study with a CV rat.[3,13]

Bacterial sepsis has previously been linked with multiple organ failure, although the evidence is not conclusive. It is, however, possible to induce multiple organ failure and the clinical syndrome of sepsis aseptically in GF animals. The cause may be excessive activation of endogenous humoral mediators and inflammatory cells.[77] The GF hairless mutant mouse is a useful model in the study of the bacterial strains responsible for nosocomial skin infections and their treatment.[23]

GF mice have been used in the study of *Neisseria gonorrhoeae*, the only animal model other than chimpanzees in which sustained mucosal colonization has been demonstrated.[39] Another investigation looked at local defence mechanisms against microbial invasions of the normal nasal mucosa using GF, SPF, and CV mice.[26]

Monoclonal antibody production is currently an important scientific project worldwide, but it is difficult to prepare monoclonal antibodies against certain bacteria, such as *E. coli*. The elimination of intestinal flora antigens in GF mice permits production of hybridomas of improved specificity with less frequent cross reactions.[38]

Gnotobiotic rats have been used as a source of tracheal organ cultures. Using such cultures, a murine mycoplasma isolated from fish, M. *mobile 1633 K*, was studied and shown to colonize and damage epithelial cells.[78] In a second study 11 seal Mycoplasma strains from three Mycoplasma species were shown to have different cytopathological activities.[16]

The GF rat has also been used in dental research. A study has been conducted to investigate the possible carigenicity of Streptococcus bovis. The results obtained demonstrated that the fissures of the teeth were colonized by three different strains of the organisms and that these caused caries.[21] The gnotobiotic rat model has been used for research into the development of an oral vaccine that was shown to reduce caries and coincidentally the amount of *S. mutans* in the oral cavity.[7]

Nutrition

The influence of gut flora on the metabolism of various nutrients and additives has been studied by comparing GF and CV rats.[1,10,11,14,19,20,79] GF male rats have been used in food restriction studies, where it was shown that food restriction in a GF rat retarded the development of pituitary gonadotroph nodules, but did not prevent their formation.[15]

In the newborn child and patients on antibiotic treatment vitamin K deficiency has been recorded. The mechanism of the induction of this deficiency has been studied in a GF and CV mouse model.[30,35]

Body Temperature

The gut flora possibly has a tonic stimulatory effect on the body temperature of rodents. One investigation found evidence of lowered body temperature in GF mice compared to CV mice regardless whether the measurements were taken during daytime or nighttime. It was further found that activity did not influence the findings.[8] In studies on GF rats and mice it has been demonstrated not only that the presence of microorganisms influences the body temperature, but also that the Gr+ organisms are the major source of the stimulatory effect.[24]

Toxicology, Pharmacology, and Physiology

A totally standardizable animal model consisting of GF and isolator-maintained SPF animals was used to evaluate the influence of the microflora on biotransformation, pharmacokinetics, and energy metabolism in the rat. Differences in hepatic glucose metabolism between rats of the two microbial states are suggested by the author. The activities of citrate synthase and malate dehydrogenase were higher in GF than in SPF rats.[80]

NONRODENT MODELS

Although rodents account for the majority of the published reports on the use of gnotobiotic animals in research, other animals have been used successfully. The GF/CV minipig model has been used to investigate the metabolism of therapeutic substances in the treatment of portosystemic encephalopathy in humans and the possible influence of the intestinal microflora.[2] Another porcine GF/CV model has been used to study the relationship between dietary copper levels and the intestinal microflora.[52] The cellular immune system of the lung has been studied by collecting cells by bronchoalveolar lavage in pigs with pneumonia and comparing them with corresponding cells from GF pigs.[50] The GF/CV pig model has been used to study the influence of various microorganisms in the development of atrophic rhinitis in the pig.[49]

GF calves have been used to study virus and bacterial infection. One study investigated the possible effects of recombinant human alpha A interferon on the development of an infection with respiratory syncytial virus.[55] The pathogenicity of *Pasteurella haemolytica* has been studied in GF and CV calves.[56]

The pathogenicity of various strains of the virus causing bovine viral diarrhea has been compared in colostrum-deprived neonatal GF lambs.[58] GF dogs have been used extensively in research projects, e.g., studies of a variety of gastrointestinal problems,[60] and in investigations on shock, cancer, immunology, burns, and wound healing.[53]

GF chickens have been compared with chickens with a highly defined microbial flora in the study of the comparative infectivity of *E. coli* in the presence of infectious bronchitis virus.[46] In common with investigations in other species the interaction between diet and intestinal microflora has been studied in GF and CV chickens.[47,48] GF quail have been used in the study of human neonatal necrotizing enterocolitis. The quail were monoassociated with various *Clostridium butyricum* strains to elucidate the pathogenesis of the bacteria in this disease.[44]

TERMINOLOGY OF HYGIENIC QUALITY IN ANIMALS

A short vocabulary is presented below of some of the important expressions used to denominate the hygienic quality of laboratory animals (see also Figure 12).

Associated (colonized): Specifically infected with certain microorganisms.

Axenic: From a = without, xenos = stranger. "Individuals, free from any demonstrable life except that produced by their own protoplasm". Linguistically the term is synonymous with germ-free, but the term is sometimes used synonymously with gnotobiotic.

Colonization resistance: The phenomenon by which the normal microflora excludes pathogens from an existing colonized body site = microbial interference or antagonism.

Conventional: Harboring indigenous and undefined microbiota.

Defined flora: Microflora of animals whose microbiology is totally known.

ISOLATOR

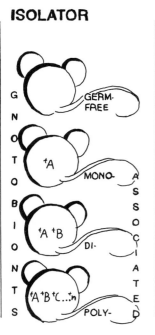

G
N   GERM-
O   FREE
T
O   †A
B   MONO-
I
O   †A †B
N   DI-
T
S   †A †B †C...†n
    POLY-

A
S
S
O
C
I
A
T
E
D

BARRIER

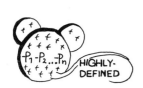

†P₁-P₂...Pₙ HIGHLY-
             DEFINED

CONVENTIONAL

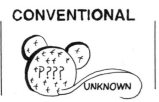

†P??? UNKNOWN

Figure 12. Microbiological quality of laboratory animals: A, B, C = nonpathogenic microbial species; P = pathogenic microbial species. (Courtesy Cecilie Cocozza, Oslo.)

Gnotobiotic: *Gnotes* meaning well known and *biota* meaning all life or the total of living organisms. The term includes germ-free as well as microbiologically associated animals. Sometimes erroneously used as a synonym for germ-free.

Gnotobiont: Animal in the gnotobiotic state.

Germ-free (GF): Free from any detectable form of life, except for its own living cells.

Highly defined barrier-maintained animals: Animals free from specified organisms considered to be pathogenic to the species. With an otherwise, principally, unknown (undefined) microflora/fauna = specified pathogen free (SPF). Originate from polyassociated animals and are kept under barrier conditions.

Mono-, di-, and polyassociated: Animals associated (purposely infected) with one, two or several micro-organisms.

REFERENCES

1. Ball, L. M., Rafter, J. J., Gustafsson, J. A., Gustafsson, B. E., Kohan, M. J., and Lewtas, J., Formation of mutagenic urinary metabolites from i-nitropyrene in germfree and conventional rats: role of the gut flora, Carcinogenesis, 12, 1, 1991.

2. Bird, S. P., Hewitt, D., Rathcliffe, B., and Gurr, M. I., Effects of lactulose and lactitol on protein digestion and metabolism in conventional and germfree animal model: relevance of the results to their use in the treatment of portosystemic encephalopathy, *Gut,* 31, 1403, 1990.

3. Flanagan, J. J. Jr., Rush, B. F. Jr., Murphy, T. F., Smith, S., Machiedo, G. W., Hsieh, J., Rosa, D. M., and Heneghan, J. B., A "treated" model for severe hemorrhagic shock: a comparison of conventional and germ-free animals, *J. Med.,* 21, 104, 1990.

4. Goodland, R. A., Ratcliffe, B., Fordham, J. P., and Wright, N. A., Does dietary fibre stimulate intestinal epithelial cell proliferation in germ free rats?, *Gut,* 30, 820, 1989.

5. Greve, J. W., Gouma, D. J., Soeters, P. B., and Buurman, W. A., Suppression of cellular immunity in obstructive jaundice is caused by endotoxins: a study with germ-free rats, *Gastroenterology,* 98, 478, 1990.

6. Ishikawa, K., Satoh, Y., Oomori, Y., Yamano, M., Matsuda, M., and Ono, K., Influence of conventionalization on cecal wall structure of germ-free Wistar rats: quantitative light and qualitative electron microscopic observations, *Anat. Embryol.,* 180, 191, 1989.

7. Jackson, S., Mestecky, J., Childers, N. K., and Michalek, S. M., Liposomes containing anti-idiotypic antibodies: an oral vaccine to induce protective secretory immune responses specific for pathogens of mucosal surfaces, *Infect. Immun.,* 58, 1932, 1990.

8. Kluger, M. J., Conn, C. A., Franklin, B., Freter, R., and Abrams, G. D., Effects of gastrointestinal flora on body temperature in rats and mice, *Am. J. Physiol.,* 258, 552, 1990.

9. Knize, M. G., Overvik, E., Midtvedt, T., Turteltaub, K. W., Happe, J. A., Gustafsson, J. A., and Felton, J. S., The metabolism of 4,8-DiMeIQx in conventional and germ-free rats, *Carcinogenesis,* 10, 1479, 1989.

10. McDevitt, J., and Goldman, P., Effect of the intestinal flora of the urinary organic acid profile of rats ingesting a chemically simplified diet, *Food Chem. Toxicol.,* 29, 107, 1991.

11. Nielsch, A. S., Ward, F. W., Coates, M. E., Walker, R., and Rowland, I. R., Influence of dietary protein and gut microflora on endogenous synthesis of nitrate induced by bacterial endotoxin in the rat, *Food Chem. Toxicol.,* 29, 387, 1991.

12. Overvik, E., Lindeskog, P., Midtvedt, T., and Gustafsson, J. A., Mutagen excretion and cytochrome P-450-dependent activity in germfree and conventional rats fed a diet containing fried meat, *Food Chem. Toxicol.,* 28, 253, 1990.

13. Rush, B. F. Jr., Redan, J. A., Flanagan, J. J. Jr., Henegan, J. B., Hsiek, J., Murphy, T. F., Smith, S., and Machiedo, G. W., Does the bacteremia observed in hemorrhagic shock have clinical significance? A study in germ-free animals, *Ann. Surg.,* 210, 342, 1989.

14. Sandler, M., Przyborowska, A., Halket, J., Watkins, P., Glover, V., and Coates, M., Urinary but not brain isatin levels are reduced in germ-free rats, *J. Neurochem.,* 57, 1074, 1991.

15. Sano, T., Kovacs, K., Stefaneanu, L., Asa, S. L., and Snyder, D. L., Spontaneous pituitary gonadotroph nodules in aging male Lobund-Wistar rats, *Lab. Invest.,* 61, 343, 1989.

16. Stadtländer, C., Hartmann, D., Binder, A., and Kirchhoff, H., Ivestigation of seal mycoplasmas for their cytotoxic potential on tracheal organ cultures of SPF and gnotobiotic rats, *Int. J. Med. Microbiol.,* 272, 216, 1989.

17. Sumi, Y., Nagura, H., and Miyakawa, M., Induction of pituitary tumors in germ-free rats exposed to Aspergillus versicolor, *Cancer Res.,* 50, 400, 1990.

18. Szentkuti, L., Riedsel, H., Enss, M. L., Gaertner, K., and Von Engelhardt, W., Pre-epithelial mucus layer in the colon of conventional and germ-free rats, *Histochem. J.,* 22, 491, 1990.

19. Tokunaga, T., Oku, T., and Hosoya, N., Utilization and excretion of a new sweetener, fructooligosaccharide (Neosugar), in rats, *J. Nutr.,* 119, 553, 1989.

20. Ward, F. W., Coates, M. E., and Walker, R., Influence of dietary protein and gut microflora on endogenous synthesis of nitrate and N-nitrosamines in the rat, *Food Chem. Toxicol.,* 27, 445, 1989.

21. Willcox, M. D., Drucker, D. B., and Green, R. M., In vivo dental plaque-forming ability and carigenicity of the bacterium Streptococcus bovis in gnotobiotic rats, *Arch. Oral Biol.,* 35, 163, 1990.

22. Sainte-Marie, G., and Peng, F. S., Formation of morphologically unusual features, associated with immunodeficiencies, in lymph-nodes of gnotobiotic rats exposed to a conventional milieu, *Arch. Histol. Cytol.,* 53, 55, 1990.

23. Barc, M. C., Tekaia, F., and Bourlioux, P., In vivo standardization of cutaneous bacterial activity of antiseptics by using monoxenic hairless mice, *Appl. Environ. Microbiol.,* 55, 1911, 1989.

24. Conn, C. A., Franklin, B., Freter, R., and Kluger, M. J., Role of Gram-negative and Gram-positive gastrointestinal flora in temperature regulation of mice, *Am. J. Physiol.*, 261, 1358, 1991.

25. Corthier, G., Muller, M. C., Wilkins, T. D., Lyerly, D., and L'Haridon, R., Protection against experimental pseudomembranous colitis in gnotobiotic mice by use of monoclonal antibodies against Clostridium difficile toxin A, *Infect. Immun.*, 59, 1192, 1991.

26. Ichimiya, I., Kawauchi, H., Fujiyoshi, T., Tanaka, T., and Mogi, G., Distribution of immunocompetent cells in normal nasal mucosa: comparison among germ-free, specific pathogen-free, and conventional mice, *Ann. Otol. Rhinol. Laryngol.*, 100, 638, 1991.

27. Isaak, D. D., Bartizal, K. F., and Caulfield, M. J., Decreased pathogenicity of murine leukemia virus-Moloney in gnotobiotic mice, *Leukemia*, 2, 540, 1988.

28. Itoh, K., and Freter, R., Control of Escherichia coli populations by a combination of indigenous clostridia and lactobacilli in gnotobiotic mice and continuous-flow cultures, *Infect. Immun.*, 57, 559, 1989.

29. Kawamura, S., Hiramaya, K., Mishima, M., Miyaji, K., Akiyma, T., and Mitsuoka, T., Endotoxic activity in faeces of mice from different microbiological environments, *Res. Microbiol.*, 141, 1095, 1990.

30. Komai, M., Shirakawa, H., and Kimura, S., Newly developed model for vitamin K deficiency in germfree mice, *Int. J. Vitam. Nutr. Res.*, 58, 55, 1988.

31. Koopman, J. P., van der Logt, J. T., Heessen, F. W., van den Brink, M. E., Scholten, P. M., Hectors, M. P., and Nagengast, F. M., Elimination of murine viral pathogens from the caecal contents of mice by anaerobic preparation, *Lab. Anim.*, 23, 76, 1989.

32. Mahé, S., and Corthier, G., Effect of toxins produced by various Clostridium difficile strains on cecum size reduction in gnotobiotic mice, *Can. J. Microbiol.*, 34, 916, 1988.

33. Norin, K. E., Persson, A. K., Saxerholt, H., and Midtvedt, T., Establishment of Lactobacillus and Bifidobacterium species in germfree mice and their influence on some microflora-associated characteristics, *Appl. Environ. Microbiol.*, 57, 1850, 1991.

34. Pecuet, S., Chachaty, E., Tancrède, C., and Andremont, A., Effects of roxithromycin on fecal bacteria in human volunteers and resistance to colonization in gnotobiotic mice, *Antimicrob. Agents. Chemother.*, 35, 548, 1991.

35. Shirakawa, H., Komai, and Kimura, S., Antibiotic-induced vitamin K deficiency and the role of the presence of intestinal flora, *Int. J. Vitam. Nutr. Res.*, 60, 245, 1990.

36. Takeda, M., Kandori, H., Itagaki, S., Hirayama, K., Hatayama, K., and Doi, K., Comparative studies of some functional and morphological parameters in the livers of germfree, conventional and ex-germfree mice, *Exp. Anim.*, 40, 537, 1991.

37. Tannock, G. W., Crichton, C, Welling, G. W., Koopman, J. P., and Midtvedt, T., Reconstitution of the gastrointestinal microflora of lactobacillus-free mice, *Appl. Environ. Microbiol.*, 54, 2971, 1988.

38. Tartera, C., Davis, K., and Colwell, R. R., Production of Escherichia coli-specific hybridomas by using gnotobiotic mice, *Appl. Environ. Microbiol.*, 56, 1397, 1990.

39. Taylor-Robinson, D., Furr, P. M., and Hetherington, C. M., Neisseria gonorrhoeae colonises the genital tract of oestradiol-treated germ-free female mice, *Microbiol. Pathol.*, 9, 369, 1990.

40. Wells, C. L., Maddaus, M. A., Jechorek, R. P., and Simmons, R. L., Role of intestinal anaerobic bacteria in colonization resistance, *Eur. J. Clin. Microbiol. Infect. Dis.*, 7, 107, 1988.

41. Whitt, D. D., and Savage, D. C., Influence of indigenous microbiota on activities of alkaline phosphatase, phosphodiesterase I, and thymidine kinase in mouse enterocytes, *Appl. Environ. Microbiol.*, 54, 2405, 1988.

42. Hamilton, H. L., Follett, D. M., Siegfried, L. M., and Czuprynski, C. J., Intestinal multiplication of Mycobacterium paratuberculosis in athymic gnotobiotic mice, *Infect. Immun.*, 57, 225, 1989.

43. Owen, D. G., Gnotobiotic, athymic mice; a possible system for the study of the role of bacteria in human amoebiasis, *Lab. Anim.*, 24, 353, 1990.

44. Bousseboua, H., Le Coz, Y., Dabard, J., Szylit, D., Raibaud, P., Popoff, M. R., and Ravisse, P., Experimental cecitis in gnotobiotic quails monoassociated with Clostridium butyricum strains isolated from patients with neonatal necrotizing enterocolitis and from healthy newborn, *Infect. Immun.*, 57, 923, 1989.

45. Boot, R., Koopman, J. P., Lankhorst, A., Stadhouders, A. M., Welling, G. W., and Hectors, M. P., Intestinal "normalization" of germ-free rabbits with rabbit caecal microflora: effect of dosing regimens, *Z. Versuchstierkd.*, 32, 83, 1989.

46. Brée, A., Dho, M., and Lafont, J. P., Comparative infectivity for axenic and specific-pathogen-free chicken of 02 Escherichia coli strains with or without virulence factors, *Avian Dis.,* 33, 134, 1989.

47. Muramatsu, T., Kodama, H., Morishita, T., Furuse, M., and Okumura, J., Effect of intestinal microflora on digestible energy and fiber digestion in chickens fed a high-fiber diet, *Am. J. Vet. Res.,* 52, 1178, 1991.

48. Perez-Ruiz, R., Wal, J. M., and Szylit, D., Histamine distribution in the gastrointestinal wall of germ free and conventional chicken: evidence of the role of the digestive microflora, *Agents Action,* 25, 273, 1988.

49. Chanter, N., Magyar, T., and Rutter, J. M., Interactions between Bordetella bronchiseptica and toxigenic Pasteurella multocida in atrophic rhinitis of pigs, *Res. Vet. Sci.,* 47, 48, 1989.

50. Gehrke, I., and Pabst, R., Cell composition and lymphocyte subsets in the bronchoalveolar lavage of normal pigs of different ages in comparison with germfree and pneumonic pigs, *Lung,* 168, 79, 1990.

51. Rothkotter, H. J., Ulbrich, H., and Pabst, R., The postnatal development of gut lamina propria lymphocytes: number, proliferation, and T and B cell subsets in conventional and germ-free pigs, *Pediatr. Res.,* 29, 237, 1991.

52. Shurson, G. C., Ku, P. K., Waxler, G. L., Yokoyama, M. T., and Miller, E. R., Physiological relationship between microbiological status and dietary copper levels in the pig, *J. Anim. Sci.,* 68, 1061, 1990.

53. Cohn, I. Jr., and Henegan, J. B., Germfree animals and techniques in surgical research, *Am. J. Surg.,* 161, 279, 1991.

54. Radin, M. J., Eaton, K. A., Krakowka, S., Morgan, D. R., Lee, A., Otto, G., and Fox, J., Helicobacter pylori gastric infection in gnotobiotic beagle dogs, *Infect. Immun.,* 58, 2606, 1990.

55. Dennis, M. J., Thomas, L. H., and Stott, E. J., Effects of recombinant human alpha A interferon in gnotobiotic calves challenged with respiratory syncytial virus, *Res. Vet. Sci.,* 50, 222, 1991.

56. Vestweber, J. G., Klemm, R. D., Leipold, H. W., and Johnson, D. E., Pneumonic pasteurellosis induced experimentally in gnotobiotic and conventional calves inoculated with Pasteurella haemolytica, *Am. J. Vet. Res.,* 51, 1799, 1990.

57. Fletcher, A. M., Hoskins, J. D., and Elkins, A. D., Germfree technique for the rearing of kittens — a research tool, *Cornell Vet.,* 81, 365, 1991.

58. Jewett, C. J., Kelling, C. L., Frey, M. L., and Doster, A. R., Comparative pathogenicity of selected bovine viral diarrhea virus isolates in gnotobiotic lambs, *Am. J. Vet. Res.,* 51, 1640, 1990.

59. Manning, D. D., and Bell, J. A., Derivation of gnotobiotic ferrets. Perinatal diet and hand-rearing requirements, *Lab. Anim. Sci.,* 40, 51, 1990.

60. Miniats, O. P., Production of germ-free animals, part 2. Farm animals, in T*he Germ-Free Animal in Biomedical Research,* Laboratory Animal Handbook 9, Coates, M. E., and Gustafsson, B. E., Eds., Laboratory Animals Ltd., London, 1984, chap. 2.

61. Boot, R., Koopman, J. P., Kruijt, B. C., Lammers, R. M., Kennis, H. M., Lankhorst, A., Welling, G. W., and Hectors, M. P., The "normalization" of germ-free guinea pigs with host-specific caecal microflora, *Lab. Anim.,* 23, 48,1989.

62. Trexler, P. C., Animals of defined microbiological status, in *The UFAW Handbook of the Care and Management of Laboratory Animals,* sixth edition, Poole, T. B., Ed., Longman Scientific & Technical, Avon, 1987, chap. 6.

63. Gamble, M. R., and Needham, J. R., Microbial assessment of a single fumigation of formaldehyde of a multi-level animal facility, in N*ew Developments in Biosciences: Their Implications for Laboratory Animal Science,* Beynen, A. C., and Solleveld, A. C., Eds., Martinus Nijhoff, Boston, 1988, 117.

64. Kraft, V., Blanchet, H.M., Deeny, A, Hansen, A.K., Hem, A., Herck, H.V., Kunstyr, I., Needham, J.J., Nichlas, W., Perrot, A., Rehbinder, C., Richard, and De Vroey, G., Federation of European Laboratory Animal Associations (FELASA): R*ecommendations for health monitoring of mouse, rat, hamster, guinea pig and rabbit breeding colonies,* May 1992. To be published.

65. Boot, R., van Knapen, F., Kruijt, B. C., and Walvoort, H. C., Serological evidence for Encephalitozoon cuniculi infection (nosemiasis) in gnotobiotic guineapigs, *Lab. Anim.,* 22, 337, 1988.

66. Gordon, H. A., and Bruckner, G., Anomalous lower bowel function and related phenomena in germ-free animals, in Th*e Germ-Free Animal in Biomedical Research,* Laboratory Animal Handbook 9, Coates, M. E., and Gustafsson, B. E., Eds., Laboratory Animals Ltd., London, 1984, chap. 9.

67. Henegan, J. B., Physiology of the alimentary tract, in T*he Germ-Free Animal in Biomedical Research,* Laboratory Animal Handbook 9, Coates, M. E., and Gustafsson, B. E., Eds., Laboratory Animals Ltd., London, 1984, chap. 8.

68. Wostmann, B. S., Other organs, in *The Germ-Free Animal in Biomedical Research,* Laboratory Animal Handbook 9, Coates, M. E., and Gustafsson, B. E., Eds., Laboratory Animals Ltd., London, 1984, chap. 10.

69. Wostmann, B. S., and Pleasants, J. R., The germ-free animal fed chemically defined diet: a unique tool, *Proc. Soc. Exp. Biol. Med.,* 198, 539, 1991.

70. Needham, J. R., *Handbook of Microbiological Investigations for Laboratory Animal Health,* Academic Press, London, 1979, 46.

71. Heidt, P. J., Koopman, J. P., Kennis, H. M., van den Logt, J. T., Hectors, M. P., Nagengast, F. M., Timmermans, C. P., and de Groot, C. W., The use of a rat-derived microflora for providing colonization resistance in SPF rats, *Lab. Anim.,* 24, 375, 1990.

72. Tannock, G. W., The normal microflora: new concepts in health promotion, *Microbiol. Sci.,* 5, 4, 1988.

73. van der Waaij, D., Evidence of immunoregulation of the composition of intestinal microflora and its practical consequences, *Eur. J. Clin. Microbiol. Infect. Dis.,* 7, 103, 1988.

74. Hirayama, K., Endo, K., Kawamura, S., and Mitsuoka, T., Comparison of the intestinal bacteria in specific pathogen free mice from different breeders, *Exp. Anim.,* 39, 263, 1990.

75. Juhr, N. C., and Stuckenberg, R., Leukocyte agglutination test for the determination of microbial burden, *Z.Versuchstierkd.,* 33, 221, 1990.

76. Henegan, J. B., Response of germfree animals to shock, *J. Med. Clin. Exp. Theoret.,* 21, 51, 1990.

77. Goris, R. J., Mediators of multiple organ failure, *Intensive Care Med.,* 16, Suppl., 3, 192, 1990.

78. Stadtländer, C., and Kirchhoff, H., Surface parasitism of the fish mycoplasma Mycoplasma mobile 163 K on tracheal epithelial cells, *Vet. Microbiol.,* 21, 339, 1990.

79. Lönnerholm, G., Midtvedt, T., Schenholm, M., and Wistrand, P. J., Carbonic anhydrase isoenzymes in the caecum and colon of normal and germ-free rats, *Acta Physiol. Scand.,* 132, 159, 1988.

80. Pelkonen, K., Implications of the germ-free state on biotransformation, pharmacokinetics and energy metabolism in the rat, Kuopio University Publications C., *Nat. Environ. Sci.,* 6, 1992.

Chapter 18

Monoclonal and Polyclonal Antibodies

Karin Erb and Jann Hau

CONTENTS

INTRODUCTION

A large number of animals are used in the production of antibodies for experimental and clinical analyses. The laboratory animal does not serve as a model for man in this instance and the use of immunization animals can be compared with the use of farm animals for milk or meat production.

The increasing use of immunochemical assays such as radioimmuno assay (RIA) and enzyme-linked immunosorbent assay (ELISA) based on specific antibodies raised in laboratory animals has been responsible for the marked reduction in the number of animals required in bioassays.

A major use of laboratory animals in immunological research is for the production of antibodies. Many experimental and clinical analyses are based upon techniques using these antibodies.

One functional aspect of the immune system is to protect the individual from invasion of foreign microorganisms. This protection is provided by collaboration between the non-acquired and the acquired immunity. The acquired or specific immune defense can be divided into cellular and humoral immune responses. This duality results from two populations of morphologically indistinguishable lymphoid cells, called the T lymphocytes and the B lymphocytes. It is the macrophages which initiate the humoral immune response, with the antigen-independent proliferation and maturation of B lymphocytes localized in the bone marrow, and the antigen-dependent proliferation and maturation localized in the peripheral lymphatic tissues.

All circulating B lymphocytes are covered by membrane-bound immunoglobulin, and the antigen-dependent maturation is stimulated by the binding of the variable site of the immunoglobulin to an antigen determinant of the foreign antigen. This binding stimulates further maturation of the lymphocyte via blast cells to plasma cells. The latter secrete antibodies of the same class and specificity as the membrane-bound immunoglobulin (i.e., monoclonal antibodies).

Every single B lymphocyte which is stimulated by an antigen gives rise to a clone of identical cells, all producing the same type of antibody. This theory was published by Burnet in 1957[1] and is called the clonal selection theory.

For many years immunologists and other scientists have used antiserum from different experimental animals for many different purposes. The antiserum obtained from the immunized animals contains immunoglobulins with different specificities and they are the products of all the different clones stimulated by the antigens (i.e. polyclonal antibodies).

MONOCLONAL ANTIBODIES

The need for better defined and more homogeneous reagents was met when Köhler and Milstein[4] introduced the hybridoma technology in 1975. These extremely important findings were acknowledged with the awarding of the Nobel Prize.

Since the acceptance of the clonal selection theory, it has been known that the key to better defined antibodies is to isolate the individual B lymphocytes activated by the antigens. However, normal mammalian cells can only be grown in vitro for a few days before dying. This is not sufficient time to allow a rational harvest of the secreted antibodies.

In the 1960s, Anderson and Potter,[2] and Potter[3] described the initializing and isolation of plasmacytoma cell lines. BALB/c mice received intraperitoneal injections of pristane (mineral oil, 2,6,10,14-tetramethylpentadecane) and obtained transplantable plasmacytoma cell lines called MOPC, Mineral Oil induced PlasmaCytomas. These cell lines could be cultured in vitro because of their malignancy, and they produced murine immunoglobulin of unknown specificity.

In the first description of the production of monoclonal antibodies, Köhler and Milstein[4] performed a fusion between spleen cells from mice immunized with SRBC (sheep red blood cells) and a myeloma cell line, P3/X63-Ag8[5] (IgG$_1$, kappa light chain), which is a mutant from MOPC-21.[6] The fusion between parental cells was performed using inactivated Sendai virus.[7] The resulting hybrids produced the MOPC-21 protein in addition to new immunoglobulin with specificities to SRBC. These hybrid cell lines obtained by fusion between immune lymphocytes and myeloma cells inherited the parental capability for both antibody production and immortality, and are therefore called hybridoma cell lines.

Selection for growth of hybridoma cells is based on the fact that unfused immune lymphocytes will die in tissue culture medium and myeloma cells will die in selective medium. Littlefield[8] introduced the selection medium containing aminopterin, hypoxanthine, and thymidine (HAT-medium). Aminopterin is an analogue of folic acid, binding very strongly to folic acid reductase, which blocks the coenzymes required for the de novo pathway of DNA synthesis. Thus, all cells will die in media containing aminopterin, but all normal mammalian cells contain the enzymes hypoxanthine-guanine phosphoribosyltransferase (HGPRT) and thymidine kinase (TK), so hypoxanthine and thymidine can be utilized via the "salvage" pathway of DNA synthesis. Myeloma cells are deficient in HGPRTase and will die in HAT selection medium, therefore, only hybrids between spleen cells and myeloma cells will survive. The HGPRT-deficient cell lines can be isolated by growing the plasmacytoma cells in the presence of a purine analogue, 8-azaguanine or 6-thioguanine. HGPRTase enzyme catalyses the incorporation of the purine analogue into DNA where it will interfere with normal protein synthesis, and the cell will die (Figure 1).

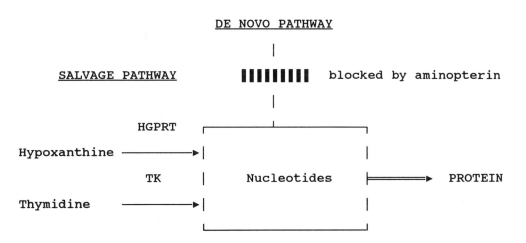

Figure 1. The principle of HAT-selection.

Many steps are involved in the production of monoclonal antibodies, and several methods have been described and excellently reviewed by a number of authors.[9-20] The goal of this chapter is to focus on the problems and techniques associated with the handling of animals during the production of monoclonal antibodies. Specific methods of culturing and screening the resulting hybridomas must therefore be sought elsewhere.[21-26]

IMMUNIZATION
Choice of Animal

The choice of animal species and strains as immune spleen cell donors for fusion is largely dependent on the myeloma cell line available and the origin of the immunogen. The mouse is the animal most commonly used for immunization; first, because there are various murine myeloma cell lines available, and second, because mice are easy to keep and handle, and generally respond better than rats. The BALB/c inbred strain of mice is preferred since many of the myeloma cell lines have a BALB/c background. If spleen donor and fusion partner have the same background, the preparation of large quantities of immunoglobulin in ascites causes no problems in BALB/c mice. Other strains of inbred mice can alternatively be used for immunization if the BALB/c strain responds poorly to the antigen. The ascites production should then be carried out in the respective F1 hybrid, or in immunologically incompetent mice, i.e., irradiated mice, athymic mice, nude mice or SCID mice.

Rats are recommended when monoclonal antibodies against murine antigens[27] or large quantities of ascites are needed.[28,29] For still unknown reasons the efficiency of successful rat x rat hybridomas is often less compared to mouse x mouse hybridomas. Therefore many groups have produced heterohybridomas instead; for example, rat-mouse,[30] rabbit-mouse,[31] goat-mouse,[32] or mink-mouse[33] interspecific hybridomas. The disadvantage of heterohybridomas is genetic instability, resulting in loss of chromosomes coding for immunoglobulin production.

Choice and Preparation of Immunogen

One major advantage of the hybridoma technique is the variety of possible immunization procedures. Immunization can be achieved by the methods below.

Purified antigens — Purified antigens have been used extensively in classical xenogeneic immunization protocols for the production of polyclonal antibodies. A major advantage of working with monoclonal antibodies is that the purity of the immunogen is not important, provided an assay system is available to detect the specific antibodies.

Whole cells, cell homogenates, or unpurified mixtures of antigens — This approach represents an attractive feature of the hybridoma technology and is probably its greatest advantage over the standard xenogeneic immunization procedure. Immunization with whole cell preparations applied to tumor immunology allows the production of monospecific antibodies directed to known as well as unknown tumor antigens.

Chemically modified antigens — Not all antigens are immunogenic to the same extent. Compounds of low molecular weight, monomeric antigens, and water-soluble substances are likely to be poor immunogens. Increasing the immunogenicity is possible by binding low-molecular-weight antigens to larger carrier molecules or by denaturation of the antigens with glutaraldehyde or formaldehyde. In the latter case the specific antibodies will react with the denatured antigen and not with the native one. This can make it difficult to prepare reagents for clinical and diagnostic applications because the immunogens must be isolated so as to ensure that they are present in the same form as the antigens are present in the final assay.[34]

Fused splenic or lymph node lymphocytes without intentional preimmunization — This procedure has been used extensively in the study of autoimmune disorders.

Immunization with Soluble Antigens

Protocols for immunization of mice vary widely. They are empirical and must be adjusted to individual antigens in order to achieve the best immunization conditions.

To stimulate a good response to a soluble antigen, the use of adjuvant is usually necessary. All adjuvant procedures used for the preparation of antisera are potentially useful in the hybridoma area. Even though Freund's adjuvant was first described about 50 years ago, it is still the most effective non-specific immunopotentiator known for stimulating both humoral and cellular immunity. *Bordetella pertussis* is also used as an adjuvant, and is claimed to stimulate a blast cell response before fusion.[14,22,35] Freund's complete adjuvant (FCA) is a mixture of mineral oil (Bayol F) and emulgator (mannide mono-oleate), containing killed *Mycobacterium tuberculosis*. The incomplete adjuvant (FIA) is a mixture of oil and emulgator without a bacterial component. Preparation of antigen in adjuvant is a water-in-oil emulsion.

At our laboratory, soluble antigen preparations are made by dissolving 1 mg of antigen in 1 ml of phosphate-buffered saline (PBS), and then adding the protein solution drop by drop to 1 ml of Freund's incomplete adjuvant (FIA). The preparation of the water-in-oil emulsion is made on a shaking table to ensure the formation of a creamy white solution after each drop. The antigen-adjuvant emulsion is checked by carefully placing drops in saline in a petri dish. If the emulsion is stable, the first or the second drop will not disperse. It is important to perform the drop-in-water test to be sure that the preparation is not made as an oil-in-water solution, which gives no adjuvant effect. The adjuvant preparation must be handled with care.

The site of injection is of crucial importance, not for the stimulation of the immune system, but for the well-being of the animal. Intradermal injections often cause large painful ulcers, and the intra-footpad route is also very painful and completely unnecessary. Adequate priming can usually be achieved by subcutaneous, intraperitoneal, or intramuscular routes. A typical volume of emulsion is between 50 and 200 µl per mouse. Our routine immunization schedule for priming mice is as follows: every mouse receives 100 µl of the emulsion intraperitoneally (i.p.) as the primary immunization. The following (1-3) booster immunizations are injected i.p. every 3 weeks. The final boost 2 to 4 days prior to fusion is given intravenously in an aqueous form without any use of adjuvant.

Immunization with Intact Cells

Intact cells are highly immunogenic and do not usually require the use of adjuvant. The cells are harvested from cell cultures and washed extensively by centrifugation in PBS or serum-free culture medium (RPMI-1640). The cells are counted, and resuspended at a concentration of 10^8 cells per ml. The immunization is performed by i.p. injection of 100 µl. The following 1–3 booster injections are given every 3 weeks, and the final boost before fusion is also administered i.p.

It is recommended to monitor the immune response in the immunized animal. This is done by taking a blood sample, and analyzing the antibody response in an adequate assay. Normally we use 4-5 mice for every immunization schedule to be able to select the animal with the best response. If all the mice are good responders, we prepare the spleen cells from all of them, pool the cells and carry out fusion with one portion while the rest are frozen and stored at -135°C. This makes it possible to repeat fusion with similarly stimulated spleen cells.

Antigens with a very low molecular weight must be prepared in a different manner. One way is to use glutaraldehyde for conjugation of the small haptenic antigens with a highly immunogenic carrier such as keyhole limpet hemocyanin,[36] or to perform the Alum precipitation, described by Hudson and Hay.[26] If only small amounts of immunogen are available, the intrasplenic immunization protocol is useful,[37-38] or, as described by Raymond and Suh,[39] small amounts of immunogen can elicit an immune response when injected into a lymph node.

Mirza et al.[40] state that administration of antigen in the footpads of mice followed by fusion of popliteal and inguinal lymph node lymphocytes results in a higher frequency of hybridomas secreting specific antibody, compared to conventional immunization. In spite of their comments that no swellings or ulcerations of the footpads were observed, we still find that this administration route should be avoided, because it must be considered painful.

MYELOMA CELL LINES

Numerous myeloma cell lines have been used successfully for the generation of hybridomas. Many of today's mouse myeloma cell lines are descendants of Potter's original MOPC-213 which have been selected for HAT sensitivity and the loss of immunoglobulin. Tables 1 and 2 list the commonly used murine and rat myeloma cell lines. In choosing the myeloma line, both the species of origin and the immunoglobulin production of the myeloma cell line should be considered, as both have great influence on the desired end product.

It is preferable to choose myeloma cells that are non-secretors, as the hybrid cells generated will produce the immunoglobulin chains from both the parental cells. The choice of non-secretor myeloma cell lines depends upon the doubling time, fusion efficiency, need for feeder cells, and cloning efficiency. Most of the murine plasmocytoma cell lines are available from the American Type Tissue Culture Collection (ATCC), 12301, Parklawn Drive, Rockville, MD 20852.

FUSION AGENTS

Fusion of somatic cells to produce cell hybrids can be achieved by viruses or chemicals. The fusion process involves three stages: (1) agglutination, (2) membrane fusion between adjacent cells, and (3) osmotic swelling.[41] Köhler and Milstein used inactivated Sendai virus to produce the first hybridoma cells described.[4] Via the envelope hemagglutinin spikes the virus binds to sialic acid-containing receptors on the surface of the spleen cells. This cross-linking causes agglutination and fusion. Recently Nagata et al.[42] described hybridoma generation by means of Vesicular stomatitis virus as the fusion agent. They state that this fusion method has considerable influence on the isotypes of the antibodies obtained, and suggest the advantage of obtaining IgG monoclonal antibodies by means of virus fusion. However, virus preparation is laborious, and the activity of various batches is variable and liable to decay. The disadvantages led to the search for chemical fusogens. Pontecorvo[43] first demonstrated that polyethylene glycol (PEG) in high concentrations was a useful fusion agent for mammalian cell hybridization.

Since then nearly all hybridoma protocols describe the use of PEG (molecular weight 1000 to 6000). Although the membrane fusion efficiency increases with increasing PEG concentration, the viability of the cells drops sharply with PEG concentrations above 50%. Exposure time is also a very critical factor: too short a time results in too few hybrids, too long a time causes too toxic an effect of the PEG, so the optimal time is between 1 and 2 min. It is also very important to dilute PEG slowly at the termination of the fusion. It has been reported that the addition of dimethylsulfoxide allows the PEG concentration to be reduced, thus lowering the toxicity but maintaining the same fusion efficiency.[44,45]

PREPARATION OF CELLS FOR FUSION
Feeder Cells

Many of the available myeloma cell lines depend on feeder cells in order to obtain acceptable fusion frequencies. It must be noted that cloning of established hybridomas sometimes provides feeder cells.[12] Feeder cells improve the yield of hybridomas by adding unknown growth factors to the medium. Several different cell types have been used as feeder cells. The most widespread are murine peritoneal exudate cells, among which especially the macrophages are effective.

Alternative sources of feeder cells are mouse thymocytes,[46] rat thymocytes,[47] mouse spleen cells from unimmunized mice,[48] irradiated human fibroblasts,[49] lymphokines from mixed thymocyte culture,[50,51] and conditioned medium.[52]

Adult, untreated BALB/c mice (of the same genetic background as the hybridoma) are killed by cervical dislocation, rinsed in 70% alcohol, transferred to a sterile work area and dissected with sterile instruments. The cleaned mouse is crucified on a soft board with needles. A small hole in the abdominal skin is cut with scissors and the abdominal skin is removed. The peritoneum is washed with alcohol and 10 ml of serum-free cell culture medium (RPMI-1640) is injected into the abdominal cavity directly above the symphysis with a 25-gauge, 1.6-cm needle. After gentle massage of the abdomen, the medium is

Table 1. Murine Cell Lines Available for Fusion Procedures

Cell line	Short name	Ig class	Derived from
P3.X63-Ag8[2]	X63	IgG$_1$,kappa	MOPC-21
P3.X63-Ag8U.1[58]	—	kappa	X63
P3.X63-Ag8.653[59]	X63-Ag8.653	None	X63
P3/NS1/1-Ag4-1[60,61]	NS-1	kappa	X63
NS0/1[24]	NS0	None	NS-1
Sp2/0-Ag14[62]	SP2	None	Sp2/HLGK
FO[12]	F0	None	SP2/0
FOX-NY[63]	FOX-NY	None	NS-1
MPC11-X45.6TG.1.7[64]	45.6.TG1.7	IgG$_{2a}$,kappa	MPC-11
S194/5XXO-1[5]	—	None	S-194/5
XS63[5]	XS63	None	S63

All the above-mentioned mouse myeloma cell lines are of BALB/c origin.

XC1.5/51[5]	XC1.5/51	None	C1.18

(C1.18 is a cell line derived from the tumor X-5563, which arose spontaneously in a C3H mouse)

Table 2. Rat Cell Lines Available for Fusion Procedures

Cell line	Short name	Ig class	Derived from
210-RCY3-Ag1[24]	—	kappa	S210
Y3-Ag1.2.3[28]	—	kappa	210-RCY3-Ag1
YB2/3HL[24]	—	Ig	Y3-Ag1.2.3
YB2/0[65]	—	None	YB2/3HL
IR983F[66]	—	None	LOU/c

removed by inserting an 18-gauge, 4-cm needle just under the lower right rib. Aspiration of the medium should be stopped when the back pressure becomes too high. If the medium becomes turbid, indicating bleeding or contamination, it must be discarded. Normally it is possible to withdraw 8 ml of peritoneal washing medium, containing about 5×10^6 peritoneal exudate cells. The cell harvest is transferred to a 50-ml Nunc centrifugation tube and topped up with serum-free medium. Centrifuged at 400 g for 10 min, the cell pellet is resuspended in medium and counted. The cells are diluted to 2×10^5 cells per ml in serum containing culture medium. Fifty µl of the feeder cell suspension is transferred into each well of a microtiter plate, to be used for fusion. It is recommended to prepare the feeder cells one day prior to fusion to let the feeder cells adhere to the plastic. If bacterial contamination has occurred, it will be possible to discover this and discard the plates. Normally, we use five microplates per fusion and a feeder cell concentration of 10^4 per well. It is sufficient to prepare feeder cells from two mice.

Spleen Cells

The immunized mouse is killed by cervical dislocation, rinsed in 70% alcohol and placed on a board in a sterile cabinet, and the spleen is removed under aseptic conditions. The abdominal skin is cut and pulled aside to expose the peritoneum. An incision is then made just over the spleen on the left side of the mouse. The spleen is pulled out carefully with forceps, and released from the mesentery by means of a scalpel. The spleen is transferred to a petri dish containing serum-free RPMI-1640, and the exterior of the spleen is washed before transfer to another petri dish containing RPMI-1640, 10% fetal calf serum. Single cells are obtained by carefully scraping the spleen with a scalpel. The cell suspension is sucked in and out with a pasteur pipette and transferred into two 10-ml tipped tubes. The mixture is allowed to settle for approximate 2 min, and the supernatant is transferred to a 50-ml Nunc centrifugation tube. The spleen cells are washed by centrifugation and counted.

FUSION PROCEDURE

A variety of procedures for provoking fusion of immunized spleen cells and myeloma cells exists. The following protocol has proven consistently successful in our hands, and has been adopted, with minor modifications, from the protocol originally described by Köhler.[23]

Immune spleen cells (10^8) and myeloma cells (10^7) are mixed and washed by centrifugation. All the supernatant is aspired, the cell pellet is loosened by flicking the tube, and 0.5 ml 50% PEG (Merck MW 4000) is added drop by drop to the cell pellet for a period of 1 min. The tube is shaken for another minute, after which 10 ml of serum-free RPMI-1640 is added slowly (initially by drops) over a period of 5 min to dilute the PEG. The mixture is incubated at 37°C in a CO_2 incubator for 10 min, further diluted to 50 ml with serum-free RPMI-1640, and centrifuged for 5 minutes at 400 g. The supernatant is discarded and the cell pellet is resuspended in 75 ml HAT-medium. The fusion product is seeded on 96-well flat bottom microculture plates (Nunc) with 150 μl per well. The culture plates were seeded with feeder cells (50 μl per well) the day before fusion. Every 3 days the cultures are fed by aspirating half of the culture fluid and replacing it with prewarmed, fresh HAT-medium. Ten to 14 days post-fusion the HAT-medium is replaced by HT-medium, and the cultures are inspected for hybrid cell growth. When macroscopical colonies are seen at around days 7 to 8, or the color of the medium has changed to yellow, the supernatants are removed for screening of antibody activity. Positive clones are propagated and cloned by limited dilution[14] (0.5 cells per well using feeder cells).

MASS PRODUCTION OF ANTIBODIES *IN VITRO* OR *IN VIVO*

Production of large quantities of antibodies *in vitro* is based on normal culturing of hybridoma cell lines in culture bottles, roller bottles, hollow fiber units, or fermentors. Murine hybridomas normally produce between 10 and 100 μg per ml in *in vitro* culture. If larger quantities of antibodies are needed, *in vivo* production is most often used.

Hybridomas derived from BALB/c origin can be propagated in primed BALB/c mice. The antibody recovery will reach between 1 and 5 mg per ml ascites fluid.

PREPARATION OF ASCITES FLUID

Mice are primed by i.p. injection of 37°C prewarmed pristane (2,6,10,14-tetramethylpentadecane, Aldrich Chemical Co., Milwaukee, WI), at a volume of 0.25 to 0.5 ml per mouse.[53,54] A long-lasting analgesic, like Temgesic, should be given at the same time as pristane is administered, since pristane seems to cause pain. Seven to 10 days later the hybridoma cell line in the log phase of growth is washed, counted, and resuspended at a concentration of 1×10^6 to 1×10^7 cells per ml culture medium (RPMI-1640, unsupplemented), and 0.5 ml is injected i.p. into each mouse. The animals are monitored twice daily for abdominal swelling, which can occur rapidly, and the volume should be sufficient after 10 to 12 days. The ascitic fluid can be collected from anesthetized mice by inserting an 18-gauge, 4-cm needle into the peritoneal cavity and allowing the ascites to drain into 10-ml sterile tubes. The amount collected from one mouse varies between a few ml to about 10 ml per day. It is possible to collect ascites fluid from the same mouse every day for 3 to 4 days, but for welfare reasons the number of collections should be limited to two.

Problems in the ascites production can occur: the primed mouse may not develop sufficient ascites or the hybridoma cell line may grow as a solid tumor. The recommended way is to prime 5 to 10 mice for each cell line, and when the first ascites is collected, to inject 0.5 ml of the ascites into preprimed mice. These "second-generation" mice will respond more quickly and with larger volumes of ascites. When ascites production is well established, some ascitic fluid is collected aseptically for isolation of ascites cells, and the standard freezing procedure is carried out. If more antibodies are needed, these ascites cells will produce larger quantities of ascites fluid more quickly, sparing time and trouble.

Each collection of ascites fluid is incubated at 4°C overnight, centrifuged at 10,000 g for 15 min to remove clots, cells, and other debris, before storage at -80°C. At the end of the ascites production the collections are thawed, pooled, and filtrated through a prefilter and a 0.22 μm filter (Millipore, Bedford, MA). Sterilized material is aliquoted and kept frozen at -80°C until use.

Jones et al.[55] report the use of Freund's incomplete adjuvant as a priming agent instead of pristane, stating that the number of hybridoma cells and the time interval between the priming and the hybridoma inoculation can be reduced. This method has not been successful in our hands.

Witte and Ber[56] have reported that an improved efficiency of ascites production is seen with intrasplenic inoculation. This method is stated to be simple and to have the advantage over the normally used i.p. inoculation by requiring only a low number of hybridoma cells (10^4).

Rat hybridomas can be propagated as ascites cells in rats just as described for mice. Heterohybridomas or human hybridoma cell lines can only be grown as ascites cells in immunologically incompetent mice. Irradiated mice can be used, but during the last decade nude mice have proved to be more suitable for ascites production. The nude mouse has an incomplete immune system due to its missing thymus. This immune defect allows acceptance of xenogeneic transplants. If the ascites production fails in the nude mouse, the hybridoma cell line can be inoculated subcutaneously to establish a solid tumor. When the tumor propagates, the mouse is sacrificed, and the tumor mass removed, suspended and placed back into culture. After 2 to 3 weeks in culture approximately 10^7 subcutaneously adapted hybridoma cells can be injected and accepted in pristane-primed nude mice, and ascites can be collected as described above.[57]

GUIDELINES FOR THE PRODUCTION OF MONOCLONAL ANTIBODIES

ROUTE OF INJECTION

The route of injection is i.p. for both soluble immunogen and whole cells followed by i.p. booster injections. The final booster injection with soluble immunogen is administered i.v.

DOSE VOLUME

The total dose volume with or without adjuvant is 0.1 ml.

ADJUVANT

FIA adjuvant is used only for i.p. injections with soluble immunogen, while injections with whole cells and i.v. injections are performed without any form of adjuvant.

TIME INTERVALS

Immunizations:

1. Day 0: i.p. injection of antigen with or without adjuvant
2. Day 21: i.p. booster injection
3. Day 42: final i.v. injection of soluble antigen and final i.p. injection of whole cells

Fusion:

4. Day 44: (one day before fusion) untreated mice are killed by cervical dislocation and the peritoneal cells are harvested
5. Day 45: (three days after the final booster injection) the immunized mouse is killed by cervical dislocation and the spleen is aseptically removed

ASCITES PRODUCTION

6. Day 0: a mouse is primed with 0.5 ml Pristane (37°)
7. Day 8: 10^7-10^8 cells are injected i.p. into the primed mouse
8. Day 18: ascites fluid collected from the mouse during anesthesia
9. Day 19: procedure from Day 18 is repeated

POLYCLONAL ANTIBODIES

IMMUNIZATION
Choice of Animal

The rabbit is by tradition the most widely used species for production of polyclonal antibodies. The rabbit breeds used for immunization tend to be quite big, the animals are gentle, easy to handle, and their husbandry is simple. Blood sampling from the marginal ear veins is unproblematic and the antibodies precipitate well like most other mammalian antibodies. Being the most frequently used species for antibody production, the rabbit accounts for the majority of commercial second antibodies of various kinds. However, the rabbit should not automatically be the first choice when the production of antisera is considered. Other species may be more suitable for an individual project, and the way rabbits are housed solitarily in fairly small cages is ethically questionable if the animals are kept for a long period, which is often the case for immunization animals.

Other suitable species for antibody production include goats and sheep. Both of these species have many advantages as antibody producers. They are easy to handle and maintain, they are available in many sizes, and blood sampling from the jugular vein is easier and quicker than blood sampling from rabbits' ear veins. The larger size of sheep and goats should also make it feasible to use very lenient immunization methods and still obtain sufficient quantities of antibodies.

If only small amounts of antisera are needed there are good reasons for choosing mice or rats. A major advantage is the minimal interindividual variation in antibody response when raising the antibodies in inbred rodents, whereas rabbits exhibit remarkable interindividual variation, even within closed colonies.[67] Animal species differ in their immune response to different antigens and adjuvants,[68] and perhaps the most generally appropriate species for production of polyclonal antibodies is the domestic hen. One of the advantages associated with the use of birds for production of antibodies against proteins of mammalian origin is the phylogenetic distance between the species. A rabbit will synthesize few or no antibodies of low avidity if it is immunized with rabbit proteins. It can also be deduced from this that chicken antisera are very useful when employed for demonstrating immunological cross reactions between analogous proteins in different mammalian species.[69,70]

Because of the transovarian passage of specific antibodies it is possible to purify antibodies from egg yolk. The immunoglobulin concentration in the chicken egg yolk is higher than in chicken or rabbit serum, and the productivity is approximately 6000 ml of egg yolk per chicken per year as compared to approximately 500 ml of serum per year from a rabbit in an intensive immunization protocol. Purification of immunoglobulins from the egg yolk is fairly simple and several methods have been published.[71] Avian IgG possesses certain characteristics which are often advantageous for their later use, such as no mammalian complement binding, no binding to mammalian Fc receptors, and no binding to proteins A and G.

The use of chickens for production of antibodies is attractive from an ethical viewpoint, and with respect to the 3 Rs.[72] Mammals can thus be replaced by a species with a lower degree of neurophysiological sensitivity. The number of animals needed can be reduced with a factor of 10 to 20, and since the use of egg yolk antibodies does not require handling, restraint and blood sampling, it must be considered a more refined way of producing polyclonal antibodies.

Cell lines for the production of monoclonal chicken antibodies have now also been successfully developed, although there seem to be problems associated with the longevity of the cells.[73]

Immunogens

Immunogens are defined as substances that are able to induce an immune response, whereas an antigen is a substance which can react immunologically with the antibody. The two are not always synonymous but very often no distinction is made in the literature.

In order for a molecule to be immunogenic and able to provoke an immune reaction in an animal, it generally has to have a molecular weight greater than 3000 to 4000 Daltons,[74] and a rule of thumb is the bigger the molecule, the better the antibody response. The molecule should be biodegradable and at the same time have a certain structural stability, and be present in more or less the same form in different injections. In polypeptides and proteins an antigenic site or epitope is usually made up of approximately six amino acids. In order to be a good immunogen the molecule must possess at least one epitope that can be recognized by the cell surface antibody found on B cells, and it must have at least one surface structure that can be recognized simultaneously by a class II protein and by a T cell receptor. Small peptides and steroid hormones are usually poor immunogens or not immunogenic at all and have to be coupled to a carrier molecule if antibodies are to be raised against them as described in the section on monoclonal antibodies.

When raising polyclonal antisera, as opposed to the production of monoclonal antibodies, the purity of the immunogen is of major importance. It can be time-consuming and laborious to purify the antigen, but usually the time is well spent, as it is much easier to render an antiserum only weakly contaminated with antibodies against other molecules monospecific, than to remove a lot of unwanted specificities by extensive absorption procedures. The later use of the antibodies may also limit the choice of method used for their absorption. If the antibodies are to be used in tissue localization studies, for instance, solid-phase absorption must be used. Liquid-phase absorption would result in addition of foreign molecules to the antiserum, causing the risk of unreliable results.

Adjuvants

As adjuvants constitute a cornerstone in the production of polyclonal antibodies, and the traditional use of adjuvants often results in reduced animal welfare, the description of adjuvants has been given ample space in this chapter.

The most commonly used immunological adjuvants can be classified into one or more of four groups: oil-based adjuvants, mineral adjuvants, saponins, and microbial products.[75] For experimental purposes the oil-based adjuvants are the most frequently used. The most potent adjuvants are the oil-based adjuvants containing bacterial material. Oil-based adjuvants are not used in human vaccines because of severe local reactions with granuloma and abscess formation.[76]

Oil-based adjuvants are usually not used in animals for human consumption, since the oil may penetrate through fascial planes and spoil the meat. Freund's complete adjuvant is quite unacceptable in food animals, not only because of the mineral oil, but also because the mycobacteria in the adjuvant render animals positive to tuberculin, a critical feature in areas where tuberculosis is under control.

Adjuvants were defined in 1926 by Ramon[77] as immunity-stimulating substances that in combination with specific antigen vaccines enhance immunity levels above those obtained without the adjuvant. The most widely used adjuvants in commercial veterinary vaccines are the mineral adjuvants which employ mineral gels such as aluminum hydroxide, aluminum phosphate, or aluminum potassium sulfate (alum). These adjuvants are produced in colloidal suspensions to which the immunogenic material is adsorbed.[78] They can be stored for relatively long periods, which is a feature not generally found in oil-based adjuvants once they have been emulsified with the immunogen in water preparation.

In experimental immunology and production of antisera for experimental or diagnostic use the restrictions to the adjuvant mentioned under meat-producing animals do not apply. This is why the very potent and aggressive oil-based adjuvants, and in particular Freund's adjuvants,[79] are still very commonly used for production of polyclonal antisera.

The detailed reactions involved in the adjuvant stimulation of the immune system are complex and vary from one species to another. They have been the subject of many excellent review papers,[80,81] and will not be dealt with in detail here.

One of the features that makes oil-based adjuvants so efficient is their depot effect. When antigenic material in a water solution is injected into an animal, a prompt and rapid dissemination of the injected material occurs. Alum precipitation of antigens causes only slight retention of antigen. However, if the same material is injected in a water-in-oil emulsion, with or without mycobacteria, the oil vesicles are retained at the site of injection for many months while the material undergoes very slow absorption. The rate of antigen elimination from the injection site has been reported to have a half-life of approximately 14 days. The antibody response to emulsified protein antigens seems to be relatively constant for up to a year.[82]

Antigenic stimulation may arise not only at the site of injection, where an epithelioid-macrophage granuloma reaction is formed, but also in other foci when antigens are injected in FCA.[83] Adjuvants containing mycobacterial material have been found to be maximally effective when the antigen is rapidly catabolized. Raised ambient temperature or a high carbohydrate diet were demonstrated to slow down catabolism and work against the adjuvant effect.[84]

Usually FCA is found to be more potent than FIA; if FCA is used at all, it should only be used once and in the first injection. Repeated injections of FCA lead to very severe tissue reactions and may result in anaphylactic shock.

Some studies have indicated that FIA is as potent as FCA,[85] but FCA must be regarded as a definitely more aggressive and potent adjuvant than FIA. The antibodies formed against the bacterial components of complete adjuvants can disturb the use of the antiserum, which is an additional reason for avoiding the use of these types of adjuvants.

Freund's adjuvants and animal welfare considerations

Few publications focus on lesions induced by Freund's adjuvant alone; however, it is evident that subcutaneous or intravenous application of FCA in rabbits, rats, mice, hamsters, and guinea pigs results in focal necrosis, ulceration, fistulous tracts, and trauma.[86] Moreover, a common finding is the presence of disseminated granulomas in lungs, liver, kidney, heart, lymph nodes, and skeletal muscle[87,88] and the possibility of inducing a number of different autoimmune diseases.

There is marked species variation in the response to Freund's adjuvants, and chickens, whose lymphoid tissues are not organized in lymph nodes, exhibit a slightly delayed response compared with mammals.[89]

Several reports demonstrate that the use of Freund's adjuvants, in particular FCA, causes pain in animals. Indeed, Freund's adjuvant-induced arthritis constitutes the only laboratory animal model of chronic pain that has been validated to a significant extent.[90] Pathological changes in the joints of immunized animals do not seem to be restricted solely to the use of oil adjuvants. Rheumatoid-like joint lesions have also been found in rabbits immunized with serum or milk proteins by intraperitoneal injection of alum-precipitated proteins. Different breeds of rabbit were shown to develop different incidences of lesions, suggesting a genetic influence on the development of these lesions.[91] There is evidence to suggest that FCA may be carcinogenic, and the use of this adjuvant is now questioned in many countries not only because of animal welfare considerations but also because of the extremely unpleasant complications for personnel who accidentally injure themselves while immunizing the animals. Even if the skin is pricked accidentally and no injection is made, this can be very painful and result in dramatic swelling of the area, and the wound may heal very slowly and still discharge two years after the incident.[92]

The Canadian Council on Animal Care decided in 1988 that all routes of administration of FCA other than subcutaneous and (deep) intramuscular would fall under the category "highly questionable or unacceptable".[93]

Alternative adjuvants

Many adjuvants that are less harmful than Freund's are commercially available, and some of the most promising alternatives seem to be different derivatives of the synthetic N-acetyl-muramyl-L-alanyl-D-isoglutamine (muramyl dipeptide, MDP). MDP represents the minimal structure which can replace the mycobacterial cells in FCA, and it enhances the antibody response when administered with the immunogen in aqueous solution in mice.[94] The adjuvant effect of MDP has been demonstrated to be genetically controlled in mice and influenced by genes inside and outside the major histocompatibility complex.[95]

Other oil-based adjuvants are used as oil-in-water emulsions instead of the Freund's water-in-oil system. Modern examples of this are RIBI containing squalene, monophosphoryl lipid A (MPL), and trehalose dimycolate (TDM). In mice RIBI has been found to be more immunopotentiating than FCA, but having quite severe side effects also.[96] Unfortunately, studies in rabbits of the effect of RIBI yielded less encouraging results.[97]

Saponins are a class of adjuvants which can be extracted from a number of plant families. Saponin adjuvants have been used in veterinary vaccines for decades. The most popular saponin is termed Quil-A, a potent adjuvant for membrane-derived or particulate antigens, whereas its adjuvant activity for water-soluble proteins is poor or lacking.[98]

Dextran polymer particles (Sephadex G-200), which form a gel matrix used in column size chromatography, has been found to be as potent an adjuvant as FIA in a study using bovine serum albumin as the antigen.[99]

Inert polymer pellets (ethylene-vinyl acetate copolymer) have also been used successfully instead of traditional adjuvants. These pellets, which are sometimes less than 1 mm in diameter, are implanted subcutaneously and release the antigen over a period of 6 months,[100] and in some rabbit immunization schemes the pellets have been found to be as potent an adjuvant as FCA.[101]

GENETIC CONTROL OF ANTIBODY RESPONSE, INFLUENCE OF SEX AND AGE

The antibody response to most antigens seems to be genetically determined and under polygenic control, involving H-2 genes.[102,103] In certain instances the genetic control of the immune response seems to be dependent on antigen dose and increasing doses can transform a poorly responding mouse strain into a good responder.[104]

A sex difference in the magnitude of antibody response within inbred strains has frequently been observed.[105]

Young animals have been shown to be better antibody producers than old animals in standard immunization schemes;[106] the length of the immunization period should therefore be as short as possible, also for the sake of the welfare of the animals. Rabbits may conveniently be started in an immunization scheme on weaning at the age of 1 month. There are many advantages in using young animals, the most important being that they are less likely to be affected by previous infections.

IMMUNOGEN DOSE AND SITE OF INJECTION

The immunogen dose is usually not a critically limiting factor for the production of a good antibody response, but in the production of antisera as well as in the development of vaccines increasing doses of both immunogen and adjuvant often result in an increased response.[107] Adam and coworkers[108] found a near-linear relation between the adjuvant dose and the amount of antibody produced. However, in general, the relation between immunogen dose and subsequent antibody titer is far from directly proportional.

Both antigen dose and timing of injections have been demonstrated to influence the immune response to malignant ascites cells,[109] and the relative proportion of the antigen-specific immunoglobulin classes (IgA, IgE, IgG, and IgM) has been demonstrated to vary according to antigen dose.[110] Larger doses are usually associated with the production of higher titers against impurities and consequently moderate doses should be chosen. During the first 6 to 12 months of the immunization scheme in rabbits and goats a gradual increase in both antibody titer and antibody avidity is usually recorded. Thus, if the antibodies are to be used in, e.g., immunospecific purification of the antigen by affinity chromatography, it is not advantageous to use antibodies from animals that have been immunized for a long time. Another good reason for not employing very long immunization periods is that simultaneous with the increase in titer of the wanted antibodies there is also an increase in the titer of antibodies with specificities against the impurities which are always present.

Many different injection sites have been used in attempts to raise antibodies. Most of these sites, however, must be considered more uncomfortable, if not painful, for the animal than the standard intramuscular and subcutaneous injection sites. When immunizing rabbits subcutaneously, the traditional way is to deposit the immunogen mixture at several sites in the neck region. Studies have shown, however, that the response is not diminished by depositing the material subcutaneously in the flank region more posteriorly.[111] The advantage is that when the rabbit is lifted out of the cage by gripping the scruff of its neck, the immunization site, which might be sore because of abscess formation, etc. is not touched. Horne and co-workers[112] found that intra-articular administration of antigen in complete adjuvant failed to induce an adjuvant effect on the immune response, just like intra-lymph node injection failed to prove superior to the footpad route at several dose levels also including a complete adjuvant.[113]

In human studies of the efficacy of influenza vaccination of adults intradermal inoculation was found not to be more efficient in terms of the resulting increase in antibody titer than the subcutaneous route of administration. The antibody rise in children was somewhat greater when intradermal inoculation was used instead of subcutaneous injection.[114] However, it is obvious that very good scientific arguments must be required in order to allow future painful injection procedures.

GUIDELINES FOR THE PRODUCTION OF POLYCLONAL ANTIBODIES

The following guidelines[88,115] can be used for rabbit-size and larger animals and for most immunogens to obtain a good antibody response obtained with minimal distress to the animals.

ROUTES OF INJECTION

The route and recommended site of injection is subcutaneous on the back region of the animal, lateral to the spine, at a site with good movability of the skin, or small volumes (0.1 to 0.5 ml) intramuscularly. For i.m. inoculation muscles of the hind limbs are the preferred site. FIA or FCA must not be injected into lumbar muscles. Not recommended are footpad, intradermal, intravenous, and intraperitoneal routes with either FIA or FCA.

DOSE VOLUME

For i.m. or s.c. injections of FIA or FCA, the recommended volume is 0.1 to 0.2 ml per site for a total dose of max. 1.0 ml.

ADJUVANT

Alternatives to Freund's adjuvants are encouraged, e.g., various derivatives of MDP. If FCA is used, it should be for the initial injection only. Booster injections should never be made with FCA.

TIME INTERVALS

1. Day 0: s.c. antigen-adjuvant injections
2. Day 14: s.c. or i.v. booster injection with antigen
3. Day 28: procedure for day 14 is repeated
4. Day 42: analysis of antiserum

Exsanguination during anesthesia or collection of 40 ml of blood (4-kg rabbit) every 28 days. Booster injections may be given if necessary. Exsanguination should not be later than 12 months.

REFERENCES

1. Burnet, F. M., A modification of Jerne's theory of antibody production using the concept of clonal selection, *Austr. J. Sci., 20, 67, 1957.*

2. Anderson, P. N. and Potter, M., Induction of plasma cell tumours in BALB/c mice with 2,6,10,14-tetramethylpentadecane (Pristane), *Nature, 222, 994, 1969.*

3. Potter, M., Immunoglobulin-producing tumors and myeloma proteins of mice, *Physiol. Rev., 52, 631, 1972.*

4. Köhler, G. and Milstein, C., Continuous cultures of fused cells secreting antibody of predefined specificity, *Nature, 256, 495, 1975.*

5. Horibata, K. and Harris, A. W., Mouse myelomas and lymphomas in culture, *Exp. Cell Res., 60, 61, 1970.*

6. Cotton, R. G. H., Secher, D. S. and Milstein, C., Somatic mutation and the origin of antibody diversity. Clonal variability of the immunoglobulin produced by MOPC21 cells in culture, *Eur. J. Immunol., 3, 135, 1973.*

7. Harris, H. and Watkins, J. F., Hybrid cells derived from mouse and man: artificial heterokaryons of mammalian cells from different species, *Nature, 205, 640, 1965.*

8. Littlefield, J. W., Selection of hybrids from matings of fibroblasts in vitro and their presumed recombinants, *Science, 145, 709, 1964.*

9. Melchers, F., Potter, M. and Warner N. L., Preface, *Curr. Top. Microbiol. Immunol., 81, IX, 1978.*

10. Milstein, C., Galfre, G., Secher, D. S. and Springer, T., Monoclonal antibodies and cell surface antigens, *Cell Biol. Int. Rep., 3, 1, 1979.24*

11. Kennett, R. H., Monoclonal antibodies. Hybrid myelomas. A revolution in serology and immunogenetics, *Am. J. Hum. Genet., 31, 539, 1979.*

12. Fazekas de St. Groth, S. and Scheidegger, D., Production of monoclonal antibodies: strategy and tactics, *J. Immunol. Meth., 35, 1, 1980.*

13. Milstein, C., Monoclonal antibodies, *Sci. Am, 243, 56, 1980.*

14. Goding, J. W., Antibody production by hybridomas, *J. Immunol. Meth., 39, 285, 1980.*

15. Secher, D. S., Monoclonal antibodies by cell fusion, *Immunol. Today, 22, July 1980.*

16. Diamond, B. A., Yelton, D. E. and Scharff, M. D., Monoclonal antibodies. A new technology for producing serologic reagents, *N. Engl. J. Med., 304, 1344, 1981.*

17. Galfre, G. and Clark, M. R., Strategies in the derivation of hybrid myelomas, in *Monoclonal antibodies and development in immunoassay*, Albertini, A. and Ekins, R., Eds., Elsevier/North-Holland Biomedical Press, Amsterdam, 1981, 23.

18. Westerwoudt, R. J., Improved fusion methods. IV. Technical aspects, *J. Immunol. Meth., 77, 181, 1985.*

19. Waldmann, M. C. H., Production of murine monoclonal antibodies, in *Methods in hematology: "Monoclonal antibodies"*, Beverley, P. C. L., Ed., Churchill Livingstone, Edinburgh, 1986, chap. 1.

20. Pirofski, L., Casadevall, A., Rodriguez, L., Zuckier, L. S. and Scharff, M. D., Current state of the hybridoma technology, *J. Clin. Immunol., 10, 5S, 1990.*

21. Kennett, R. H., Fusion protocols, in *Monoclonal antibodies, hybridomas, a new dimension in biological analyses*, Kennett, R. H., McKean, T. J. and Bechtol, K. B., Eds., Plenum Press, New York, 1980, 365.

22. Oi, V. T. and Herzenberg, L. A., Immunoglobulin-producing hybrid cell lines, in *Selected methods in cellular immunology*, Mishell, B. B. and Shiigi, S. M., Eds., Freeman and Company, San Francisco, 1980, chap. 17.

23. Köhler, G., The technique of hybridoma production, in *Immunological Methods II*, Academic Press, Orlando, 1981, chap. 17.

24. Galfrè, G. and Milstein, C., Preparation of monoclonal antibodies: Strategies and procedures, in *Methods in enzymology, 73*, Langone, J. J. and Van Vunakies, H., Eds., Academic Press, Orlando, 1981, chap. 1.

25. Morrow, K. J., Ünüvar, E., King, S. W. and Mleczko, J. B., Techniques for the production of monoclonal and polyclonal antibodies, in C*olloidal gold: Principles, methods and applications*, Academic Press, Orlando, 1991, chap. 2.

26. Hybridoma cells and monoclonal antibody, in *Practical Immunology*, Hudson, L. and Hay, F. C., Eds., Blackwell Scientific Publications, Oxford, 1980, chap. 11.

27. Leptin, M. and Melchers, F., A monoclonal antibody with specificity for murine μ heavy chain which inhibits the formation of antigen-specific direct IgM plaques, *J. Immunol. Meth., 59, 53, 1983.*
28. Galfrè, G., Milstein, C. and Wright, B., *Nature (London), 277, 131, 1979.*
29. Clark, M., Cobbold, S., Hale, G. and Waldmann, H., Advantages of rat monoclonal antibodies, *Immunol. Today, 4, 100, 1983.*
30. Kayano, T., Motoda, R., Usui, M., Ando, S., Matuhasi, T. and Kurimoto, M., Growth of rat-mouse hybridoma cells in immunosuppressed hamsters, *J. Immunol. Meth., 130, 25, 1990.*
31. Yarmush, M. L., Gates, F. T., Weisfogel, D. R. and Kindt, T. J., Identification and characterization of rabbit-mouse hybridomas secreting rabbit immunoglobulin chains, *Proc. Natl. Acad. Sci. U.S.A., 77, 2899, 1980.*24
32. Capparelli, R., Del Sorba, G. and Iannelli, D., Goat-mouse hybridomas secreting goat immunoglobulins, *Hybridoma, 9, 149, 1990.*
33. Ufimtseva, E. G., Galakhar, N. L., Matjakhina, L. D., Khlebodarova, T. M. and Djatchenko, S. N., Mink-mouse interspecific hybridomas, *Hybridoma, 10, 517, 1991.*
34. Pancino, G. F., Osinaga, E., Vorauher, W., Kakouche, A., Mistro, D., Charpin, C. and Roseto, A., Production of a monoclonal antibody as immunohistochemical marker on paraffin embedded tissues using a new immunization method, *Hybridoma, 9, 389, 1990.*
35. Stähli, C., Staehelin, T., Miggiano, V., Schmidt, J. and Hring, P., High frequencies of antigen-specific hybridomas: Dependence on immunization parameters and prediction by spleen cell analysis, *J. Immunol. Meth., 32, 297, 1980.*
36. French, D., Fischberg, E., Buhl, S. and Scharff, M. D., The production of more useful monoclonal antibodies, *Immunol. Today, 7, 344, 1986.*
37. Spitz, M., Spitz, L., Thorpe, R. and Eugui, E., Intrasplenic primary immunization for the production of monoclonal antibodies, *J. Immunol. Meth., 70, 39, 1984.*
38. Nielsson, B. O., Svalander, P. C. and Larsson, A., Immunization of mice and rabbits by intrasplenic deposition of nanogram quantities of protein attached to sepharose beads or nitrocellulose paper strips, *J. Immunol. Meth., 99, 67, 1987.*
39. Raymond, Y. and Suh, M., Lymph node primary immunization of mice for the production of polyclonal and monoclonal antibodies, *J. Immunol. Meth., 93, 103, 1986.*
40. Mirza, I. H., Wilkin, T. J., Cantarini, M. and Moore, K., A comparison of spleen and lymph node cells as fusion partners for raising of monoclonal antibodies after different routes of immunization, *J. Immunol. Meth., 105, 235, 1987.*5.
41. Knutton, S. and Pasternak, C. A., The mechanism of cell-cell fusion, *TIBS, 220, October 1979.*
42. Nagata, S., Yamamoto, K., Ueno, Y., Kurata, T. and Chiba, J., Preferential generation of monoclonal IgG-producing hybridomas by use of vesicular stomatitis virus-mediated cell fusion, *Hybridoma, 10, 369, 1991.*
43. Pontecorvo, G., Production of mammalian somatic cell hybrids by means of polyethylene glycol treatment, *Somatic Cell Genet., 1, 397, 1975.*
44. Norwood, T. H., Zeigler, C. J. and Martin, G. M., Dimethyl sulfoxide enhances polyethylene glycol-mediated somatic cell fusion, *Somatic Cell Genet., 2, 263, 1976.*
45. Lane, R. D., A short-duration polyethylene glycol fusion technique for increasing production of monoclonal antibody-secreting hybridomas, *J. Immunol. Meth., 81, 223, 1985.*
46. Gustafsson, B., Jondal, M. and Sundqvist, V.-A., SPAM-8, a mouse-human fusion partner in the production of human monoclonal antibodies. Establishment of a human monoclonal antibody against cytomegalovirus, *Hum. Antibod. Hybridomas, 2, 26, 1991.*
47. Holmdahl, R., Moran, T. and Andersson, M., A rapid and efficient immunization protocol for production of monoclonal antibodies reactive with autoantigens, *J. Immunol. Meth., 83, 379, 1985.*
48. Zola, H. and Brooks, D., Techniques for the production and characterization of monoclonal hybridoma antibodies, in *Monoclonal hybridoma antibodies. Techniques and applications,* Hurrell, G. R., Ed., CRC Press, Boca Raton, FL, 1982, chap. 1.
49. Brodsky, F. M., Bodmer, W. F. and Parham, P., Characterization of a monoclonal anti-beta$_2$-microglobulin antibody and its use in the genetic and biochemical analysis of major histocompatibility antigens, *Eur. J. Immunol., 9, 536, 1979.*
50. Micklem, L. R., McCann, M. C. and James, K., The use of rat mixed-thymocyte culture-conditioned medium for hybridoma production, cloning and revival, *J. Immunol. Meth., 104, 81, 1987.*

51. Reading, C. L., Theory and methods for immunization in culture and monoclonal antibody production, *J. Immunol. Meth., 53, 261, 1982.*

52. Sugasawara, R. J., Cahoon, B. E. and Karu, A. E., The influence of murine macrophage-conditioned medium on cloning efficiency, antibody synthesis, and growth rate of hybridomas, *J. Immunol. Meth., 79, 263, 1985.*

53. Brodeur, B. R., Tsang, P. and Larose, Y., Parameters affecting ascites tumour formation in mice and monoclonal antibody production, *J. Immunol. Meth., 71, 265, 1984.*

54. Hoogenraad, N., Helman, T. and Hoogenraad, J., The effect of pre-injection of mice with pristane on ascites tumour formation and monoclonal antibody production, *J. Immunol. Meth., 61, 317, 1983.*

55. Jones, S. L., Cox, J. C. and Pearson, J. E., Increased monoclonal antibody ascites production in mice primed with Freund's incomplete adjuvant, *J. Immunol. Meth., 129, 227, 1990.*

56. Witte, P. L. and Ber, R., Improved efficiency of hybridoma ascites production by intrasplenic inoculation in mice, *J. Natl. Cancer Inst., 70, 575, 1983.*

57. Truitt, K. E., Larrick, J. W., Raubitschek, A. A., Buck, D. W. and Jacobson, S. W., Production of human monoclonal antibody in mouse ascites, *Hybridoma, 3, 195, 1984.*

58. Yelton, D. E., Diamond, B. A., Kwan, S.-P. and Scharff, M. D., Fusion of mouse myeloma and spleen cells, *Curr. Top. Microbiol. Immunol., 81, 1, 1978.*

59. Kearney, J. F., Radbruch, A., Liesegang, B. and Rajewsky, K., A new mouse myeloma cell line that has lost immunoglobulin expression but permits the construction of antibody-secreting hybrid cell lines, *J. Immunol., 123, 1548, 1979.*

60. Cowan, N. J., Secher, D. S. and Milstein, C., Intracellular immunoglobulin chain synthesis in non-secreting variants of a mouse myeloma: Detection of inactive light-chain messenger RNA, *J. Mol. Biol., 90, 691, 1974.*

61. Köhler, G. and Milstein, C., Derivation of specific antibody-producing tissue culture and tumor lines by cell fusion, *Eur. J. Immunol., 6, 511, 1976.*

62. Köhler, G. and Shulman, M. J., Cellular and molecular restrictions of the lymphocyte fusion, *Curr. Top. Microbiol. Immunol., 81, 143, 1978.*

63. Taggart, R. T. and Samloff, I. M., Stable antibody-producing murine hybridomas, *Science, 21, 1228, 1983.*

64. Margulies, D. H., Kuehl, W. M. and Scharff, M. D., Somatic cell hybridization of mouse myeloma cells, *Cell, 8, 405, 1976.*

65. Clark, M. R. and Milstein, C., Expression of spleen cell immunoglobulin phenotype in hybrids with myeloma cell lines, *Somatic Cell Genet., 7, 657, 1981.*

66. Bazin, H., Production of rat monoclonal antibodies with the LOU rat nonsecreting IR983F myeloma cell line, in *Protides of the biological fluids*, Peeters, H., Ed., Pergamon Press, New York, 1982, 615.

67. Harboe, N.M.G. and Ingild, A., Immunization, isolation of immunoglobulins and antibody titre determination, *Scand. J. Immunol., 17, Suppl. 10, 245, 1983.*

68. Long, D.A., The influence of the thyroid gland upon immune responses of different species to bacterial infection, *CIBA Found. Colloq. Endocrinol., 10, 287, 1957.*

69. Hau, J., Westergaard, J.G., Svendsen, P., Bach, A., and Teisner, B., Comparison between pregnancy-associated murine protein-2 (PAMP-2) and pregnancy specific beta-1 glycoprotein (SP-1), *J. Reprod. Fertil., 60, 115, 1980.*

70. Hau, J., Westergaard, J.G., Svendsen, P., Bach, A., and Teisner, B., Comparison of pregnancy-associated murine protein-1 and human pregnancy zone protein, *J. Reprod. Immunol., 3, 341, 1981.*

71. Jensenius, J.C., Andersen, I., Hau, J., Crone, M. and Koch, C., Eggs: conveniently packaged antibodies, methods for purification of yolk IgG, *J. Immunol. Meth., 46, 63, 1981.*

72. Russell, W.M.S. and Burch, R.L., *The principles of humane experimental technique, UFAW Special Edition*, Universities Federation for Animal Welfare, Potters Bar, England, 1992.

73. Nishinaka, S., Suzuki, T., Matsuda, H. and Murata, M., A new cell line for the production of chicken monoclonal antibody by hybridoma technology, *J. Immunol. Meth., 139, 217, 1991.*

74. Poulsen, O.M. and Hau, J., Murine passive cutaneous anaphylaxis test (PCA) for the "all or none" determination of allergenicity of bovine whey proteins and peptides, *Clin. Allergy, 17, 75, 1987.*

75. Lindblad, E.B. and Sparck, J.V., Basic concepts in the application of immunological adjuvants, *Scand. J. Lab. Anim. Sci., 14, 1, 1987.*

76. Stewart-Tull, D.E.S., Mineral oil adjuvants, *Vaccine, 3, 152, 1985.*

77. Ramon, G., Procedes pour accroitre la production des antitoxines, *Ann. Inst. Pasteur, 40, 1926.*

78. Drescher, J., Grutzner, L. and Godgluck, G., Immunogenic activity of aqueous and aluminium oxide absorbed poliovirus vaccines in Macaca mulatta, *Int. Symp. on Adjuvants of Immunity,* Utrecht 1966; Symp. Series Immunobiol. Standard, 6, 157 (Karger, Basel/New York) 1967.

79. Freund, J. and McDermott, K., Sensitization to horse serum by means of adjuvants, *Proc. Soc. Exp. Biol. NY, 49, 548, 1942*

80. Stewart-Tull, D.E.S., The immunological activities of bacterial peptidoglycans, *Annu. Rev. Microbiol., 34, 311, 1980.*

81. Stewart-Tull, D.E.S., Immunopotentiating activity of peptidoglycan and surface polymers, in *Immunology of the Bacterial Cell Envelope*, Stewart-Tull, D.E.S. and Davies, M., Eds. John Wiley & Sons, New York, 1985.

82. Talmage, D.W. and Dixon, F.J., The influence of adjuvants on the elimination of soluble protein antigens and the associated antibody responses, *J. Infect. Dis., 93, 176, 1953.*

83. Freund, J. and Lipton, M.M., Experimental allergic encephalomyelitis after the excision of the injection site of antigen-adjuvant emulsion, *J. Immunol., 75, 454, 1955.*

84. Stark, J.M., Rate of antigen catabolism and immunogenicity of BGG in mice, *Immunology, 19, 457, 1970.*

85. Stewart, D.J., Clark, B.L., Peterson, J.E., Griffiths, D.A., Smith, E.F. and O'Donnell, I.J., Effect of pilus dose and type of Freund's adjuvant on the antibody and protective reponses of vaccinated sheep to Bacteroides nodusus, *Res. Vet. Sci., 35, 130, 1983.*

86. Kittell, C.L., Banks, R.E. and Hadick, C.L., Raised skin lesions in rabbits after immunization, *Lab. Anim., 1991.*

87. Schiefer, B. and Stunzi, H., Pulmonary lesions in guinea pigs and rats after subcutaneous injection of complete Freund's adjuvant or homologous pulmonary tissue, *Zbl. Vet. Med., 26, 1, 1979.*

88. Hau, J., The rabbit as antibody producer — advantages and disadvantages, in *Symposium uber Zucht, Haltung, und Ernhrung des Kaninchens.* Das Kaninchen als Modell in der Biomedizinischen Forschung, Altromin, Tierrztliche Fortbildung, Lage, Germany, 1988.

89. White, R.G., Adjuvant stimulation of antibody synthesis, in *Immunopathology, VIth Int. Symp.* Grindelwald, Switzerland P. Miescher, Ed., Schwabe and Co., Basel, 1970, 91.

90. Colpaert, F.C., Evidence that adjuvant arthritis in the rat is associated with chronic pain, *Pain, 28, 201, 1987.*

91. Oldham, G. and Coombs, R.R.A., Early rheumatoid like joint lesions in rabbits injected with foreign serum or milk proteins, *Int. Arch. Allergy Appl. Immunol. 61, 81, 1980.*

92. Chapel, H.M. and August, P.J., Report of nine cases of accidental injury to man with Freund's complete adjuvant, *Clin. Exp. Immunol., 24, 358, 1976.*

93. Anon, Freund's adjuvant, *Resource, 12, 1988.*

94. Ellouz, F., Adam, A., Ciorbaru, R. and Lederer, E., Minimal structural requirements for adjuvant activity of bacterial peptidoglycan derivatives. *Biochem. Biophys. Res. Commun., 59, 1317, 1974.*

95. Staruch, M.J. and Wood, D.D., Genetic influences on the adjuvanticity of muramyl dipeptide in vivo, *J. Immunol., 128, 155, 1982.*

96. Lipman, N.S., Trudel, L.J., Murphy, J.C. and Sahali, Y., Comparison of immune response potentiation and in vivo inflammatory effects of Freund's and RIBI adjuvants in mice, *Lab. Anim. Sci., 42, 193, 1992.*

97. Johnston, B.A., Eisen, H. and Fry, D., An evaluation of several adjuvant emulsions regimens for the production of polyclonal antisera in rabbits, *Lab. Anim. Sci., 41, 15, 1991.*

98. Dalsgaard, K., The saponin adjuvant Quil-A, *Vaccine, 3, 155, 1985.*

99. Ernst, T.M., Gillert, K.E. and Mueller, S., Influence of dextran polymer particles (Sephadex G-200) on humoral immune responses, *Int. Arch. Allergy Appl. Immunol., 62, 463, 1980.*

100. Preis, I. and Langer, R.S., A single-step immunization by sustained antigen release, *J. Immunol. Meth., 28, 193, 1979.*

101. Niemi, S.M., Fox, J.G., Brown, L.R. and Langer, R., Evaluation of ethylene-vinyl acetate copolymer as a non-inflammatory alternative to Freund's complete adjuvant in rabbits, *Lab. Anim. Sci., 35, 609, 1985.*

102. Cannat, A., Feingold, N., Caffin, J.C. and Serre, A., Studies on the genetic control of murine humoral response to immunization with a peptidoglycan-containing fraction extracted from Brucella melitensis, *Ann. Immunol. 130c, 675, 1979.*

103. Lifshitz, R., Schwartz, M. and Mozes, E., Specificity of genes controlling immune responsiveness to (T,G)-A-L and (Phe, G)-A-L, *Immunology, 41, 339, 1980.*

104. Young, C.R. and Atassi, M.Z., Genetic control of the immune response to myoglobin. IX. Overcoming genetic control of antibody response to antigenic sites by increasing the dose of antigen used in immunization, *J. Immunogenet., 9, 343, 1982.*

105. Borel, Y. and Stollar, B.D., Strain and sex dependence of carrier-determined immunologic tolerance to guanosine, *Eur. J. Immunol., 9, 166, 1979.*

106. Kaplan, P.J., Caperna, T.J. and Garvey, J.S., Bovine serum albumin humoral immune response in aged Fischer 344 rats, *Mech. Ageing Dev., 16, 61, 1981.*

107. Solyom, F., Makar, A., Fazekas, A., Roith, J. and Czelleng, F., Immunogenicity. Studies of foot and mouth disease vaccines at different concentrations of antigen and saponin, *Ann. Rech. Vet.,11, 35, 1980.*

108. Adam, A., Ciorbaru, R., Petit, J.-F. and Lederer, E., Isolation and properties of a macromolecular, water-soluble, immunoadjuvant fraction from the cell wall of Mycobacterium smegmatis, *Proc. Natl. Acad. Sci. U.S.A. 69, 851, 1972.*

109. Laursen, M.L. and Laursen, K., Dependence on antigen dose and timing in the immune responses of C3H mice to malignant ascites cells, *Immunology, 40, 403, 1980.*

110. Cozad, G.C., Al-Naib, S.M. and Murphy, J.W., Effects of cryptococcal capsular polysaccharide on the immune response, in *Proceedings of the second international specialized symposium on yeasts,* Tokyo 1972 (Ed. K. Iwata), 1976, 160.

111. Stewart, J.D., A comparison of intradermal and subcutaneous routes of administration of antigen in the rabbit. MSc dissertation, The Royal Veterinary College, London, 1990.

112. Horne, C.H.W., Herbert, W.J. and White, R.G., Evaluation of the method of direct injection of antigen into a joint cavity for the production of humoral and cell-mediated immunity in the guinea-pig, *Immunology, 18, 551, 1970.*

113. Horne, C.H.W. and White, R.G., Evaluation of the direct injection of antigen into a peripheral lymph node for the production of humoral and cell-mediated immunity in the guinea-pig, *Immunology, 15, 65, 1968.*

114. Bruyn, H.B., Meiklejohn, G. and Brainerd, H.D., Influenza vaccination: a comparison of antibody response obtained by various methods of administration, *J. Immunol., 62, 1, 1949.*

115. Hau, J., Retningslinier for immunisering af forsøgsdyr, *Dyreforsøgstilsynets (DK) årsberetning 1989, 66, 1990.*

Chapter 19

Laboratory Animal Anesthesia

Per Svendsen

CONTENTS

INTRODUCTION

Anesthesia in laboratory animals is essential for preventing pain during surgery. It is also important for the result of the operation and the experiment that the animal is under complete control and makes no sudden movements during the surgical procedure. Whenever possible, physiological experiments should be performed while the animal is under anesthesia. This, however, requires control of side effects that might interfere with the experiment and the interpretation of the results.

The animal experimenter is confronted with the problem of using anesthetics in different species and strains of animals in which the reaction to a given drug may differ considerably. The anesthetic that is efficient in one species may be harmful to another.

Full surgical anesthesia includes sedation with decreased perception of external stimuli, analgesia, suppression of reflex activity and skeletal muscle tone. This situation may be accomplished by depression of the central nervous system. Provided the depression is deep enough, the animal is rendered unconscious, relaxed and unresponsive to painful stimuli. However, this method will inevitably cause depression of respiratory, cardiovascular and other centers, and result in severe side effects or death.

Surgical anesthesia can often be accomplished by combining several different types of drugs, for instance by combining a sedative with a central or a local analgesic. This type of anesthesia is a balanced combination of sedation, analgesia, hypnosis and muscle relaxation. Depending on the animal species and the extent of the surgical intervention, different combinations are used.

Many drugs act synergistically on the central nervous system, and a combination of such drugs allows a reduction of the dose of each agent, thus decreasing the risk of a toxic reaction and minimizing side effects.

Different species of animals may vary in their response to anesthetic drugs due to metabolic differences. Small animals like mice, hamsters and rats have relatively high metabolic rates, and need relatively larger doses of anesthetics compared to larger species. More specific differences also exist between species in their qualitative response to certain drugs. Morphine generally has a depressive action in animals, but in cats morphine causes excitation and in mice convulsions, if given in the same dose as that of the dog. Similarly, ketamine hydrochloride is a potent sedative in primates, but a very poor one in rats and guinea pigs.

Within the same species of animal variations occur between stocks and inbred strains. These differences reflect differences in liver and plasma enzyme activity.

The effect of anesthetics differs between the sexes, e.g., female rats are more susceptible to drugs like pentobarbitone and *d*-tubocurarine than male rats. The action of anesthetics may also be related to the age of the animal. Usually young animals are more sensitive than older. This is either due to differences in enzyme activity or to varying amounts of body fat.

Repeated dosage of drugs like barbiturates or phenothiazines results in increased activity of the drug-degrading enzymes of the hepatocytes producing a significant reduction of the time of action of the drugs.

ADMINISTRATION OF ANESTHETICS

ADMINISTRATION BY INJECTION

The advantage of injectable anesthetics is the simplicity of the equipment — basically a syringe and a needle. The disadvantages are the slow onset of the drug action and the difficulty in controlling the level of anesthesia. Administration by intramuscular and intraperitoneal routes is relatively simple in most laboratory animal species. However, the rate of absorption and the anesthetic effect vary considerably. When choosing intramuscular or intraperitoneal administration, drugs with a wide safety margin should be preferred. Intravenous administration is technically more difficult, but it makes it possible to give the anesthetic so as to provide the desired depth of anesthesia.

Intravenous injections are best administered using a flexible indwelling catheter rather than a metal hypodermic needle. The most useful type consists of a flexible plastic catheter placed on the outside of a metal needle. The needle acts as an introducer for the plastic catheter. Different sizes are available to fit most laboratory animal species. During anesthesia the intravenous catheter should be connected to an infusion bottle with isotonic saline to secure continued intravenous access.

ADMINISTRATION BY INHALATION

The main advantages of inhalation anesthesia are that the depth of anesthesia can be altered rapidly and that the animal recovers rapidly. The main disadvantages are the necessity for sophisticated equipment and the risk of environmental pollution with anesthetic vapor, posing a health hazard to personnel.

The essential requirements of inhalation anesthesia are the supply of oxygen to the lung alveolar membrane, the removal of carbon dioxide from the lungs, and the supply of anesthetic gas at a controlled partial pressure to the alveolar membrane. The precondition for satisfying these three requirements is sufficient alveolar ventilation. Since most anesthetics depress the respiratory center and therefore cause a reduction in alveolar ventilation, artificial ventilation is necessary to achieve a stable condition with normal oxygenation and acid-base balance.

The alveolar concentration of the anesthetic is, however, governed by both alveolar ventilation and cardiac output. An increase in alveolar ventilation without an increase in cardiac output will result in a rise in alveolar concentration until a state of equilibrium with the tissues is reached.

The potency of different inhalation anesthetics is defined by their minimal alveolar concentration (MAC). The MAC is the alveolar concentration of the compound at a pressure of 1 atm which will prevent response to a specified stimulus in 50% of the animals. For every inhalation anesthetic studied, MAC has proven to be constant for different species of animals, but differs 10 to 20% between species. Hypoxia does not alter MAC, whereas hypotension causes a 20% reduction in halothane MAC in dogs. Release of central nervous system catecholamines increases MAC and thus the anesthetic requirement. Factors like age, body temperature and pregnancy all reduce MAC and anesthetic requirement. Sedatives and analgesics also reduce MAC, and surgical anesthesia is reached at a lower dose.[1]

Inhalation anesthesia should not be used unless the animal is intubated, so as to avoid the risk of polluting the environment with anesthetic gases. The practice of inducing anesthesia by inhalation via a face mask is not recommended as the animal will resist the treatment and become stressed.

The simplest anesthetic apparatus is Ayre's T-piece. It consists of a piece of corrugated tubing with a volume about one third of the tidal volume, a T-piece connected to the endotracheal tube and a supply of oxygen and anesthetic gas. The anesthetic mixture enters the T-piece at a flow rate of about twice the minute volume.

Magill's attachment consists of a non-return expiratory valve located close to the animal, corrugated tubing with a volume to ensure that exhaled gases do not return to the reservoir bag, and a reservoir bag with a capacity of at least 8 times the tidal volume of the animal, with the anesthetic gas supply flowing past the reservoir. The gas inflow should equal the animal's minute volume.

The to-and-fro system consists of a soda-lime CO_2 absorber with a pop-off valve and a closed rebreathing bag into which the anesthetic gas is introduced. The advantage of this system is a low flow of anesthetic gas.

These open or semi-open systems have the disadvantage of a relatively large waste of anesthetic gas, and a considerable risk to the personnel. In case of respiratory arrest it is difficult to assist ventilation.

The closed circle absorption system is the most widely used. The advantages are an efficient removal of CO_2 and the maintenance of inspired anesthetic concentrations. Assisted ventilation is possible by manual compression of the rebreathing bag.

Artificial ventilation is essential for maintaining normal pO_2, pCO_2, and acid-base balance of the blood. As a rule artificial ventilation should be used whenever physiological experiments are performed on anesthetized animals.

COMMONLY USED ANESTHETIC DRUGS

SEDATIVES

The most commonly used sedatives in laboratory animal anesthesia are the phenothiazine derivatives, the butyrophenones, and the benzodiazepines. These drugs all produce neurolepsis, which is a state of depressed awareness of the surroundings. In some species the sedatives will cause drowsiness, but the animals are easily aroused by sharp noises or handling. Used as a preanesthetic these drugs reduce the required amount of other anesthetics (anesthetic potentiation). In combination with analgesics some of the sedatives mentioned below will act as anesthetics (neuroleptanalgesia).

Phenothiazines

The following phenothiazines are used in veterinary anesthesia: acepromazine, chlorpromazine, promazine, propionylpromazine, methotrimeperazine, and promethazine. Most frequently used in laboratory animal anesthesia is acepromazine (Plegicil®).[2-8] Acepromazine produces optimal sedation at a certain dose, and the effect is not increased by increasing the dose.

The main side effect of acepromazine is to produce hypotension, mainly through peripheral alpha-sympathetic blockade. In healthy animals this effect is well tolerated, whereas hypovolemic and shocked animals may develop a fatal fall in arterial blood pressure following treatment with acepromazine. Intravenous injection of acepromazine may occasionally cause excitation in horses. Whether this may occur in laboratory animals is not known.

Apart from propionylpromazine (Combelene®),[9] used as a sedative in mini-pigs, the other phenothiazines mentioned are rarely used in laboratory animal anesthesia.

Butyrophenones

The butyrophenones used in laboratory animal anesthesia are azaperone, droperidol, and fluanisone. Azaperone (Sedaperone®, Suicalm®, Stressnil®) produces good sedation in pigs following intramuscular injection. If the pig is disturbed during the first 20 min following injection, excitation may occur. In laboratory animal anesthesia azaperone is used as a preanesthetic in pigs prior to or in combination with metomidate.[10-12]

Cardiovascular and respiratory effects of azeperone on pigs are minor provided the drug is administered by intramuscular injection. Following intravenous injection of azaperone the pig becomes excited, and a significant fall in systolic blood pressure occurs.[13] In man the butyrophenones may cause very unpleasant side effects including hallucinations, restlessness, mental agitation and aggression. It is not known whether this is also the case in animals.

Droperidol (Dehydrobenzperidol®) and fluanisone (Haloanisone®) are both potent neuroleptic agents with an action of 6 to 8 h. They are potent antiemetics and antagonize respiratory depression caused by opiates. They decrease peripheral resistance and markedly increase peripheral blood flow, eliciting a minor decrease in blood pressure.[14] Both compounds are used in combination with fentanyl to produce neuroleptanalgesia in pigs, dogs, rabbits, hamsters, and rats.[15-25]

Benzodiazepines

The benzodiazepines show sedative, hypnotic properties and muscle relaxing properties. Diazepam (Valium®, Aposepam®, Diazemuls®) is a potent sedative and muscle relaxant in most animal species. It potentiates the action of opiates, barbiturates, and halothane. The main site of the tranquilizing effect is the hippocampus, whereas the site of muscle relaxing is independent of sedation and found in the spinal cord. Diazepam is not commonly used in ordinary veterinary anesthesia, but has found important use as a muscle relaxant in laboratory animal anesthesia, especially in combination with neuroleptanalgesics.[20,22,26-29] Diazepam in combination with azaperone provides excelent sedation in pigs. The effect of the diazepam analogues midazolam and zolazepam have been tested in several laboratory animal species.[30]

Xylazine Hydrochloride

The alpha-2-agonist xylazine (Rompun®) is a potent sedative and hypnotic with central muscle relaxant and possibly analgesic properties. Xylazine causes a dose-dependent, progressive depression of the central nervous system. There is a great variation in sensitivity to the drug between different species of laboratory animals. Small ruminants are very susceptible, whereas pigs are resistant to xylazine. The action of other anesthetics is potentiated by xylazine. The compound is very useful for sedation of a number of laboratory animals.[29]

The side effects of xylazine include a dose-related depression of the respiratory center and the cardiovascular center.[31] The latter effect, however, is modified by complex effects on both the sympathetic and parasympathetic systems. The final result on blood pressure, heart rate, and cardiac output depends on the animal species, dose, and route of administration. As xylazine causes contractions of the pregnant uterus, the compound should not be used late in pregnancy. Dogs and cats frequently vomit following injection of xylazine.

ANALGESICS

Opiates are the most effective analgesics. They are used to produce balanced anesthesia, neuroleptanalgesia and relief of postoperative pain. Opiate analgetics may stimulate or depress the central nervous system depending on the dose given and the animal species treated. Depression of the central nervous system includes analgesia, respiratory depression, and sedation, whereas stimulation causes excitement and vomiting. In general a low dose will cause depression and a high dose excitement. Cats are more sensitive than other species of commonly used laboratory animals. The opiate analgetics act via the opiate receptors in the brain and the spinal cord. Certain agents like naloxone and diprenorphine will antagonize the effect of opiate analgesics and reverse their action.

Fentanyl Citrate

Fentanyl is a potent analgesic. It is rapidly absorbed after intramuscular injection, and analgesia and depression develop after a few minutes. Intravenous injection produces bradycardia and respiratory arrest and should not be attempted. Atropine sulfate should always be administered to prevent vagal inhibition of the heart. Respiratory depression can be rapidly reversed by administration of the antagonist naloxone.

Fentanyl is commonly administered with a sedative to produce a state of neuroleptanalgesia.

Etorphine Hydrochloride

Etorphine is an extremely potent analgesic used extensively to immobilize wild animals. The preparation Immobilon® is a combination of acepromazine and etorphine commonly used to produce neuroleptanalgesia in dogs in veterinary practice. It has been tested in laboratory rats, but rejected due to severe depression of respiration.[24] The effect is reversed by the specific antagonist diprenorphine (Revivon®).

Etorphine is extremely toxic to humans and should not be used by inexperienced laboratory personnel. The antagonist diprenorphine should always be available and administered intravenously in case of accidental self-injection.

Buprenorphine

Buprenorphine (Temgesic®) is a partial agonist with very potent analgesic properties. Buprenorphine is effective for 8 to 10 h after administration, and is therefore the agent of choice in post-operative pain treatment, whereas it is not used as an anesthetic.

HYPNOTICS

The most commonly used hypnotics are barbiturates, propanidid, saffan, metomidate and alpha-chloralose. Short-acting hypnotics are useful for induction of anesthesia which is to be continued by an inhalation method. The hypnotic compounds have little or no analgesic properties, and should only be used in combination with analgesic drugs.

Thiopental Sodium

Thiopental (Pentothal®) is the most common induction compound used in dogs, ruminants, and pigs.[32-35] Thiopental is a dry substance to be dissolved immediately before use to form a 2.5% solution. It must be administered strictly intravenously due to the alkaline pH. The action of thiopental depends on the amount injected, the speed of injection, the rate of distribution of the drug in the non-fatty tissues, and the rate of uptake in fatty tissues. Thiopental appears to cross the blood-brain barrier very rapidly, and therefore a small amount injected rapidly will produce a high concentration in the brain and an almost immediate state of deep narcosis. The drug will, however, soon be distributed in the non-fatty tissues of the body, resulting in a rapid decrease in the depth of narcosis. If, on the other hand, a larger dose is given by slow intravenous injection, the drug is distributed throughout the body tissues, and the plasma concentration will be maintained for a longer period. The recovery period then depends on the rate at which thiopental is taken up by the fatty tissues, since the concentration in the non-fatty tissues is already high at the end of the injection. It is common practice to give half the calculated dose by rapid intravenous injection, and the remaining half in small increments over 1 to 2 min until full effect.

Induction of anesthesia with thiopental is followed by a period of apnea caused by central nervous depression after the initial high plasma concentration. The sensitivity of the respiratory center is reduced and ventilation diminished resulting in respiratory acidosis. Following rapid injection of thiopental there is a fall in arterial blood pressure, which subsequently returns to near normal levels. There is an increase in laryngeal and bronchial reflexes under light thiopental narcosis, and tracheal intubation should not be attempted until the thiopental narcosis is sufficiently deep.

Thiamylal

Thiamylal (Surital®) resembles thiopental in chemical structure and anesthetic action. It has found some use in dogs as an inducer of inhalation anesthesia.[35]

Inactin

Inactin is chemically related to thiopental, but less potent. It has found only limited use in anesthesia of laboratory animals.[36] In hamsters a significant rise in the blood sugar concentration occurs under inactin narcosis.[37]

Propanidid

Propanidid (Sombrevin®) is a eugenol, chemically related to oil of cloves. Following rapid intravenous injection there is a brief period of hyperventilation and loss of consciousness. The drug is used almost only for short-acting anesthesia of nude mice used for tumor transplantation. Following intraperitoneal injection the mouse is unconscious for 2 to 3 min. Recovery is very fast, and the animal is alert after another 2 to 3 min. The advantage of this method is that the nude mouse does not develop hypothermia during anesthesia.

Alphaxolone-Alphadolone

The steroid compound alphaxolone in combination with alphadolone (Saffan®, Althesin®) is a useful short-acting narcotic in cats. It should be given by rapid intravenous injection to prevent vomiting. The drug has been tested in rats and guinea pigs, but found unsuitable due to respiratory and cardiovascular depression.[16,38] Alphaxolone-alphadolone may cause edema of the ears and paws.

Metomidate Hydrochloride

Metomidate hydrochloride (Hypnodil® vet) is an imidazole derivative with strong hypnotic and muscle relaxant activity but weak analgesic properties. The solution should be prepared shortly before use and administered either intravenously or intraperitoneally. Metomidate is a very useful compound for induction of anesthesia in pigs. The peak effect of metomidate lasts for about 25 min.

The injection of metomidate is followed by slight hypertension and decreased heart rate. Respiration and blood gas tensions are maintained at a near normal level.[33]

Pentobarbital Sodium

Pentobarbital sodium (Mebumal®, Nembutal®) is a long-acting barbiturate. Despite several disadvantages it is still used extensively in laboratory animal anesthesia. It has only weak analgesic properties and a relatively large dose must be given to secure surgical anesthesia. Following intravenous injection the drug crosses the blood-brain barrier slowly, and the injection rate must therefore be slow, too, if the effect is to be assessed while the drug is being administered. Intraperitoneal injection can be used in rats and mice, but there is a risk of overdosing. In dogs pentobarbital is a useful compound in combination with a sedative and an analgesic. Recovery from pentobarbital anesthesia is always slow, especially in dogs, pigs, and cats.

The most important side effect is depression of the respiratory center and a fall in blood pressure due to peripheral vasodilatation.[24]

Alpha-Chloralose

Alpha-chloralose is a white, crystalline chemical. A 1 to 2% solution is prepared by dissolving the compound in warm water (40°C) immediately before use. Alpha-chloralose is a hypnotic and muscle relaxant without any analgesic properties.[39] It has proved to be very valuable in physiological experiments where stable cardiovascular parameters are essential.[16,40]

Urethane

Urethane is the ethyl ester of carbaminic acid. Like alpha-chloralose it produces light hypnosis and muscular relaxation without analgesia. The compound is used in combination with alpha-chloralose to suppress muscular activity.[16,36,41,42] However, the compound is carcinogenic, and may present a health risk to laboratory workers.

DISSOCIATIVE ANESTHETICS
Ketamine Hydrochloride

The cyclohexamine derivative ketamine hydrochloride (Ketalar® vet, Vetalar®) produces a state of dissociative anesthesia in which complete analgesia is combined with superficial hypnosis. This state is associated with a functional dissociation between the thalamoneocortical and limbic systems, with depression of the former before there is any effect on the latter. The animal will show hypertonus, muscle movements and laryngeal reflexes, and its eyes will remain open.[43] In man ketamine is known to produce hallucinations during recovery. Whether this is the case in animals is unknown, but the animal should be allowed to recover in a quiet environment. In veterinary practice the drug is used in combination with xylazine for anesthesia of cats.[44,45] For experimental purposes ketamine has been used either alone, or in combination with other drugs, in several species.[29]

Ketamine causes a mild respiratory depression with an increased respiratory rate and reduced tidal volume, and a fall in arterial blood pressure and heart rate.[24] Repeated injections of ketamine causes no change in the blood chemistry of primates.[46]

VOLATILE INHALATION ANESTHETICS
Halothane

Halothane (Fluothane®) is a fluorinated hydrocarbon. It is a clear, colorless, non-irritating liquid. The MAC is 0.91 for pigs and 1.01 for guinea pigs,[47,48] making it a very potent anesthetic agent. In combination with nitrous oxide the MAC is reduced by 65%. In properly sedated animals anesthesia can be induced with halothane concentrations of 2 to 4%, and anesthesia is maintained by inhalation of 1 to 2% halothane vapor. Recovery is usually completed in 10 to 20 min.

Halothane causes depression of the respiratory center, leading to decrease in the tidal volume and respiratory acidosis. Administration of halothane provokes an immediate fall in arterial blood pressure and heart rate caused by a direct depressant effect on the myocardium and a central depressant effect on the vasomotor center. Halothane increases the sensitivity of the myocardium to adrenaline, causing ventricular fibrillation.

Halothane is metabolized by the liver, and there is a marked microsomal liver enzyme induction following halothane anesthesia. Recovery from halothane anesthesia is accompanied by shivering, and animals must be kept warm and well oxygenated during this phase.

In susceptible pigs halothane can induce malignant hyperthermia.[49-52]

Halothane is an excellent anesthetic for animals used for experimental surgery. It should, however, always be administered using a calibrated halothane vaporizer to prevent dangerously high concentrations. Halothane should never be used with an open system due to the health hazard for the laboratory staff.

Enflurane

Enflurane is a fluorinated ether with physical properties similar to halothane. The MAC for guinea pigs is 2.17.[47] Administration of 3 to 5% enflurane will induce anesthesia in all species of laboratory animals, and depending on the sedatives given, anesthesia can be maintained with inspired concentrations of 1 to 3%. In pigs enflurane anesthesia leads to a moderate fall in blood pressure and respiratory rate. In dogs no cardiovascular effect is observed, but respiratory depression and acidosis occur.[35,53]

Very little enflurane is metabolized by the liver, and the drug is largely eliminated via the lungs. In models requiring minimal liver enzyme induction, there seems to be an advantage in using enflurane rather than halothane.

Isoflurane

Isoflurane is chemically related to enflurane. The MAC for pigs is 1.57, for guinea pigs 1.15, and for rats varying between 1.20 and 1.57 depending on the strain.[47,54,55] Administered together with nitrous oxide MAC is reduced up to 42% in pigs.[54] Respiratory depression is slightly more severe than with halothane, but there is less cardiovascular depression.[56]

Isoflurane is less metabolized than enflurane by the liver. This may be an advantage in studies on drug metabolism and toxicity.

Methoxyflurane

Methoxyflurane is a halogenated ethyl methyl ether. The MAC for most laboratory species is 0.22. Respiratory and cardiovascular depression is less than with halothane. Methoxyflurane has a strong affinity for the body fat depots, and the compound persists in the blood for up to 24 h after apparent recovery from anesthesia. Metabolism of methoxyflurane causes the release of fluorine in the urine of humans, which may cause renal damage. Methoxyflurane has very potent analgetic properties after a slow rate of induction. The compound is therefore best used after induction with a short-acting injectable agent or in combination with halothane. Induction of methoxyflurane anesthesia in small laboratory animals in an inhalation chamber[57-59] is slow, and appears stressful to the animals. The use of open masks[6,60-63] should be avoided due to the health hazard for laboratory staff. Instead the animals should be intubated.

Diethyl Ether

Diethyl ether is a colorless volatile fluid. The inflammable and explosive vapor is 2.6 times heavier than air, and is therefore likely to accumulate close to the floor. Diethyl ether irritates the respiratory tract, and may produce laryngospasm, coughing and apnea during induction of anesthesia. The MAC value is between 2 and 3 in different species. Cardiovascular functions are well maintained under diethyl ether anesthesia due to a balance between the direct myocardial depressant effect and the effect of reflexly released adrenaline and noradrenaline. During diethyl ether anesthesia the spleen contracts and the intestines dilate. The blood sugar concentration rises as a result of the increase in adrenaline release. Bile secretion from the liver and kidney function are also depressed, and remain so for up to 24 h after recovery.

Although diethyl ether is a safe anesthetic it has so many disadvantages that it is not recommended for use in laboratory animals.

Nitrous Oxide

Nitrous oxide is a colorless gas that liquefies when compressed at 40 atm. The MAC for nitrous oxide is between 200 and 255 in dogs, cats, and monkeys, and the anesthetic effect is less than that reported for man.[64] Nitrous oxide will, however, reduce the MAC for halothane, methoxyflurane, isoflurane, and the dose of pentobarbital in pigs, rabbits, and guinea pigs.[54,57,65-68]

Nitrous oxide has little effect on the respiratory and cardiovascular systems, and no adverse effects are reported on hepatic or renal function.

Nitrous oxide is very useful in combination with other anesthetics. It should be used in a mixture with oxygen not exceeding 50%.

MUSCLE RELAXANTS

Varying degrees of muscle relaxation can be achieved according to the drug(s) chosen and in some cases the dose needed may produce deep generalized depression of the central nervous system. The consequence is depression of the respiratory and vasomotor centers, resulting in hypoxia, hypercapnia, respiratory acidosis, and hypotension. The respiratory side effects can be counteracted by artificial ventilation, whereas the cardiovascular depression persists.

Relaxation can also be produced by drugs that have a local effect at the neuromuscular junction. These drugs have little effect on the central nervous system. The neuromuscular junction can either be blocked by agents that compete with the neurotransmitter acetylcholine for the end plate receptors and occupy them without producing depolarization, or by agents that cause persistent depolarization of the end plate membrane and thus prevent the passage of excitation from the motor nerve to the muscle fiber.

Muscle relaxants can be used in laboratory animal anesthesia to facilitate artificial respiration and relax skeletal muscles during surgery. Endotracheal intubation is also facilitated, but intubation is usually easily performed without relaxation.

It should be emphasized that muscle relaxants must never be administered unless facilities for intubation and artificial ventilation are present. It must also be recognized that muscle relaxants are neither anesthetics nor are they analgesics, and an animal should never be given a muscle relaxant unless it is already under full surgical anesthesia. These drugs should never be used unless the animal is under constant surveillance, including continuous monitoring of heart rate and blood pressure to ensure that painful procedures are not carried out without sufficient analgesia.

Gallamine Triethiodide

Gallamine triethiodide (Flaxedil®) is a non-depolarizing compound. Following intravenous injection in dogs and pigs the heart rate increases by 10 to 20% and there is a rise in blood pressure. In dogs an intravenous dose of 1 mg/kg causes complete muscle relaxation within 2 min. In pigs the necessary dose is 4 mg/kg. The effect lasts for 20 to 40 min after intravenous injection.

The action of gallamine triethiodide can be reversed by neostigmine, which prevents the breakdown of acetylcholine in the synaptic cleft, thus allowing acetylcholine to displace gallamine from the end plate receptors.

Pancuronium Bromide

Pancuronium bromide (Pavulon®) has a non-polarizing activity similar to that of gallamine. After intravenous injection of 0.05 to 0.15 mg/kg it produces complete relaxation for 40 to 80 min.[32,69] Malignant hyperthermia has been reported in pigs following administration of pancuronium bromide.

Suxamethonium Bromide

Suxamethonium produces depolarization of the end plate and prevents passage of the action potential. It produces relaxation of striated muscle 10-15 seconds after intravenous injection, and the effect lasts for about 5 min. Repeated injections may cause hypotension and bradycardia if the animal has not previously been treated with atropine sulfate. Muscular relaxation is followed by muscle fasciculations, which in humans are known to be extremely painful.

Administration of suxamethonium is indicated to facilitate endotracheal intubation.

ANTICHOLINERGICS

Anticholinergic agents are not anesthetics as such. Their main action is to antagonize the effects of acetylcholine and thus block transmission at parasympathetic postsynaptic nerve endings.

Atropine Sulfate

Atropine sulfate is the anticholinergic drug most commonly used in laboratory animal anesthesia. Following intramuscular or subcutaneous injection, salivation and bronchial secretion are reduced and bronchial muscles are relaxed. In ruminants atropine causes a change in the viscosity of the saliva resulting in a more viscid saliva. In the cardiovascular system the main action of atropine is to increase the heart rate. Arterial blood pressure is unchanged after atropine administration except if already depressed by vagal stimulation, when it will increase. Atropine sulfate is metabolized differently in different species of laboratory animals and the dose therefore varies.

LOCAL ANALGESICS
Lidocaine Hydrochloride

Local analgesic procedures are frequently used in veterinary practice, whereas they have found little application in laboratory animal anesthesia. Lidocaine hydrochloride is well absorbed through mucous membranes, and spraying of the pharynx and larynx regions may facilitate endotracheal intubation.[70] Local analgesic creams may also be useful to prevent minor pain and discomfort in connection with venal puncture in dogs, cats, and rabbits.[71] Infiltration of lidocaine is useful for suturing minor wounds or for taking muscle biopsies.

Regional analgesia is performed by injecting the analgesic compound around the nerve trunk. The advantages of this method are that the surgical field itself is left undisturbed and that relatively small volumes of the drug are needed to secure a good analgesia. The analgesic solution must, however, be brought into the closest possible contact with the nerve, and special care must be taken to ensure that there is no sheath of fascia between the nerve and the solution.

Epidural analgesia is performed by injecting the analgesic extradurally, thereby desensitizing the nerve roots as they emerge from the spinal cord. The injection is given in the lumbo-sacral foramen, and the extension of the anesthesia can be varied by the volume injected. This technique is rarely used in laboratory animals.

MONITORING THE ANESTHETIZED ANIMAL

A careful clinical assessment of the anesthetized animal is essential to the welfare of the animal and the outcome of the experiment. As the experimenter can seldom rely on having professional assistance from an anesthetist, it is important to make a habit of continuously assessing the clinical condition of the animal. Most important are the rate and pattern of respiration, the color of visible mucous membranes, the pulsation of visible arteries, and the vascular tone of organs in the surgical field.

Extensive surgery, especially when muscle relaxants are administered to the animals, requires more objective recordings of the clinical state. Cardiovascular function is best monitored by electrocardiography and direct measurement of the arterial blood pressure. The electrocardiogram gives information about the electrical events in the heart, the heart rate and rhythm, but no information about the cardiac output. The leads can be placed on the sternum after careful shaving and cleaning of the skin. The most useful information derived from the electrocardiogram is the rate and rhythm of the heart. If anesthesia is insufficient and the animal can recognize pain, heart rate may increase before the animal reacts or wakes up.

The arterial blood pressure is best recorded by direct measurement in a suitable artery. In the rabbit percutaneous cannulation of the central aureal artery is easily performed using an indwelling catheter. In the dog percutaneous cannulation is also possible using the saphenous artery. In pigs and sheep a transverse incision is made on the medial surface of the femur and the gracilis and sartorius muscles are separated to locate the femoral artery. Cannulation is best performed using the "Seldinger technique" where a guide wire replaces the introduced needle. The catheter is threaded over the guide wire into the artery. Arterial pressure is the product of cardiac output and peripheral resistance. Cardiac output is the product of heart rate and stroke volume. The only measurable parameters are the heart rate and the arterial pressure. A low arterial blood pressure may be related to either peripheral dilatation or reduced cardiac output. It is thus not possible to predict anything about the essential parameter, i.e., the cardiac output. Arterial blood pressure is primarily important to ensure the correct anesthetic level. Most anesthetics cause depression of the cardiovascular center, and arterial blood pressure is related to the depth of anesthesia.

The central venous pressure is measured in the cranial vena cava via a catheter introduced into the jugular vein. A high central venous pressure indicates reduced cardiac output or fluid overload, and a low central venous pressure reflects reduced blood volume or high cardiac output.

The respiratory function is usually evaluated by counting the respiratory frequency and observing the characteristics of the breathing pattern. This gives no indication of the level of oxygenation in the tissues or the removal of carbon dioxide from the lungs. It is necessary to measure arterial pO_2, pCO_2, and acid-base balance to ensure correct respiration during anesthesia. If the animal is maintained on artificial respiration, the minute volume can be regulated to compensate for irregularities. If the animal breathes spontaneously, respiratory acidosis and hypoxia indicate too deep an anesthesia, and administration of anesthetic should be reduced.

General anesthesia interferes with the animal's ability to control body temperature, and evaporative heat loss from the surgical field leads to a fall in body temperature. A fatal rise in body temperature may occur in pigs during halothane anesthesia due to malignant hyperthermia. Body temperature should therefore always be monitored during anesthesia, and the external temperature regulated to ensure that the body temperature of the animal is kept near the normal level. Thermostat-regulated heating pads are available for small rodents. Electrical heating pads should not be used since they may cause heat stroke in small animals and severe burns in large animals. A heating pad based on circulating hot water is preferable.

PREANESTHETIC TREATMENT

CLINICAL ASSESSMENT

Most laboratory animals are healthy and in good condition before an experiment involving anesthesia is carried out, and extensive clinical examination is usually not necessary. However, it is advisable to examine the respiratory system for abnormal respiratory sounds and increased secretion, and the digestive system for signs of diarrhea. The animal should also be examined for signs of dehydration (reduced elasticity of the skin).

FEEDING PRIOR TO ANESTHESIA

Dogs, cats, pigs, and monkeys should not be fed 12 h before undergoing anesthesia to prevent vomiting. Sheep and goats are ruminants and will develop ruminal tympany (bloat) if they are anesthetized and placed in dorsal or lateral recumbency, due to accumulation of fermentation gases in the rumen. These animals should therefore not be fed for at least 24 h prior to anesthesia. Ewes late in pregnancy should not, however, be deprived of feed too long, as this may provoke ketosis. Rabbits and small rodents do not vomit and can be fed without restriction. Drinking water should always be available at all times before anesthesia to prevent dehydration during surgery.

SEDATION OF THE ANIMAL

Sedation of the animal prior to induction of anesthesia is important for several reasons. Sedatives reduce fear and the animal can be handled without the use of force. This reduces the output of catecholamines and thus the anesthetic dose. Most sedatives act synergistically with the hypnotic and analgesic agents, resulting in a reduction of the amounts of these drugs.

The sedative should be administered in surroundings known to the animal and by a person it has confidence in. The animal can be given an anticholinergic agent together with the sedative to reduce salivation and stimulate heart action. After administration the animal should be left alone in quiet surroundings for sufficient time for the drugs to take action. It is important not to disturb the animal during this phase as it may become excited.

ANESTHETIC MANAGEMENT

INDUCTION OF ANESTHESIA

When the sedatives have taken full action, the animal should be gently brought to a separate preparation room where anesthesia is induced and the animal prepared for surgery. It is important not to use the

322

operation room or laboratory for this purpose, as the animal may be unnecessarily disturbed by the activity that is commonly seen there.

In the preparation room the first procedure is to insert a venous catheter. It is important to use a flexible catheter to prevent accidental damage to the vein if the animal makes a sudden move. In dogs, cats, and small ruminants the cephalic vein is used, in pigs and rabbits intravenous injection is given in the aureal vein. The catheter is secured with adhesive tape. Before injecting, the correct placement of the catheter should be checked to prevent perivascular injection. Several intravenous preparations are alkaline and may cause pain and tissue damage if not injected correctly into the blood stream.

Once the animal has been brought into reflexless anesthesia, the trachea is intubated to secure a free airway. Artificial ventilation is now possible. Endotracheal intubation is easily performed in large animals like dogs, pigs, and sheep. The animal should be anesthetized to the level where the mouth can be opened without resistance. The animal is best placed in lateral recumbency on its left side. The assistant stands facing the back of the animal, holding the upper jaw with his left hand and the lower jaw and tongue with his right hand. The tongue is pulled forward and the neck extended. The tip of the epiglottis is usually positioned behind the soft palate. The anesthetist places a laryngoscope with a straight blade approximately 20 cm long at the base of the tongue. The endotracheal tube is used to depress the epiglottis forward onto the base of the tongue, and the tip of the laryngoscope blade is placed on the epiglottis to bring the arytenoid cartilages into view. The tube is now advanced into the trachea, the cuff insufflated, and the tube fixed to the upper jaw with adhesive tape.[10,70,72,73]

Small animals like rabbits, guinea pigs, and rats are more difficult to intubate due to the limited size of the mouth. The rabbit can be intubated using a neonatal laryngoscope blade (Miller # 0–2). The animal is placed in dorsal recumbency with the neck extended to keep the mouth, larynx, and trachea in linear alignment. The mouth of the rabbit is long (3.5 to 5 cm along the cephalo-caudal axis). The epiglottis is large, U-shaped, soft and flexible. The vocal cords are extremely anterior and run in dorso-ventral direction at an angle. A tube with a diameter of no more than 3.5 mm is used. The laryngoscope blade is placed to the left of the upper incisors and parallel to the floor of the mouth. The tongue is maintained in the midline, and the laryngoscope is moved to permit a view of the larynx. Insertion of the tube is performed during inspiration when the vocal cords are open.[74,75] A somewhat similar technique is described for guinea pigs.[76] Rats are intubated in dorsal recumbency with the nose extended slightly over the edge of the table. The upper jaw is pulled below the table with an elastic band behind the incisors. Using a fiberscope or head-mounted mirror, the epiglottis can be viewed. Intubation is performed with a flexible 16-gauge intravenous polyethylene catheter.[77,78]

Respiration can be supported if necessary once the animal is intubated. The animal is now ready for preparation for surgery, including clipping of the hair coat, washing of the skin, and disinfection. When the preparation is complete, the animal is brought to the operation room where intravenous infusion of isotonic saline is established and the anesthetic equipment, including surveillance equipment, is connected.

ANESTHETIC MAINTENANCE

Anesthesia with injectable agents is maintained by repeated doses whenever the animal reacts to painful stimuli. Anesthesia with short-acting compounds can be maintained by continuous intravenous infusion at a rate equal to the metabolism of the compound.[79]

The use of volatile anesthetics requires a supply of oxygen and a vaporizer that is capable of delivering the anesthetic at the correct concentration. Since all anesthetic agents depress the respiratory center, it is essential to prevent acid-base disturbances by assisting respiration. This can be done manually by compression of the reservoir bag or by means of a mechanical ventilator.

The depth of anesthesia should be determined by the respiratory pattern and the presence and absence of reflexes. The respiratory movements are composed of an elevation of the costae and a contraction of the diaphragm. As anesthesia deepens, the intercostal muscles are paralyzed first, followed by the diaphragm. The anesthetist should therefore follow the respiratory pattern as anesthesia develops. If the respiration becomes abdominal, the anesthetic stage has become too deep, and respiratory arrest will soon follow if futher anesthetic agent is administered. The most important reflexes are the pedal reflex, the corneal reflex, and the palpebral reflex. The pedal reflex is tested by applying a pinch to the interdigital skin of the hind leg. If the reflex is present the animal will withdraw its leg. The corneal reflex is tested by a slight touch of the cornea with a small piece of moistened cotton wool or tissue paper, and the palpebral reflex by a slight touch of the eye lid. If the reflexes are present the animal will blink.

As anesthesia progresses the animal passes through the different anesthetic stages. Shortly after the anesthetic agent is given the animal becomes excited, it then passes a transitory normal stage before entering a stage of general depression resulting in surgical anesthesia. As the animal wakes up again it will pass the same stages in opposite order. It is important to note that the animal will also pass through an excitatory phase before it has completely recovered. This stage is particularly dangerous in ruminants, as the animal may regurgitate and aspirate rumen contents causing aspiration pneumonia or even suffocation. The anesthetic stages will vary according to species and the anesthetic agent used. As the animal reaches the stage of surgical anesthesia, reflexes can no longer be observed and there is no response to a skin incision.

ANESTHETIC EMERGENCIES
Respiratory failure

Respiratory failure due to insufficient ventilation is a result of depression of the respiratory center by an anesthetic overdose or by hypoxia, or it is caused by obstruction of the respiratory tract by bronchial secretions, blood, or vomit. In ruminants ventilation can be suppressed by ruminal tympany (bloat) due to inability to eructate ruminal fermentation gases during anesthesia. Paralysis of the respiratory muscles following administration of muscle relaxants can also cause insufficient ventilation if artificial respiration is inadequate.

Treatment of respiratory failure includes a halt to further administration of anesthetics, suction of the respiratory tract, supply of pure oxygen, and artificial respiration. If the animal is intubated, artificial respiration is achieved by squeezing the rebreathing bag. If the animal is not fitted with an endotracheal tube, pressing on the sternum rhythmically can help movement of gas to and from the lungs. If possible an anesthetic antagonist should be given. Insufficient gas exchange across the alveolar membrane is most commonly caused by pulmonary edema and alveolar collapse. The treatment consists in increasing cardiac output and changing the position of the animal on the operation table.

Cardiovascular Failure

Cardiovascular failure leads to insufficient tissue perfusion and cellular hypoxia. There are two major factors leading to cardiovascular failure during anesthesia of laboratory animals: hemorrhage and depression of cardiac function. If the condition is not corrected a vicious circle is initiated in which tissue hypoxia leads to increased lactic acid formation in the tissues, increased capillary permeability, edema formation, and fatal acidosis. The symptoms of cardiovascular failure are paleness of skin and mucous membranes due to vasoconstriction. The pulse becomes weak and rapid, and the arterial blood pressure drops. The heart rate is initially elevated in an attempt to compensate for the low cardiac output. As hypoxia develops the myocardium is depressed and bradycardia develops. Respiration becomes rapid and superficial.

Cardiovascular failure is treated by removing the anesthetic agent if the primary cause is cardiac depression, or controlling the hemorrhage if fluid loss is the cause. Artificial ventilation with pure oxygen should be established in order to secure sufficient oxygenation. The circulating blood volume should be expanded by intravenous infusion of isotonic saline or Ringer's solution. If the condition does not improve and the central venous pressure remains high, cardiac failure is likely to be the cause. Continuous infusion of isoprenaline (1:5000 5% dextrose) at a rate of 1 ml/min for 10 min stimulates heart rate and cardiac output. Vasopressor agents will effectively increase blood pressure but at the expense of increased cardiac work and oxygen consumption.

Malignant hyperthermia

Malignant hyperthermia, a well-known condition in humans, was first described in 1969 in pigs subjected to anesthesia with halothane, nitrous oxide, and oxygen.[49,52] The clinical symptoms develop with dramatic speed within minutes after exposure to halothane. Tachycardia, stiffness of the muscles, tachypnea, and hyperventilation which rapidly progresses to apnea, cyanosis of the skin, and a rapid rise in body temperature to as much as 45°C are seen. The condition is hereditary. When exposed to halothane, blood lactate concentration increases first. Whole body oxygen consumption increases two- to threefold followed by respiratory and metabolic acidosis and marked hyperkalemia. Increases in catecholamines and temperature occur secondarily accompanied by progressive cardiovascular failure.[50] Malignant hyperthermia is identical to the disease known as the porcine stress syndrome, which occurs when pigs are exposed to severe stress during transport.[51,80]

Malignant hyperthermia can be prevented by intravenous injection of dantrolene (3.5 to 5.0 mg/kg) prior to the administration of halothane.[32,81-83] If the condition has developed, intravenous injection of 7.5 mg/kg dantrolene has shown good curative effect.[50,82,84]

Fluid and Electrolyte Disturbances

Changes in fluid and electrolyte balance are the result of hemorrhage and evaporation from exposed inner surfaces during surgery, and fever, diarrhea, or vomiting during recovery from anesthesia. Dehydration, expressed as a percentage of body weight, can be diagnosed clinically by examining skin elasticity. At approximately 5% dehydration, increased skin turgor with a doughy, inelastic consistency is noted. At 7% dehydration, definite changes in skin consistency are present. At 10% dehydration the animal is depressed, has sunken eyes, and dry skin and mucous membranes. The animal may move around or rest in sternal recumbency. When dehydration has reached 15% the animal is moribund, it often lies on its side and has a lowered body temperature. The water needs can roughly be calculated as a percentage of the body weight:

$$body\ weight\ (kg)\ x\ dehydration\ (\%) = replacement\ (l)$$

As an example, a 3.5-kg rabbit with an estimated 5% dehydration will need: $3.5 \times 5/100 = 0.175$ l of fluid.

A more precise estimation of dehydration is obtained by measuring the hematocrit value. Table 1 shows the relationship between hematocrit value and extracellular fluid volume.

The sodium balance is estimated from the serum sodium concentration and the hematocrit. Sodium is the major cation in the extracellular fluid, which is approximately 20% of the body weight. As the normal sodium concentration is 143 mEq/l, the deficit can be calculated as follows:

$$Na^+\ deficit = 20\%\ x\ body\ weight\ x\ (normal\ Na^+ - actual\ Na^+)$$

This equation, however, is only valid when the animal is in fluid balance. As both sodium balance and water balance are frequently disturbed at the same time, the sodium deficit is calculated using the following equation:

$$Na^+\ deficit = extracellular\ fluid\ x\ (normal\ Na^+ - actual\ Na^+)$$

As an example: a dog weighing 12 kg with a hematocrit value of 54% and a serum Na^+ of 123 mEq/l. The fluid deficit is 60 ml/kg or a total of 720 ml. The sodium deficit is $143-123 = 20$ mEq/l of extracellular fluid. The extracellular fluid volume at a hematocrit of 54% is 140 ml/kg or a total of 1680 ml. The dog thus has a deficit of $1.680 \times 20 = 32.4$ mEq Na^+ and 720 ml H_2O. Isotonic saline contains 154 mEq Na^+/l. The sodium deficit is thus replaced by intravenous infusion of 210 ml isotonic saline. The remaining water deficit of 510 ml is replaced by infusion of isotonic glucose.

The hydrogen ion concentration in the organism is regulated by several buffer systems, of which the bicarbonate-carbonic acid system is the most important. The buffer system is expressed by the Henderson-Hasselbalch equation:

$$pH = pK + (HCO_3^-)/0.03\ x\ pCO_2)$$

The bicarbonate concentration is calculated at a fixed pCO_2 by a measurement of the pH. This bicarbonate value is known as the standard bicarbonate. The normal concentration is 24 mEq/l. Values above 24 mEq/l indicate base excess, values below indicate base deficit. As an example: a mini-pig weighing 20 kg has a hematocrit value of 51% and a standard bicarbonate of 16 mEq/l. The pig has a water deficit of 40 ml/kg or a total of 800 ml. The extracellular fluid is $160 \times 20 = 3.2$ l. The base deficit is $24 - 16 = 8$ mEq/l or a total of $8 \times 3.2 = 25.6$ mEq HCO_3^-. The isotonic bicarbonate solution contains 167 mEq HCO_3^- per liter. The base deficit is thus corrected by infusion of 153 ml isotonic bicarbonate solution. The remaining water deficit is replaced by infusion of 647 ml isotonic glucose.

RECOVERY FROM ANESTHESIA

The recovery period after anesthesia poses several risks for the animal. At the transition between unconsciousness and consciousness the animal may pass through a period of excitation. The animal may hurt itself during this stage if left unattended. In small ruminants it is important not to remove the endotracheal tube until the excitation is over, as the animal is unable to control regurgitation at this stage, and aspiration of rumen content may result.

Table 1. The approximate relationship between hematocrit value and extracellular fluid volume.

	Hematocrit (%)	Extracellular vol. (ml/kg)
Overhydrated	37	280
	38	260
	41	240
	43	220
Normal	42 ± 3	200 ± 20
Dehydrated	48	180
	51	160
	54	140
	58	120

Recovery should always take place in a separate room, and not in a cage or pen with other animals, as they may attack the unconscious or semiconscious animal. The temperature should be approximately 25°C for larger animals and about 35°C for rats and mice, and neonates of all species. An infrared lamp above the cage is an excellent way to provide satisfactory environmental conditions for large animals. Small animals are conveniently placed in a cabinet in which temperature is regulated by one or more electrical bulbs.

If recovery is expected to take a long time, the animal should be turned over every 15 min to prevent lung congestion. Ruminants should be placed in sternal recumbency and supported in this position to facilitate gas eructation from the forestomachs. Analgesic treatment should not be instituted until the danger of respiratory depression is over.

STAFF SAFETY

It is important to be aware of the health hazards to laboratory personnel involved with animal anesthesia. The most obvious risk is exposure to volatile anesthetics. As a general rule these agents should be used only in closed systems, and surplus anesthetic vapor should be removed by a ventilation system which secures that no gas accumulates in the operation room or laboratory.[85,86]

Diethyl ether is highly inflammable and mixtures of ether and oxygen or air are explosive. This agent should therefore be used only if special safety precautions are taken, including spark-proof electrical fittings and efficient ventilation. Diethyl ether should never be used in open systems or in ordinary laboratory rooms.

Several anesthetic drugs are highly poisonous or addictive to humans, and should only be handled by competent persons. The analgesic etorphine is extremely toxic, and accidental self-injection can be fatal. An opiate antagonist should always be available if this drug is used. Compounds like urethane and alpha-chloralose are believed to be carcinogenic, and should only be handled by experienced personnel wearing protective gloves.

ANESTHETIC METHODS IN DIFFERENT SPECIES

Numerous anesthetic methods have been suggested and described, and it would not be possible to mention them all in this chapter. All the methods described below are, however, well documented and several of them used routinely by the author. It is important to stress that a well-established anesthetic method with which the experimenter is confident, should not be replaced without a very good reason. A new method will inevitably cause changes in the experimental conditions, leading to systematic errors. It is therefore important to develop and refine one method and stay with that method throughout the whole experiment.

ANESTHESIA OF PIGS

The pig, especially the mini-pig, is the animal of choice when it comes to experimental surgery of the digestive system and the cardiovascular system. It is also the animal of choice for surgical training of medical and veterinary surgeons. The digestive physiology of the pig is comparable to that of humans, and the pig is an ideal model for comparative studies of hepatic and pancreatic physiology.

Pigs tolerate anesthesia very well. The disadvantages are the difficulty in performing venous puncture and the difficulty in handling large pigs.

Premedication and Sedation

Pigs should always be pretreated with atropine sulfate to reduce the profuse salivation and to stimulate heart action.[11,87] The dose for pigs is 0.05 mg/kg (s.c. or i.m.).

The following sedatives are recommended for pigs: azaperone,[9-13,88] acepromazine,[12] propionylpromazine,[9] xylazine,[29,79,89] diazepam [29] and metomidate.[33]

Inhalation Anesthetics

The most convenient method for sedating the pig is by intramuscular injection of atropine sulfate (0.05 mg/kg), azaperone (4 mg/kg), and diazepam (0.5 mg/kg). The pig is left undisturbed for 20 to 30 min, after which time it is deeply sedated. It can now be brought to the preparation room, where a catheter is placed in the aureal vein and metomidate is given intravenously until the animal is in reflexless anesthesia (approximately 4 mg/kg). The pig can now be intubated, prepared for surgery and brought to the operation room. Anesthesia is continued with halothane (1 to 2%) and nitrous oxide (40%). Using this method the respiratory rate is reduced from 20 to 14 breaths per minute, resulting in a pCO_2 between 45 and 50 mmHg and a moderate acidosis. The mean arterial blood pressure is reduced to about 80% of the level in non-anesthetized pigs. If artificial ventilation is applied at a rate of 20 breaths per minute and a minute volume of 150 ml/kg/min acid-base balance is normalized.[33]

Injectable Anesthesia

Injection anesthesia using azaperone, diazepam, and metomidate is a useful method for minor surgery and experimental procedures. After premedication similar to that described above, repeated doses of metomidate are given every 15 min or as a continuous infusion of 0.04 mg/kg/min. In practice this is performed by dissolving 1 g metomidate in 1 l isotonic saline. The dose for a 25-kg mini-pig is then 1 ml (17 drops) per minute. Using this method, respiration is stimulated, causing a slight reduction in pCO_2. There is considerable individual variation in arterial blood pressure, but pronounced hypotension is not seen.[33]

When ketamine alone is given to pigs at dosages of from 10 to 20 mg/kg, the animals respond in 1 to 2 min. They first become ataxic with muscle tremors and extensor rigidity. Respiratory rate and heart rate increase, and the animals lie on their sides panting and salivating. The body temperature falls up to 5°C after 10 min. Combining ketamine with diazepam (1 mg/kg) or xylazine (2 mg/kg) produces sedation with excellent muscular relaxation lasting 90 and 40 min, respectively.[29] The combination of xylazine (1 mg/kg) and ketamine (10 mg/kg) given intravenously results in a 15% decrease in heart rate, a transient fall in arterial blood pressure and a 43% fall in cardiac output. Respiration is unchanged by the anesthesia, and acid-base balance remains within the normal range.[89]

Xylazine-ketamine anesthesia can be prolonged by continuous drop infusion of sodium thiopental. After premedication with xylazine-ketamine the animal is intubated and sodium thiopental (50 ml of a 2.5% solution dissolved in 500 ml isotonic saline) is infused at a rate of about 30 drops per minute.[79]

Alpha-chloralose is a very useful agent in terminal experiments where stable cardiovascular parameters are essential. It is, however, important to note that alpha-chloralose has no analgetic properties, and painful procedures must not be performed in an animal under the influence of alpha-chloralose alone. The recommended dose is 100 mg/kg i.v. Alpha-chloralose can be given to the animal while initial surgical preparation is carried out under the influence of a volatile anesthetic (e.g., halothane). After completion of the surgical procedure, the inhalant can be removed, and after about 30 to 40 min, the animal will be under the sole influence of alpha-chloralose, and the experiment can proceed. If the animal is allowed to breathe spontaneously hypercapnia and respiratory acidosis will develop, while blood pressure and heart rate remain within the normal range. Artificial ventilation with a minute volume of 150 ml/kg/min and a frequency of 20 breaths per minute acid will normalize acid-base balance.

It should be noted that metabolic abnormalities due to halothane and other anesthetics may persist longer than the anesthetic action of these agents.[40]

ANESTHESIA OF SMALL RUMINANTS

The sheep is a very useful animal model in reproductive and fetal physiology. Surgery on the fetus, including catheterization of arteries and veins, is tolerated. In addition sheep are frequently used in the study of ruminant physiology involving cannulation of the forestomachs and the intestinal tract.

Premedication and Sedation

Atropine sulfate causes secretion of a thick viscid saliva in small ruminants and is not very useful for premedication. Several sedatives are used. Xylazine is very potent in these animals; sheep are deeply sedated by intramuscular injection of 0.2 mg/kg. Goats are much more sensitive to xylazine, and injection of 0.05 mg/kg i.m. results in up to 12 h of sedation. Xylazine should never be given to animals late in pregnancy. Diazepam in doses between 1 and 2 mg/kg is an effective sedative in both sheep and goats. Acepromazine is usually given to sheep at a dose ranging from 0.05 to 0.1 mg/kg. In goats the dose is 0.1 mg/kg. Acepromazine provides a safe and effective sedative in both species after 20 to 30 min.

Inhalation Anesthesia

The sheep is sedated with acepromazine (0.5 mg/kg) i.m. After 20 to 30 min the animal is usually in sternal recumbency. The animal is moved to the preparation room, and an indwelling plastic catheter is introduced into the cephalic vein. Thiopental sodium (2.5%) at a dose of approximately 10 mg/kg is injected i.v. Half the volume is injected rapidly, and the remaining volume is given slowly until the mouth can be opened without resistance. The animal is intubated, and respiration is assisted. After completion of skin preparation the animal is brought to the operation room and anesthesia is continued with halothane (1%), nitrous oxide (40%), and oxygen (60%), using artificial ventilation with a minute volume of 6 to 8 l and a respiratory frequency of 20 breaths per minute. This method has proven to be safe for fetal surgery in sheep.

Injectable Anesthesia

The response to ketamine alone in both sheep and goats is extremely variable and characterized by tremors and rigidity. Sedation with xylazine or diazepam 10 min prior to ketamine injection results in an excellent anesthesia.

Sheep are given 0.1 mg/kg xylazine i.m., and 10 min later 4 mg/kg ketamine i.v. Surgical anesthesia lasts for approximately 25 min. Anesthesia is accompanied by transient respiratory acidosis and a significant decrease in arterial blood pressure and vascular resistance. This method should not be used in goats due to the unpredictable effect of xylazine in this species.

Ketamine combined with diazepam has proven safe in both sheep and goats. The animal is sedated with diazepam at 2 mg/kg i.v. some 15 min before an initial dose of ketamine (4 mg/kg i.v.). Anesthesia lasts about 15 min, but can be extended with repeated doses of ketamine. Anesthesia is accompanied by respiratory acidosis, a significant increase in vascular resistance, and arterial blood pressure within the normal range.[26,29]

ANESTHESIA OF DOGS

Premedication and Sedation

Atropine at a dose of 0.02 to 0.1 mg/kg i.m. is useful in dogs in counteracting bradycardia caused by some agents, e.g., halothane. It is also useful in reducing the volume of saliva in breeds which tend to produce large amounts of saliva.

The sedatives most often used in dogs are acepromazine and xylazine. Fluanisone or droperidol in combination with fentanyl (Hypnorm® and Innovar®) is used to induce neuroleptanalgesia in dogs.

Inhalation Anesthesia

The sedated dog is given an intravenous injection of thiopental sodium (5 to 10 mg/kg). Half the dose is given rapidly, the remainder over 30 s until the animal is completely relaxed. After endotracheal intubation, anesthesia is maintained with an inhalant anesthetic (halothane, methoxyflurane, isoflurane, etc.) with 40% nitrous oxide and 60% oxygen. Blood pressure and respiration are reduced by halothane. Artificial ventilation with a frequency of 20 to 30 breaths per minute and a minute volume of approximately 150 ml/kg will maintain a normal pO^2 and acid-base balance.

Injectable Anesthesia

Pentobarbital is still widely used in dog anesthesia in spite of the respiratory depression and the slow recovery. The dog is sedated with acepromazine (0.5 mg/kg) i.m. or fentanyl/fluanisone (Hypnorm®) (0.1 ml/kg) i.m. A dose of 5 to 10 mg/kg pentobarbital (2.5%) is given i.v. The first half is injected rapidly to prevent excitation, the rest slowly to effect. Anesthesia lasts up to 60 min, and can be prolonged by repeated doses of 5 mg/kg. Pentobarbital should never be used as the sole agent due to respiratory depression.

Basal anesthesia lasting 6 to 8 h with minimal physiological disturbance can be established with a combination of fentanyl/fluanisone (0.1 ml/kg) i.m., pentobarbital (5 mg/kg) i.v. and pancuronium (0.05 mg/kg) i.v., The dog is intubated and ventilated artifically. Pentobarbital is diluted 1 g/l isotonic saline, and given as a continuous infusion at a rate of 5 ml/kg/h.

Cardiovascular studies are frequently performed in dogs anesthetized with alpha-chloralose (80 to 100 mg/kg), either employed as the sole anesthetic agent or in combination with analgesic or hypnotic compounds. The advantage of this anesthetic method is that the animals demonstrate cardiovascular responses that are virtually indistinguishable from those of a resting conscious animal. This, however, is only true if the animal is not exposed to any painful stimuli.

The effect of different doses of alpha-chloralose in combination with morphine sulfate has been examined.[90] Dogs were given an initial dose of morphine sulfate (5 mg/kg) and alpha-chloralose (80 mg/kg), and maintained anesthetized for 12 h by repeated doses of alpha-chloralose ranging between 16 and 100 mg/kg/h. The study concludes that the hourly infusion of 28 mg/kg in artificially ventilated animals provided the least hemodynamic variability. The highest doses were toxic, causing death within 8 h.

Alpha-chloralose is generally recommended for terminal experiments only. One study, however, has investigated the use of alpha-chloralose for repeated anesthetic procedures in dogs between the ages of 80 and 300 days. Anesthesia was induced by intravenous thiopental sodium (5 mg/kg) and alpha-chloralose (80 mg/kg), and additional doses of alpha-chloralose were given to maintain anesthesia (118 ± 19 mg/kg). Recovery lasted approximately 4 h in each experiment, and the dogs exhibited normal health and growth as compared with non-treated dogs. There were no indications of acute renal, hepatic, pancreatic, or cardiac toxicity immediately after anesthesia, and no evidence of chronic toxicity following completion of the study.[91]

Combinations of neuroleptic agents and opiate analgesics are widely used in veterinary practice for sedation, premedication, and for carrying out minor surgical procedures.[92,93] Three combination preparations are available for veterinary use: Hypnorm® (fluanisone and fentanyl), Innovar-vet® (droperidol and fentanyl), and Immobilon® (acepromazine and etorphine). The advantage of using these agents is the possibility of reversing the effect by antagonistic compounds. The disadvantage of Hypnorm® and Innovar® is that the dogs remain very sensitive to noise. Supplementary anesthesia should be administered by inhalation, as intravenous drugs may produce severe respiratory depression. Injection of Immobilon® produces a profound and prolonged state of unconsciousness and analgesia. Respiration is severely depressed, and the dog may become cyanotic if oxygen is not administered.

Doses for dogs are Hypnorm® and Innovar®, 0.1 ml/kg, and Immobilon® 0.05 ml/kg. As previously mentioned etorphine is extremely toxic to humans, and the antagonist Revivon® or Naloxone® should always be injected in case of accidental self-injection.

Ketamine given in doses ranging from 5 to 10 mg/kg often causes excitation and convulsion, and this agent cannot be recommended for dogs.

ANESTHESIA OF CATS

Cats object to being exposed to unfamiliar proceedings and handled by unfamiliar persons, and it may be difficult to give intravenous injections. Therefore, sedation and induction of anesthesia often have to be performed by intramuscular injection, increasing the risk of overdosing the animal.

Sedation and Premedication

Anticholinergic agents should always be given to cats both to prevent bronchial secretions from obstructing the narrow airway, and to block vagal reflexes. The dose of atropine sulfate for a cat is high, up to 1 mg/kg, due to the presence of liver atropine esterase, which rapidly metabolizes the agent.

Phenothiazine derivatives are frequently used in cats, but the sedation they produce is very variable. The dose of acepromazine (Plegicil®) is 0.25 to 0.5 mg/kg i.m. Diazepam and other drugs of the benzodiazepine group do not produce sedation in cats, but they may be used to produce muscle relaxation. The most effective sedative for cats is xylazine (Rompun®), but even this compound may produce variable results. The dose is 1 to 2 mg/kg i.m. Cats usually vomit after administration, and react to sharp noise.[29] The effect of xylazine can be reversed by the alpha-2 adrenergic blocking agent yohimbine at a dose of 0.1 mg/kg.[44]

Inhalation Anesthesia

Anesthesia is induced by intravenous injection of thiopental sodium at a dose of up to 10 mg/kg in the sedated cat. Before endotracheal intubation the laryngeal mucous membrane is desensitized by spraying it with a local analgesic drug to prevent laryngeal spasm. The outer diameter of the uncuffed tube should be 5 or 5.5 mm. A tight seal can be ensured by packing the mouth and pharynx with gauze sponges. Anesthesia is maintained using halothane (1 to 2%) or methoxyflurane (0.1 to 0.2%) and nitrous oxide (40%) and oxygen (60%).

Injectable Anesthesia

The most commonly used method of anesthesia in the cat is by i.m. injection of ketamine hydrochloride (25 mg/kg) in combination with sedation with xylazine (0.5 mg/kg) and atropine sulfate (1 mg/kg). Ketamine produces a slight stimulation of the cardiovascular system and a minimal respiratory depression. During anesthesia the eyes remain open, and measures should be adopted to prevent drying of the cornea. The maximal effect is reached 10 to 15 min after intramuscular injection and lasts for 30 to 40 min. Further ketamine increments of 5 to 10 mg/kg i.m. or 2 mg/kg i.v. are given to prolong anesthesia. Recovery time is 8 to 12 h depending on the total dose given.

Ultra-short anesthesia can be achieved with alphaxolone-alphadolone. The dose is 9 to 12 mg/kg, half of which is given rapidly i.v. and the remainder slowly to effect. Surgical anesthesia develops within 30 s and lasts for about 10 min. Recovery is uneventful if the cat is not disturbed. Intubation can be performed under alphaxolone-alphadolone anesthesia.

ANESTHESIA OF PRIMATES

Primates should preferably be anesthetized when handled, as they can inflict severe bites and transfer diseases pathogenic to man. Anesthetic drugs must be given as injections while the monkey is physically restrained in a crush-back cage or in a net.

Premedication and Sedation

Atropine sulfate (0.05 mg/kg) s.c. should routinely be given as premedication to all primate species. The most commonly used sedatives for monkeys are xylazine (0.6 to 2.0 mg/kg),[94-97] diazepam (7.5 mg/kg)[28] and acepromazine (0.55 mg/kg).[7]

Injectable Anesthesia

Surgical anesthesia is achieved by i.m. injection of ketamine in doses between 10 and 20 mg/kg in several primate species pretreated with a sedative. Ketamine used without a sedative results in poor muscle relaxation and slow grasping movements of limbs and hands during surgery.[29]

The ketamine-xylazine combination depresses the heart rate and arterial blood pressure by 40 to 50%, whereas respiration, blood gases, and acid-base balance are virtually unaffected.[94]

Surgical anesthesia of baboons lasting up to 6 h can be achieved by continuous i.v. infusion of alphaxolone-alphadolone at a dose rate of 0.2 mg/kg/min after induction with ketamine.[98]

ANESTHESIA OF RABBITS

The rabbit is a useful animal model for experimental surgery, including transplantation experiments. It is frequently quoted that rabbits are difficult animals to anesthetize. This may be because rabbits often suffer from subclinical pulmonary infection without showing clear symptoms. If respiration is suppressed by anesthesia, lethal hypoxia may result. The use of healthy animals is of great importance.

Premedication and Sedation

Rabbits should be treated with atropine sulfate 20 to 30 min prior to administration of other agents. Excellent sedation and muscle relaxation is accomplished by i.v. injection of 1 mg/kg diazepam. The time to effect is a few seconds after i.v. injection and the duration is 2 to 6 h.

Acepromazine (1 mg/kg) i.m. sedates rabbits in 10 min lasting 1 to 2 h. Fentanyl/fluanisone in a low dose (0.1 ml/kg) provides excellent sedation in rabits. It also causes vasodilation, and is a very useful medication during blood sampling.

Inhalation Anesthesia

Anesthesia is induced in the sedated rabbit by i.v. injection of thiopental, 1.25% at a dose of 20 to 30 mg/kg, half of which is given rapidly and the remainder slowly till effect. Intubation af the rabbit is possible using a neonatal laryngoscope.[74] Anesthesia can be maintained by methoxyflurane[6,62,75,99] or halothane.[66] Induction with methoxyflurane alone without sedation should not be attempted as the animals will show markedly increased motor activity and a prolonged stage of excitement.[6]

Halothane in combination with nitrous oxide[66] or halothane alone[74] provides a safe anesthesia in rabbits. Cardiac output is, however, decreased, resulting in hypotension.

Injectable Anesthesia

Pentobarbital is still commonly used for rabbit anesthesia although the method carries a high risk for the rabbit because of the narrow margin between surgical anesthesia and respiratory arrest. If pentobarbital is to be used as the sole agent, the solution should be diluted to a concentration of 2 mg/ml. Anesthesia is induced with an initial dose of 10 mg/kg (5 ml solution/kg). Increments of 2 to 10 mg are then administered until a satisfactory anesthetic level is reached.[100] If pentobarbital is combined with acepromazine (1 mg/kg), the dose necessary to reach surgical anesthesia can be reduced and the safety margin increased.

Anesthesia using ketamine hydrochloride has frequently been described. Ketamine alone in doses in the range of 10 to 60 mg/kg results in a variable and inconsistent sedation lasting 30 to 60 min. Analgesia is poor, and the animals will respond to painful stimuli irrespective of the dose of ketamine used. Immediately after ketamine administration the respiratory frequency and blood oxygenation decrease in a dose-dependent manner. At doses ranging from 6 to 18 mg/kg moderate hypotension due to peripheral vasodilatation is observed.[29,101] The sedative and analgesic effects of ketamine are greatly improved when combined with a sedative like xylazine (3 to 5 mg/kg),[102-105] promazine (5.6 mg/kg)[106] or acepromazine (0.75 mg/kg).[3]

The combination of fentanyl and fluanisone (Hypnorm®) or droperidol (Innovar®) is very efficient in producing neuroleptanalgesia in rabbits. Muscle relaxation, however, is insufficient for major surgery to be performed. Full surgical anesthesia with good muscle relaxation can be achieved by Hypnorm® or Innovar® (0.3 ml/kg) i.m. and diazepam (5 mg/kg).[22]

Neuroleptanalgesia using etorphine hydrochloride (Immobilon®) is not recommended in rabbits, due to severe depression of the respiratory center.[93]

Light to medium surgical anesthesia lasting for 8 to 10 min can be produced in rabbits by i.v. injection of alphaxolone-alphadolone (12 mg/kg). Analgesia, however, is not sufficient for very painful manipulations.[107]

ANESTHESIA OF GUINEA PIGS

Guinea pigs are considered difficult to anesthetize for several reasons: the body weight is difficult to estimate since the gastrointestinal content may contribute 30 to 40% of the total body weight; responses to anesthetic agents vary with the dietary status of the animal (ascorbic acid deficiency or blood glucose level); the airways are relatively narrow and may be obstructed by mucous secretions; and finally the guinea pig has no superficial veins that allow easy intravenous injection.

Premedication and Sedation

Atropine sulfate (0.05 mg/kg) s.c. should be given 30 min prior to other agents. Sedation of guinea pigs is best achieved by i.p. injection of diazepam (5 mg/kg). Xylazine (1.8 mg/kg) is also an efficient sedative in guinea pigs, but it results in a marked decrease in blood pressure.[21]

Inhalation Anesthesia

Endotracheal intubation of guinea pigs is possible using a tracheal tube made from an 8-cm length of polyethylene tubing with an outer diameter of 2.42 mm. The tip of the tube is tapered and smoothed by heating the tubing and gently drawing it out. The tube is fitted with a metal stylet. Insertion of the tube is done blindly during inspiration using a small "laryngoscope" made from acrylic plastic.[76]

Induction of anesthesia in the guinea pig is difficult due to the lack of suitable veins for injection. The most frequently described method is by inhalation of methoxyflurane on an open mask or in an inhalation chamber.[57,59,60,108,109] With the current knowledge of the dangers of exposure to anesthetic gases, these methods should be avoided except if carried out in a ventilated hood.

Injectable Anesthesia

The most frequently quoted method for guinea pig anesthesia is by i.m. injection of ketamine hydrochloride. Used as the sole agent analgesia is poor even in doses as high as 250 mg/kg.[10,17] The ketamine dose recommended ranges between 20 and 44 mg/kg in combination with xylazine (0.15 to 5 mg/kg),[16,110] droperidol (2.5 mg/kg),[111] acepromazine (2 mg/kg),[4] or pentobarbital (6 mg/kg).[112] The combination that appears most acceptable with regard to analgesia, and maintenance of near normal cardiovascular and respiratory parameters appears to be: premedication with atropine sulfate (0.04 mg/kg), sedation with xylazine (5 mg/kg) and anesthesia by i.m. injection of ketamine (20 mg/kg).[16]

Neuroleptanalgesia using fentanyl-fluanisone or fentanyl-droperidol in guinea pigs sedated with midazolam or diazepam provides good analgesia and muscle relaxation. The respiratory rate, however, is reduced by approximately 50%.[23]

ANESTHESIA OF RATS

Rats are commonly used for experimental procedures requiring surgery. Anesthesia and surgery are well tolerated in rats provided they are free from respiratory disease. Doses of different anesthetics may differ between strains, and females are more sensitive to certain agents than males. The correct dose for a given group of animals should therefore be checked in a pilot experiment.

Premedication and Sedation

Atropine sulfate (0.05 mg/kg) s.c. should always be given to rats 20 to 30 min before anesthesia. The most efficient sedative for rats is diazepam (2.5 mg/kg). Following i.p injection the rat is deeply sedated within 10 min. Midazolam is a water-soluble benzodiazepine that produces excellent sedation at a dose of 3.75 mg/kg. Xylazine as a sole sedative agent cannot be recommended in rats.[113]

Inhalation Anesthesia

Endotracheal intubation of rats is possible following induction with pentobarbital (30 mg/kg) i.p. A flexible 16-gauge i.v. polyethylene catheter is suitable as a tube. The needle stylette of the catheter is filed down to be 1 mm shorter than the catheter and bent at a 30° angle 2 cm from the end. The rat is placed in dorsal recumbency with its nose projecting slightly over the edge of the table. The upper jaw is pulled below the board with an elastic band. A fiber-optic light is used for illumination. By upward traction on the tongue with the thumb and forefinger and downward pressure on the trachea with the middle finger, it is possible to see the epiglottis and vocal cords, and introduce the tube.[77,78] Anesthesia masks for delivering anesthetic gases have been described.[61,85,114] However, these devices should be used only in a ventilated hood to protect laboratory staff from exposure to anesthetic gases.

Injectable Anesthesia

Pentobarbital has been used extensively as an anesthetic agent in rats. For long periods of surgical anesthesia an initial dose of 50 mg/kg for males and 25 mg/kg for females i.p. is given. Anesthesia can be prolonged by an additional oral dose of a similar amount of pentobarbital diluted with water to a final volume of 3 ml/kg.[115] The disadvantage of pentobarbital as the sole agent is the narrow range between surgical anesthesia and respiratory depression.[36] Pentobarbital produces a profound hypothermia in rats, and temperature support is always required when using this anesthetic method.[18]

Ketamine hydrochloride in combination with diazepam or pentobarbital provides anesthesia with a rapid superficial respiration, which increases during the anesthetic period, resulting in hypoxia and acidosis. Blood pressure declines during anesthesia from a normal level of 130 mmHg to about 90 mmHg.[17,24]

Neuroleptanalgesia using fentanyl-fluanisone (Hypnorm®) (0.3 ml/kg) or fentanyl-droperidol (Innovar® vet) (0.2 to 0.4 ml/kg) in combination with diazepam (2.5 mg/kg) provides excellent anesthesia and muscle relaxation in rats. Mean arterial blood pressure is reduced to approximately 80 mmHg, and remains stable throughout a 2-h period. This fall in blood pressure is partly counteracted by an increase in heart rate, indicating that the predominant effect is on the peripheral circulation.[24,25] The effect of fentanyl on body temperature is minimal compared to other anesthetic combinations.[18] Respiratory rate, pCO_2, acid-base balance, and pO_2 are practically undisturbed during neuroleptanalgesia provided the dose does not exceed 0.3 ml/kg.[17,24]

Subcutaneous injection of etorphine hydrochloride (0.0125 to 0.05 mg/kg), acepromazine (0.04 to 0.16 mg/kg) and atrophine sulfate (0.075 to 0.3 mg/kg), has been suggested as an effective anesthetic for rats.[116] Respiratory depression is, however, so profound that acidosis and hypoxia reach unacceptable levels.[24]

ANESTHESIA OF MICE

Two factors contribute to the difficulties of anesthetizing mice: the low body weight and the different genetic background of inbred strains. The low body weight increases the risk of overdosing the mouse, and the high body surface:weight ratio easily leads to heat loss and hypothermia. The different inbred strains have different metabolic rates and pathways, and anesthetic agents are metabolized differently. This makes it impossible to use standardized doses, and any anesthetic drug must be tested whenever a new strain of mouse is used.

Premedication and Sedation

Atropine sulfate (0.04 mg/kg) reduces salivation in mice exposed to diethyl ether anesthesia. The best sedative agent in this species is diazepam (5 mg/kg) i.p.

Inhalation Anesthesia

Diethyl ether-soaked cotton wool under a grid in a simple glass container with a lid has been the favorite method of anesthetizing mice. However, the method has several disadvantages: it appears to be very unpleasant for the animal, which becomes excited and tries to escape from the container. The method also involves a risk for the laboratory staff of exposure to the volatile compound, and of explosion. A similar technique using methoxyflurane has the same disadvantages. If inhalation methods are to be used in mice, they should be performed in a ventilated hood.

Injectable Anesthesia

Ultra-short anesthesia in mice is best achieved by i.p. injection of propanidid (Sombrevin®). A dose of approximately 0.3 ml will produce anesthesia for 2 to 3 min.

The most widely used method for medium-length anesthesia of mice is neuroleptanalgesia.[23,113] In practice a solution is made containing 1 part Hypnorm®, 1 part diazepam (5 mg/ml) and 2 parts isotonic saline. The standard dose for outbred mice is 0.1 ml/10 g. For inbred strains the dose should be tested in a pilot experiment. This method provides 20 to 40 min of surgical anesthesia. It is important to maintain the body temperature by external heat supply.

Long-term anesthesia of mice can be achieved by an initial i.v. injection of alphaxolone-alphadolone of 20 mg/kg followed by repeated i.v. doses of 6 mg/kg every 15 min.[107]

Pentobarbital and ketamine are not recommended anesthetics in mice due to a marked variation in response to these agents.

REFERENCES

1. Quasha, A.L., Eger, E.I. and Tinker, J.H., Determination and Applications of MAC, *Anesthesiology*, 53, 315, 1980.
2. Gray, K.N., Raulston, G.L., Flow, B.L., Jardine, J.H. and Huchton, J.I., Repeated Immobilization of Miniature Swine with an Acepromazine-Ketamine Combination, *Southwest. Vet.*, 31, 27, 1978.
3. Lipman, N.S., Marini, R.P. and Erdman, S.E., A Comparison of Ketamine/Xylazine and Ketamine/ Xylazine/Acepromazine Anesthesia in the Rabbit, *Lab. Anim. Sci.*, 40, 395, 1990.
4. Shucard, D.W., Andrew, M. and Beauford, C., A Safe and Fast-Acting Surgical Anesthetic for Use in the Guinea Pig, *J. Appl. Physiol.*, 38, 538, 1975.
5. Brown, C.M. and Layman, D.K., Use of Ketamine-HCl Anesthesia in Studies of Chylo-micron-Triglyceride Metabolism in the Rat, *Lab. Anim. Sci.*, 40, 183, 1990.
6. McCormick, M.J. and Ashworth, M.A., Acepromazine and Methoxyflurane Anesthesia of Immature New Zealand White Rabbits, *Lab. Anim. Sci.*, 21, 220, 1971.
7. Connolly, R. and Quimby, F.W., Acepromazine-Ketamine Anesthesia in the Rhesus Monkey (Macaca mulatta), *Lab. Anim. Sci.*, 28, 72, 1978.
8. Cronin, M.F., Booth, N.H., Hatch, R.C. and Brown, J., Acepromazine-Xylazine Combination in Dogs: Antagonism with 4-Aminopyridine and Yohimbine, *Am. J. Vet. Res.*, 44, 2037, 1983.

9. Ellendorff, F., Parvizi, N., Elsaesser, F. and Smidt, D., The miniature pig as an animal model in endocrine and neuroendocrine studies of reproduction, *Lab. Anim. Sci.*, 27, 822, 1977.

10. Gasthuys, F., Pollet, L., Simoens, P., Lauwers, H. and De Laey, J.J., Anaesthesia for flourescein angiography of the ocular fundus in the miniature pig, *Vet. Res. Commun.*, 14, 393, 1990.

11. Pfenninger, E., Grünert, A., Müller, W. and Siegler, W., Die Buprenorphin-Lachgas-Sauerstoff-Narkose am Tiermodell Hausschwein, *Z. Versuchstierkd.*, 26, 67, 1984.

12. Becker, M. and Reglinger, R., Die vergleichende Betrachtung der Vitalfunktionen nach Neuroleptika- und Narkosemittelapplikation beim Schwein, *Berl. Münch. Tierärztl. Wochenschr.*, 87, 165, 1974.

13. Clarke, K.W., Effect of Azaperone on the Blood Pressure and Pulmonary Ventilation in Pigs, *Vet. Rec.*, 85, 649, 1969.

14. Parker, J.L. and Adams, H.R., The Influence of Chemical Restraining Agents on Cardiovascular Function: a Review, *Lab. Anim. Sci.*, 28, 575, 1978.

15. Klöcking, H.-P. and Sedlarik, K., Influence of Anaesthetics on the Fibrinolytic Activity in Minipigs, *Folia Haematol.*, 115, 132, 1988.

16. Brown, J.N., Thorne, P.R. and Nuttal, A.L., Blood Pressure and Other Physiological Responses in Awake and Anesthetized Guinea Pigs, *Lab. Anim. Sci.*, 39, 142, 1989.

17. Wixson, S.K., White, W.J., Hughes, H.C., Jr., Lang, C.M. and Marshall, W.K., The Effect of Pentobarbital, Fentanyl-Droperidol, Ketamine-Xylazine and Ketamine-Diazepam on Arterial Blood pH, Blood Gasses, Mean Arterial Blood Pressure and Heart Rate in Adult Male Rats, *Lab. Anim. Sci.*, 37, 736, 1987.

18. Wixson, S.K., White, W.J., Hughes, H.C., Jr., Lang, C.M. and Marshall, W.K., The Effects of Pentobarbital, Fentanyl-Droperidol, Ketamine-Xylazine and Ketamine-Diazepam on Core and Surface Body Temperature Regulation in Adult Male Rats, *Lab. Anim. Sci.*, 37, 743, 1987.

19. Wixson, S.K., White, W.J., Hughes, H.C., Jr., Marshall, W.K. and Lang, C.M., The Effect of Pentobarbital, Fentanyl-Droperidol, Ketamine-Xylazine and Ketamine-Diazepam on Noxious Stimulus Perception in Adult Male Rats, *Lab. Anim. Sci.*, 37, 731, 1987.

20. Ferguson, J.W., Anaesthesia in the Hamster Using a Combination of Methohexitone and Diazepam, *Lab. Anim.*, 13, 305, 1979.

21. Flynn, A.J., Dengerink, H.A. and Wright, J.W., Blood Pressure in Resting, Anesthetized and Noise-Exposed Guinea Pigs, *Hear. Res.*, 34, 201, 1988.

22. Peeters, M.E., Gil, D., Teske, E., Eyzenbach, V., Brom, W.E.V.D., Lumeij, J.T. and de Vries, H.W., Four Methods for General Anaesthesia in the Rabbit: A Comparative Study, *Lab. Anim.*, 22, 355, 1988.

23. Flecknell, P.A. and Mitchell, M., Midazolam and Fentanyl-Fluanisone: Assessment of Anaesthetic Effects in Laboratory Rodents and Rabbits, *Lab. Anim.*, 18, 143, 1984.

24. Svendsen, P. and Carter, A.M., Influence of Injectable Anaesthetic Combinations on Blood Gas Tensions and Acid-Base Status in Laboratory Rats, *Acta Pharmacol. Toxicol.*, 57, 1, 1985.

25. Skollenborg, K.C., Grönbech, J.E., Grong, K., Åbyholm, F.E. and Lekven, J., Distribution of Cardiac Output during Pentobarbital Versus Midozalam/Fentanyl/Fluanisone Anaesthesia in the Rat, *Lab. Anim.*, 24, 221, 1990.

26. Coulson, N.M., Januszkiewicz, A.J., Dodd, K.T. and Ripple, G.R., The Cardiorespiratory Effects of Diazepam-Ketamine and Xylazine-Ketamine Anesthetic Combinations in Sheep, *Lab. Anim. Sci.*, 39, 591, 1989.

27. Wixson, S.K., White, W.J., Hughes, H.C., Jr., Lang, C.M. and Marshall, W.K., A Comparison of Pentobarbital, Fentanyl-Droperidol, Ketamine-Xylazine and Ketamine-Diazepam Anesthesia in Adult Male Rats, *Lab. Anim. Sci.*, 37, 726, 1987.

28. Woolfson, M.W., Foran, J.A., Freedman, H.M., Moore, P.A., Shulman, L.B. and Schnitman, P.A., Immobilization of Baboons (Papio anubis) Using Ketamine and Diazepam, *Lab. Anim. Sci.*, 30, 902, 1980.

29. Green, C.J., Knight, J., Precious, S. and Simpkin, S., Ketamine Alone and in Combination with Diazepam or Xylazine in Laboratory Animals: a 10 Year Experience, *Lab. Anim.*, 15, 163, 1981.

30. Silverman, J., Huhndorf, M., Balk, M. and Slater, G., Evaluation of a Combination of Tiletamine and Zolazepam as an Anesthetic for Laboratory Rodents, *Lab. Anim. Sci.*, 33, 457, 1983.

31. Kumar, A. and Thurmon, J.C., Cardiopulmonary, Hemocytologic and Biochemical Effects of Xylazine in Goats, *Lab. Anim. Sci.*, 29, 486, 1979.

32. Ehler, W.J., Mack, J.W., Brown, D.L. and Davis, R.F., Avoidance of Malignant Hyperthermia in a Porcine Model for Experimental Open Heart Surgery, *Lab. Anim. Sci.*, 35, 172, 1985.

33. Svendsen, P. and Carter, A.M., Blood Gas Tensions, Acid-Base Status and Cardiovascular Function in Miniature Swine Anaesthetized with Halothane and Methoxyflurane or Intravenous Metomidate Hydrochloride, *Pharmacol. Toxicol.*, 64, 88, 1989.

34. Rugh, K.S., Zinn, G.M., Paterson, J.A. and Thorne, J.G., Inhalation Anesthesia in Adult Cattle, *Lab. Anim. Sci.*, 35, 178, 1985.

35. White, G.L., Holmes, D.D. and Hinshaw, L.B., Physiological Changes in the Dog Anesthetized with Thiamylal and Enflurane, *Lab. Anim. Sci.*, 27, 383, 1977.

36. Buelke-Sam, J., Holson, J.F., Bazare, J.J. and Young, J.F., Comparative Stability of Physiological Parameters During Sustained Anesthesia in Rats, *Lab. Anim. Sci.*, 28, 157, 1987.

37. Turner, T.T. and Howards, S.S., Hyperglycemia in the Hamster Anesthetized with Inactin (5-Ethyl-5-(1-Methyl Propyl)-2-Thiobarbiturate), *Lab. Anim. Sci.*, 27, 380, 1977.

38. Sage, M.D., West, E.J. and Gavin, J.B., Cardiac Performance of Isolated Beating Hearts Obtained from Rats Anesthetized by Three Different Agents, *Lab. Anim. Sci.*, 35, 153, 1985.

39. Holtzgrefe, H.H., Everitt, J.M. and Wright, E.M., Alpha-Chloralose as a Canine Anesthetic, *Lab. Anim. Sci.*, 37, 587, 1987.

40. Svendsen, P., Ainsworth, M.A. and Carter, A.M., Acid-Base Status and Cardiovascular Function in Pigs Anaesthetized with alpha-Chloralose, *Scand. J. Lab. Anim. Sci.*, 17, 89, 1990.

41. Collando, P.S., Poso-Andrada, M.J., Gonzáles, J., Jimérez, R. and Esteller, A., Effect of Pentobarbital or Urethane on Bile Secretion and Chemical Composition of Blood in the Rabbit, *Lab. Anim.*, 21, 11, 1987.

42. Reid, W.D., Davies, C., Pare, P.D. and Pardy, R.L., An Effective Combination of Anaesthetics for 6-hours Experimentation in the Golden Syrian Hamster, *Lab. Anim.*, 23, 156, 1989.

43. Wright, M., Pharmacological Effects of Ketamine and its use in Veterinary Medicine, *J. Am. Vet. Med. Assoc.*, 180, 1462, 1982.

44. Hsu, W.H. and Lu, Z.-X., Effect of Yohimbine on Xylazine-Ketamine Anesthesia in Cats, *J. Am. Vet. Med. Assoc.*, 185, 886, 1984.

45. Brown, M.J., McCarthy, T.J. and Bennett, B.T., Long Term Anesthesia Using a Continuous Infusion of Guaifenesin, Ketamine and Xylazine in Cats, *Lab. Anim. Sci.*, 41, 46, 1991.

46. Hawkey, C.M., Dean, S. and Hart, M.G., The Influence of Anaesthetics on the Haematology of the Patas Monkey, Erythrocebus patas, *Lab. Anim.*, 12, 167, 1978.

47. Seifen, A.B., Kennedy, R.H., Bray, J.P. and Seifen, E., Estimation of Minimum Alveolar Concentration (MAC) for Halothane, Enflurane and Isoflurane in Spontaneously Breathing Guinea Pigs, *Lab. Anim. Sci.*, 39, 579, 1989.

48. Tranquilli, W.J., Thurmon, J.C., Benson, G.J. and Steffy, E.P., Halothane potency in pigs (Sus scrofa), *Am. J. Vet. Res.*, 44, 1106, 1983.

49. Harrison, G.G., Saunders, S.J., Biebuyck, J.F., Hickman, R., Dent, D.M., Weaver, V. and Terblanche, J., Anaesthetic-induced Malignant Hyperthermia and a Method for its Prediction, *Br. J. Anaesth.*, 41, 844, 1969.

50. Gronert, G.A. and Theye, R.A., Halothane-Induced Porcine Malignant Hyperthermia: Metabolic and Hemodynamig Changes, *Anesthesiology*, 44, 36, 1976.

51. Nelson, T.E., Jones, E.W., Henrickson, R.L., Falk, S.N. and Kerr, D.D., Porcine Malignant Hyperthermia: Observations on the Occurrence of Pale, Soft, Exudative Musculature Among Susceptible Pigs, *Am. J. Vet. Res.*, 35, 347, 1974.

52. Sybesma, W. and Eikelenbloom, G., Malignant Hyperthermia Syndrome in Pigs, *Neth. J. Vet. Sci.*, 2, 155, 1969.

53. Becker, M. and Beglinger, R., Hämodynamische, kardiale und respiratorische Veränderungen unter Enfluran-Mononarkose beim Göttinger Miniaturschwein, *Anaesthesist*, 31, 145, 1982.

54. Eisele, P.H., Talken, L. and Eisele, J.H., Jr., Potency of Isoflurane and Nitrous Oxide in Conventional Swine, *Lab. Anim. Sci.*, 35, 76, 1985.

55. Cole, D.J., Marcantonio, S. and Drummond, J.C., Anesthetic Requirement of Isoflurane is Reduced in Hypertensive and Wistar-Kyoto Rats, *Lab. Anim. Sci.*, 40, 506, 1990.

56. Eisele, P.H., Woodle, E.S., Hunter, G.C., Talken, L. and Ward, R.E., Anesthetic, Preoperative and Postoperative Considerations for Liver Transplantation in Swine, *Lab. Anim. Sci.*, 36, 402, 1986.

57. Bett, N.J., Hynd, J.W. and Green, C.J., Successful Anaesthesia and Small-Bowel Anastomosis in the Guinea Pig, *Lab. Anim.*, 14, 225, 1980.

58. Heidt, G.A., A Portable Anesthesia Chamber for Intractable Small Mammals, *Lab. Anim. Sci.*, 28, 212, 1978.

59. Watson, R.T. and McLeod, K., Inhalation Anesthesia With Methoxyflurane for Guinea Pig Ear Surgery, *Arch. Otolaryngol.*, 104, 179, 1978.

60. Mulder, J.B. and Hauser, J.J., A Closed Anesthetic System for Small Laboratory Animals, *Lab. Anim. Sci.*, 34, 77, 1984.

61. Levy, D.E., Zwies, A. and Duffy, T.E., A Mask for Delivery of Inhalation Gasses to Small Laboratory Animals, *Lab. Anim. Sci.*, 30, 868, 1980.

62. Kent, G.M., General Anesthesia in Rabbits Using Methoxyflurane, Nitrous Oxide, and Oxygen, *Lab. Anim. Sci.*, 21, 256, 2192.

63. Wass, J.A., Keene, M.S. and Kaplan, H.M., Ketamine-Methoxyflurane Anesthesia for Rabbits, *Am. J. Vet. Res.*, 35, 317, 1974.

64. Steffey, E.P., Gillespie, J.R., Berry, J.D., Eger, E.I., II, and Munson, E.S., Anesthetic Potency (MAC) of Nitrous Oxide in the Dog, Cat, and Stump-Tail Monkey, *J. Appl. Physiol.*, 36, 530, 1974.

65. Merin, R.G., Verdouw, P.D. and de Jong, J.W., Dose-dependent Depression of Cardiac Function and Metabolism by Halothane in Swine (Sus scrofa), *Anesthesiology*, 46, 417, 1977.

66. Sartick, M., Eldrige, M.L., Johnson, J.A., Kurz, K.D., Fowler, W.L., Jr., and Payne, C.G., Recovery Rate of the Cardiovascular System in Rabbits Following Short-Term Halothane Anesthesia, *Lab. Anim. Sci.*, 29, 186, 1979.

67. Sawyer, D.C. and Lumb, W.V., Halothane Anesthesia in Miniature Swine, *Anesth. Analg., (Cleveland)*, 49, 616, 1970.

68. Roberts, F.W., Anaesthesia in Pigs, *Anaesthesia*, 26, 445, 1971.

69. Swindle, M.M., Horneffer, P.J., Gardner, T.J., Gott, V.L., Hall, T.S., Stuart, R.S., Baumgartner, W.A., Borkon, A.M., Galloway, E. and Reitz, B.A., Anatomic and Anesthetic Considerations in Experimental Cardiopulmonary Surgery in Swine, *Lab. Anim. Sci.*, 36, 357, 1986.

70. Becker, M., Anesthesia in Göttingen Miniature Swine Used for Experimental Surgery, *Lab. Anim. Sci.*, 36, 417, 1986.

71. Flecknell, P.A., Liles, J.H. and Williamson, H.A., The Use of Lignocaine-Prilocaine Local Anaesthetic Cream for Pain-Free Venepuncture in Laboratory Animals, *Lab. Anim.*, 24, 142, 1990.

72. Marshall, M., Intubationsspatel für Miniaturschweine, *Zbl. Vet. Med.*, 21, 84, 1974.

73. Kissinger, J.T. and Hughes, H.C., Fabrication Methods for Endotracheal Tubes for Sheep, Goats, and Calves, *Lab. Anim. Sci.*, 34, 97, 1984.

74. Davis, N.L. and Malinin, T.I., Rabbit Intubation and Halothane Anesthesia, *Lab. Anim. Sci.*, 24, 617, 1974.

75. Lindquist, P.A., Induction of Methoxyflurane Anesthesia in the Rabbit after Ketamine Hydrochloride and Endotracheal Intubation, *Lab. Anim. Sci.*, 22, 898, 1972.

76. Kujime, K.K. and Natelson, B.H., A Method for Endotracheal Intubation of Guinea Pigs (Cavia porcellus), *Lab. Anim. Sci.*, 31, 715, 1981.

77. Alpert, M., Goldstein, D. and Triner, L., Technique of Endotracheal Intubation in Rats, *Lab. Anim. Sci.*, 32, 78, 1982.

78. Thet, L.A., A Simple Method for Intubating Rats Under Direct Vision, *Lab. Anim. Sci.*, 33, 368, 1983.

79. Kyle, O.C., Novak, S. and Bolooki, H., General Anesthesia in Pigs, *Lab. Anim. Sci.*, 29, 123, 1979.

80. Wagner, A.J., The Porcine Stress Syndrome, *Vet. Med. Rev.*, 1, 68, 1972.

81. Gronert, G.A., Milde, J.H., Theye, R.A. and Bahlman, S.H., Dantrolene in Porcine Malignant Hyperthermia, *Anesthesiology*, 44, 488, 1976.

82. Flewellen, E.H. and Nelson, T.E., Dantrolene Dose Response in Malignant Hyperthermia-Susceptible (MHS) Swine, *Anesthesiology*, 52, 303, 1980.

83. Harrison, G.G., The Prophylaxis of Malignant Hyperthermia by Oral Dantrolene Sodium in Swine, *Br. J. Anaesth.*, 49, 315, 1977.

84. Hall, G.M., Lucke, J.N. and Lister, D., Treatment of Porcine Malignant Hyperpyrexia. The Successful Use of Dantrolene in the Pietrain Pig, *Anaesthesia*, 32, 472, 1977.

85. Glen, J.B., Cliff, G.S. and Jamieson, A., Evaluation of a Scavenging System for Use with Inhalation Anaesthesia Techniques in Rats, *Lab. Anim.*, 14, 207, 1980.

86. Green, C.J., Anaesthetic Gasses and Health Risks to Laboratory Personel: a Review, *Lab. Anim.*, 15, 397, 1981.

87. Kumar, A. and McCullough, N., General Anesthesia for Newborn Pigs, *Lab. Anim. Sci.*, 29, 251, 1979.

88. Hoyt, R.F., Hayre, M.D., Dodd, K.T. and Phillips, Y.Y., Long-Acting Intramuscular Anesthetic Regimen for Swine, *Lab. Anim. Sci.*, 36, 413, 1986.

89. Trim, C.M. and Gilroy, B.A., Cardiopulmonary Effects of a Xylazine and Ketamine Combination in Pigs, *Res. Vet. Sci.*, 38, 30, 1985.

90. Rubal, B.J. and Buchanan, C., Supplemental Chloralose Anesthesia in Morphine Premedicated dogs, *Lab. Anim. Sci.*, 36, 59, 1986.

91. Grad, R., Witten, M.L., Quan, S.F., McKelvie, D.H. and Lemen, R.J., Intravenous Chloralose is a Safe Anesthetic for Longitudinal Use in Beagle Puppies, *Lab. Anim. Sci.*, 38, 422, 1988.

92. Flecknell, P.A., Hooper, T.L., Fetherstony, G., Locke, T.J. and McGregor, C.G.A., Long-Term Anaesthesia with Alfentanil and Midazolam for Lung Transplantation in the Dog, *Lab. Anim.*, 23, 278, 1989.

93. Blane, G.F., Boura, A.L.A., Fitzgerald, A.E. and Lister, R.E., Actions of Etorphine Hydrochloride, (M99): A Potent Motphine-Like Agent, *Br. J. Pharmacol. Chemother.*, 30, 11, 1967.

94. Reutlinger, R.A., Karl, A.A., Vinal, S.I. and Nieser, M.J., Effects of Ketamine HCl-Xylazine HCl Combinations on Cardiovascular and Pulmonary Values of the Rhesus Macaque (Macaca mulatta), *Am. J. Vet. Res.*, 41, 1453, 1980.

95. April, M., Tabor, E. and Gerety, R.J., Combination of Ketamine and Xylazine for Effective Anaesthesia of Juvenile Chimpanzees (Pan troglodytes), *Lab. Anim.*, 16, 116, 1982.

96. Naccarto, E.F. and Hunter, W.S., Anaesthetic Effects of Various Ratios of Ketamine and Xylazine in Rhesus Monkeys (Macaca mulatta), *Lab. Anim.*, 13, 317, 1979.

97. Bankneider, A.R., Phillips, J.M., Jackson, K.T. and Vinal, S.I., Jr., Comparison of Ketamine with the Combination of Ketamine and Xylazine for Effective Anesthesia in the Rhesus Monkey (Macaca mulatta), *Lab. Anim. Sci.*, 28, 742, 1978.

98. Cookson, J.H. and Mills, F.J., Continuous Infusion Anaesthesia in Baboons with Alpha-xolone-Alphadolone, *Lab. Anim.*, 17, 196, 1983.

99. Kisloff, B., Ketamine-Paraldehyde Anesthesia for Rabbits, *Am. J. Vet. Res.*, 36, 1033, 1975.

100. Morgan, W.W., Morlan, S.L., Krupp, J.H. and Rosenkrantz, J.G., Pentobarbital Anesthesia in the Rabbit, *Am. J. Vet. Res.*, 27, 1133, 1966.

101. Dhasmana, K.M., Saxena, P.R., Prakash, O. and Van Der Zee, H.T., A Study on the Influence of Ketamine on Systemic and Regional Haemodynamics in Conscious Rabbits, *Arch. Int. Pharmacodyn.*, 269, 323, 1984.

102. Wyatt, J.D., Scott, R.A.W. and Richardson, M.E., The Effects of Prolonged Ketamine-Xylazine Intravenous Infusion on Arterial Blood pH, Blood Gases, Mean Arterial Blood Pressure, Heart and Respiratory Rates, Rectal Temperature and Reflexes in the Rabbit, *Lab. Anim. Sci.*, 39, 411, 1989.

103. Brown, R.H. and Ferner, W.T., The Use of Xylazine-Ketamine Anesthetic for Intraocular Surgery on Rabbits, *Am. J. Ophthalmol.*, 99, 614, 1985.

104. Popilskis, S.J., Oz, M.C., Gorman, P., Florestal, A. and Kohn, D.F., Comparison of Xylazine with Tiletamine-Zolazepam (Telazol) and Xylazine-Ketamine Anesthesia in Rabbits, *Lab. Anim. Sci.*, 41, 51, 1991.

105. Ludders, J.W., Thomas, C.B., Sharp, P. and Sedgwick, C.J., An Anesthetic Technique for Repeated Collection of Blood from New Zealand White Rabbits, *Lab. Anim. Sci.*, 37, 803, 1987.

106. Mulder, J.B., Anesthesia in the Rabbit Using a Combination of Ketamine and Promazine, *Lab. Anim. Sci.*, 28, 321, 1978.

107. Green, C.J., Halsey, M.J., Precious, S. and Wardley-Smith, B., Alphaxolone-Alphadolone Anaesthesia in Laboratory Animals, *Lab. Anim.*, 12, 85, 1978.

108. Olson, M.E., A Simple Anesthetic Chamber, *Lab. Anim. Sci.*, 36, 703, 1986.

109. Franz, D.R. and Dixon, R.S., A Mask System for Halothane Anesthesia of Guinea Pigs, *Lab. Anim. Sci.*, 38, 743, 1988.

110. Hart, M.V., Rowles, J.R., Hohimer, A.R., Morton, M.J. and Hosenpud, J.D., Hemodynamics in the Guinea Pig after Anesthetization with Ketamine/Xylazine, *Am. J. Vet. Res.*, 45, 2328, 1984.

111. Mårtensson, L. and Carter, A.M., Distribution of Cardiac Output in the Late Pregnant Guinea Pig During Anaesthesia with Ketamine, *Z. Versuchstierkd.*, 26, 175, 1984.

112. Rosso, P. and Bassi, J.A., Ketamine-Pentobarbital Maternal Anesthesia and Fetal Survival in the Guinea Pig, *Anesth. Analg., (Cleveland),* 56, 472, 1977.
113. Green, C.J., Neuroleptanalgesic Drug Combinations in the Anaesthetic Management of Small Laboratory Animals, *Lab. Anim.,* 9, 161, 1975.
114. Ventrone, R., Baan, E. and Coggins, C.R.E., Novel Inhalation Device for the Simultaneous Anaesthesia of Several Laboratory Rodents, *Lab. Anim.,* 16, 231, 1982.
115. Matthews, H.B., A Simple Method for Extending the Period of Surgical Anesthesia in Rats, *Lab. Anim. Sci.,* 28, 720, 1978.
116. Fisker, A.V., Stage, I. and Philipsen, H.P., Use of Etorphine-Acepromazine and Diprenorphine in Reversible Neuroleptanalgesia of Rats, *Lab. Anim.,* 16, 109, 1982.

Chapter 20

The Treatment of Pain and Suffering in Laboratory Animals

Adrian J. Smith

CONTENTS

INTRODUCTION

Our ethical commitments embodied in the three Rs of Russell and Burch,[1] working for the *R*eplacement, *R*eduction, and *R*efinement of animal experiments, demand strict standards for the prevention of pain and suffering. There is little point in striving for top microbiological and genetic quality if laboratory animals experience their surroundings as stressful, in the widest sense of the word.

DEFINITION OF PAIN AND SUFFERING

Many experiments on laboratory animals have, as the British Animals (Scientific Procedures) Act of 1986[2] states, "the effect of causing pain, suffering, distress or lasting harm". Defining such terms, which have such strong subjective overtones in humans, is an awesome task. Some of the problems associated with defining pain in animals have recently been reviewed by Wall.[3] The International Association for the Study of Pain has defined pain as "an unpleasant sensory and emotional experience associated with actual or potential tissue damage or described in terms of such damage".[4] In addition to variations in severity, pain may be acute or of chronic duration. Pain is also a perception, not just a physical phenomenon, and therefore requires a functional cerebral cortex and a state of consciousness.[5]

The word "suffering" originates from the Latin indicating the carriage of a burden, implying the endurance of a condition that is painful, distressing or injurious. Suffering implies a degree of continuing mental distress, which may, but not necessarily, come as an added burden to a pathological lesion.[6]

Satisfactory management of pain and suffering in laboratory animals is first achieved when all components of a state of *dis*-ease have been removed.

Society often exhibits highly inconsequent attitudes to animals, consciously or otherwise, which can easily prejudice the treatment the animals in question receive. This may lead, for example, to better pain control in the larger or more vociferous laboratory animals, or those we often keep in our homes. Companion animals are, perhaps, all other things being equal, *less* likely to suffer in the laboratory than other species, since it is likely that these human-animal bonds will be especially well nurtured. It may indeed be necessary to remind researchers that mice and rats have, despite traditional prejudice about the spread of disease and difficulty of handling, an ability to feel pain and to suffer that is comparable with other vertebrates. Species variations among vertebrates probably consist more of variations in the animals' ability to feel anxiety about the risk of an unpleasant experience as yet in the future. This potential for suffering can be assumed to be related to the size of the cerebral cortex, or to the degree of what has been called encephalization.[7]

Our understanding of pain and suffering in non-mammals is woefully inadequate. Research suggests that fish can experience pain and fear.[8] Attitudes to the possibility of pain perception in invertebrates are also under revision.[9] Cephalopods and some higher invertebrates are now believed to have nervous systems that are as well developed as some vertebrates, thereby warranting their inclusion in categories of invasiveness normally reserved for vertebrate species. Indeed, the Universities Federation for Animal Welfare in Britain has published a handbook on the care and management of cephalopods in the laboratory.[10] Furthermore, Wigglesworth states that it should be assumed that insects feel pain and that they should be narcotized for potentially painful experiments.[11]

A result of this laudable interest in the welfare of species to whom we have previously given little thought, is that they may be afforded better protection as laboratory animals than that they might experience in the wild.

THE PHYSIOLOGY OF PAIN

Accurate and repeatable observations on the physiology of pain and the effects of nociceptive stimuli are still equally inaccessible as a scientific instrument ("dolorimeter") that can measure pain objectively. Human experience teaches us that different organs are sensitive to different pain thresholds, and differences in sensitivity have been described in connection with assessing the severity of scientific procedures on laboratory animals.[12] Human studies show also that the perception of pain is not necessarily related to the external appearance or extent of the injury.[13] Perception of pain involves:[3]

1. Injury or tissue damage that stimulates nerve impulses in specialized sensory fibers
2. The entry of these nerve impulses into the central nervous system where they provoke:
   a. Local muscle reflexes
   b. Autonomic reflexes affecting among other things blood pressure, heart rate and respiration
   c. Endocrine responses in, among other organs, the pituitary and adrenal glands
   d. Ascending afferent impulses to the thalamus and cerebral cortex
3. A "pure sensation" of pain provoked by the arrival of these impulses in the thalamus and cortex
4. The assessment by the mind of the meaning of this sensation in terms of past experience, the present situation and future expectations, which together results in behavioral events, including vocalization

More extensive coverage of the subject is available.[14-17]

ASSESSMENT OF PAIN AND SUFFERING

A rapid and correct diagnosis is always a prerequisite for efficient treatment. Accurate diagnosis is dependent upon regular observation by personnel who are trained in the characteristic behavioral patterns of each species. Symptoms of distress can vary markedly between species, depending in part upon whether the species is naturally aggressive or vociferous. Several noteworthy efforts at producing both guidelines for recognizing and assessing pain in animals[18,19] and estimates of the likely severity of scientific procedures[12] have been prepared. Methods of scoring changes in variables associated with pain have also been designed, such as the Disturbance Index for assessing the severity of procedures in rodents.[20] There can, however, be considerable variations between assessors in the assignment of scores.[21] Ultimately, there is no substitute for the regular observation of laboratory animals by personnel trained for the species in question. In the context of pain research, it has been suggested that investigators should be subjected to the same degree of pain inflicted by the nociceptive test to be employed.[22]

SIGNS OF ACUTE PAIN

Considerable variations may be seen between species, and also within species depending upon the individual's pain threshold. The degree of vocalization in a stressful situation can, for example, vary considerably between species, without this necessarily being a reflection of differences in pain perception.[12] Observations should therefore be carried out without the animal being aware that it is being observed, since fear or arousal provoked by the presence of humans can stimulate behavior that will mask signs of pain.

In general, signs of pain may include:

- Hyperactivity, inactivity, recumbency, social withdrawal
- An increase or decrease in vocalization
- Changes in feed and water intake, and feeding patterns
- Aggressive or defensive behavior, directed towards other individuals, offspring (cannibalism), or the individual itself (self-mutilation)
- Changes in behavioral patterns such as foraging, grooming, exercising, sexual activity, and sleep
- Changes in body temperature

Detailed descriptions of signs of pain and distress in the individual species are provided in the reports mentioned above. Many laboratory animal species are originally nocturnal and may therefore naturally appear sleepy in the daytime, but both pain and boredom can result in abnormal lethargy.

CHRONIC PAIN AND SUFFERING

Chronic pain and discomfort may induce only subtle changes that are difficult to detect without running specific tests.[12] Here it is especially important for animal caretakers to have a good knowledge of the species under their care. In addition to suffering brought about by somatic pain, animals may suffer because of less obvious changes in the environment such as changes in cage type, the number of animals housed together, or vicinity to species with which they naturally interact (predators or competitors). The ability, particularly in companion animals, to communicate sensations to its handler may also improve the animal's situation, in the same way as human distress can be alleviated by the mere act of sharing one's feelings with others.

In conclusion, although our knowledge of animals' experience of pain and distress is woefully inadequate, we should be sufficiently anthropomorphic to give the animal the benefit of the doubt, and ask ourselves if we would feel pain in a similar situation. We must also be prepared to change our standards regularly, as our understanding of how animals perceive their environment improves.

THE PREVENTION OF PAIN AND SUFFERING IN LABORATORY ANIMALS

Stressors likely to cause pain or suffering in laboratory animals may be broadly divided into environmental conditions and experimental techniques.

ENVIRONMENTAL CONDITIONS

Modern laboratory animal practice often involves the acquisition of purpose-bred animals from an external breeding establishment. Animals therefore stand the risk of experiencing a wide range of potentially stressing events even before the experiment starts. These may include:

- Transport to the laboratory animal unit
- Changes in group size, disturbing established social hierarchies
- The stress of isolation
- New and unfamiliar human contacts with technicians and research workers
- Changes in housing such as temperature, humidity and lighting
- Changes in feeding routines and diet

Stress felt by one animal can rapidly be communicated to other animals by means of olfactory stimuli (pheromones) and behavioral cues such as rapid movement and vocalization. Sudden or persistent noise sources, such as bells, computers, fans and water pipes, particularly those generating ultrasound, should be avoided. Researchers should only have access to their own animals, and as much routine work as possible should be performed by technicians with whom the animals are familiar. An acclimatization period of 7 to 10 days before the experiment should always be provided. This period should be used actively to familiarize the animals to their new environment, among other things by regular handling. This positive reinforcement may even reduce the necessity for pain-killers in minor manipulations during the experiment itself.

EXPERIMENTAL TECHNIQUES

Animal handling — The "element of surprise" should be made use of whenever possible. Drug injection need not involve more disturbance to the animal than a rapid fixation of the injection site with virtually simultaneous injection. Preparatory work, such as filling syringes, should be performed out of the animal's sight and hearing. Where possible, procedures should be carried out in the animal's own environment, and it should often be unnecessary to remove it from its cage. However, it is important to consider the possibility of a treatment disturbing other animals in the room, via the sight, sound or smell of the individual being treated. This potential for fear is perhaps greatest in the case of small laboratory animals, where it is more difficult for the animal handler to induce a calming effect than when handling, for example, dogs and cats. Treatment should therefore if possible be undertaken in an adjoining room to which the animal's cage can easily be moved. Some animal handlers undoubtedly induce a greater sense of calm and confidence in animals than others. The use of tranquilizers should be considered, even for relatively painless procedures such as blood sampling and close inspection of the body, since restraint can be a potent stressor, particularly in rodents. Frequent handling can often be avoided by the use of catheterization or radiotelemetry to collect physiological data. These techniques will in addition give more physiologically normal measurements of parameters such as heart rate, body temperature and plasma hormone concentrations.

Injection techniques and blood sampling — The intramuscular and intraperitoneal injection routes should be avoided wherever possible, since these are likely to be more painful than subcutaneous injections. The area around the injection site should be lightly massaged afterwards to reduce pain. The volume injected must be compatible with the space available, to avoid overstretching muscle, the subcutaneous space or peritoneum. Injectables should be warmed to body temperature if their volume is significant, and they must be administered at correct osmotic pressure and be non-irritant wherever possible. A single blood sample from a healthy animal should not exceed 10% of the animal's blood volume, which is in turn approximately 7% of its body weight. If repeated sampling is indicated, the animal's hematological status must be monitored closely. Cardiac puncture should only be performed on an animal that is fully anesthetized and which does not awake from that anesthesia. Retro-orbital puncture should not be used. These two techniques convey a risk of leakage of blood to the surrounding space which can probably cause considerable pain and, in the case of cardiac puncture, be fatal.

Anesthesia — The effective use of anesthetics, and the unhesitating use of methods of euthanasia that rapidly produce unconsciousness, will abolish much pain in laboratory animals. It is of paramount importance, however, that the animal concerned is capable of relaying its feelings to the observer. Thus, neuromuscular blockers that paralyze the animal without depressing its consciousness must never be used except in conjunction with an anesthetic regime that has been proven to provide satisfactory anesthesia *without* the blocker. Premedication can alleviate a lot of anxiety and pain and will often result in a smoother recovery from anesthesia. Agents that have an analgesic component should always be preferred. Provision should always be made during an operation for the rapid administration of pain-killers: surface veins may become difficult to enter due to low blood pressure resulting from shock or deep anesthesia, so catheters should be inserted in advance.

Surgery — Surgical intervention is a major potential cause of pain. The need for postoperative analgesia can, however, be minimized by reducing physical trauma to the animal during surgery and maintaining it under adequate anesthesia. The attainment of these conditions is discussed in more detail elsewhere in this book.

Postoperative care — Good postoperative care, planned in advance, can spare animals much suffering. It is important to make realistic estimates of the time taken to undertake a procedure, so that this work is not neglected or handed over to inexperienced personnel. The administration of fluids at body temperature, attention to electrolyte balance, rest and a calm and comfortable, warm environment will all contribute to a less painful postoperative period. Administration of certain antibiotics under anesthesia may, however, unduly prolong the anesthesia.[23] Postoperative analgesics, on the other hand, *should* be administered before the animal recovers, so that it is free from pain from the moment it wakes up. It must also be remembered that chemical reversal of sedation or anesthesia, which is nowadays often part of an operative procedure, may lead to a simultaneous reversal of analgesia: adequate pain relief must then be provided using other drugs if there is any chance of pain being present.

Specific techniques — Antibody production, and in particular the raising of polyclonal antibodies, has often been carried out using techniques that owe more to established practice than scientifically justified method. Antibody production is potentially a cause of considerable pain and suffering, dependent upon, among other things, the choice of injection site and adjuvant. Monoclonal antibody production *in vivo* should be strictly limited to those situations where *in vitro* production is impossible. Freund's adjuvant should only be used where it is essential. Detailed guidelines for both monoclonal and polyclonal antibody production should be an integral part of good laboratory practice. Similar considerations apply to the use of laboratory animals in cancer research. Guidelines such as those developed by the United Kingdom Coordinating Committee on Cancer Research (UKCCCR)[24] should be implemented locally.

Many of the animal models described in this book involve procedures which have the potential for inducing pain or suffering. Each model must be scrutinized before use, and followed closely at the individual laboratory.

The control of pain and suffering in laboratory animals demands much of the individual experimenter and animal technician in the form of ethical awareness. A major part of the treatment of pain and suffering is the planning of experiments that minimize or eradicate the possibility of pain.

DRUGS USED FOR THE TREATMENT OF PAIN

Unfortunately, the relief of pain and suffering in animals is one of the areas of veterinary medicine that is most in need of attention. The specific suggestions given below will undoubtedly need some revision as our knowledge in this field increases. No one drug will satisfy all requirements for analgesia in laboratory animal medicine. Interspecies differences in anatomy, physiology, pharmacology, nutritional needs, and, not least, temperament must all be taken into account. Within a species, the individual's biological rhythms and stage of life will also be of importance. It is essential to be familiar with basic data on physiological parameters such as body temperature, respiration rate, pulse, appearance and behavior, and their normal variation limits even when the animal is not stressed. Inbred strains of laboratory animals may show remarkably different values.

GENERAL CONSIDERATIONS IN THE USE OF ANALGESICS

Many analgesics relevant to laboratory animal medicine may not be readily available. It is therefore imperative to plan potentially painful procedures well in advance. Standard Operating Procedures (SOPs) with details of standard analgesic regimens should be made available to the staff. Animal houses should always display the names and telephone numbers of at least two veterinarians or other qualified staff members in case of an acute need for analgesia. This information must be available not only to animal caretakers who may feel unable to cope with the situation themselves, but also to other staff members such as security officers and cleaning personnel who may coincidentally discover unacceptable situations.

CHOICE OF ANALGESIC

The use of analgesics in laboratory animal science is occasionally questioned by researchers who are afraid that such drugs may interfere with the results they are attempting to obtain. The primary responsibility of the animal caretaker is, however, to provide adequate analgesia. It must be the researcher's responsibility, not that of the animal caretaker, to examine the literature for possible evidence that the proposed analgesic cannot be used. The possible side-effects of *postoperative* analgesia should, anyway, have little bearing on the experiment, since an adequate postoperative period of several days should be provided before the animal is subjected to the experiment itself, during which time the effects of these analgesics will have worn off.

Pain-killing drugs can broadly be divided into three categories:

Narcotic analgesics: These cause a certain amount of depression of the central nervous system (CNS), depending on the species, at the same time as being potent analgesics. The group includes the opioids morphine, pethidine, etorphine, fentanyl, and buprenorphine.

Antipyretic analgesics: These are also known as non-steroidal anti-inflammatory drugs (NSAIDs) and include acetylsalicylic acid (aspirin), flunixin, paracetamol and phenacetin.

Nociceptive blockers: Local anesthetics and alpha-2 adrenoceptor agonists such as xylazine and medetomidine block impulses from pain receptors (nociceptors). Some, such as the alpha-2 agonists, are also CNS depressants, the degree of depression depending upon the species concerned and dosage. CNS depression in itself is, however, no guarantee of pain relief.

METHODS APPLIED TO THE DIFFERENT SPECIES

TREATMENT OF ACUTE PAIN

Many excellent reviews of analgesics for laboratory animal use are available.[25-29] Table 1 gives a list of relevant drugs for laboratory animal purposes, and suggested doses. The choice of drug will be determined, among other things, by the degree of analgesia needed, its required duration, experimental design and the user's personal experience with analgesic drugs in the relevant species. Pure μ agonists such as morphine are to be preferred in cases of severe pain.[26] Buprenorphine is recommended in particular because of its potent analgesic effect and long duration. Care should be taken, however, not to administer opioids to animals that are not in pain, as they may depress them unnecessarily, which can lead to reduced food intake.[30] There is little data available, particularly for the small laboratory animal species, to give firm recommendations as to which NSAID should be used, or to their dosing frequency. Estimates must therefore often be based on experience from other species. Flunixin appears to be more potent and longer-lasting, but it has primarily been tested in non-rodents.[31]

Local anesthetics are frequently used for surgical purposes, for example where opioids are contraindicated, by infiltrating the incision site or by blocking the sensory nerves from that area. Their value is that they give minimal disturbance to the animal's physiology. The animal can, however, feel pain when the local nerve block wears off, and an NSAID should be administered 6 hours postoperatively to provide analgesia.[26] Local anesthestics can, however, also be used to provide effective short-term analgesia. For example, local anesthetic cream can be applied to the skin over a blood vessel before venipuncture.[32]

The provision of continuous analgesia necessitates an adequate number of trained staff in the animal unit. As an alternative to frequent injections, which themselves can be painful, infusion pumps can be used, either fastened to the animal or attached by a catheter. Administration of analgesics in the feed or water is simple and inexpensive, assuming that the animal has not reduced its consumption because of immobility caused by pain.[26]

TREATMENT OF CHRONIC PAIN

Repeated administration of NSAIDs is recommended if the experimental protocol does not preclude them.[26] Treatment should be kept at a low dose to avoid side effects. They may be administered in the drinking water, and appropriate doses can be calculated if water intake is monitored. Prolonged analgesia can also be achieved by administering buprenorphine in drinking water,[33] but tolerance to opioids can develop. Drug administration in the drinking water may, however, pose problems since it has been observed (Liles and Flecknell, personal communication) that rats may limit their water intake to the dark periods of the diurnal cycle, opening the possibility of periods without adequate analgesia.

EUTHANASIA

INDICATIONS, EVALUATION OF METHODS AVAILABLE

Euthanasia is an acceptable resort in the treatment of animal suffering. The treatment of pain in animals is therefore not complete without a discussion of methods of euthanasia for the different animal species. These methods must ensure a *rapid, irreversible, loss of consciousness*, the time thereafter taken to kill the animal being of less importance.

Euthanasia usually necessitates some form of physical control over the animal, to minimize the risk of the animal suffering during the euthanasia and of human onlookers being harmed. The degree of control will be dependent upon the species, breed, size, degree of tameness, presence or absence of painful disease or injury, the animal's degree of excitation and the method of euthanasia. It is, however, a

Table 1. Suggested analgesics for use in laboratory animals.

	Mouse	Rat	Guinea pig	Rabbit
Aspirin	120 mg/kg per os 4 hourly	100 mg/kg per os 4 hourly	85 mg/kg per os ? 4 hourly	100 mg/kg per os ? 4 hourly
Buprenorphine	0.05-0.1 mg/kg s.c. 8-12 hourly	0.01-0.05 mg/kg s.c. 8-12 hourly	0.05 mg/kg s.c. 8-12 hourly	0.01-0.05 mg/kg s.c., i.v. 8-12 hourly
Butorphanol	1-5 mg/kg s.c. 4 hourly	2.0 mg/kg s.c. 4 hourly		0.1-0.5 mg/kg i.v. 4 hourly
Codeine	60-90 mg/kg per os or 20 mg/kg s.c. 4 hourly	60 mg/kg 4 hourly		
Diclofenac	8 mg/kg per os	10 mg/kg per os	2.1 mg/kg per os	
Flufenamic acid		5 mg/kg per os	30 mg/kg per os	
Flunixin	2.5 mg/kg s.c. ? 12 hourly	2.5 mg/kg s.c. 12 hourly		1.1 mg/kg s.c. ?12 hourly
Ibuprofen	30 mg/kg per os ? 4 hourly	15 mg/kg per os ? 4 hourly	10 mg/kg i.m.	10 mg/kg i.v. ? 4 hourly
Indomethacin	1 mg/kg per os	2 mg/kg per os	2.5-8.8 mg/kg per os	12.5 mg/kg per os
Mefenamic acid			224 mg/kg per os	
Morphine	2–5 mg/kg s.c. 2–4 hourly	2–5 mg/kg s.c. 2–4 hourly	2–5 mg/kg s.c. 4 hourly	2–5 mg/kg s.c. 2–4 hourly
Nalbuphine	4–8 mg/kg s.c. ?4 hourly	1–2 mg/kg s.c. 3 hourly		1–2 mg/kg i.v. 4–5 hourly

Table 1. Suggested analgesics for use in laboratory animals (continued)

	Mouse	Rat	Guinea pig	Rabbit
Naproxen			14.9 mg/kg per os	
Paracetamol	200 mg/kg per os 4 hourly	200 mg/kg per os 4 hourly		
Pentazocine	10 mg/kg s.c. 3–4 hourly	10 mg/kg s.c. 3–4 hourly		5 mg/kg i.v. 2–4 hourly
Pethidine	10–20 mg/kg s.c. 2–3 hourly	10–20 mg/kg s.c. 2–3 hourly	10–20 mg/kg s.c. 2–3 hourly	10–20 mg/kg s.c. 2–3 hourly
Phenylbutazone	30 mg/kg per os	20 mg/kg per os	40 mg/kg per os	
Piroxicam	3 mg/kg per os	3 mg/kg per os	5.7 mg/kg per os	
Suprofen	25 mg/kg per os			
Tenoxicam		10 mg/kg per os	7.2 mg/kg per os	

	Cat	Dog	Pig	Sheep	Primate
Aspirin	Toxic	10 mg/kg per os 6 hourly			20 mg/kg per os 6 hourly
Buprenorphine	0.005–0.01 mg/kg s.c., i.v. 8–12 hourly	0.01–0.02 mg/kg s.c., i.v. 8–12 hourly	0.005–0.01 mg/kg i.m. 8–12 hourly	0.005–0.01 mg/kg i.m. 4–6 hourly	0.01 mg/kg i.m., i.v. 8–12 hourly
Butorphanol	0.4 mg/kg s.c. 3–4 hourly	0.4 mg/kg s.c. 3–4 hourly			

Codeine	0.25-0.5 mg/kg per os 6 hourly with Paracetamol				
Flunixin	1 mg/kg s.c. daily for up to 5 days	1 mg/kg per os daily	?1 mg/kg s.c. daily	?1mg/kg s.c. daily	?2.5-10.0 mg/kg i.m. daily
Ibuprofen		5-10 mg/kg per os 24-48 hourly			
Morphine	0.1 mg/kg s.c. 4 hourly	0.5-5.0 mg/kg s.c. 4 hourly	up to 20 mg total dose i.m. 4 hourly	10 mg s.c. 4 hourly	1-2 mg/kg s.c. 4 hourly
Nalbuphine	1.5-3.0 mg/kg i.v. 3 hourly	0.5-2.0 mg/kg s.c. 3-8 hourly			
Paracetamol	Toxic	10-20 mg/kg per os 6 hourly with Codeine			
Pentazocine	8 mg/kg i.p. 4-6 hourly		2 mg/kg i.m. 4 hourly		2-5 mg/kg i.m. 4 hourly
Pethidine	10 mg/kg s.c. 2-3 hourly		2 mg/kg i.m. 4 hourly	200 mg total dose i.m. 4 hourly	2-4 mg/kg i.m. 3-4 hourly

Dose rates are based upon data from analgesiometry and from clinical experience. The data are taken with permission from Flecknell[26] and Liles and Flecknell.[27] It is emphasized that many of these dose rates need further clinical evaluation before full recommendation can be given. In some cases there is considered to be too little data available to be able to recommend dosing intervals. Intramuscular (i.m.) administration should be avoided, since it is likely to be more painful than, for example, the subcutaneous (s.c.) route, but it is nonetheless mentioned in the table where there is considered to be insufficient work to support recommendation of the s.c. route at this time.

prerequisite in most cases of euthanasia that the operator has a good working knowledge of methods of restraint of the species concerned.

Criteria that need to be considered in assessing a method of euthanasia include:

1. The ability of the method to kill the animal without inflicting pain or distress, i.e., ensuring a negligible delay before the induction of unconsciousness
2. The reliability of the method, i.e., absence of risk that the animal may awaken later
3. Security for personnel administering the euthanasia and onlookers, and the emotional effects on them
4. Compatibility of the method with the experiment, if animal tissue is to be examined after death
5. Economic considerations, and the time taken to carry out the procedure, especially if large numbers of animals are to be euthanized
6. The physical availability of the chemicals or mechanical aids required
7. The danger of drug abuse when using chemical methods

The time taken for a given method to kill the animal is of less importance, as long as the animal is rendered instantaneously (and irreversibly) unconscious (see 1 and 2 above), but for practical purposes it is obviously an advantage if this time interval is relatively short.

The methods available for euthanasia have been discussed widely.[34-36] These have been summarized below.[34]

Methods Causing Hypoxemia

Direct hypoxemia results from inhalation of gases such as nitrogen and carbon monoxide in the absence of oxygen. Indirect hypoxemia can also be caused by paralysis of the respiratory muscles so that the animal is incapable of inhaling. *Agents such as neuromuscular blockers that cause such a paralysis must never be used on animals that are not fully unconscious.* The same applies to agents causing cardiac arrest without cerebral depression (e.g., the i.v. injection of calcium and potassium salts).

Methods Designed to Cause a Depression of Central Nervous Function

These include anesthetic gases and injectable anesthetic agents. Choice of anesthetic should be limited to proven agents, and here the longer-acting barbiturates such as pentobarbitone are recommended. Combinations with neuromuscular blockers are not recommended for fear of paralyzing the respiratory muscles before full unconsciousness is reached. Similar constraints apply to chemicals causing cardiac arrest without affecting cerebral function. Once the animal is fully unconscious, however, any form of euthanasia may be employed. Since rather high and prolonged concentrations of anesthetic gases are often needed to produce death, it is often an advantage to kill the animal with another method after induction of anesthesia by gas.

Carbon dioxide is frequently used for euthanasia of small rodents and birds. The gas is easily available, causes no chemical contamination of tissue and is not dangerous to the operator. However, different results are often obtained by different operators, probably due to design differences in the apparatus which lead to varying gas concentrations. To ensure rapid death, the container in which the animals are gassed should be completely filled with carbon dioxide before the animals are placed there. In that case unconciousness appears within seconds, and death within minutes. Ether and chloroform are in this author's opinion no longer compatible with good laboratory practice and should not be used either as anesthetics or for euthanasia.

Methods Causing Physical Injury to the CNS

These include the oldest forms of euthanasia such as blows to the head, cervical dislocation and decapitation, and also shooting, electrical shock and rapid freezing by immersion in liquid nitrogen. The latter can only be used for extremely small organisms where one is guaranteed almost immediate loss of function. Physical insults to the CNS must be carried out in such a way that the animal is rendered immediately unconscious. For example, electrical stunning must be designed so that the electrical current passes directly and immediately through the cerebral hemispheres, concussing the animal before halting cardiac activity. It has been debated as to whether or not decapitation and cervical dislocation of rodents and rabbits are humane methods of euthanasia.[37-40] Prior use of an anesthetic, or sedation if this is not incompatible with the research protocol, is recommended when using these techniques. Decapitation by itself is not believed to produce unconsciousness in the severed heads of reptiles and amphibians.[36]

It is important to remember that the presence of movement does not necessarily mean perception of pain, and equally that the absence of movement does not necessarily mean that the animal is free from pain, as can be the case under the influence of neuromuscular blockers.

The use of sedatives, or an element of surprise, without risking injury to the animal or bystanders, should always be considered, to reduce the possibility of anxiety. Finally, the animal must not be abandoned until all doubt about its ability to recover from the euthanasia has been removed. This is best achieved by waiting until *rigor mortis* has set in. Alternatively, cardiac and respiratory function may be irreversibly impeded, such as by opening the thoracic cavity to prevent lung inflation or by severing the major blood vessels.

SUGGESTED METHODS FOR THE DIFFERENT SPECIES

Cat — Sedation with 3 to 5 mg/kg xylazine s.c. followed by i.v. injection of 1 ml/kg of a 10% solution of pentobarbitone.

Dog — Sedation with 0.3 to 0.5 mg/kg propionylpromazine s.c. followed by i.v. injection of 1 ml/kg of a 10% solution of pentobarbitone.

Guinea pig — Sedation with 0.02 mg fentanyl and 1 mg fluanisone/100 g s.c. followed by i.p. injection with 0.1 ml/100 g of a 10% solution of pentobarbitone. Alternatively, a blow to the head using a hard blunt object, after sedation, may be administered by personnel who have trained on anesthetized or dead animals. Other methods include exposure to a high concentration of halothane (5%) and the use of a physical form of euthanasia or overdose of pentobarbitone while the animal is still unconscious.

Mouse — Sedation with 0.002 mg fentanyl and 0.1 mg fluanisone/10 g s.c. followed by i.p. injection of 0.5 ml of a 10% solution of pentobarbitone. Alternatively, cervical dislocation, preferably after sedation with fentanyl/fluanisone or halothane.

Rabbit — Sedation with 0.02 mg fentanyl and 1 mg fluanisone/kg s.c. followed by i.v. injection of 1 ml/kg of a 10% solution of pentobarbitone. If adequate sedation is not achieved by the s.c. injection of fentanyl/fluanisone, the dose can be supplemented after 10 minutes by an i.v. injection of 0.02 mg fentanyl and 1 mg fluanisone (total dose, not per kilogram).

Rat — Sedation with 0.01 mg fentanyl and 0.5 mg fluanisone/100 g s.c. followed by i.p. injection of 0.2 ml/100 g of a 10% solution of pentobarbitone. Cervical dislocation after sedation with fentanyl/fluanisone may be used on rats weighing less than 50 g, but on larger animals it is difficult to ensure rapid separation of the vertebrae; the technique is, however, to be recommended under anesthesia.

CONCLUDING REMARKS

1. The treatment of pain and suffering in animals is often a case of *preventing* pain and suffering.
2. All mammals should be assumed to have the same ability to feel pain.
3. The laboratory animal must be given the benefit of the doubt when evaluating the need for analgesics or designing a research protocol. The rule must be that if a given treatment would cause pain or distress in humans, then it must be assumed that the same reaction will be provoked in animals.
4. Guidelines should be drawn up for specific procedures that have the potential to cause pain. Such guidelines are, however, never a substitute for personal assessment of the individual animal.
5. Literature studies should be performed in case the procedure has been carried out elsewhere. Experimental procedures should be reviewed regularly in the light of new experience and new literature: the acceptable, not the accepted, should always be the aim!
6. Pilot studies should be performed if there is any doubt about the pain or distress a procedure may induce. Many experimental models may be satisfactorily developed under an anesthesia from which the animals do not awaken.
7. Experienced staff recognize signs of distress and pain at an early stage. There is an ethical obligation to train animal staff and to establish clear lines of action in the event of unforeseen animal pain.
8. The question should always be asked: does the unit have the necessary competence, facilities and equipment for what is being planned?
9. The end-point of an experiment should only exceptionally be mortality or a state of continuing pain or discomfort.
10. The option of humane euthanasia exists in laboratory animal medicine. At least one, and preferably several, humane methods of euthanasia for each species being employed in the laboratory should always

be available. Availability includes the provision of staff who are competent and emotionally prepared to administer the euthanasia so that the procedure can be carried out swiftly and painlessly for the animal.

In conclusion, we can extend Jane Smith's remarks on invertebrates[9] to all animal species that they should be "kept in the best and most appropriate conditions during their lives in the laboratory; given the benefit of the doubt in procedures which have the potential to cause pain and distress; and, when the time comes, killed in the most humane manner possible". And as Polly Taylor has so aptly put it:[41] "there is no reason for an animal to tolerate pain simply because it does not complain".

ACKNOWLEDGMENT

The author wishes to express his thanks to Dr. Paul Flecknell for providing the analgesic doses and for valuable comments on the manuscript.

REFERENCES

1. Russell, W. M. S. and Burch, R. L., The *Principles of Humane Experimental Technique*, Charles C. Thomas, Springfield, Illinois, 1959.
2. Animals (Scientific Procedures) Act 1986: Act Eliz II. Ch. 14. Her Majesty's Stationery Office, London, 1986.
3. Wall, P. D., Defining "Pain in Animals", in *Animal Pain*, Short, C. E. and Van Poznak, A., Eds., Churchill Livingstone, New York, 63, 1992.
4. Merskey, H., Classification of chronic pain, *Pain*, suppl. 3, 1, 1983.
5. Spinelli, J. S., Reducing pain in laboratory animals, *Laboratory Animal Science*, 18, 65, 1987.
6. Fraser, A.F., An Analysis of Suffering, in *The Experimental Animal in Biomedical Research, Volume 1: A Survey of Scientific and Ethical Issues for Investigators*, Rollin, B. E. and Kesel, M. L., Eds., CRC Press, Boca Raton, Florida, 217, 1990.
7. Short, R. V., Primate ethics, in *Primates, The Road to Self-Sustaining Populations*, Benirschke, K., Ed., Springer-Verlag, Berlin, 1, 1986.
8. Pickering, A. D., *Stress and Fish*, Academic Press, New York, 1981.
9. Smith, J. A., A question of pain in invertebrates, *ILAR News (Institute of Laboratory Animal Resources)*, 33, 25, 1991.
10. Boyle, P. R., *The UFAW Handbook on the Care and Management of Cephalopods in the Laboratory*, Universities Federation for Animal Welfare, Potters Bar, 1991.
11. Wigglesworth, V. B., Do insects feel pain?, *Antenna*, 4, 8, 1980.
12. Report of the Laboratory Animal Science Association Working Party, The assessment and control of the severity of scientific procedures on laboratory animals, *Laboratory Animals*, 24, 97, 1990.
13. Melzack, R., Wall, P. D. and Ty, T. C., Acute pain in an emergency clinic, *Pain*, 14, 33, 1982.
14. Wall, P. D. and Melzack, R., Eds., *Textbook of Pain*, Churchill Livingstone, New York, 1984.
15. Short, C. E. and Van Poznak, A., Eds., *Animal Pain*, Churchill Livingstone, New York, 1992.
16. Rollin, B. E. and Kesel, M. L., Eds., *The Experimental Animal in Biomedical Research, Volume 1: A Survey of Scientific and Ethical issues for Investigators*, CRC Press, Boca Raton, Florida, 1990.
17. Kitchell, R. L. and Erickson, H. H., Eds., *Animal Pain: Perception and Alleviation*, American Physiological Society, Bethesda, Maryland, 1983.
18. Morton, D. B. and Griffiths, P. H. M., Guidelines on the recognition of pain, distress and discomfort in experimental animals and a hypothesis for assessment, *Veterinary Record*, 116, 431, 1985.
19. Working Party of the Association of Veterinary Teachers and Research Workers, *Guidelines for the Recognition and Assessment of Pain in Animals*, Universities Federation for Animal Welfare, Potters Bar, England, 1989.
20. Barclay, R. J., Herbert W. J., and Poole, T. B., *The Disturbance Index: A Behavioural Method of Assessing the Severity of Common Laboratory Procedures on Rodents*, Universities Federation for Animal Welfare, Potters Bar, England, 1988.
21. Beynen, A. C., Baumans, V., Bertens, A. P. M. G., Havenaar, R., Hesp, A. P. M. and van Zutphen, L. F. M., Assessment of discomfort in gallstone-bearing mice: a practical example of the problems encountered in an attempt to recognize discomfort in laboratory animals, *Laboratory Animals*, 21, 35, 1987.

22. Zimmermann, M., Ethical guidelines for investigations of experimental pain in conscious animals, *Pain*, 16, 109, 1983.

23. Adams, H. R., Teske, R. H., and Mercer, H. D., Anesthetic-antibiotic interrelationships, *Journal of the American Veterinary Medical Association*, 168, 409, 1976.

24. United Kingdom Coordinating Committee on Cancer Research (UKCCCR), Guidelines on the welfare of animals used in experimental neoplasia, *Laboratory Animals*, 22, 195, 1988.

25. Flecknell, P. A., *Laboratory Animal Anaesthesia*, Academic Press, London, 1987.

26. Flecknell, P. A., Pain reduction and pain relief in laboratory animals, *Scandinavian Journal of Laboratory Animal Science*, 18, 147, 1991.

27. Liles, J. H. and Flecknell, P. A., The use of non-steroidal anti-inflammatory drugs for the relief of pain in laboratory rodents and rabbits, *Laboratory Animals*, 26, 241, 1992.

28. Green, C. J., *Animal Anaesthesia*, Laboratory Animal Handbooks No. 8, Laboratory Animals Ltd., London, 1979.

29. Yoxal, A. T., Pain in small animals — its recognition and control, *Journal of Small Animal Practice*, 19, 423, 1978.

30. Flecknell, P. A. and Liles, J. H., Evaluation of locomotor activity and food and water consumption as a method of assessing post-operative pain in rodents, in: *Animal Pain*, Short, C. E. and Van Poznak, A., Eds., Churchill Livingstone, New York, 482, 1992.

31. Reid, J. and Nolan, A. M., A comparison of the postoperative analgesic and sedative effects of flunixin and papaveretum in the dog, *Journal of Small Animal Practice*, 32, 603, 1992.

32. Flecknell, P. A., Liles, J. H. and Williamson, H. A., The use of lignocaine-prilocaine local anaesthetic cream for pain-free venepuncture in laboratory animals, *Laboratory Animals*, 24, 142, 1990.

33. Kistler, P., *Zur Schmerzbekämpfung im Tierversuch (Attenuation of Pain in Animal Experimentation)*, dissertation ETH no. 8568, University of Bern, Zurich, 1988.

34. American Veterinary Medical Association Panel Reports, Euthanasia in laboratory animals, *Journal of the American Veterinary Medical Association*, 188, 252, 1986.

35. Rowsell, H. C., Euthanasia: acceptable and unacceptable methods of killing, in *The Experimental Animal in Biomedical Research, Volume 1: A Survey of Scientific and Ethical Issues for Investigators*, Rollin, B. E. and Kesel, M. L., Eds., CRC Press, Boca Raton, Florida, 381, 1990.

36. Universities Federation for Animal Welfare/World Society for the Protection of Animals, *Euthanasia of Amphibians and Reptiles*, UFAW, Potters Bar, 1989.

37. Allred, J. B. and Berntson, G. C., Is euthanasia of rats by decapitation humane?, *Journal of Nutrition*, 116, 1859, 1986.

38. Carney, J. A. and Walker, B. L., Mode of killing and plasma corticosterone concentration in the rat, *Laboratory Animal Science*, 23, 675, 1973.

39. Klemm, W. R., Correspondence, *Laboratory Animal Science*, 37, 148, 1987.

40. Mikeska, J. A. and Klemm, W. R., EEG evaluation of humaneness of asphyxia and decapitation euthanasia of the laboratory rat, *Laboratory Animal Science*, 25, 175, 1975.

41. Taylor, P., Analgesia in the dog and cat, *In Practice*, 7, 5, 1985.

Chapter 21

Surgical Procedures

H. P. Olesen

CONTENTS

INTRODUCTION

Experimental surgery is necessary for the development of new surgical methods and highly valuable in the testing of the biocompatibility of new biomaterials. Physiological and pharmacological research often requires surgical preparation before animal experiments can be performed.

Any surgical intervention is traumatic for the organism. To minimize the trauma, it is important that the surgeon has access to a well-organized and well-equipped surgical facility and that he uses the proper surgical technique.

The aim of this chapter is to give a short description of the laboratory for experimental surgery and the basic principles of surgical procedure. The reader who needs more detailed information on these subjects should consult more comprehensive texts.[1-6]

SURGICAL FACILITIES AND EQUIPMENT

Besides the operating room, the laboratory for experimental surgery should include an area for preparation and care of the animal, areas for cleaning, sterilization and storage of instruments, and X-ray facilities, laboratories and offices for investigators and staff (Figure 1).

THE OPERATING ROOM

The operating room must be located centrally in the laboratory area so that it is unnecessary to pass it to gain access to other parts of the building. The floor and wall surfaces should be constructed of a smooth, easily cleaned material and be free of pipes and other dust-gathering installations. There should be a floor outlet drain, thermostatic heat, controlled filtered ventilation and humidity. Wall outlets for oxygen, nitrous oxide, compressed air and vacuum should be provided. The room should be well lighted, and electrical outlets should be abundant, as experimental surgery often requires several recording instru-

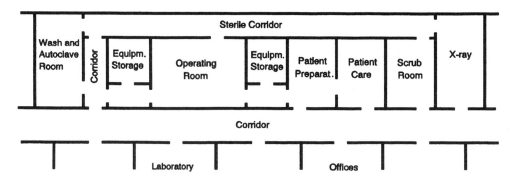

Figure 1. Plan of the experimental surgical department at the Panum Institute, University of Copenhagen.

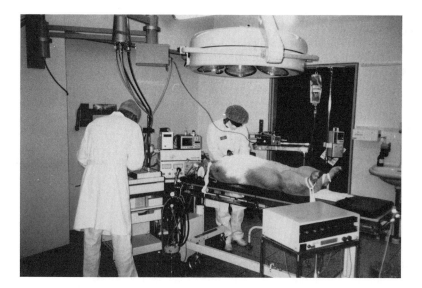

Figure 2. The operation room should be well lighted and well equipped.

ments. The room ought to be at least 40 m2 (Figure 2). The operating room should be equipped with an adjustable operating table. To minimize heat loss from the animal the table should be covered with a thermostated mattress.

An anesthetic machine and an artificial ventilator to maintain general anesthesia and normocapnia during surgery are necessary if surgery has to be performed on large laboratory animal species. An operating lamp should be installed above the operation table to illuminate the operation area. A number of portable stainless steel tables are suitable for instruments and recording equipment. A diathermy unit with both monopolar and bipolar systems is very useful for incision and hemostasis in major surgery. A portable suction unit should be accessible for aspirating fluid, e.g., from the abdominal or thoracic cavity.

During experimental investigations a number of physiological parameters are measured. Equipment for recording such parameters should be available in the experimental unit. Most essential is equipment for recording cardiovascular and respiratory parameters such as electrocardiogram, pulse rate, blood pressure, cardiac output, blood flow, expired carbon dioxide concentration, arterial partial pressures of oxygen and carbon dioxide, etc. Furthermore, instruments for continuous recording of body temperature and for infusion should be available.

A special room close to the operating room for storage of this equipment is desirable.

THE PREPARATION ROOM

The preparation room should be adjacent to the operating room. Preparation of the animal for experimental surgery includes anesthesia, clipping, washing, and disinfection of the surgical area. The room must contain necessary drugs and equipment for these purposes, i.e., a metal table covered with an isolating, easily cleanable mattress, anesthetic drugs, a laryngoscope, endotracheal tubes, an anesthetic machine, an oxygen outlet, a resuscitation bag, a stethoscope, different sizes of sterile needles, syringes and indwelling cannulas, gauze sponges, adhesive tape, a clipper, a vacuum cleaner, soap and antiseptic solution for preparing the surgical area.

THE RECOVERY ROOM

A recovery room adjacent to the preparation room with suitable cages for the operated animals should be available. Here the animals may be observed and treated during the postoperative period. The room should be well heated, have controlled ventilation, and be equipped for infusions and oxygen treatment.

OTHER FACILITIES AND EQUIPMENT

The cleaning and sterilization area must have a hot and cold water supply, a washing machine, an ultrasonic cleaner, and dry and steam autoclaves. Adjacent to this area there should be a storage room, where the sterilized surgical trays, linen packs, and other items can be stored. X-ray and fluoroscopic equipment are necessary or useful in many experimental procedures. It should be possible to use them not only in the specific X-ray room, but in the operating room, too.

SURGICAL INSTRUMENTS

There exist a great number of highly specialized instruments, but it is outside the scope of this chapter to give a description of them all. For most purposes a limited range of standard instruments is adequate and some of them are mentioned below.

Scalpel handles and blades — The scalpel handle size 3 of medium length and blade size 10 are useful for most purposes. The scalpel blades are packed in sterile peel-open packets. The blades should only be used for one operation and then discarded (Figure 3d).

Scissors — Operating scissors are available in many sizes and forms designed for special purposes. The most common types for general use are curved or straight scissors with sharp and/or blunt points. Surgical scissors are made for cutting tissue and should never be used to cut gauze, adhesive tape, or other materials (Figure 3a, b, c).

Forceps and clamps — The tissue forceps known as the rat-tooth forceps is used for holding fascia and skin during wound closure. When more gentle tissue handling is necessary, the atraumatic forceps or dissection forceps with serrated tips should be used (Figure 3e, f). Hemostatic forceps or clamps are found in various sizes and in straight, curved, and angled shapes and are equipped with a ratchet lock. They have serrated blades and are used for clamping vessels to secure hemostasis. The angled ones are suitable for passing ligatures around vessels and other tubular structures. The Kocker clamp is toothed at the tip and ought only to be used in tissue that will be removed. There exist many specialized atraumatic clamps, e.g., for use in vascular and gastrointestinal surgery. Towel forceps or clamps are used to hold drapes in position on the skin (Figure 4).

Retractors — Retractors are necessary basic instruments. There are two main types available: the manual and the self-retaining, but they come in many variations with sharp or blunt blades (Figure 5).

Needle holders — Needle holders have hardened, toothed jaws and are found in many lengths and forms constructed for special surgical procedures. The Mathieu needle holder has an open ratchet lock that is released by pressing the lock past the point of maximum closure. For general use a 15-cm straight needle holder is suitable (Figure 6).

Needles — The surgical needle may be straight or curved, eyed or eyeless and with a taper point or a cutting point.[7] The body of the needle is flattened to improve stability in the needle holder. The taper point needle is primarily used on easily penetrated tissue, e.g., the peritoneum and viscera. The cutting needle is of a triangular shape with three cutting edges. It is used for tough tissues such as fascia and skin (Figure 7). The eyeless needle is the most frequently used. It has the suture swaged to the needle, which ensures high consistency between needle and suturing material (Figure 8). This atraumatic suture causes a minimum of tissue damage during penetration, as no double strand has to pass through the tissue (Figure 9).

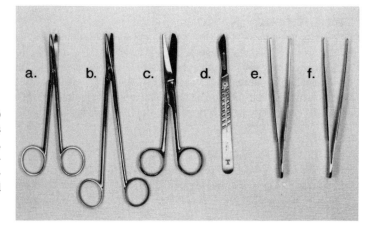

Figure 3. Surgical instruments: (a) Metzenbaum dissecting scissors (curved, blunt-blunt); (b) (straight, blunt-blunt); (c) Mayo dissecting scissors (straight, sharp-blunt); (d) scalpel; (e) tissue forceps (rat-tooth); and (f) dissecting tissue forceps.

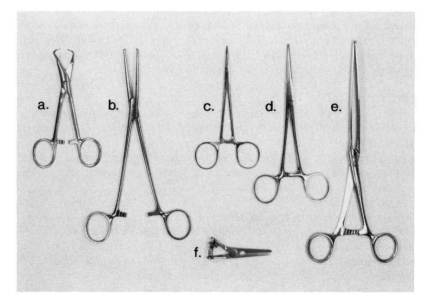

Figure 4. Surgical instruments: (a) towel forceps; (b) Kocker forceps; (c) hemostatic forceps (mosquito); (d) hemostatic forceps; (e) intestinal forceps; and (f) vessel forceps (bulldog clamps).

SUTURE MATERIALS

Sutures can be classified as absorbable, non-absorbable, monofilament or multifilament. They are made of either natural or synthetic materials. Sutures come in various sizes. The strengths and dimensions of all suture materials are standardized in the United States Pharmacopeia (USP) and in the European Pharmacopeia (EP). The EP standard employs a metric classification in which diameters are given in tenths of a millimeter (Table 1).

Absorbable sutures — The absorbable sutures are either of organic origin (catgut) or synthetic origin (polyesters). They disintegrate in the tissues by phagocytosis or hydrolysis. Catgut is prepared from the submucosal layer of sheeps intestine. Plain catgut causes a marked foreign-body tissue response and is absorbed with loss of tensile strength in about 10 days. By treating the surface of catgut with chromic acid the absorption is slowed, and about 50% of the tensile strength is maintained for up to 2 weeks (Figure 10). The knot security is unstable, especially when wet. The synthetic absorbable suture material disintegrates by hydrolysis and is absorbed with minor tissue reaction. It is commonly braided, which gives excellent handling properties and a higher coefficient of friction, ensuring good knot stability.[8]

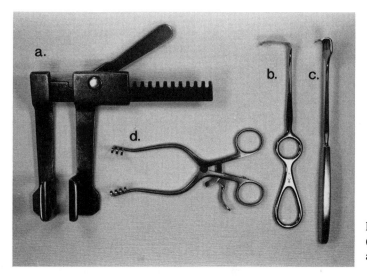

Figure 5. Retractors: (a) rib spreader; (b) manual (blunt); (c) manual (sharp); and (d) self-retaining.

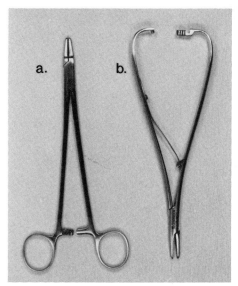

Figure 6. Needle holders: (a) Mayo-Hegar needle holder; (b) Mathieu needle holder.

Tensile strength is maintained for several weeks (Figure 10). The multifilament suture has interstices that can harbor microorganisms and capillarity, i.e., the suture acts as a wick along which tissue fluid and microorganisms move. This causes local inflammatory tissue reaction.

Non-absorbable sutures — The only non-absorbable suture of natural origin to be mentioned here is silk. It is braided, has excellent handling properties, acceptable tensile strength and high knot stability, but it often causes local tissue reaction.[9-11] The synthetic non-absorbable sutures are made from different polymeric materials. They are available in both monofilament and multifilament forms. Many of the monofilaments cause little tissue reaction, are non-capillary, and have high tensile strength. As knot stability is relatively poor, four or more throws are necessary. Stainless steel and other non-corrosive metals are used as sutures for wound closure and as clips to ligate vessels.

PREPARATION OF THE SURGICAL PACKS

The instruments and supplies that are to be used for a surgical procedure must be wrapped or packed so that they maintain their sterility until use, and it should be possible to open the pack without contaminating the contents. Standard surgical packs needed for one operation should contain gowns and hand towels, skin drapes, a tray with general surgical instruments, and gauze sponges. Special instruments and equipment should be wrapped individually using the commercially available plast paper tube system.

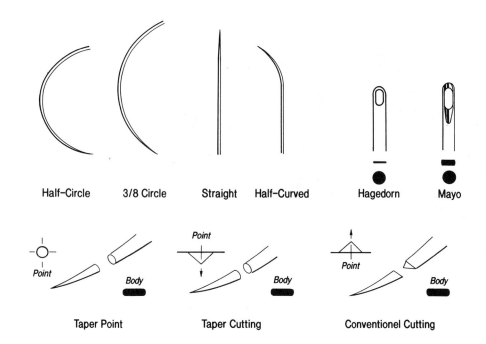

Half-Circle   3/8 Circle   Straight   Half-Curved   Hagedorn   Mayo

Taper Point   Taper Cutting   Conventionel Cutting

Figure 7. The basic needle shapes and components (courtesy Ethicon).

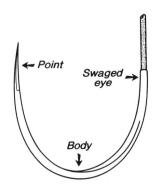

Figure 8. The eyeless atraumatic needle (courtesy Ethicon).

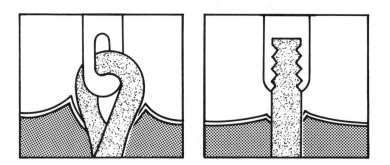

Figure 9. The eyed needle (left) with double strand causes more tissue damage than the eyeless needle (right) with a single strand (courtesy Ethicon).

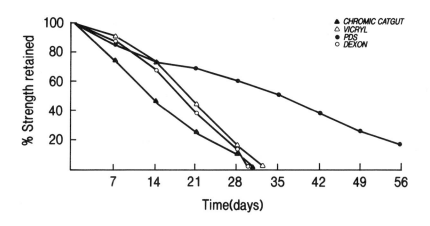

Figure 10. Comparative loss in tissue of tensile strength of catgut, Dexon (homopolymer of glycolide), Vicryl (copolymer of glycolide and lactide), and PDS (polyioxanone). (Courtesy Ethicon.)

Other supplies such as gloves, catheters, syringes, etc. are available in sterile packs for single use, as are surgical gowns and drapes.

STERILIZATION OF INSTRUMENTS AND SUPPLIES

The instruments and equipment used in a surgical procedure or entering the operative field must be sterilized, especially when the animal is to survive for further experiments and observation. Physical sterilization by dry or moist heat is the most commonly used method. Dry heat is an effective method of sterilizing sharp metallic instruments because it does not dull the edges. However, dry heat sterilization requires one to two hours at a temperature of 150 to 177°C (300 to 350°F) to be effective.

Steam autoclaves provide sterilization at 121°C (250°F) (1 kg/cm²) or at 133°C (270°F) (2 kg/cm²). As the steam must completely penetrate the package to ensure sterilization, the packages must be porous to steam. The time necessary to produce sterilization is at least 15 minutes at a temperature of 121°C or 3 minutes at 133°C for single instruments or small packs. The time must be increased for sterilization of larger packs. Boiling for 20 to 30 minutes has been used for sterilization of instruments, but it should only be used in an emergency situation.[12] Heat-sensitive materials can be sterilized by using either ethylene oxide gas in a closed container or ionizing radiation. Instruments and materials must be clean and dry prior to packing for sterilization by any of the methods mentioned. To check that the proper temperature is reached autoclave tape should be used. As the tape only indicates temperature and not sterilization as such, biological tests must occasionally be made.

Properly wrapped and sterilized packs will remain sterile for up to 6 months when stored in a clean, dry environment.

CARE AND PREPARATION OF THE ANIMAL BEFORE SURGERY

Successful experimental surgery requires that the animal is in good health. It should be conditioned in the animal department for a few weeks prior to its intended use. During that period clinical and hematological examinations should be performed. Abnormalities should be corrected or the animal excluded.

The animal should be fasted 12 to 24 hours prior to surgery, but have free access to water to avoid dehydration. After the animal has been anesthetized, the surgical site is clipped and the hairs are removed with a vacuum cleaner. The area is then washed using brush, soap and warm water, wiped and re-washed with an antiseptic solution and wiped again with dry sterile sponges — always first at the incision line and then towards the periphery. The animal is moved to the surgical room and restrained on the operating table with soft ropes or tapes and if necessary supported with sandbags. Intravenous admission should be established and the animal should be connected to an electrocardiograph. A final application of an antiseptic solution — 0.5% iodine in 70% ethyl alcohol — on the operation site is made with sterile sponges,[13-14] and sterile drapes can be applied.

360

Table 1. Suture Diameter Eqivalences - Comparison of USP and EP Suture Standards

USP size codes		EP size codes (mm)	Suture diameter (mm)
Organic absorbable materials	Non-absorbable materials and synthetic absorbable materials	Organic and synthetic absorbable material. Non-asorbable materials	Min. Max.
	11/0	0.1	0.01-0.019
	10/0	0.2	0.02-0.029
	9/0	0.3	0.03-0.039
	8/0	0.4	0.04-0.049
8/0	7/0	0.5	0.05-0.069
7/0	6/0	0.7	0.07-0.099
6/0	5/0	1	0.10-0.14
5/0	4/0	1.5	0.15-0.19
4/0	3/0	2	0.20-0.24
3/0	2/0	2.5	0.25-0.29
2/0	0	3	0.30-0.39
0	1	4	0.40-0.49
1	2	5	0.50-0.59
2	3	6	0.60-0.69
3	4	7	0.70-0.79
4	5	8	0.80-0.89
5	6	9	0.90-0.99
6	7	10	1.00-1.09

(Courtesy Davis and Geck).

PREPARATION OF THE SURGICAL TEAM

When entering the surgical area the members of the surgical team should wear surgical caps covering all their hair and surgical masks. Before the scrubbing procedure rings, watches, etc. are removed from hands and arms. The surgeon's fingernails should be trimmed and cleaned under running warm water after the hands have been soaped. Hands and forearms are scrubbed methodically with a sterile brush, a scrubbing agent and warm water. Suitable for this purpose are sterile single-use brushes/sponges prepared with jodophor/detergent solution. The scrubbing time is at least five minutes or ten brush strokes of the entire surface of the fingers, hands and forearms. The hands are held higher than the elbows during scrubbing, rinsing and drying to prevent contamination from water running from the unsterile surface of the upper arms to the forearms and hands. The surgeon now takes a sterile towel from a pack just opened by an assistant and dries hands and arms, carefully avoiding contamination from unscrubbed surfaces. The surgical gown is unfolded and the surgeon's arms are inserted into the armholes, bare hands touching only the inner surface. The gown may be pulled on and tied by an assistant. Finally the surgeon pulls on sterile gloves without touching the outer surfaces of the gown and the gloves (Figure 11).

DRAPING

Draping serves to prevent contamination of the surgical site and the surgeon from the surrounding skin (Figure 12). Consequently the drapes must be sterile and cloth drapes should be double layer. Draping for operations of the body trunk requires one adhesive skin drape and four cloth drapes. First the adhesive skin drape is placed on the skin of the operative site, then cloth drapes are placed, one on either side, followed by one over the cranial and another over the caudal part. This arrangement prevents the side drapes from slipping down, and requires only four towel clamps to retain them in position (Figure 13).

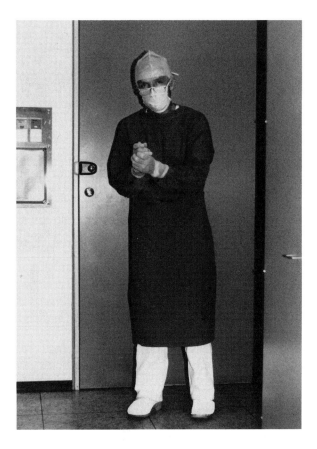

Figure 11. The surgeon correctly dressed for surgical work.

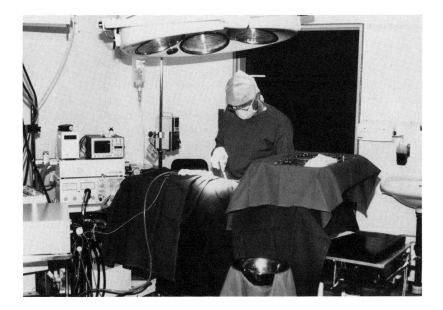

Figure 12. The entire draping of the animal, table, and instrument stand.

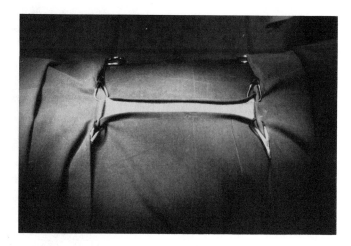

Figure 13. The primary drapes placed and secured with towel forceps.

The drapes should not be of plastic or other impervious material because of the danger of overheating the patient.

SURGICAL TECHNIQUE

Proper attention to the fundamental principles of surgical technique forms the basis of good surgical practice. Strict attention should be paid to asepsis. Tissue should be handled gently. Skin incisions should be made with sharp blades, as the crushing of tissue causes delayed healing. The incisions should permit proper access to the surgical area, placed if possible along the muscle and fascia fibers, and in a manner that causes a minimum of trauma to nerves, blood supply and muscles. Natural cleavages should be used to gain access to deeper structures. In careful operative technique unnecessary opening of tissue plane is avoided, as is also the crushing and devitalizing of tissue by holding with clamps for retraction. Hemostasis should be carried out continuously during incision. Minor capillary hemorrhage can be controlled by gentle pressure with sponges. Bleeding vessels are grasped with mosquito forceps and ligated with a thin absorbable suture or coagulated by electrocautery. Large bleeding surfaces may be controlled with coagulants such as gelatin foam, fibrin adhesive or topical thrombin. The incision should be closed layer by layer and the edges approximated without undue tension. Dead spaces should be eliminated; if allowed to remain, they may give rise to accumulation of blood and fluid, and wound infection may ensue.

HANDLING OF INSTRUMENTS

For cutting the skin and similar tissues the scalpel is held like a table knife. In order to cut with a minimum of tissue damage, the whole length of the blade must be drawn over the tissue with a single smooth motion and a constant pressure on the knife. Only for delicate dissection of fine structures is the scalpel held like a pencil. For accurate handling of scissors the thumb is placed in one ring of the handle and the ring finger in the other, with the middle finger curled round the outside of the ring and the index finger pulp placed on the joint of the instrument. Tissue forceps are normally held in the opposite hand in the same way as a pencil. When applying hemostatic forceps the fingers are placed as for scissors. The vessels are grasped with the tip of the instrument and clamped with one or two clicks of the ratchet lock. Releasing the forceps should be done with one hand. For the right hand, the forceps are held in the same manner as when applying them. For the left hand, the ring farthest away is grasped between the thumb on top and the index and middle fingers underneath, while the ring finger and little finger push the other ring until the ratchet lock opens.

WOUND CLOSURE

The purpose of the suture is to hold the wound together in good apposition until the natural wound healing process is sufficient to make support from the suture material unnecessary (Figure 14). Each layer is closed separately, and the edges should be approximated without undue tension. The sutures should include the same amount of tissue on either side of the wound; if the needle is inserted at different depths

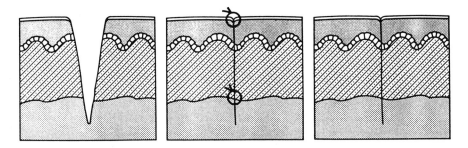

Figure 14. Correct apposition of the wound. (Courtesy Davis and Geck.)

on opposing sides of the wound, the edges will overlap when the suture is tied. Portions of fat and muscle should not protrude between the layers sutured and no "dead space" should be allowed to remain. The strength of the sutured wound depends on the tissue being sutured, and the tensile strength and knot stability of the suture used. Closure of the peritoneum may be achieved by using a simple interrupted or continuous suture (Figures 15b and e), and a fine absorbable suture is to be preferred. Fascia is the strongest tissue in the abdominal wall and many other sites in the body. As sutures in the fascia bear the maximum stress of the wound, care must be taken when suturing and simple interrupted sutures are recommended (Figure 15b). In spite of the slow healing time of fascial tissue, both synthetic absorbable and synthetic non- absorbable sutures can safely be used.[15,16]

Sutures in the muscles and fat do not contribute to the strength of the wound; the edges should be apposed by suturing surrounding fascia and connective tissue sheaths, but if necessary a few absorbable interrupted sutures may be placed in the muscle and fat. A few subcutaneous simple interrupted sutures including the subcuticular layer will bring the skin edges close together.

The skin sutures should bring the edges into a precise or slightly everting apposition without interposition of underlying tissue. Skin closure can be achieved with a continuous or interrupted suture, but the interrupted vertical mattress suture is best (Figure 15c). The stitches must be tied gently and loosely, taking into account the edema that will occur during the next few days. A thin non-absorbable monofilament suture is preferable, because the capillarity of the multifilament suture facilitates the penetration of microorganisms from the skin surface to the deeper layers.

Closure of wounds in the viscera should be done with an inverting suture to ensure apposition of serosa to serosa (Figure 16). When leakage and contamination from the lumen may occur, many surgeons prefer a two-layer closure, the first layer with a simple interrupted suture and the second layer with an inverting suture.[17-19]

The purse-string suture is a circular inverting suture used for inversion of visceral stumps, and for securing tubes and catheters (Figure 17).

THE KNOT

The general principles of knot-tying apply to all suture materials. The knot should be secured so that slippage is impossible, but not so tight that the tissue is strangulated. The only exception to this is the application of ligatures for hemostasis.

In tying knots, a sawing or seesaw motion should be avoided as friction between strands can weaken the integrity of the suture. Buried knots should be small and suture ends cut as short as possible to minimize the amount of foreign material introduced to the wound. The square knot is the most reliable for tying most suture materials. The friction or surgeon's knot should only be used when tissue tension is such that use of the square knot would result in poor apposition (Figures 18 and 19).

In general three throws are sufficient for multifilament sutures and four or more throws for monofilament sutures to prevent knot slippage.

The two-handed and instrument knotting techniques are illustrated in Figures 20 and 21.

CATHETERIZATION

Most experimental animal model studies require catheterization of tubular structures for infusion, collection of samples or measurement of flow rates and other physiological parameters.[20-30] Chronic indwelling catheters are particularly helpful in long-term studies in conscious animals. Only catheterization that needs surgical intervention will be mentioned here. Tubes used for catheters should be inert to the

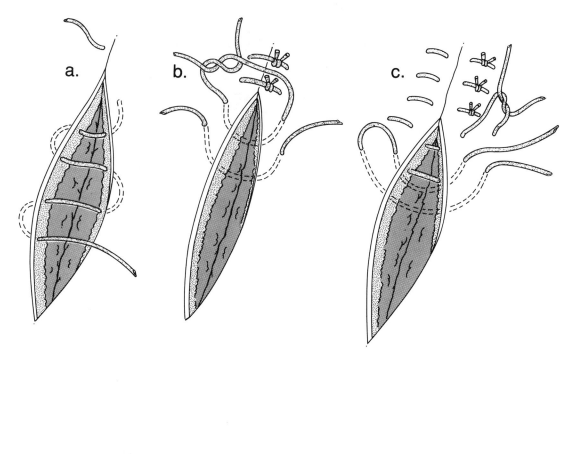

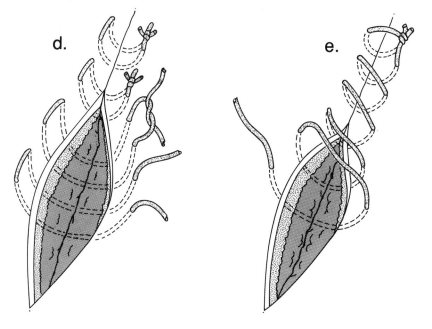

Figure 15. Suture techniques: (a) Subcuticular suture; (b) simple interrupted suture; (c) interrupted vertical mattress suture; (d) interrupted horizontal mattress suture; (e) simple continuous suture. (Courtesy Davis and Geck.)

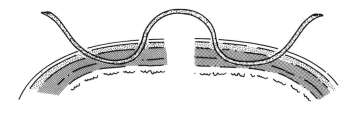

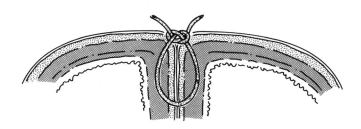

Figure 16. Lembert's inverting suture.

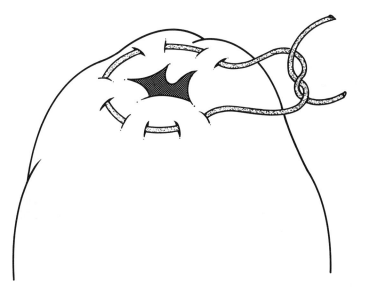

Figure 17. Purse-string suture.

organism, have smooth inner and outer surfaces, be relatively flexible and kink-free, and resistant when exposed to body fluids. Plastic materials with most of these properties are, e.g., polyethylene, silastic and polyurethane.

Polyethylene tubing is relatively cheap and useful in acute experiments, but in chronic experiments commercially available catheters for special purposes are preferable. In many aspects the surgical technique is identical no matter which tubular structure is to be cannulated. The description below is the technique used for cannulation of the jugular vein and/or carotid artery. A 6- to 8-cm long skin incision is made parallel to the vessel. The structures below are separated by alternating blunt and sharp dissection, and when possible, natural cleavage is used. The vessel is identified and isolated for 3 to 4 cm.

Two ligatures are placed around the vessel about 2 cm apart. The cranial one can now be tied, while the caudal one is used to control hemorrhage during introduction of the catheter. A transverse cut through one third of the vessel is made with a pair of micro-scissors. The edge of the hole is grasped with a straight

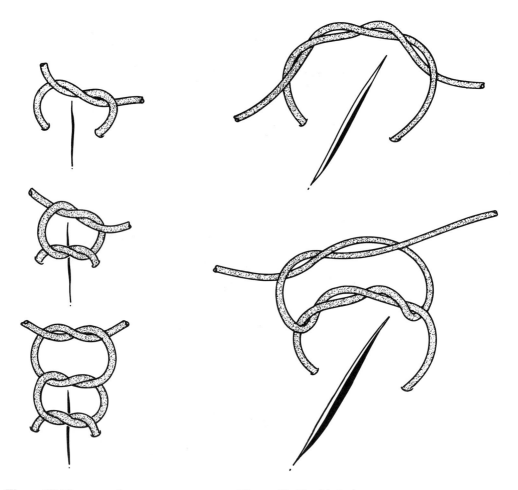

Figure 18. The square knot.   **Figure 19.** The friction or surgeon's knot.

mosquito hemostat to ensure that the intima will not loosen, which would make it impossible to introduce the catheter (Figure 22). The catheter is inserted until the tip is in the desired position, and both ligatures are tied round the vessel and the catheter to ensure hemostasis and fixation.

In chronic studies in conscious animals it is necessary to prevent the catheter from being pulled out or damaged by the animal. This is best done by leading it from the skin incision subcutaneously to the neck region, where the animal is least likely to pull it out (Figure 23). A long cannula with an internal diameter a little bigger than the external diameter of the catheter is passed from the skin incision subcutaneously to the desired position. The catheter is then passed back through the cannula to the site of the vein puncture and the cannula is removed. The catheter is mounted with a stopcock and flushed and filled with heparinized saline (50 U/ml) to prevent thrombosis. The exterior part of the catheter and the stopcock can be protected by an elastic tube bandage. The catheter should be flushed daily with heparinized saline to ensure patency.

Catheterization of the portal and hepatic veins is often of interest in both acute and chronic experiments, and is therefore mentioned here.[31-36] The portal vein is usually catheterized via the splenic vein, and the hepatic vein via the caval vein.

A quick method, useful in both short- and long-term experiments, is performed through a midline superior laparotomy. A lobe of the liver is partly exposed. For fixation and hemostasis an intestinal clamp is applied approximately 5 cm from the apex of the lobe. An incision is made at a slight angle to the clamp until 1 to 2 mm wide vessels are found, and the catheter is passed 10 to 15 cm into the hepatic venous system, placing the tip close to the bifurcation with the inferior vena cava. A small portal vein branch is found beside a branch of the hepatic artery. The catheter is inserted until it can be palpated in the

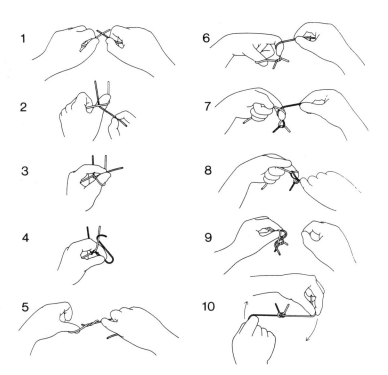

Figure 20. The two-hand tying technique. (Courtesy Davis and Geck.)

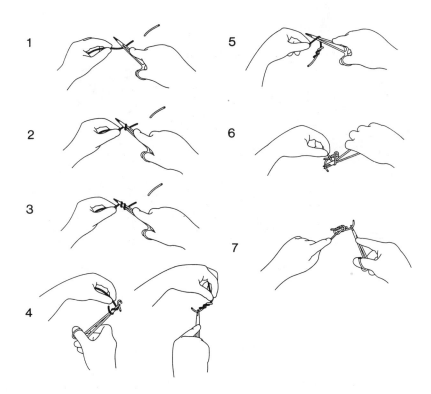

Figure 21. The instrument tying technique. (Courtesy Davis and Geck.)

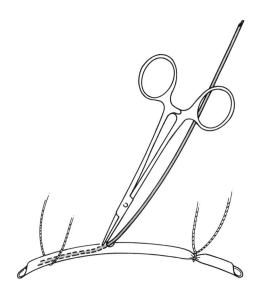

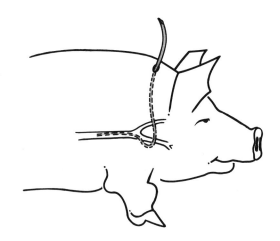

Figure 22. Insertion of a catheter into a vessel.

Figure 23. Exteriorization of the catheter.

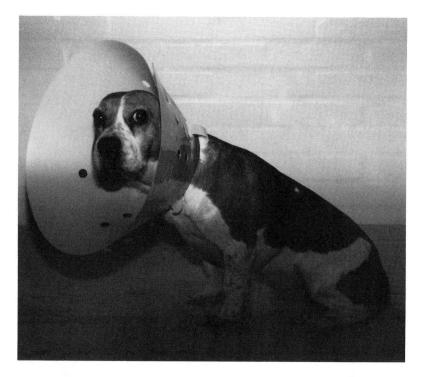

Figure 24. Dog with collar for prevention of self-mutilation.

hepatoduodenal ligament. The fixation of the catheters should be performed with a suture ligature through the liver tissue.

POSTOPERATIVE TREATMENT

The animals used in experimental surgery are generally young and in good condition, which facilitates rapid wound healing. If fundamental principles of surgical technique and asepsis have been followed, the surgical wound will heal with primary intention, and wound complications are seldom seen. Poor healing and disruption of the surgical wound may occur following local factors such as poor hemostasis, strangulation of large pieces of tissue, disturbance of blood supply, and wound infection.

As herniation may occur following improper suturing or knot loosening, interrupted sutures are recommended in all layers, bearing in mind that animals move around a few hours after surgery. Wound bandaging is usually unnecessary in most animals, but some restrictive or protective devices may be necessary to avoid self-inflicted trauma to the operation wound (Figure 24).

Usually antimicrobial treatment is unnecessary after proper surgery; only following operations entering the gastrointestinal tract should prophylactic treatment with a suitable combination of antimicrobial drugs against both aerobic and anaerobic micro-organisms be applied. For analgetic treatment, the chapter concerning this subject should be consulted.

In the postoperative period great attention must be given to the water requirements of the patient. Parenteral fluid administration of isotonic saline solution may be necessary to avoid dehydration until the animal has recovered from anesthesia. Surgical patients with specific electrolyte requirements or imbalance should be treated after close assessment of the fluid balance.

REFERENCES

1. De Boer, J., Archibald, J., and Downie, H. G., *An Introduction to Experimental Surgery,* American Elsevier Publishing Company, New York, 1975.
2. Van Dongen, J. J., Remie, R., Rensema, J. W., and Van Wunnik, G. H. J., *Manual of Microsurgery on the Laboratory Rat,* Elsevier, Amsterdam, 1990.
3. Dougherty, R. W., *Experimental Surgery in Farm Animals*, Iowa State University Press, 1981.
4. Hecker, J. F., *Experimental Surgery on Small Ruminants,* Butterworth & Co., Southampton, 1974.
5. Knecht, C. D., Allen, A. R., Williams, D. J., and Johnson, J. H., *Fundamental Techniques in Veterinary Surgery,* W.B. Saunders Company, Philadelphia, 1981.
6. Slatter, D. H., *Textbook of Small Animal Surgery,* W.B. Saunders Company, Philadelphia, 1985.
7. Swindler, M. M., *Basic Surgical Exercises Using Swine,* Praeger Scientific, 1986.
8. *Suture Use Manual, Use and Handling of Sutures and Needles,* Ethicon, 1977.
9. Tera, H. and Åberg, C., The strength of suture knots after one week in vivo, *Acta Chir. Scand.* 142, 301, 1976.
10. Craig, P. H., Williams, J. A., Davis, K. W., Magoun, A. D., Levy, A. J., Bogdansky, S., and Jones, J. P., A biologic comparison of polyglatin 910 and polyglycolic acid synthetic absorbable sutures, *Surgery,* 141, 1, 1975.
11. Postlethwait, R. W., Willigan, D. A., and Ulin, A. W., Human tissue reaction to sutures, *Ann. Surg.,* 181, 144, 1975.
12. Salthouse, T. N. and Matlaga, B., Significance of cellular enzyme activity at nonabsorbable suture implant sites: silk, polyester and polypropylene, *J. Surg. Res.,* 19, 127, 1975.
13. Eshleman, J. R., Methods used for sterilization or disinfection of instruments, *J. Dent. Educ.,* 32, 330, 1968.
14. Collins, C. H., Allwood, M. C., Bloomfield, S. F.. and Fox, A., *Disinfectants: Their Use and Evaluation of Effectiveness,* Academic Press, London, 1981.
15. Ghosh, J., Maisels, D. O. and Woodcock, A. S., Preoperative skin disinfection, *Br. J. Surg.,* 54, 551, 1967.
16. Irvin, T. T., Koffman, C. G., and Duthie, H. L., Layer closure of laparotomy wounds with absorbable and non-absorbable suture materials, *Br. J. Surg.,* 63, 793, 1976.
17. Kjærgaard, J., Laursen, N. P., Madsen, C. M., Tilma, A., and Zimmermann-Nielsen, C., Comparison of dexon and mersilene sutures in the closure of primary laparotomy incisions, *Acta Chir. Scand.,* 142, 315, 1976.
18. Westaby, S., *Wound Care,* William Heinemann Medical Books Ltd., London, 1985.
19. Zederfeldt, B. H. and Hunt, T. K., *Wound Closure,* Davis & Geck, New Jersey, 1990.
20. Bailie, M.B., Vascular-access-port implantation for serial blood sampling in conscious swine, *Lab. Anim. Sci.,* 36, 431, 1986.
21. Barnstein, N.J., Gilfillan, R.S., Pace, N. and Rahlmann, D.F., Cronic intravascular catheterization, *J. Surg. Res.,* 6, 6-11, 1966.
22. Berlo, C. L. H., van den Bogaard, A. E. J. M., Bost, M. C. F., and Soeters P. B., A technique to study splanchnis metabolism in the unrestrained conscious pig, *Lab. Anim. Sci.,* 38, 463, 1988.

23. Brown, C. S., and Hardenbergh, E., A technique for sampling lymph in unanesthetized dogs by means of an exteriorized thoracic duct- venous shunt, *Surgery,* 29, 502, 1951.

24. Girardet, R. E. and Benninghoff, D. L., Surgical techniques for long-term effects of thoracic duct lymph circulation in dogs, *J. Surg. Res.,* 15, 168, 1973.

25. Jensen, L. T., Olesen, H. P., Risteli, J., and Lorenzen, I., External thoracic duct-venous shunt on conscious pigs for long term studies of connective tissue metabolites in lymph, *Lab. Anim. Sci.,* 40, 620, 1990.

26. Manolas, K. J., Farmer, H. M., Cussen, M., and Welbourn, An experimental model for simultaneous chronic sampling of portal and systemic blood and gastrointestinal lymph via cannulae in conscious swine, *Cornell Vet.,* 73, 333, 1983.

27. Nelson, A. W. and Swan, H., Long-term catheterization of the thoracic duct in the dog, *Arch. Surg.,* 98, 83, 1969.

28. Staub, N. C., Bland, R. D., Brigham, K. L., Demling, R., Erdmann, A. J., and Woolverton, W. C., Preparation of chronic lung lymph fistulas in sheep, *J. Surg. Res.* 19, 315, 1975.

29. Snow, H. D. and Tyner, J. G., Chronic arterial and venous catheterization in sheep, *Am. J. Vet. Res.,* 30, 2241, 1969.

30. Witzel, D. A., Littledike, E. T., and Cook, H. M., Implanted catheters for blood sampling in swine, *Cornell Vet.,* 63, 432, 1973.

31. Farins, L. R., Woodle, E. S., Frey, C. F., Nakayama, S. I., and Ward, R. E., A simple technique for experimental hepatic vein catheterization in swine, *Lab. Anim. Sci.,* 36, 406, 1986.

32. Faulkner, R. T., Czajkowski, W. P., Rayfield, E. J., and Hickman, R. L., Technique for portal catheterization in Rhesus monkey (Macaca mulatta), *Am. J. Vet. Res.,* 37, 473, 1976.

33. Hand, M. S., Philips, R. W., Miller, C. W., Mason, R. A., and Lumb, W. V., A method for quantitation of hepatic, pancreatic, and intestinal function in conscious yucatan miniature swine, *Lab. Anim. Sci.,* 31, 728, 1981.

34. Olesen, H. P., Sjøntoft, E., and Tronier, B., Simultaneous sampling of portal, hepatic and systemic blood during intragastric loading and tracer infusion in conscious pigs, *Lab. Anim. Sci.,* 39, 429, 1989.

35. Santiesteban, R., Hutson, D., and Dombro, R. S., Chronic catheterization of the portal vein in dogs, *Lab. Anim. Sci.,* 33, 373, 1983.

36. Sirek, A., and Sirek, O. V., A new technique for hepatic portal sampling in the conscious dog, *Proc. Soc. Exp. Biol. Med.,* 172, 397, 1983.

Chapter 22

Microsurgical Procedures in Experimental Research

Daniel A. Steinbrüchel

CONTENTS

INTRODUCTION

The history and development of microsurgical procedures essentially reflects recurrent attempts over several decades to solve the problem of establishment or reestablishment of vascular continuity in vessels of decreasing diameter. At the same time it illustrates the mutual beneficial influence of clinical experience and experimental microsurgical results, where clinical data initiated detailed investigations in microsurgical animal models, while experimental experience could directly be applied to clinical procedures.

Carrel and Guthrie were the first who demonstrated the feasibility of vascular anastomosis.[1-3] Before this time, a major vascular lesion in an extremity usually resulted in amputation. In spite of the introduction of the microscope to clinical use in 1921[4] and a gradual development of specialized instruments and accessories (clamps, suture material), successful vascular anastomosis of vessels in the 2- to 3-mm range was technically not feasible until 1960, when Jacobson and Suarez[5] demonstrated the successful anastomosis of blood vessels of 1 mm in external diameter.

Subsequently, the application of microsurgical/microvascular procedures rapidly progressed, both clinically and experimentally. Successful replantation of amputated extremities[6-9] and the transfer of free skin flaps as composite grafts were reported,[10-16] and a variety of microsurgical models were described from different laboratories, focusing on the transplantation of primary vascularized organs in rodents.[17-26]

Today, microsurgical techniques are widely used in ophthalmologic, otologic, reconstructive and plastic surgery. Experimentally, microsurgical models are applied in studies focusing on physiological aspects and processes in the microvasculature subsequent to free tissue transfer, and in transplantation research where microvascular models (performed as routine procedures) form the basis of testing new immunosuppressing/immunomodulating treatment strategies, and permit a more detailed study of the processes involved in allogenic and xenogeneic rejection of transplanted organs.

BASIC REQUIREMENTS FOR EXPERIMENTAL MICROSURGICAL PROJECTS

Performing microsurgical procedures with success, in terms of valid and relevant experimental data, is dependent on several factors, including not only the necessary technical equipment, but also research assistants with motivation, a certain persistence, and a genuine scientific interest. It needs training, qualified supervision and a positive attitude to teamwork, since scientifically interesting projects which include microsurgery will consist of an interdisciplinary approach to often complex problems, in cooperation with immunologists, pathologists, physiologists, and clinicians.

TECHNICAL REQUIREMENTS

Microscopes — Preference has to be given to the operating microscope compared to magnifying glasses. It offers the advantage of greater magnification (stepwise or zoom function), built-in illumination and possibility of documentation (video, photograph). On the other hand, the field of view is limited and the depth of focus moderate, which can partly be compensated for, however, by foot switch control. The cost is clearly a disadvantage, but it will prove to be a good investment in the long run. Furthermore, diploscopes make the performance of complex microsurgical procedures easier and allow detailed training supervision.

Microsurgical instruments and accessories _ A few high-quality instruments with which the user is familiar and can use automatically are sufficient. An extensive variety of different instruments usually has no beneficial effect on technical accuracy and efficiency. As a rule, as simple as possible is best. The choice of optimal clamps, suture material and needles for different vessel and tissue types must be taken into account. Figure 1 illustrates a simple set of essential microsurgical instruments, consisting of a needle holder, a pair of dissecting scissors and a pair of microsurgical forceps. A satin finish to avoid glare is an advantage and the instruments should have a sufficient length to make a convenient pen grip possible. Two single clamps and a twin-clip approximating clamp are shown in Figure 2, and the size is illustrated by the match. Microsurgical instruments are rather expensive and very delicate, but appropriate use and care guarantees excellent function for many years (for further reading concerning more detailed instrument description see References 27 and 28).

Laboratory facilities — The importance of optimal facilities for observation and housing of animals (with respect to microsurgical models, most often rodents) must not be underestimated. Advanced projects often include intensive monitoring, not only limited to the immediate postoperative period, but for several months. Qualified full-time technical assistance is therefore necessary to achieve optimal benefit in terms of valid, complete and reproducible experimental results.

BASIC TECHNIQUES OF MICROSURGICAL VASCULAR ANASTOMOSIS

Atraumatic technique is an essential prerequisite for successful microsurgical procedures. The preparation of arteries and veins includes dissection from surrounding tissue, where a sharp division of structures (with scissors) on the basis of knowledge of natural cleavages is the principle. Blunt dissection and unnecessary manipulation of the vessels must be avoided. The choice of clamps has to be adapted to the type and size of vessel; an optimal clamp exerts a minimal necessary degree of compression, diminishing the risk of endothelial damage. After division of the vessel, with one clear cut, the stumps are rinsed with saline solution. Addition of heparin is not decisive; the important factor for a successful anastomosis is the surgical technique. Subsequently, adjacent adventitia is removed and the stumps can, if necessary, be gently dilated. Any instrumental manipulation with risk of intimal damage during preparation as well as suturing increases the possibility for thrombosis of the anastomosis.

END-TO-END ANASTOMOSIS

The infrarenal aorta or the femoral artery in rats are the most suitable objects for the beginner in experimental microsurgery.

Interrupted Suture Technique

Several methods have been described in the literature.

Eccentric biangulation technique — This technique, first described by Cobbet (1967),[29] is today very popular and can be recommended as the initial type of suture technique for beginners in the field of microsurgical vessel anastomosis. As illustrated in Figures 3A and 3B, the initial two-stay sutures are applied 120 degrees apart. One or two interposed sutures will finish the anterior wall, after which the vessel is rotated 180 degrees. The posterior wall can now be sutured. The use of a twin-clip approximating clamp is a clear advantage for this type of suture technique.

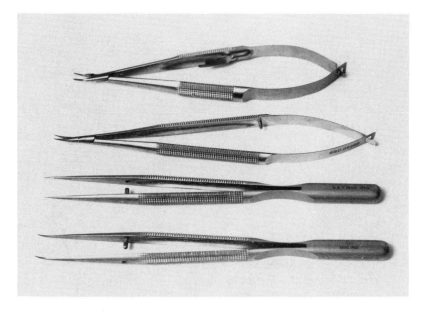

Figure 1. A basic set of microsurgical instruments with needle holder, dissecting scissor, and a pair of microsurgical forceps.

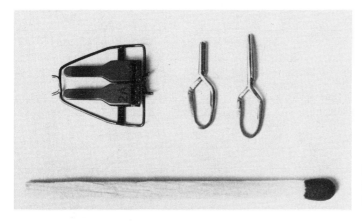

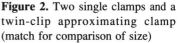

Figure 2. Two single clamps and a twin-clip approximating clamp (match for comparison of size)

Biangulation technique (Figure 4)[30] — It is not always possible to place the initial stay sutures in the exact eccentric position, especially when there is a major discrepancy between vessel diameters. The use of the biangulation technique can therefore be an advantage, where the two initial stay sutures are placed 180 degrees apart, thereby defining an appropriate adaption of the two different vessel diameters. Interpositioning of sutures in the anterior wall, and after rotation, in the posterior wall, will complete the anastomosis.

Successive interrupted sutures ("ship's wheel type") (Figure 5)[31] — The technique is especially suitable where interrupted sutures are preferred, but anatomical circumstances do not allow a free rotation of the vessel. It is an advantage to place the first suture in the posterior wall. After the suture has been tied, one end is cut near the knot, while a gentle traction of the long end will facilitate the exact positioning of the next adjacent suture. This procedure is repeated until the anastomosis is finished.

Running Suture Technique
This technique shortens anastomosis time and improves primary hemostasis, but includes the risk of stenosis in less trained hands (Figure 6).[32]

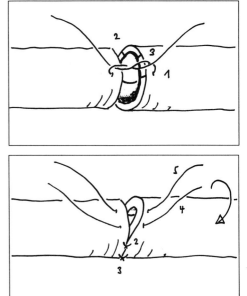

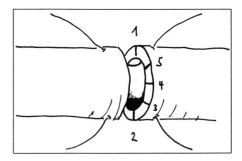

Figure 3. (A) Initial stay sutures are placed 120 degrees apart (**1,2**). (B) The vessel is turned 180 degrees and the anastomosis can be accomplished from the front.

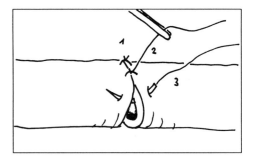

Figure 4. Initial stay sutures are placed 180 degrees apart (**1,2**); remaining sutures are interposed thereafter.

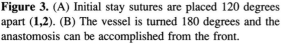

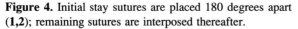

Figure 5. The former stay suture is used to assist the placement of the next suture in a continuous way.

END-TO-SIDE ANASTOMOSIS

The principles of suture technique are basically identical to those of end-to-end anastomosis. Interrupted or running sutures can be used. However, as microsurgical organ transplantation models usually do not permit a free rotation of vessels, anastomosis technique includes suturing of the posterior wall from the luminal side, which is done more easily using a running type of suture. The technique is illustrated in Figure 7.

VEIN ANASTOMOSIS

Veins are very fragile in rodents and must be handled very carefully. The technique of anastomosis is essentially the same as applied in arteries.

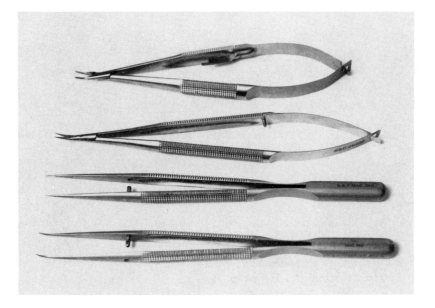

Figure 1. A basic set of microsurgical instruments with needle holder, dissecting scissor, and a pair of microsurgical forceps.

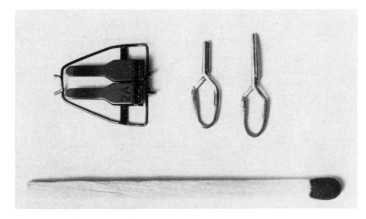

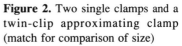

Figure 2. Two single clamps and a twin-clip approximating clamp (match for comparison of size)

Biangulation technique (Figure 4)[30] — It is not always possible to place the initial stay sutures in the exact eccentric position, especially when there is a major discrepancy between vessel diameters. The use of the biangulation technique can therefore be an advantage, where the two initial stay sutures are placed 180 degrees apart, thereby defining an appropriate adaption of the two different vessel diameters. Interpositioning of sutures in the anterior wall, and after rotation, in the posterior wall, will complete the anastomosis.

Successive interrupted sutures ("ship's wheel type") (Figure 5)[31] — The technique is especially suitable where interrupted sutures are preferred, but anatomical circumstances do not allow a free rotation of the vessel. It is an advantage to place the first suture in the posterior wall. After the suture has been tied, one end is cut near the knot, while a gentle traction of the long end will facilitate the exact positioning of the next adjacent suture. This procedure is repeated until the anastomosis is finished.

Running Suture Technique
This technique shortens anastomosis time and improves primary hemostasis, but includes the risk of stenosis in less trained hands (Figure 6).[32]

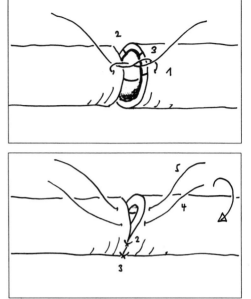

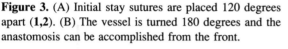

Figure 3. (A) Initial stay sutures are placed 120 degrees apart (**1,2**). (B) The vessel is turned 180 degrees and the anastomosis can be accomplished from the front.

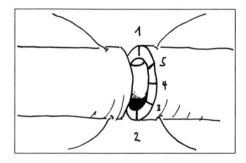

Figure 4. Initial stay sutures are placed 180 degrees apart (**1,2**); remaining sutures are interposed thereafter.

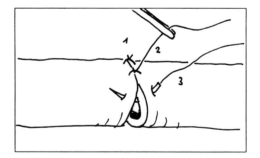

Figure 5. The former stay suture is used to assist the placement of the next suture in a continuous way.

END-TO-SIDE ANASTOMOSIS

The principles of suture technique are basically identical to those of end-to-end anastomosis. Interrupted or running sutures can be used. However, as microsurgical organ transplantation models usually do not permit a free rotation of vessels, anastomosis technique includes suturing of the posterior wall from the luminal side, which is done more easily using a running type of suture. The technique is illustrated in Figure 7.

VEIN ANASTOMOSIS

Veins are very fragile in rodents and must be handled very carefully. The technique of anastomosis is essentially the same as applied in arteries.

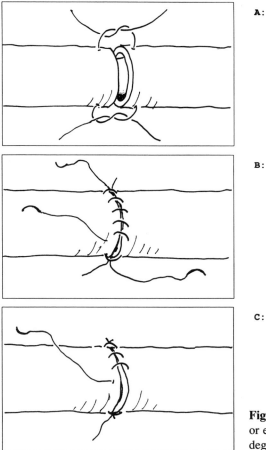

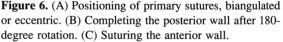

Figure 6. (A) Positioning of primary sutures, biangulated or eccentric. (B) Completing the posterior wall after 180-degree rotation. (C) Suturing the anterior wall.

CUFF TECHNIQUE

This is an alternative, non-suture method for vascular anastomosis (Figure 8).[33-35] In principle, one vessel end is everted over a polyethylene cuff, the other is pulled over the endothelialized cuff, and the anastomosis is secured by a circular ligation.

SPLINT TECHNIQUE

This very useful method has preferably been used for ureter and bile duct end-to-end anastomosis, or the insertion of a stented ureter or choledochus into the recipient bladder or duodenum respectively.[36,37]

The suture and anastomosis techniques illustrated here are the basic approach to microvascular surgery, which will naturally be the object of modifications, preferences and improvements in accordance with personal experience and increasing surgical skill.

SELECTION OF OFTEN-USED MICROSURGICAL MODELS FOR TRANSPLANTATION RESEARCH

The introduction of microsurgical procedures to organ transplantation research has made the investigation of specific immunological questions and immunosuppressing or immunomodulating treatment strategies possible.

The use of inbred rodent strains (mainly rats) combines the possibility of technically feasible whole organ transplantation in donor-recipient combinations, where the genetic disparity in respect to major histoincompatibility is identical between random individuals from the same strain. The outcome of an organ transplantation between two, for all practical reasons genetically identical, rodent strains is therefore reproducible and predictable.[38]

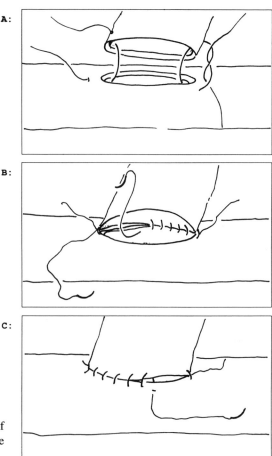

Figure 7. (A) Placing of angle sutures. (B) Suture of the posterior wall from the inside. (C) Completing the anastomosis from the front.

At the same time rats have a size making it possible for trained microvascular surgeons to achieve patency rates (preferably >95% for more simple procedures) which satisfy the statistical and scientific demands for reproducible and valid results, where technical failure does not cover real observation data.

Transplantation research using microsurgical animal models will often include the use of polyclonal or monoclonal antibodies, different sera, immunological reagents, and a variety of methods and procedures, applied as organ recipient treatment, as well as for immunological and histological analysis. Many of these reagents are commercially available for rats and mice, which is an enormous advantage when planning transplantation research projects in laboratories that initially do not have the possibility of producing these reagents.

From a more practical but no less important point of view: rats are cheap, housing is uncomplicated, the animals seem to tolerate surgical and anesthesiological stress well and are highly resistant to postoperative infection.

This section will deal with the two major microsurgical transplantation models (heart and kidney), and finally a few more complex procedures will be mentioned.

HETEROTOPIC HEART TRANSPLANTATION IN THE RAT

Cardiac transplantation in rats is the most often-used model in transplantation research, and consists in principle of a short circuit of normal heart hemodynamics. The donor heart is excised after ligation of the inferior and superior caval veins, and the pulmonary veins, and after division of the aorta and pulmonary artery. On the recipient side, the donor aorta is anastomosed end-to-side to the infrarenal aorta, and the pulmonary artery end-to-side to the inferior caval vein. As recipient vessels the common carotid artery and external jugular vein can be used when preference is given to the heterotopic cervical heart transplantation model. Figure 9 illustrates the result after heterotopic heart transplantation to the recipient abdominal vessels.

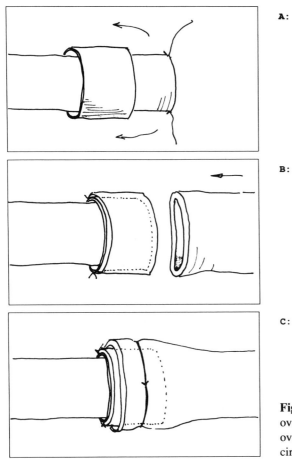

A:

B:

C:

Figure 8. (A) A plastic cuff of adequate size is pushed over the vessel end. (B) Evertion of the vessel stump over the cuff. (C) Completing the anastomosis with a circular ligation.

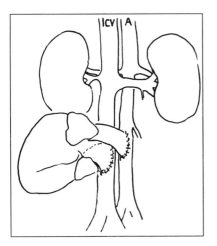

Figure 9. Heterotopic heart transplantation to recipient abdominal vessels with an aorta-to-aorta and a pulmonary artery-to-inferior caval vein anastomosis.

The transplanted heart is perfused via the coronary arteries, draining to the right atrium and through the right ventricle to the venous system of the recipient. But the left ventricle has no physiological function, since there is no ventricular inlet. The model is suitable for immunological and histological studies, or investigations focusing on cardioplegic methods and organ preservation. Graft function, in terms of palpable heart beat, is easily monitored. However, heterotopic cardiac transplantation is a less adequate model for hemodynamic or functional studies.[39,40]

Several modifications have been described using the recipient abdominal or cervical vessels for anastomosis, or placing the donor heart as left ventricular bypass.[19,24,25,33,41,42]

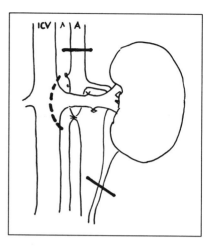

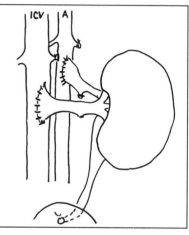

Figure 10(A) Donor nephrectomy for heterotopic left kidney transplantation with an aortic cuff and a vein patch of the inferior caval vein. (B) End-to-side anastomosis from donor to recipient aorta and from the renal vein to the inferior caval vein. Insertion of the ureter into the bladder.

KIDNEY TRANSPLANTATION IN THE RAT

In contrast to the heterotopic heart transplantation model, renal transplantation offers, besides histological and immunological monitoring, the possibility of differentiated functional assessment of a transplanted organ.[43-45] After bilateral nephrectomy of the recipient's own kidneys, renal function will depend exclusively on the graft.

Several techniques of organ harvesting and reimplantation have been described, basically differing on the site of anastomosis. In the heterotopic renal transplantation model, the donor kidney is harvested with or without an aortic/caval vein segment or patch, and anastomosed end-to-side to the recipient infrarenal aorta and caval vein.[20,21,46] The procedure is illustrated in Figure 10.

The orthotopic model makes use of an end-to-end anastomosis between the donor and recipient renal vessels, thereby replacing the recipient's own kindey with a graft (Figure 11).[47,48]

The urinary tract can be reconstituted by ureteric implantation into the recipient bladder, bladder-to-bladder anastomosis, or a direct end-to-end ureter anastomosis.

Any of these different techniques can produce excellent results. Major or minor variations are less important, compared to the necessity of atraumatic microsurgical practice and perfectionism, as well as a reduction of warm ischemia time to zero.

OTHER MICROSURGICAL TRANSPLANTATION MODELS

This section summarizes a few more complex microsurgical models which are used for transplantation research. For more detailed description of techniques and methods, see the references.

1. Lung transplantation[49,50]
2. Orthotopic liver transplantation[35,51-53]

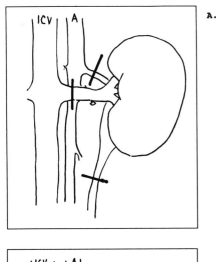

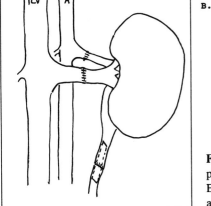

Figure 11(A) Donor nephrectomy for orthotopic left kidney transplantation with division of the renal artery, vein and ureter. (B) End-to-end anastomosis of renal vessels after recipient nephrectomy, and end-to-end ureter anastomosis using the splint technique.

3. Small intestine transplantation[26,54]
4. Pancreas transplantation[55,56]
5. Esophagus replacement[57,58]
6. Multivisceral grafts, including liver, pancreas, stomach, omentum, small intestine and colon[59]

CONCLUDING REMARKS AND COMMENTS

Technical procedures and methods used in experimental microsurgery are essentially the same as applied in the clinic; however, the basic approach is principally different. In the clinic, the surgeon faces an individual problem with a subsequent optimal solution to this problem. Experimental microsurgery tries to elucidate a specific biological question where the microsurgical procedures per se are not actually interesting, and this implies a preferably 100% standardization and reproducibility of the individual experiments. The aim of these studies is the observation and determination of biological variation, and not the monitoring of intraoperative modifications. In other words: detailed repetition of procedures is necessary and only experimental series with high success rates are scientifically acceptable.

There is no mystery about successful performance of microsurgical procedures. It is the result of training, perfectionism and persistence. The basic rule is: as simple as possible, as fast as possible.

Projects of major scientific interest and value which include microsurgical models are based on an interdisciplinary approach to often complex problems. Cooperation and team work are therefore essential. Care has to be taken with respect to animal observation and housing. Time-consuming and difficult microsurgical procedures can end up with surgical success, but disappointing and useless results from a scientific point of view, if optimal laboratory facilities and full-time technical assistance are not available or are neglected.

REFERENCES

1: Carrel, A., La technique opératoire des anastomoses vasculaire et la transplantation des viscères, *Lyon Med., 98, 859, 1902.*

2: Carrel, A., Guthrie, C. C., Complete amputation of the thigh with replantation, *Am. J. Med. Sci., 131, 297, 1906.*

3: Guthrie, C. C., Some physiologic aspects of blood vessel surgery, *JAMA, 51, 1658, 1908.*

4: Nylén, C. O., The otomicroscope and microsurgery 1921-71, *Acta Otolaryngol., 73, 453, 1972.*

5: Jacobson, J. H., Suarez, E. L., Microsurgery in anastomosis of small vessels, *Surg. Forum, 11, 243, 1960.*

6: Kleinert, H. E., Kasdan, M. L., Salvage of devascularized upper extremities including studies on small vessel anastomosis, *Clin. Orthop., 29, 29, 1963.*

7: Malt, R. A., McKhann, C. F., Replantation of severed arms, *JAMA, 189, 716, 1964.*

8: Horn, J. S., Successful reattachment of a completely severed forearm, *Lancet, 1, 1152, 1964.*

9: Bunke, H. J., Jr., Schulz, W. P., Experimental digital amputation and reimplantation, *Plast. Reconstr. Surg., 36, 62, 1965.*

10: Krizek, T. J., Tani, T., DesPrez, J. D., Kiehn, C. L., Experimental transplantation of composite grafts by microsurgical vascular anastomoses, *Plast. Reconstr. Surg., 36, 538, 1965.*

11: Strauch, B., Murray, D. E., Transfer of composite graft with immediate suture anastomosis of its vascular pedicle measuring less than 1 mm in external diameter using microsurgical techniques, *Plast. Reconstr. Surg., 40, 325, 1967.*

12: McLean, D. H., Buncke, H. J., Autotransplant of omentum to a large scalp defect with microsurgical revascularization, *Plast. Reconstr. Surg., 49, 268, 1972.*

13: McGregor, I. A., Morgan, G., Axial and random pattern flaps, *Br. J. Plast. Surg., 26, 202, 1973.*

14: Daniel, R. K., Taylor, G. I., Distant transfer of an island flap by microvascular anastomoses, *Plast. Reconstr. Surg., 52, 111, 1973..*

15: O'Brien, B. M., MacLeod, A. M., Hayhurst, J. W., Morrison, W. A., Successful transfer of a large island flap from the groin to the foot by microvascular anastomoses, *Plast. Reconstr. Surg., 52, 271, 1973 .*

16: Acland, R., Smith, P., Microvascular surgical techniques used to provide skin cover over an ununited tibial fracture, *J. Bone. Jt. Surg., 58, 471, 1976.*

17: Lee, S. H., Fisher, B., Portacaval shunt in the rat, *Surgery, 50, 668, 1961.*

18: Miller, B. F., Gonzales, E., Wilchins, L. J., Nathan, P., Kidney transplantation in the rat, *Nature, 194, 310, 1962.*

19: Abbott, C. P., Lindsey, E. S., Creech, O., Jr., DeWitt, C. W., A technique for heart transplantation in the rat, *Arch. Surg., 89, 645, 1964.*

20: Fisher, B., Lee, S., Microvascular surgical techniques in research, with special reference to renal transplantation, *Surgery, 58, 904, 1965.*

21: Lee, S., An improved technique of renal transplantation in the rat, *Surgery, 61, 771, 1967.*

22: Reemtsma, K., Gialdo, N., Depp, D. A., Eichwald, E. J., Islet cell transplantation, *Ann. Surg., 168, 438, 1968.*

23: Mikaeloff, P. P., Levrat, R., Nesmoz, P., Rassat, J. P., Philippe, M., Dubernard, L. M., Bel, A., Heterotopic liver transplantation in the rat. Value, technique, results of about 70 cases, *Lyon Chir., 68, 133, 1969.*

24: Ono, K., Lindsey, E. S., Improved technique of heart transplantation in rats, *J. Thorac. Cardiovasc. Surg., 57, 225, 1969.*

25: Lee, S., Willoughby, W. F., Smallwood, C. J., Dawson, A., Orloff, M. J., Heterotopic heart and lung transplantation in the rat, *Am. J. Pathol., 59, 279, 1970.*

26: Monchick, G., Russel, P. S., Transplantation of small bowel in the rat: technical and immunological considerations, *Surgery, 70, 693, 1971.*

27: Engemann, R., Deltz, E., Thiede, A., Nahtmaterialien und Nahttechniken in der experimentellen Mikrochirurgie, in *Nahtmaterialien und Nahttechniken,* Thiede, A., Hamelmann, H., Eds., Springer, Berlin, 1982, 90.

28: Silber, S. J., Microsurgical technique, in *Microsurgery,* Silber, S. J., Ed., Williams & Wilkins, Baltimore, 1979, 1.

29: Cobbet, J., Small vessel anastomosis, *Br. J. Plast. Surg., 20, 16, 1967.*

30: Harashina, T., Use of the untied suture in microvascular anastomosis, *Plast. Reconstr. Surg.*, *59, 134, 1977.*

31: Fujino, T., Aoyagi, F., A method of successive interrupted suturing in microvascular anastomoses, *Plast. Reconstr. Surg., 55, 240, 1975.*

32: Biemer, E., Schmidt-Tintemann, U., Anatomische und funktio nelle Grundlagen für die Wahl von Nahtmaterialien und Naht techniken in der klinischen Mikrochirurgie, in *Nahtmaterialien und Nahttechniken,* Thiede, A., Hamelmann, H., Eds., Springer, Berlin, 1982, 400.

33: Heron, I., A technique for accessory cervical heart transplantation in rabbits and rats, *Acta Pathol. Microbiol. Scand.[A], 79, 366, 1971.*

34: Dunn, D. C., Orthotopic renal transplantation in the rabbit, *Transplantation, 22, 427, 1976.*

35: Kamada, N., Calne, R. Y., Orthotopic liver transplantation in the rat, *Transplantation, 28, 47, 1979.*

36: Daniller, A., Buchholz, R., Chase, R. A., Renal transplantation in rats with use of microsurgical techniques: a new method, *Surgery, 63, 956, 1968.*

37: Zimmermann, F. A., Obermüller, K., Gokel, J. M., DornKling, S., Die Gallengangrekonstruktion bei der Ratte durch Choledocho-Choledochostomie über einen verlorenen Drain, *Z. Exp. Chir., 14, 241, 1981.*

38: Günther, E., Immunogenetic aspects of organ transplantation in the rat, in *Microsurgical Models in Rats for Transplantation Research,* Thiede, A., Deltz, E., Engemann, R., Hamel mann, H., Eds., Springer, Berlin, 1985, 83.

39: Konertz, W., Thiede, A., Bernhard, A., Heterotopic heart transplantation in rats — an improved technique of functional evaluation, *Excerpta Med. Int. Congr. Ser., 465, 359, 1980.*

40: Bernhard, A., Konertz, W., Experimental heart transplantation, *J. Thorac. Cardiovasc. Surg., 86, 314, 1983.*

41: Steinbrüchel, D. A., Madsen, H. H., Nielsen, B., Larsen, S., Koch, C., Jensenius, J. C., Hougesen, C., Kemp, E., Treatment with total lymphoid irradiation, cyclosporin A and a monoclonal anti-T-cell antibody in a hamster-to-rat heart transplantation model, *Transplant. Int., 3, 36, 1990.*

42: Konertz, W., Semik, M., Bernhard, A., Left ventricular bypass in inbred rats — a new experimental model in microsurgery. Operative technique and hemodynamic evaluation, *Thorac. Cardiovasc. Surg., 28, 277, 1980.*

43: Dieperink, H., Leyssac, P. P., Larsen, S., Steinbrüchel, D., Starklint, H., Kemp, E., Glomerulotubular function in Cyclosporin A treated rats, *Clin. Nephrol., suppl 1, 70, 1986.*

44: Steinbrüchel, D., Dieperink, H., Kemp, E., Starklint, H., Larsen, S., Rat kidney allotransplantation without warm ischemia. Postoperative recovery and glomerulotubular function. *Eur. Surg. Res., 19-S1, 80, 1987.*

45: Steinbrüchel, D. A., Larsen, S., Kristensen, T., Starklint, H., Koch, C., Kemp, E., Survival, function, morphology and serological aspects of rat renal allografts. Effect of short-term treatment with cyclosporin A, anti-CD4 and anti- interleukin-2 receptor monoclonal antibodies, *A.P.M.I.S., 100, 682, 1992.*

46: Jakubowski, H. D., Renal transplantation in the rat, in *Microsurgical Models in Rats for Transplantation Research,* Thiede, A., Deltz, E., Engemann, R., Hamelmann, H., Eds., Springer, Berlin, 1985, 47.

47: Fabre, J., Lim, S. H., Morris, P. J., Renal transplantation in the rat: details of a technique, *Austr. NZ. J. Surg., 41, 69, 1971.*

48: Kamada, N., A description of cuff technique for renal trans plantation in the rat, *Transplantation, 39, 93, 1985.*

49: Asimacopoulos, P. J., Molokiha, F. A. S., Peck, C. A. S., Lung transplantation in the rat, *Transplant. Proc., 3, 583, 1971.*

50: Mark, K. W., Wildevuur, C. R. H, Lung transplantation in the rat. I. Technique and survival, *Ann. Thorac. Surg., 34, 74, 1981.*

51: Lee, S., Charters, A. C., Chandler, J. G., Orloff, M. J., A technique for orthotopic liver transplantation in the rat, *Transplantation, 16, 664, 1973.*

52: Hansen, H. H., Kim, Y., Lie, T. S., Orthotopic liver transplantation in the rat — special reference to arterialization, *Excerpta Medica Int. Congr. Ser., 465, 394, 1979.*

53: Houssin, D., Gigou, M., Franco, D., Szekely, A. M., Bismith, H., Spontaneous long-term survival of liver allografts in inbred rats, *Transplant. Proc., 11, 567, 1979.*

54: Deltz, E., Thiede, A., Microsurgical technique for small intestine transplantation, in *Microsurgical Models in Rats for Transplantation Research,* Thiede, A., Deltz, E., Engemann, R., Hamelmann, H., Eds., Springer, Berlin, 1985, 51.

55: Lee, S., Tung, K. S. K., Koopmans, H., Chandler, J. G., Orloff, M. J., Pancreaticoduodenal transplantation in the rat, *Transplantation, 13, 421, 1972.*

56: Nolan, M. S., Lindsey, N. J., Savas, C. P., Herold, A., Beck, S., Slater, D. N., Fox, M., Pancreatic transplantation in the rat. Long-term study following different methods of management of exocrine drainage, *Transplantation, 36, 26, 1983.*

57: Parsa, F. D., Spira, M., Experimental oesophagal reconstruction in rats with a free groin flap, *Plast. Reconstr. Surg., 62, 271, 1978.*

58: Uchida, L., Harii, K., Experimental replacement of the cervical oesophagus in rats with a jejunal free transplantation, *Laryngoscope, 99, 837, 1989.*

59: Murase, N., Demetris, A. J., Kim, D. G., Todo, S., Fung, J. J., Starzl, T. E., Rejection of multivisceral allografts in rats: a sequential analysis with comparison to isolated orthotopic small-bowel and liver grafts, *Surgery, 108, 880, 1990.*

Chapter 23

Postmortem Procedures

Ricardo Ernesto Feinstein

CONTENTS

INTRODUCTION

Postmortem procedures (PMP) include necropsy, collection of samples and tissue specimens, and recording of lesions observed. The major uses of PMP are in diagnosis, health quality control, and toxicology studies. In biomedical research PMP are essential to many experiments, not merely as techniques for collecting samples and specimens for examination but also as a means for improving experimental reliability. Sampling techniques may considerably influence the results of an experiment. The protocols for the sacrifice and necropsy of the animals, priorities in the tissue sampling sequence, time required to perform PMP, type of fixatives, and fixation times, are some of the topics that must be thoroughly considered in the design of animal experiments. Necropsies should follow a standard operating procedure (SOP), which should be available when PMP are being performed. Obviously, any deviation from the SOP must be documented.[1,2]

In laboratory animals, lesions and infections by pathogenic organisms are uncontrollable variables which should always be investigated. The additional costs to research of diagnostic necropsies would probably be very low, compared to the adverse effects of a permissive attitude (see Chapters 11 and 12). Diagnostic necropsies, however, should be entrusted to diagnostic laboratories, because diseases cannot be investigated without knowledge of lesions, causative factors, and disease mechanisms. Although most diagnostic necropsies are prompted by detection of sick or dead animals during the course of experiments, clinical signs may or may not be observed. Apparently healthy animals are not necessarily free from lesions that could hamper procedures or influence experimental results.[3] The impact of lesions and infections will depend on the nature and aims of experiments, but researchers should be aware that a careful postmortem examination of the animals, including seemingly healthy individuals, is the most effective way to answering the question whether complicating lesions are present. The systematic use of PMP in diagnosis and health quality control will result in better laboratory animals. Defined, high-quality animals and modern toxicological methods, such as the Fixed Dose Method-Acute Oral Toxicity, show that PMP can be used to reduce further the number of animals required for experimentation and testing.

NECROPSY AND LABORATORY SAFETY

Necropsies should be performed in a specially equipped room, since cadavers and tissue specimens are potential sources of infection to man and animals.[4] Due to the risk of microbial contamination, but also of exposure to allergens and high concentrations of harmful substances, such as anaesthetics, fixatives, solvents, etc., containment facilities and strict adherence to hygiene practices are necessary. Methods of decontamination, cleansing routines, and personal hygiene should be described in the SOP of the necropsy laboratory. PMP should be performed according to Good Laboratory Practice (GLP).[5,6] It is not within the scope of this chapter to provide a complete list of safety measures in necropsy work, but some such measures will be described.

Briefly, in necropsy work, closed-front protective clothing and rubber gloves should be worn, and also protective glasses, when working very close to the surface of organs. Wrist-watches, bracelets, or rings should not be worn. Instruments and all other necessary equipment should be prepared before starting the necropsy. The exterior of tubes, containers, plastic bags, etc., must be protected from contamination and spills. These items should be placed within reach, but not beside the cadaver. Other objects, such as telephone, door-knobs, pencils, etc. should not be touched during the necropsy. No one performing a necropsy should ever pipette by mouth, touch unprotected areas of his/her body, apply contact lenses, or wear them without goggles. Nor should he/she eat, drink, smoke, or apply cosmetics. After the necropsy hands should be washed thoroughly. Protective clothing and gloves must always be taken off when leaving the necropsy room.[5,6]

Local regulations regarding destruction procedures and labeling of containers of biological material should be consulted. Cadavers and tissues can be autoclaved or incinerated. Contaminated, disposable items, such as gloves, scalpel blades, and needles should be sterilized or transported in leak-proof containers to an appropriate plant for sterilization and destruction.

INSTRUMENTS AND MATERIALS

Surgical instruments are appropriate for most necropsies, although certain procedures, such as dissection of very small organs, require microsurgical instruments. Tubes and containers for samples must be identified clearly and indelibly (not on the covers!). If necessary use a code number. The following materials and instruments are commonly used:

- Sharp knife, scalpel blades and handle
- Dissecting scissors and small operating scissors
- Bone-cutting forceps, serrated forceps and toothed forceps
- Syringes (1 ml, 2 ml, 5 ml, and 10 ml) and needles
- Tubes for liquid samples (3 ml, 5 ml, and 12 ml)
- Container of fixative (for routine fixation in 10% buffered neutral formaldehyde solution)
- Leak-proof containers for tissue specimens (bacteriology, mycology, parasitology, virology, chemistry)
- Squeeze bottle of 70% alcohol and squeeze bottle of saline
- Swabs, for sampling purposes (see sampling techniques)
- Plastic bags of various sizes, and paper towels

An electric drill with a cutting disk is a practical aid to opening the cranium or cutting bone structures and teeth (protective glasses must always be worn when using such drills). During the necropsy instruments may be placed in a stainless steel instrument holder with 70% alcohol. Used needles and scalpel blades should be placed in a container with disinfectant.

DESCRIPTION OF LESIONS

The description of lesions should allow a reader to form a mental picture of the changes. The location, appearance, number and severity of the lesions should be described in a precise and concise manner. The location of lesions must be described according to the organ and lobe, area of the skin, portion of the intestines, etc. Anatomical structures are used as reference points. For paired organs, it should be mentioned which of them is affected. Lesions are described in terms of size, shape, color, appearance of the surface and of the cut surface, consistency, demarcation from surrounding tissues, and severity. The size should be measured in two or three dimensions in linear units (mm, cm), or in volume (ml), weight (g), or relative weight. In hollow organs and lesions the amount, appearance, and odor of the contents should be described.[7,8] Photographing of tissue specimens is a most useful aid for description, documentation, and teaching purposes. Correct photographs of medical specimens can be obtained using rather simple equipment.[9]

GUIDELINES FOR THE NECROPSY OF RODENTS AND RABBITS

The anatomical differences between rodents and rabbits do not hinder using a similar necropsy technique. The protocol can be modified, depending on the aims of the studies, but changes of the protocol must always be documented. It is convenient to examine the organs in the following order: external examination, skin and subcutaneous tissues; pelvis, abdomen, mouth, neck, and thorax; head, spinal cord, muscles and joints. After removal from the body, the organs should be laid out on the necropsy table for further examination and sampling.

EXTERNAL EXAMINATION, SKIN AND SUBCUTANEOUS TISSUES

The necropsy is started by inspecting the cadaver. The animal species, strain, animal identity (i.e., necropsy number, ear tags, tattoos, etc.), sex, and body weight are recorded. Postmortem changes are scored: in a scale ranging from one to five, one corresponds to mild decomposition of tissues, such as observed in animals sacrificed immediately before the necropsy, and five corresponds to a pronounced disintegration of tissues. The appearance of the skin, hair coat, body openings, and visible mucous membranes is observed. Loss of hair, changes in the color of the skin or mucous membranes (icterus, cyanosis, etc.), presence of discharges from natural orifices, tumors, etc. are noted. In hamsters, the flank organs, which represent a male secondary sexual characteristic, are inspected. The skin and subcutaneous tissues are palpated for lesions.

The cadaver is placed on its back and pinned to a dissection board (in rabbits this is not necessary). The skin is moistened with alcohol and a midline incision is made, from the symphysis of the mandible to the anus, avoiding the penis in male animals. The skin is reflected on both sides of the incision (Figure 1). The subcutaneous tissues are inspected. The amount of fat in the body depots and the muscular volume are observed. Skinning of the cadaver can be completed at the end of the necropsy, or at this stage. In guinea pigs and autolysed cadavers the stomach and the intestines may rupture during the skinning procedure. The mandibulary and cervical lymph nodes, the salivary glands (mandibular, parotid and sublingual) and the extraorbital lacrymal glands are observed. The mammary glands are inspected (mice have five pairs of mammary glands, rats six, hamsters six or seven, guinea pigs one, and rabbits four pairs). In female rodents the clitoral glands are inspected (Figure 1). In males the penis, prepuce and the preputial glands are examined. The inguinal lymph nodes, which are usually embedded in the subcutaneous fat tissues, are observed.

PELVIS AND ABDOMEN

The abdomen is opened by a midline incision through the abdominal wall, from the sternum to the pelvis, and by two cuts through the muscles along the costal arcs (Figure 2). The floor of the pelvis is removed, after making a sagittal cut on each side of the middle line (Figure 3). The abdominal and pelvic organs are examined *in situ*. The appearance of the serous membrane and the occurrence of abnormal contents, such as serous fluid, blood, fibrin, adhesions between organs, etc. are observed. The fat depots are examined and the nutritional condition is scored: 1, obese animal; 2, good nutritional condition; 3, poor nutritional condition; 4, undernourished, bad nutritional condition; 5, emaciation, absence of fat in the body depots.

386

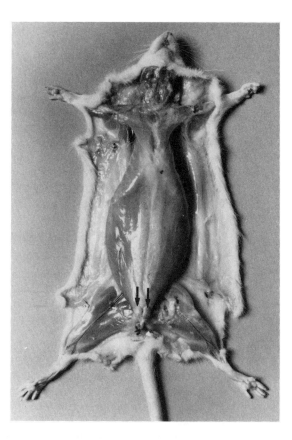

Figure 1. The arrows point at the clitoral glands.

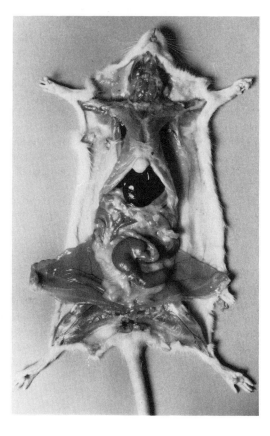

Figure 2. The abdominal cavity with the organs *in situ*. Cultural samples should be taken before handling the viscerae.

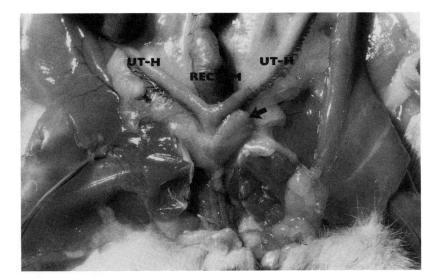

Figure 3. Pelvis with the organs *in situ*. UT-H: Uterine horn. The arrow points at the urinary bladder.

Male Genital Organs and Urinary Bladder

The scrotum is cut open and the testicles and epididymides are extracted. The fibrous ligaments anchoring the tail of the epididymis to the scrotum are cut. The vas deferens is cut, and the testicles and epididymides are removed for inspection. The ureters are cut and the remaining genital organs are removed in block, i.e., seminal vesicles, coagulating glands, bulbo-urethral glands, prostate gland, urethra, and penis. The urine is collected from the urinary bladder. Rabbit and guinea pig urine is normally turbid due to its high concentration of mineral crystals. In rodents the urethral plug, a whitish, rather hard cast, located in the lumen of the proximal urethra and sometimes extending into the bladder, is regarded as a (normal) male secondary sex characteristic.[10]

Female Genital Organs and Urinary Bladder

In young animals the female genital organs are entirely located in the pelvis, whereas in adult animals the ovaries with the oviducts are located caudally to the kidneys. The genital organs and supporting ligaments are partly embedded in fat, but the ovaries stand out from the fat tissues, being more reddish in color. The vulva and vagina are dissected free from the skin and rectum. The vagina is caught with a forceps, and the supporting ligaments of the vagina, uterus, oviduct and ovary are cut. The genital organs and the urinary bladder are opened for examination of mucous membranes.

Spleen and Pancreas

The spleen is removed by cutting the omentum and the ligamentum gastrolienalis along the greater stomach curvature. The pancreas is examined. It is a rather diffuse and richly lobulated organ, located in the supporting ligaments of the stomach and the small intestine. It is firmer and more greyish than fat tissues.

Stomach and Intestines

In mice, rats, hamsters and gerbils the stomach is divided into two distinct regions, the cutaneous or proventicular region, and the glandular region. The glandular region has a thicker wall than the cutaneous region. In the guinea pig these regions are not clearly demarcated. The rabbit stomach is not divided into special areas.[11] The intestines of rodents show no special features (in guinea pigs the cecum is a thin-walled, voluminous organ). Rabbits have long intestines, with most of the gut-associated lymphoid tissues located in the last portion of the small intestine (sacculus rotundus or ileocecal tonsil) and in the appendix vermiformis, a cecal diverticulum. The intestinal wall is thicker at the level of the sacculus rotundus and the appendix than in the rest of the intestines.

To remove the gastrointestinal tract, the anus is dissected free from the surrounding skin. The rectum is caught with a forceps and the mesentery and the supporting ligaments are cut. The supporting ligaments along the whole length of the large intestine, the small intestine, and the stomach are cut. It is convenient

388

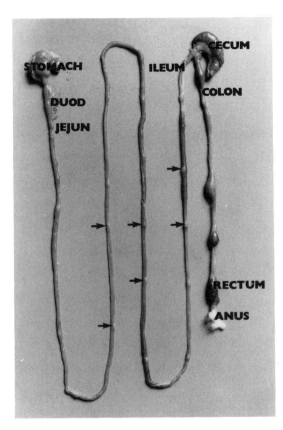

Figure 4. DUOD: Duodenum; JEJUN: jejunum. The arrows point at some of the Peyer's patches.

to cut the supporting ligaments as close to the intestines as possible. The cardia is cut with a forceps, and while the stomach is gently pulled away from the diaphragm, the esophagus is cut. Then the whole gastrointestinal tract is removed and placed on the necropsy table for examination (Figure 4). After all the other organ examinations are finished, the stomach is opened along the greater curvature. The whole length of the intestines is opened, and the gastrointestinal contents are collected and examined. The digestive mucosa is inspected, including the Peyer's patches. Lesions in the mucosa, such as erosions, can be covered by adherent contents. The surface is rinsed with saline or tap water to remove contents. The mesentery is removed including the mesenteric lymph nodes.

Liver, Kidneys and Adrenal Glands
The liver is removed by cutting the hepatic ligaments and the hepatic tissues are examined by deep cuts in different lobes. The gallbladder and its contents are examined (rats do not have this organ).

The right and left adrenals, which are located cranially and medially to the respective kidney, are removed. Both kidneys are removed by cutting the urethers and the renal vessels at the level of the renal hilus. If possible, the adrenals and kidneys are cut longitudinally, and the cortex, medulla, and the renal pelvis are examined. The renal capsule is removed and the appearance of the cortical surface is observed.

MOUTH, NECK, AND THORAX
The mandibulary muscles are cut on both sides, and the mandible is pulled backwards and if necessary removed. The oral cavity is inspected. The larynx, trachea, and esophagus are dissected by cutting the muscles in the ventral part of the neck. To open the thorax, the xiphoid cartilage is lifted with a forceps and the sternum removed by cutting on both sides along the costochondral junctions (Figure 5). The sternum is a convenient organ for histological examination of the bone marrow. The thorax and its organs are inspected *in situ*. In mice, hamsters, and rabbits the thymus is located in the anteroventral portion of the thorax, close to the middle line. Rats, in addition, have a smaller cervical portion, which lies ventrally to the trachea. In guinea pigs the thymus is entirely located in the ventral part of the neck. The tongue is caught with a forceps and pull backwards, and the soft palate and pharynx are cut with a scalpel. The tongue, esophagus, larynx, trachea with thyroid and parathyroid glands, thymus, mediastinal and bron-

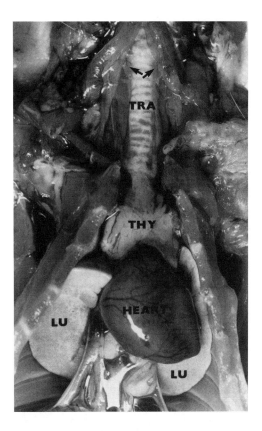

Figure 5. The thyroids are marked by arrows. TRA: Trachea; THY: thymus; LU: lung.

chial lymph nodes, lungs and heart are removed in block by gently pulling backwards and after severing the thoracic aorta and the caudal vena cava at the level of the diaphragm.

The pericardial sac is opened and the heart examined. Before the heart is opened, the left and right sides should be identified. The right atrium may be opened by making an incision from the sinus venosus into the auricle. The incision is prolonged into the right ventricle, by cutting its wall parallel to the interventricular septum towards the apex, and from the apex to the pulmonary artery. The left atrium is opened, starting the incision at the entrance of the pulmonary veins. The wall of the auricle is cut and the incision is prolonged into the left ventricle along the interventricular septum towards the apex, and from the apex into the aortic artery. The myocardial cut surface, the heart cavities, and the atrioventricular and semilunar valves are inspected. Clots are removed and the endocardium is inspected. The aortic trunk is opened, and if necessary the whole length of the aorta. The whole length of the esophagus, larynx, trachea, and the major bronchi are opened, and the mucosae of these organs and also the cut surface of the lungs are examined.

HEAD AND SPINAL CORD.

The skin is cut transversally over the neck, and the cranium is skinned and severed caudally to the occipital protuberance. The cranium of young animals and of adult mice can be opened with scissors. For adult animals of other species bone cutters are preferable. An electric drill with a cutting disk is also practical. The cranium is opened by first making two cuts from the foramen magnum to the medial part of both orbits. Then the frontal bone is cut transversally at a level just behind the orbits, which coincides with the anterior border of the cranial cavity. The lid of the skull is removed (Figure 6). To extract the brain and cerebellum from the cranium, cut the olfactory lobes with small operating scissors inserted under the anterior part of the brain. Then the optic nerves and the remaining cranial nerves on both sides are cut.

The brain and cerebellum are removed (artifacts produced by the manipulation of fresh brain tissues can be avoided by fixation of the brain *in situ)*. After removal of the brain, the pituitary gland appears on the floor of the cranium, attached to the sella turcica (Figure 7). In rodents there is a thin layer of dura mater covering the pituitary gland. The dura around the gland is cut with a scalpel. Using the scalpel blade

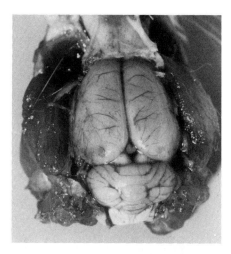

Figure 6. Cranium with the brain *in situ*. The lid of the skull was removed by making two lateral cuts, from the foramen magnum to the medial part of both orbits, and a transversal cut just behind the orbits.

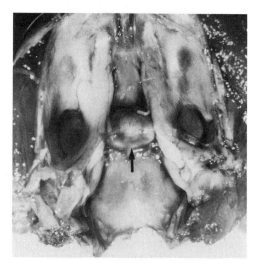

Figure 7. Dorsal endocranial view of the skull after removal of the brain and cerebellum. The pituitary gland in the sella turcica is marked by an arrow.

as a shovel, the gland is lifted out of the sella turcica. In rabbits the pituitary gland is covered by a bony projection (dorsum sellae), which has to be removed prior to removal of the gland.

The tympanic cavity is inspected. The wall of the tympanic bulla is thin and can be opened ventrally with scissors (rodents) or bone cutters (rabbits), after disinfection of the surface. The middle ear can be examined histologically after decalcification of the skull.

Using small operating scissors or a scalpel inserted in the orbit, the eyeball is freed from the surrounding tissues and the optic nerve is cut. A forceps is used to lift the eyeball, with the Harder's gland and the smaller, intraorbital lacrymal gland, out of the orbit. In guinea pigs the zygomatic salivary gland, which is located ventral to the globe of the eye is also collected.

To inspect the nasal cavity the cranium can be divided by a midline cut, in aboral-oral direction. However, if the nasal region is to be examined histologically, it had better be cut transversally together with palatine structures, for reference points, after fixation and decalcification.[12]

The spinal cord should be fixed *in situ,* because it is easily damaged if removed from the vertebral canal. In adult animals, except for mice, the spinal cord can be removed with small operating scissors or bone cutters. Starting at the first cervical vertebra, incisions are made alternately on the right and left side to remove the vertebral arches, and then the roots of the spinal nerves are cut. An alternative is to approach the spinal cord ventrally by removing the vertebral bodies (Figure 8).

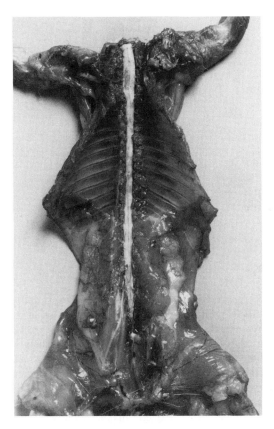

Figure 8. Ventral view of the spinal cord *in situ*, after removal of the vertebral bodies.

MUSCLES AND JOINTS

The sublumbar muscles and the muscles of the thigh region are inspected by longitudinal and transversal cuts. The major limb joints are examined. The periarticular muscles are removed and the articular capsule is swabbed with alcohol and the joints are opened with a scalpel. Samples for culturing may be obtained by scraping and swabbing the articular surfaces. If necessary, joints can be removed and fixed for histological examination.

SAMPLING TECHNIQUES

Once an animal study is completed, all that remains are the records, samples, and specimens.[13] A correct sampling technique is essential to postmortem studies. The results obtained depend on the care with which specimens are collected.

SAMPLING FOR MORPHOLOGICAL EXAMINATIONS
Histology

Cadavers should be refrigerated until the moment of necropsy, but specimens obtained from a recently killed animal are preferable. Freezing of cadavers or specimens should be avoided. It causes marked histological disruption. Tissue specimens should be obtained with a scalpel or a sharp knife, and should be handled carefully, to avoid artifacts caused by stretching or compression of tissues. Artifactual distortion of tissues can destroy, alter, mimic, or mask experimental changes. Specimens should include lesions and their surrounding tissues. Even macroscopically normal tissues should be collected, in order to reveal changes demonstrable only by microscopical examination. For routine histology, tissue specimens are fixed by immersion in 10% buffered neutral formaldehyde solution for 24 h. The volume of fixative should exceed that of the specimens at least ten times (formaldehyde solution) or twenty times (alcohol-based fixatives). For an adequate penetration of the fixative tissue specimens should not be thicker than 6 mm (Figure 9). For diagnostic electron microscopy, specimens, not thicker than 3 mm, can be fixed in glutharaldehyde or Karnovsky fluid.

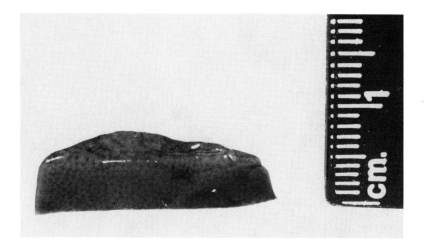

Figure 9. Liver specimen for histology.

The postmortal decomposition of tissues is a hindrance to microscopical studies. It occurs very rapidly in the intestines.[14,15] Intestinal specimens are best preserved by injecting formalin into the lumen of an unopened intestinal segment.[16] The lungs can be fixed by immersion or by perfusion with fixative via the trachea.[15] An optimal preservation of tissue morphology, or of tissue antigens, or both can be achieved by perfusion fixation. The animal is anaesthetized and the fixative is injected into the vascular system. The type and amount of fixative, perfusion pressure and injection site will depend on various factors, such as the aim of the study, the animal species, and body weight.[17-19] A different method, for small tissue specimens, based on freeze substitution and low temperature plastic embedding, also results in high-quality morphology and optimum antigen preservation.[20] The use of a microwave oven can considerably shorten the time required for fixation and subsequent histological procedures.[21] In addition, microwave oven heating of tissue sections often improves tissue antigen detection by immunohistochemistry in formalin-fixed, paraffin-embedded tissues.[22]

Vital staining, i.e., the use of colored substances injected into the vascular system, has been variously employed to investigate vascular permeability to different substances. In addition, the vital dye, Evans blue, has been found useful in the search for delicate or very small organs, such as the thoracic duct, or the paraganglia.[23-27]

Parasitology

The sampling site is important in parasitological examinations because parasites have predilection sites. In addition, simultaneous infection with various types of parasites is not uncommon. Thus, skin scrapings for parasitology should be obtained from different areas. If possible, the whole skin should be examined, including ears, eyelids, and nasal cavity. The skin should be placed in a hermetically sealed container or in a plastic bag, and refrigerated until the moment of examination. For endoparasites, samples from gastrointestinal contents should be collected during the necropsy. Samples should be placed in clean, leak-proof containers. Fresh samples are always preferable. Microscopical examination of gastrointestinal contents or feces (wet preparation) permits the identification of parasites, larvae, and eggs. Specimens examined immediately after collection are appropriate for the demonstration of motile protozoans or trophozoite stages of protozoans. Samples for examination of protozoan oocysts, helminth eggs, and adult helminths may be refrigerated. Most endoparasites located in other organs than the intestine are diagnosed by microscopical examination of tissue sections. For certain parasites, such as the protozoans *Toxoplasma gondii* and *Encephalitozoon cuniculi,* serological methods and immunohistochemical techniques are also available.[28,29] Blood smears are useful for examining for blood parasites. Smears should be of a good quality, as no diagnostic skill can compensate for a poorly made blood film.[30] Preferably, smears should be prepared from fresh blood, recently obtained without anticoagulants. Films that are not stained immediately should be fixed and stored in a protected place. Techniques for preparing smears have been described.[31]

SAMPLING FOR CULTIVATION

The results from postmortem cultures depend on the care with which specimens are collected. The diagnostic laboratory should be consulted regarding which tissues to examine and the conditions of transport of the specimens.

Bacteria

Most bacterial infections are diagnosed by bacterial culture. The successful isolation of bacteria depends on various factors, but a correct sampling technique is essential. Inadequate sampling techniques can result in the overgrowth of a causative agent by contaminant bacteria. Therefore, specimens for bacterial culture should be obtained before the organs are handled, i.e., as early as possible during the necropsy (Figure 10). Other factors of importance for culturing results are the sampling site, type of disease, its duration, whether the animals have been treated with antibiotics, etc. The period elapsed after death should also be considered, because the viability of pathogenic bacteria and mycoplasma in tissues decreases, while bacteria of the normal flora rapidly invade the tissues and may overgrow pathogenic agents. The agonal or postmortem invasion of tissues by resident bacteria must be distinguished from an infection occurring before death. Therefore, culture results must be evaluated together with necropsy findings, such as the presence of lesions compatible with the bacteria isolated.[6,32-35]

Tissue specimens for bacterial culture should be obtained with sterile instruments. The surface of the tissues can be seared with a red-hot spatula or a flame, or it can be washed with 70% alcohol. Bacterial specimens may consist of cut pieces of tissues (Figure 10). The instruments must be flamed before collecting each specimen. In the case of hollow organs (intestines, uterus), a segment is cut after ligation at both ends. Sterile swabs inserted into the tissues are also used, but the swabs should be processed within a few hours.[6,33] Cotton swabs should be avoided, as substances present in the cotton may hinder the growth of certain bacteria. Swabbing is also convenient for sampling serosal and mucosal surfaces (i.e., pericardial sac, joints, genital tract, conjunctiva, etc.). Organs having a thick capsule, but also abscesses and pustules can be opened with a scalpel after disinfection of the surface. The contents are then sampled by thorough swabbing against the capsule. Body fluids, such as urine or blood, can be aspirated with a sterile needle and syringe.

Techniques for obtaining samples for culturing mycoplasma and bacteria by washing the respiratory and the genital mucosa have been described in detail.[34] However, for respiratory bacteria washing was not as effective as swabbing or cut tissue blocks.[35] Bacterial specimens from organs and serosal or mucosal surfaces can be transferred to a culture medium using a sterile loop. For print cultures the surface of the tissues is pressed against a culture medium, or a blotting paper is pressed against the tissues and then transferred to a culture medium.[36,37] The use of transport media, and the conditions of transport of the specimens to the laboratory are of considerable importance. Swabs should not be allowed to dry, or the viability of many bacteria and mycoplasmas is rapidly reduced. Transport in sterile phosphate-buffered saline (PBS) at 4°C was found to maintain the stability of murine mycoplasmas and various pathogenic bacteria, except for *Pasteurella multocida* and *Pasteurella pneumotropica*.[38] Specimens submitted to distant laboratories should be refrigerated.

Fungi

Specimens for fungal culture, except dermatological specimens, should be kept moist with sterile distilled water or saline. Specimens should be obtained aseptically, as has been described for bacterial sampling. Dermatological specimens should be free from contamination by blood. Hairs and the base of hair shafts, and skin scrapings, can be collected in Petri dishes after washing the skin with 70% alcohol. Skin scrapings should include the center and the periphery of lesions.[39]

Virus

Necropsy specimens for virus isolation should be collected aseptically (see sampling for bacteriology), placed in leak-proof sterile containers without preservative, and chilled. Specimens, except blood, should be stored frozen, preferably at -70°C. The postmortal decomposition of tissues inactivates many viruses. Thus, specimens should be obtained shortly after death, and preferably during the early stage of infection.[40]

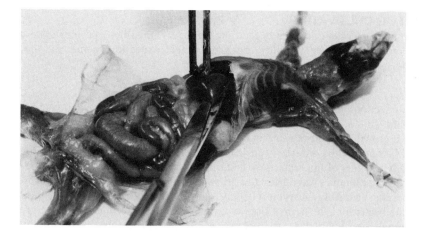

Figure 10. Cutting a piece of liver for bacteriology. The specimen is obtained before the organs are handled.

SAMPLING FOR SEROLOGY

Blood samples for serology should be obtained from live animals. Techniques to collect adequate samples have been variously described.[41-43] In recently sacrificed animals blood can be aspirated with a syringe or a Pasteur pipette from the heart, from the thorax after severing the posterior vena cava or the thoracic aorta, or from the axilar or inguinal areas, after severing the arteries at these areas. Blood samples for serology should be obtained aseptically and without additives. To avoid hemolysis the blood must be obtained and processed carefully (blood must not be forced through a small gauge needle and the separation of serum from the rest of the blood must not be delayed). Serum samples can be maintained for a short time at 4°C, or stored frozen, preferably at -70°C. Large volumes of serum should be fractioned to avoid repeated freezing and thawing.

SAMPLING FOR CHEMICAL INVESTIGATION

Fodder and bedding should be examined when deficiencies or contamination by pesticides, herbicides, heavy metals, or other substances that might influence biological processes are suspected. Serum and tissue specimens collected without chemical contamination should be placed in leak-proof, clean tubes or containers. Each organ must be sent in a separate container. Polyethylene bags are not always appropriate because they are permeable to many organic substances, and the plasticizers used in their manufacture may contaminate the sample.[44] Serum and tissue specimens should be frozen for transportation to the laboratory. Whole blood should not be frozen. Blood, collected in tubes containing fluoride and oxalate as preservative and anticoagulant, can be transported refrigerated. Specimens preferred for chemical examination are liver, kidney, blood or serum, urine, and stomach with its contents. Bone should be collected when a pesticide or metal is suspected.[45] The laboratory should be consulted about the type and amount of specimens necessary for each analysis.

ACKNOWLEDGMENT

I wish to thank Bengt Ekberg for the photographs presented in this chapter. The photographs shown were taken during the necropsy of a female Sprague-Dawley rat, aged approximately three months.

REFERENCES

1. Hildebrandt, P. K., Regulatory aspects and potential pitfalls of toxicologic pathology, in *Handbook of Toxicological Pathology,* Haschek, W. M., Rousseaux, C. G., Eds., Academic Press, San Diego, 1991, chap. 9.
2. Bucci, T. J., Evaluation of altered morphology, in *Handbook of Toxicological Pathology,* Haschek, W. M., Rousseaux, C. G., Eds., Academic Press, San Diego, 1991, 23.

3. Feinstein, R. E., and Rehbinder, C., Health monitoring of purpose bred laboratory rabbits in Sweden: Major findings. *Scand. J. Lab. Anim. Sci., 15, 49, 1988.*

4. Smith, M. W., Hazards and safety aspects of animal work, in *Laboratory Animals. An Introduction for New Experimenters,* Tuffery, A. A., Ed, John Wiley & Sons, Chichester, 1987, chap. 7.

5. Grizzle, W. E., and Polt, S. S., Guidelines to avoid personnel contamination by infective agents in research laboratories that use human tissues. *J. Tissue Culture Methods, 11, 191, 1988.*

6. Du Moulin, G. C., and Love, W., The value of autopsy microbiology. *Clin. Microbiol. Newslett., 10, 165, 1988.*

7. Feldman, D. B., and Seely, J. C., *Necropsy guide: Rodents and the Rabbit.* CRC Press, Boca Raton, Florida, 1988.

8. Strafuss, A. C., *Necropsy. Procedures and Basic Diagnostic Methods for Practicing Veterinarians.* Charles C. Thomas, Springfield, Illinois, 1988.

9. Edwards, W. D., Photography of medical specimens: experiences from teaching cardiovascular pathology. *Mayo Clin. Proc., 63, 42, 1988.*

10. Kunstyr, I., Küpper, W., Weisser, H., Naumann, S., and Messow, C., Urethral plug. A new secondary male sex characteristic in rat and other rodents. *Lab. Anim., 16, 151, 1982.*

11. Ghoshal, N. G., and Bal, H. S., Comparative morphology of the stomach of some laboratory mammals. *Lab. Anim., 23, 21, 1989.*

12. Popp, J. A., and Monterio-Riviere, N. A., Macroscopic, microscopic and ultrastructural anatomy of the nasal cavity, rat, in *Respiratory System,* Jones, T. C., Mohr, U., Hunt, R. D., Eds., Springer-Verlag, Berlin, 1985, 3.

13. Noel, R. B., Toxicity testing, hazard assessment, and data quality assurance in respect to use of laboratory animals, in *Animals in Toxicological Research,* Bartosek, I., Guaitani, A., Pacei, E., Eds., Raven Press, New York, 1982, 45.

14. Scheifele, D., Bjornson, G., and Dimmick, J., Rapid postmortem gut autolysis in infant rats: A potential problem for investigators. *Can. J. Vet. Res., 51, 404, 1987.*

15. Seaman, W.J., *Postmortem Change in the Rat: A Histologic Characterization.* Iowa State University Press, Ames, 1987, chap. 1,2,4.

16. Fenwick, B. W., and Kruckenberg, S., Comparison of methods used to collect canine intestinal tissues for histological examination, *Am. J. Vet. Res., 48, 1276, 1987.*

17. Hayat, M. A., Methods of fixation, in *Principles and Techniques of Electron Microscopy,* Hayat, A. M., Ed., Litton Educational Publishing, New York, 1970, 95.

18. Bugge, H. P., and Plöen, L., Changes in the volume of sertoli cells during the cycle of the seminiferous epithelium in the rat. *J. Reprod. Fertil., 76, 39, 1986.*

19. Siemiatkowski, M., Plöen, L., and Björkman, N., Combined perfusion and percolation of embalmed animal bodies for removing formaldehyde. *Acta Anat., 133, 251, 1988.*

20. Murray, G.I., and Ewen, S.W.B., A novel method for optimum biopsy specimen preservation for histochemical and immunohistochemical analysis. *Am. J. Clin. Pathol., 95, 131, 1991.*

21. Boon, M. E. and Kok, L. P., *Microwave Cookbook of Pathology.* Columb Press Leyden, Leiden, 1987.

22. Shi, S.-R., Key, M. E., and Kalra, K. L., Antigen retrieval in formalin-fixed, paraffin-embedded tissues: An enhancement method for immunohistochemical staining based on microwave oven heating of tissue sections. *J. Histochem. Cytochem., 39, 741, 1991.*

23. LeVeen, H. H., and Fishman, W. H., Combination of Evans blue with plasma protein: its significance in capillary permeability studies, blood dye disappearance curves, and its use as a protein tag. *Am. J. Physiol., 151, 26, 1947.*

24. Coleridge, H., Coleridge, J. C. G., and Howe, A., A search for pulmonary arterial chemoreceptors in the cat, with a comparison of the blood supply of the aortic bodies in the new-born and adult animal, *J. Physiol., 191, 353, 1967.*

25. Richardson, K. C., The fine structure of autonomic nerves after vital staining with methylene blue. *Anat. Rec., 164, 359, 1969.*

26. Clasen, R. A., Pandolfi, S., and Has, G. M., Vital staining, serum albumin and the blood-brain barrier. *J Neuropathol.Exp. Neurol., 29, 266, 1990.*

27. McDonald, D. M., and Blewett, R. W., Location and size of carotid body-like organs (paraganglia) revealed in rats by the permeability of blood vessels to Evans blue dye, *J. Neurocytol., 10, 607, 1981.*

28. Waller, T., Lyngset, A., Elvander, M., and Morein, B., Immunological diagnosis of encephalitozoonosis from post-mortem specimens, *Vet. Immunol. Immunopathol. 1, 353, 1980.*

29. Waller, T., and Bergqvist, N. R., Rapid simultaneous diagnosis of toxoplasmosis and encephalitozoonosis in rabbits by carbon immunoassay. *Lab. Anim. Sci., 32, 515, 1982.*

30. Coles, E. H., The blood film, in *Veterinary Clinical Pathology,* fourth edition, W.B. Saunders, Philadelphia, 1986, 53.

31. Schalm, O. W., Jain, N. C., and Carroll, E. J., The blood film, in *Veterinary Hematology,* Lea & Febiger, Philadelphia, 1975, 25.

32. Brooks, G. F., Butel, J. S., Ornston, L. N., Jawetz, E., Melnick, J. L., and Adelberg, E. A., Principles of diagnostic medical microbiology, in *Jawetz, Melnick & Adelberg's Medical Microbiology,* 19th edition. Prentice-Hall, London, 1991, 587.

33. Ikram, M., and Hill, E., Laboratory procedures in bacteriology, in *Microbiology for Veterinary Technicians,* American Veterinary Publications, Inc., Goleta, 1991, chap. 5.

34. Cassell, G. H., Davidson, M. K., Davis, J. K., and Lindsey, J. R., Recovery and identification of murine mycoplasmas, in *Methods in Mycoplasmology,* Tully, J. G., and Razin, S., Eds., Academic Press, San Diego, 1983, 129.

35. Needham, J. R., *Handbook of Microbiological Investigations for Laboratory Animal Health,* Academic Press, London, 1979, 14.

36. Sögaard, P., Larsen, K. E., Buhl, L., Lou, H. E., and Henriques, U., Bacteriological autopsy. I. A methodological study. *APMIS, 99, 541, 1991.*

37. Larsen, K. E., Sögaard, P., Buhl, L., Lou, H. E., and Henriques, U., Bacteriological autopsy. II. Comparison of a group of cancer patients with a control group. *APMIS, 99, 545, 1991.*

38. Shimoda, K., Maejima, K., Kuhara, T., and Nakagawa, M., Stability of pathogenic bacteria from laboratory animals in various transport media. *Lab. Anim., 25, 228, 1991.*

39. McGinnis, M. R., *Laboratory Handbook of Medical Mycology,* Academic Press, New York, 1980, chap. 3.

40. Heuschele, W. P., and Castro, A. E., Selection and submission of diagnostic specimens, in *Veterinary Diagnostic Virology. A Practicioner's Guide,* Castro, A. E., Heuschele, W. P., Eds., Mosby-Year Book, Chicago, 1992, 1.

41. Loeb, W. F., and Quimby, F.W., *The Clinical Chemistry of Laboratory Animals,* Pergamon Press, New York, 1989.

42. Flecknell, P. A., Non-surgical experimental procedures, in *Laboratory Animals. An Introduction for New Experimenters,* Tuffery, A. A., Ed., John Wiley & Sons, Chichester, 1987, chap. 13.

43. Smith, A. L., Serological tests for detection of antibody to rodent viruses, in *Viral and Mycoplasmal Infections of Laboratory Rodents. Effects on Biomedical Research,* Bhatt, P. N., Jacoby, R. O., Morse, H.C., III, New, A. E., Eds., Academic Press, Orlando, 1986, chap. 34.

44. Clarke, E. G. C., and Clarke, M. L., Analytical evidence, in *Veterinary Toxicology.* Bailliere Tindal, London, 1975, 22.

45. Sunshine, I., Analytic Toxicology, in *Casarett and Doull's Toxicology. The Basic Science of Poisons,* third ed., Klaassen, C. D., Amdur, M. O., Doull, J., Eds., Macmillan, New York, 1986, chap. 27.

Chapter 24

Isolated Organs as Replacements for Vertebrate Animals

Jens Juul Holst

CONTENTS

INTRODUCTION

Why isolate organs? The surgical isolation of an organ is generally associated with the death of the donor animal. Thus, if the purpose is to save the lives of experimental animals, the choice of organ isolation is a poor one. On the other hand, the surgical isolation can be accomplished under controlled circumstances, i.e., with adequate housing of the animal before the experiment, adequate preoperative handling and general anesthesia, so that the animal suffers minimally, regardless of the nature of the subsequent experimentation. In this respect, however, there is little difference between organ isolation and experiments performed in anesthetized animals. The use of isolated organ preparations must therefore be viewed in the light of what could otherwise have been obtained in conscious or anesthetized animals.

It may be useful to discuss briefly what could be described as levels of physiological control of organ function.

LEVELS OF PHYSIOLOGICAL CONTROL OF ORGAN FUNCTION

UNICELLULAR MECHANISMS

Obviously the function of a cell is dependent on its metabolic state and on the supplies of fuels, oxygen, etc., but in addition to these it is increasingly evident that many cells are capable of exerting so-called autocrine control of their own function.[1] This implies that they produce a signal molecule, which, after release from the cell, interacts with receptor mechanisms on the same cell and subsequently regulates its function. Growth, in particular, is believed to be influenced by autocrine control. Obviously, autocrine regulation is best studied in single cell preparations or in cell culture systems. Whether or not control exerted by metabolites, like, e.g., carbon dioxide, should be classified as autocrine regulation is a matter of opinion. In this respect it is also of interest to note that unicellular organisms to a major extent communicate and regulate each other's function by releasing signal molecules that can be received and decoded by other unicellular organisms after the binding of the signal molecule to appropriate receptors.[2]

PLURICELLULAR INTERACTION

In all pluricellular organisms, including higher organisms like mammals, direct cell-to-cell communication takes place, allowing coordination of cell functions.[3] The communication may consist of electric signals in the form of electrotonic coupling between cells, or of chemical signals, transmitted via gap junctions between the cells or released from the cell surface to reach the target cell by diffusion through the extracellular space. Metabolites may play a similar role. Release of signal molecules with regulatory functions on neighboring cells is usually called *paracrine* control.[4] Although described rather recently, there is little doubt that paracrine mechanisms play an important role in all pluricellular organisms. Certain cells have paracrine regulation as a specialized function and may have a characteristic morphology reflecting this: they typically have cytoplasmic, dendrite-like processes, which may establish close contacts with the neighboring target cells.[5] In this way the paracrine cell can effectively control the function of groups of neighboring cells. It is clear from this description that the paracrine cells may be viewed as relatives of the neurons of the *nervous* system, the difference being that the nerve cell body is located at a distance from the target. It is important for the subject of the present chapter to recall that this distance may not be very long. This is particularly true for parts of the central nervous system itself and for target organs of the parasympathetic system and the enteric nervous system. For all of such regulatory systems a distinction between *local* control as opposed to the *remote* control exerted by neurons with the nerve cell body located outside the organ in question, may be useful. An additional example of remote control is provided by the *endocrine* regulation, where the signal molelcule released from a specialized endocrine organ travels to the target organ via the blood route.

STUDIES IN CONSCIOUS ANIMALS

In the design of studies of physiological regulation these levels have to be considered. In the intact, conscious animal all regulatory mechanisms are at play simultaneously. Thus, the organ is influenced by its own metabolic state and by the metabolic state of the animal as a whole, by paracrine mechanisms within the organ, by local and central nervous control, by circulatory parameters, and by metabolites and endocrine substances reaching the organ. It may be extremely difficult to distinguish between these mechanisms in the intact, conscious animal. Almost all manipulations aimed at changing the functional state of the organ under study will almost certainly be met by counter-regulatory measures that will conceal or blur the effect of the manipulation. Logically, therefore, experiments in conscious animals should be performed only with the purpose of studying cephalic mechanisms characteristic of the awake animal by comparison with results obtained in anesthetized animals. It should be noted, however, that many central nervous regulatory mechanisms may be studied in anesthetized animals, such as vagal reflexes studied by means of 2-deoxyglucose.[6]

STUDIES IN ANESTHETIZED ANIMALS COMPARED TO ISOLATED ORGANS

With the anesthetized animal it is possible to study both local and remote regulation almost everywhere in the body. It is also possible to perform electrical nerve stimulation (which cannot be performed in conscious animals), and extensive surgical intervention is possible. What, then, is the purpose of using isolated organs?

1. When using isolated organs it is possible to obtain a maximum degree of control. Almost everything can be controlled, including: a) the exact composition of the perfusate, thereby controlling influences from metabolites, salts, oncotic presssure, and oxygen/carbon dioxide; b) the blood or perfusate flow; and c) the influence of extrinsic nerves and endocrine signals. All of these may be subject to important changes during experimental manipulations in the intact animals.

2. Another advantage is the regional restriction that may be obtained. Anything released from an isolated organ necessarily derives from the organ (if the substance in question is not previously present in the perfusate). A similar control of origin may be impossible to obtain in the intact organism, either because it is too difficult to sample venous blood or tissue fluid from the region of interest or because the arteriovenous concentration difference across the organ is below the sensitivity of the measuring system

under the prevailing perfusion conditions or otherwise too difficult to determine. In the isolated system the artificial perfusate may be concentrated and manipulated biochemically to facilitate determination.

3. An isolated organ is often perfused with a completely artificial perfusion medium. Measurements of physiologically interesting parameters are therefore often greatly facilitated. Degradation of the substance occurring in blood can thus be avoided. Interference by blood in the measuring system or influence by cross-reacting substances from other organs, all of which may occur in the intact organism, can be avoided. In addition, concentration of samples before measurement may greatly increase the sensitivity of the measuring system, as mentioned above. If the substance in question is degraded by the tissue (e.g., degradation of neurotransmitters by specific enzymes), it is often possible to add enzyme inhibitors to the perfusate and prevent degradation.[7]

4. In the isolated organ, one may use pharmacological or other active agents in amounts that could not be used in the intact animal. In the intact animal it may be difficult to obtain sufficiently high concentrations of a certain substance that is usually rapidly metabolized or available in limited amounts, or, more often, because the concentrations of the drug sufficient to cause the desired effect would be harmful to the animal. Examples would be toxins and potent neuroactive agents. Isolated organs thus naturally lend themselves to toxicology studies.

5. In isolated organs it is possible to administer drugs or other agents in a highly controlled manner. In the intact animal it is often impossible to accurately determine the concentration of the substance in question at the target organ because of redistribution, dilution and metabolism in the system. In the isolated organ the target concentration can be controlled simply by adjusting the infusion rate.

6. It is possible to accurately control the perfusion conditions of the isolated organ. This applies not only to the oxygen and substrate supply, but also to the perfusion per se. Thus, the perfusion flow may be kept constant (whereby adaptive or other changes in vascular resistance may be registered by changes in perfusion pressure), or the perfusion pressure may be kept constant (whereby determination of effluent flow will provide similar information, see Figures 1 and 2). Thus, the effect on organ perfusion of a given treatment can be determined with great accuracy in such experiments. By varying the composition of the perfusate and by adding varying amounts of blood cells, rheological aspects of organ perfusion may also be addressed.

7. The isolated organ is well suited for studies of endocrine control, because accurate dose-response relationships can easily be obtained, often with the full dose-range in the same preparation. Even if tachyphylaxis occurs, this is easier to study in the isolated preparation than in the intact animal. Differences in metabolic rates of the hormones in the intact animal, which frequently obscure determination of potencies, are avoided in the isolated system. It must, however, be emphasized that the physiological impact of an endocrine system can only be studied in the intact organism. This is typically the case in studies where physiological variations of the concentration of the hormone in blood are mimicked by infusion of exogenous hormone. In this way hormone effects can be inferred (so-called *mimicry*); or, maybe better, by interference with the actions of the endogenous hormone, either by immunoneutralization or by administration of hormone receptor antagonists.

8. Isolated systems are particularly well suited for studies of local control — paracrine or neural. The local release of the paracrine or neural transmitters can often be accurately measured. By adding the transmitter to the perfusate or by blocking the actions of the endogenous transmitter with antagonists or immunoneutralization (in the case of local transmitters, as opposed to hormones, this is not easily performed in the intact animal), it is often possible to determine the role of the local control system.[8,9] An example is shown in Figure 3.

STUDIES IN ISOLATED ORGANS VERSUS TISSUE FRAGMENTS

A number of important differences distinguish isolated organs from tissue fragments:

1. Even if tissue fragments are kept small there could still be areas of the tissue where oxygen supply (and CO_2 disposal) may not be satisfactory. More important, the fragments are incapable of convective transport, implying that all transport of substrates and metabolites must occur by diffusion. Diffusion is inversely related to molecular mass. It is evident that for molecules that diffuse less easily than respiratory gases, diffusional restriction may become very important. An example is seen in the case of peptides known to act on the same receptors and having identically active sites. These may have different potencies (also from that determined in isolated organs) according to their molecular mass simply because the smaller molecules diffuse more easily.

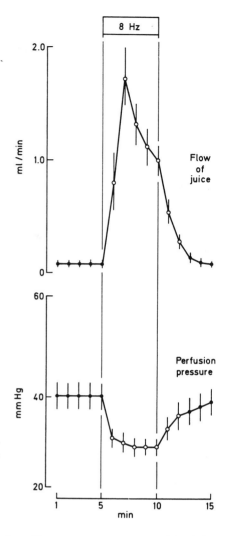

Figure 1. Isolated perfused porcine pancreas. Effect of electrical stimulation of the vagus nerves at 8 Hz on flow of juice and perfusion pressure, illustrating the profuse exocrine secretion and the vasodilation resulting from activation of the parasympathetic innervation. Mean ± SEM of 8 perfusion experiments performed as described in Reference 39.

2. The microvascular orientation of the tisssue fragment is lost. There are numerous examples of the importance of this. In the gastric oxyntic mucosa the interglandular capillaries transport bicarbonate (resulting from the parietal cell secretion of hydrogen ions) to the surface epithelium. Bicarbonate is secreted and a pH gradient across the mucous layer is maintained at the epithelial surface.[10] Obviously, in tissue fragments (isolated gastric glands) this mechanism is lost. In the pancreatic islets the arterial supply reaches the ß-cell core first and subsequently the mantle of D- and α-cells. This arrangement, which has important functional implications for the control of islet hormone secretion, is also lost.[11] In addition, by diffusing out into the incubation medium, the powerful inhibitor, somatostatin, may reach cells that it normally does not influence during vascular perfusion *in situ*.[12]

3. Polarity of tissue is often lost. Many tissues (epithelia in particular) have an important functional polarity. Unless the tissue is incubated in a half-chamber system, functions related to this polarity cannot be studied. Even if polarized tissues are mounted in half-chambers, their full functional capacity may not be appreciated, because their full capacity frequently depends on the microcirculation. For example, the capacity of transporting epithelia will be greatly underestimated without vascular perfusion.[13]

4. The role of the innervation of the tissue cannot be determined in tissue fragments. Most likely nerve elements are retained in the tissue fragments (but they may be lost). The local release of transmitter substances may influence the functions of the fragment in an unpredictable manner because the integrity of the neural supply has been disrupted. The only way to activate nerve elements is by way of electrical field stimulation or depolarization of the entire tissue (e.g., with high K+ concentrations). In both cases unspecific responses are likely to ensue. In isolated organs it is frequently possible to retain a fully functioning nerve supply (see Figures 1 to 4).

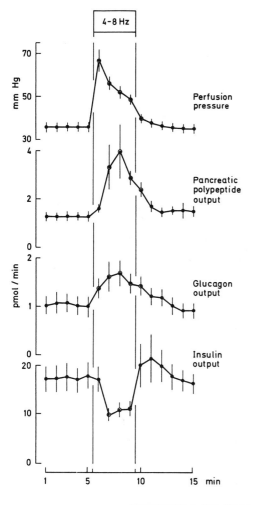

Figure 2. Isolated perfused porcine pancreas. Effect of electrical stimulation of the splanchnic nerves at 4 to 8 Hz on perfusion pressure and islet hormone secretion, illustrating the pronounced vasoconstriction and the changes in hormone secretion resulting from activation of the sympathetic innervation. Mean ±SEM of 8 perfusion experiments performed as described in Reference 40.

METHODS OF ISOLATION AND PERFUSION

Isolated organs are particularly suitable for studies of integrated neuro-hormonal and local control of organ function and for pharmacology and toxicology studies, but the method may serve numerous other purposes. The applicability of perfusion techniques is increasingly appreciated. During the last four years many publications regarding isolation and perfusion of organs have appeared. Most studies deal with liver,[14,15] heart,[16] kidney,[17,18] and lung[19] perfusion, but almost any organ may be isolated and perfused, including the pancreas,[20] placenta,[21] femur,[22] ears,[23,24] eyes,[25,26] and choroid plexus.[27]

CHOICE OF ANIMAL

Clearly the choice of animal depends on the purpose of the investigation. For biomedical research it is often hoped that the results obtained may have some relevance for human physiology/pathophysiology. When selecting the donor animals, some knowledge of differences between species regarding the organ in question is required. There are often anatomical differences; the vascular supply may differ and also the pattern of innervation. The chemical coding of the neurotransmitter content in particular may exhibit characteristic differences.[30] Financial and emotional considerations may also influence the choice. Size may be relevant simply because some surgical manipulations are more easily performed on larger laboratory animals, whereas in these some organs may be unpractically large. In our laboratory we have chosen to work mainly with young pigs. Pigs are becoming increasingly popular in biomedical research, since many of their organ systems are very similar to those of humans.[31,32] In general the vascular arrangements and the innervation of the organs also seem to be rather similar. We have also found similar coding of their autonomic nerves (in particular with respect to neuropeptides), and the chemical structures of transmitter molecules are often the same. Presumably, therefore, the receptors also show a high degree

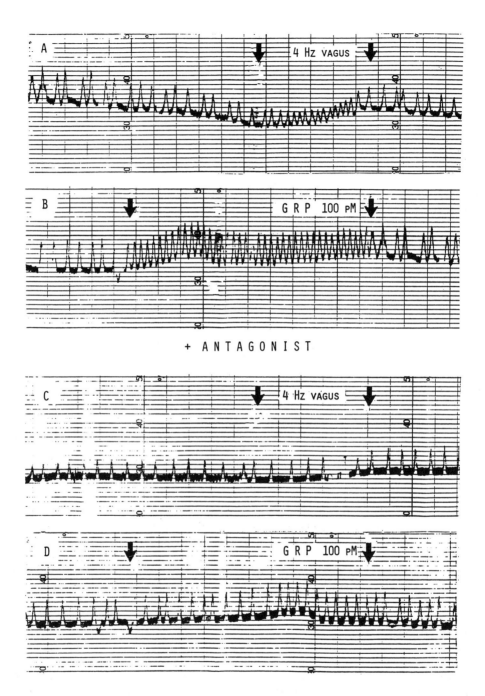

Figure 3. Isolated perfused porcine antrum. Effect of 5 min of electrical vagus stimulation (4 Hz) and 10 min of intra-arterial infusion of the neuropeptide, gastrin-releasing peptide (GRP, 10^{-10} mol/l) without and with intraarterial infusion of a GRP antagonist, Leu^{13}-y-CH$_2$NH-Leu^{14}-bombesin, on antral motility recorded by means of a traction transducer. Direct recording from a single experiment of the series described in Reference 9. The experiment illustrates the increasing frequency of antral contractions (upward deflections) resulting from both treatments and the disappearance of this effect after antagonist infusion. Ordinate scale in arbitrary units. The vertical lines demarcate 1-min periods.

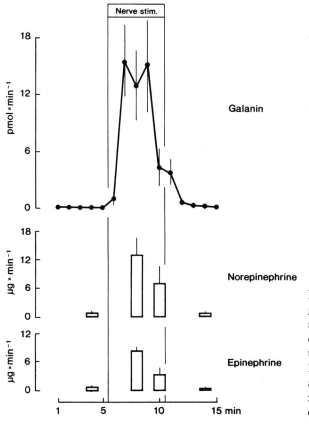

Nerve stim.

Galanin

Norepinephrine

Epinephrine

Figure 4. Isolated perfused porcine adrenal glands. Effects of electrical stimulation of the splanchnic nerves (8 to 16 Hz) on the secretion of epinephrine, norepinephrine and the neuropeptide, galanin, illustrating the pronounced stimulation of the chromaffin cells of the medulla by activation of the sympathetic innervation. Mean ± SEM of 8 experiments performed as in Reference 46.

of homology. The fact that most peptide hormones and neurotransmitters were orginally isolated from pigs also makes pigs a natural choice of experimental animal. We mostly use pigs weighing between 9 and 20 kg, simply because with larger pigs, and therefore larger organs, the perfusion experiments become prodigal of material. In addition, the young pigs usually have little fat around the organs, which facilitates surgical preparation.

ANESTHESIA

The reader should consult the anesthesia chapter for a general discussion of this subject. It should be considered, however, that many agents used in anesthesia may influence organ function. This is particularly important for agents with a high affinity for adipose tissue and/or when experiments involving nervous control are performed. Premedication may also influence organ function. With young pigs of the size used in our laboratory premedication is not necessary. With gentle handling the pig can be carried to the operating room where anesthesia may be induced with, e.g., 2% halothane in O_2/N_2O using a snout mask. The pig usually remains calm and unstressed during this procedure. As soon as the animal is asleep, halothane is substituted by intravenous chloralose. We usually dissolve 1 g of chloralose (Merck, Darmstadt, Germany) in a small volume of ethanol with heating. As soon as the solution is clear, it is transferred to a 500-ml saline drip, and infused slowly via an ear vein. After a few minutes the animal reaches surgical anesthesia. The infusion is usually continued for 0.5 to 1 h and the anesthesia lasts for several hours. O_2/N_2O is continued throughout. If necessary, chloralose may be supplemented. One of the effects of chloralose is inhibition of central temperature regulation.[33] For longer operations some sort of heating device may therefore be needed. For operations in the thorax or the abdomen, fluid loss (through evaporation and swabbing) may be extensive and a continuous saline drip is recommended. Endotracheal intubation is frequently required but may demand some skill. If necessary a tracheotomy is easily performed.

SURGERY

Medically trained personnel will find pigs remarkably similar to humans in many respects. Access to large vessels is easily gained in the neck (carotid arteries, jugular veins, and the subclavian vein) or in the groin (the femoral artery and vein). Access to the abdomen is easily gained through the midline, and to the thorax after a sternum split.

ISOLATED ORGAN PREPARATIONS ROUTINELY USED IN THE AUTHOR'S LABORATORY

STOMACH

These preparations are used for studies of gastric exocrine secretion (hydrochloric acid, pepsin, mucus),[34] endocrine secretion (gastrin, somatostatin),[35] and motility. Because the control of somatostatin secretion in particular shows marked regional differences,[36] we usually do not perfuse whole stomach preparations but remove the antrum. Motility in the two regions of the stomach is also quite different.

The stomach[34] is isolated by surgical removal of the pancreas from the gastroduodenal and the splenic vessels; isolation of a fragment of the aorta that contains the outlet of the celiac trunk; and isolation of the portal vein at the hilus of the liver. The vagus nerves may be isolated from the esophagus and mounted in electrodes for stimulation. The spleen is retained in this preparation because we consider it impossible to preserve the vascular supply to the greater curvature after removal of the spleen. Antrectomy, when relevant, is performed by dissection as close to the stomach wall as possible, whereby the vascular arcades remain intact. After transsection of the stomach the stoma is closed around a large-bore draining tube by continuous suturing in two layers. Catheters are introduced into the aorta and into the portal vein for vascular perfusion, and the lumen is perfused by means of a catheter introduced into the esophagus with drainage through the large catheter. The preparation is suspended in a water bath with the large draining catheter attached to an outlet at the bottom, draining the preparation by gravity. Motility may be recorded by transducers attached to the stomach wall or by luminal manometry.

PANCREAS[37,38]

First the spleen is removed, and the root of the mesentery is isolated and divided. Next, after removal of the left crus of the diaphragm and the left adrenal, a segment of the aorta that includes the celiac and anterior mesenteric outlets is isolated. Then, the hepatoduodenal ligament is divided, leaving the portal vein intact. The duodenum is removed while preserving both the superior and the inferior pancreaticoduodenal vessels (this is actually easy), and the duct is catheterized (baby feeding tube, french 5 to 8). We have never observed more than a single pancreatic duct in pigs. Finally, the gastrosplenic/gastropancreatic ligaments are divided, and the pancreas plus the aortic segment are isolated from the posterior abdominal wall and the inferior caval vein.

The complete vagal innervation of the pancreas may be included in the preparation in the following way.[39] The vagus nerves are identified at the level of the esophagus and isolated from the stomach together with the lesser omentum (in which the right vagus runs), and the equivalent of the gastrosplenic ligament (in which the left vagus runs), by dissection as close to the stomach wall as possible. When this dissection is completed, the whole stomach can be removed and the vagal nerves are left behind attached to the pancreas. Successful isolation of the vagus nerves is documented if electrical stimulation of the nerves causes a decrease in perfusion pressure and profuse exocrine secretion[39] (see Figure 1). The sympathetic innervation to the pancreas can be preserved by including the splanchnic nerves in the preparation.[40] The splanchnic nerves on both sides (thus far we have only been able to identify a single nerve trunk on each side) are identified on the posterior wall of the thorax and followed beneath the diaphragmatic crura. When the splanchnic nerves are included, great care must be exercised when the left adrenal is removed, because the left splanchnic nerve passes immediately beneath the anterior part of this gland. Successful isolation of the splanchnic nerves is documented if electrical stimulation causes pronounced increases in perfusion pressure[40] (see Figure 2).

GASTRIC ANTRUM

This model is an extension of the vagally innervated pancreas preparation.[41] Surgery proceeds as described above, but the isolation of the vagi (with the ligaments) is terminated at the transition zone between the corpus and the antrum. The animal is now heparinized and a catheter (soft polyethylene, preferably french 8) is inserted retrogradely into the right gastroepiploic vein where it emerges from the gastroduodenal vein. The stomach is then transsected well within the antral region, whereupon the proximal part of the stomach can be removed (after division of the esophagus). The catheter in the gastroepiploic vein now drains the antrum exclusively, whereas the portal vein drains the pancreas plus the remaining part of the antrum. The motility of the antrum may be recorded (see Figure 3) after attachment of appropriate transducers to the antral wall.[9] It is possible to isolate the antrum completely using the technique for removal of the pancreas from the gastroduodenal vessels. Vagal innervation can be omitted. Sympathetic innervation can be preserved using the technique described for the pancreas.

DUODENUM

We consider it impossible to isolate the duodenum alone and therefore always include the pancreas in this preparation, which is, therefore, identical to the pancreatic preparation except that the duodenum is not removed.[42] In this case, however, one has to be very careful with the isolation of the mesenteric root in order to preserve the posterior duodenal vessels intact.

Perfusate derived exclusively from the duodenum may be sampled after puncture of the small veins draining the duodenum with small-bore needles or catheters. Duodenal hormones may be measured in the portal venous effluent. Motility may be recorded by manometry; duodenal secretion/absorption may be studied by luminal perfusion of the preparation, which may also be used for studies of duodenal hormone secretion. Naturally, both the vagal and the splanchnic innervation can be included.

SMALL INTESTINE

Segments of the small intestine are easily isolated after isolation of a suitable artery and draining vein in the mesentery. Extrinsic nerves to the preparation may be included and stimulated either by isolation of suitable nerve trunks, which may be threaded through a stimulation electrode, or by placing a hook-shaped electrode around the supplying artery, which is frequently entangled in a network of nerve fibers.[43,44] Secretion/absorption may be measured by luminal perfusion. Motility may be measured by manometry, attachment of transducers, or by measuring the net hydrodynamic propulsive activity, simply by measuring the aboral outflow rate resulting from a slow orad infusion of an appropriate fluid.[45]

ADRENAL GLANDS[46]

Isolation starts with careful nephrectomy, followed by isolation and division of the root of the mesentery, identification and isolation of the splanchnic nerves as above (if they are to be included), after which an appropriate segment of the aorta can be isolated from the posterior abdominal wall, isolation and division of the anterior mesenteric artery and the celiac trunk. By this procedure the pancreas and the stomach and duodenum are removed from the field. A segment of the inferior caval vein that comprises the inlets of the renal veins is finally isolated. The preparation is then perfused through the aortic segment and drained through the caval vein. Preserved activity of the splanchnic nerves is documented if stimulation causes a massive increase in catecholamine (see Figure 4) or chromogranin secretion.[46,47]

COMPOSITION OF PERFUSATE

A lengthy discussion of this subject has been given by Ross.[29] We have obtained the best results (judged from performance of the isolated organ as compared to the organ *in situ*) with a Krebs Ringer bicarbonate solution supplemented with the following: glutamate, fumarate and pyruvate (5 mmol/l each), to provide excess substrates for energy metabolism; Dextran T 70 (Pharmacia, Uppsala) 5% to provide adequate oncotic pressure. Possibly, albumin would have been preferable, but a purified preparation would be required, which would be extremely costly. We do add 0.1% of highly purified albumin (human, Behringwerke, Marburg, Germany) but mainly as a carrier for regulatory peptides to be secreted or infused. Red blood cells are added to all preparations except for the adrenal gland preparation and the pancreas when only endocrine secretion is to be studied. For these preparations blood cells are not necessary,[48] whereas for gastric secretion, gastrointestinal motility and all studies involving nerve stimulation blood cell addition seems indispensable.[42]

The histological appearance of the mucosa in the gastrointestinal preparations is superior after perfusion with blood cells, partly due to improved oxygenation, and partly because of improved rheological properties of blood-cell containing perfusate.[42] Judging from oxygen consumption, hematocrit values never need to exceed 20% if the preparations are perfused at a rate of 0.3 to 0.5 ml $\times$ min^{-1} $\times$ g^{-1}, resulting in a median perfusion pressure around 30 to 40 mm Hg. We have used outdated human blood cells, but

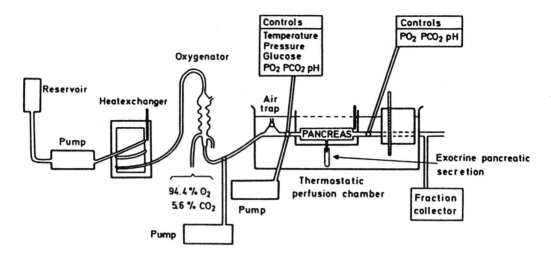

Figure 5. The perfusion arrangement routinely used in the author's laboratory.[37]

their oxygen affinity may be too high to allow adequate oxygen delivery.[49] Presently, we use fresh, thoroughly washed, bovine blood cells, obtained from a slaughter-house. Thorough washing is essential. Fluorocarbon emulsion can be used as an oxygen carrier instead of blood cells but may have untoward effects.[50] We use pulsatile pumps for perfusion (finger pumps). Documentation that this is essential is scarce.[28] When blood cells are used, we routinely add indomethacine or piroxicam to prevent formation of prostaglandins in the blood cells. This is particularly important for studies of gastric secretion.[34] It is clear, however, that other processes influenced by prostaglandins in the tissues may also be affected by this addition.

We routinely add a mixture of amino acids (pt. Vamin, Pharmacia, Sweden, to a total concentration of 5 mmol/l) to all large preparations to allow biosynthesis to proceed, and because it is believed that gastrointestinal tissues may preferentially combust certain amino acids.[51] Obviously, this addition may have specific effects on certain functions, such as hormone secretion.[48] We frequently add enzyme inhibitors to the perfusate, mostly aprotinin (Trasylol®, Bayer, Leverkusen, Germany, 100,000 kallikrein-inhibiting units) to further prevent any degradation of peptides. The beneficial effects of this addition have not been documented. Glucose is considered an experimental variable, but is always present in at least 3.5 mmol/l. We have experimented with addition of insulin (100 pmol/l), but have thus far not seen any differences compared to experiments without insulin.

Using multiple bulb glass oxygenators,[29] gassed with a mixture of 5% CO_2 in O_2, and the described perfusate flow rates, it is possible to produce oxygen tension up to 500 mmHg. This obviously fully saturates any hemoglobin present. Filters and bubble traps along the arterial line are very helpful. Our routine perfusion arrangement is illustrated in Figure 5.

CONCLUSION AND FUTURE ASPECTS

Thus, integrity of tissue, including polarity, microvascular structure and innervation distinguishes isolated organs perfused *in vitro* from other experimental models. Immediate access to the organ and its vascular and neural supply, and the possiblity of directly measuring metabolites and transmitters in fluids leaving the object of study is another important factor. Experimental studies on isolated organs are essential in order to understand regulatory, integrated physiology. It follows that isolated organs are also valuable models for the evaluation of the actions and mechanisms of actions of new drugs. There has been an exponential rise in the number of regulatory factors that have been isolated and identified in recent years, including endocrine, paracrine and neurocrine transmitters, immune hormones, growth factors, and endothelial regulators. The recent recognition of the widespread regulatory functions of nitric oxide have made such studies even more pertinent than ever before, since only in isolated perfused organs can the relative importance of each of these factors be determined. Finally, isolated organs may turn out to be particularly useful in pharmacology and toxicology studies.

REFERENCES

1. Sporn, M. B., and Roberts, A. B., Autocrine growth factors and cancer. *Nature* 313, 745, 1985.
2. Sprague, G. F., Blair, L. C., and Torner, J., Cellular interactions and regulation of cell type in the yeast Saccharomyces cerevisiae. *Annu. Rev. Microbiol.* 37, 623, 1983.
3. Gilula, N. B., Reeves, O. R., and Steinbach, A., Metabolic coupling, ionic coupling and cell contacts. *Nature* 235, 262, 1972.
4. Yamada, T., Local regulatory actions of gastrointestinal peptides, in *Physiology of the Gastrointestinal Tract*, Johnson, L. R., Ed., Raven Press, New York, 1987, chap. 5.
5. Larsson, L.-I., Goltermann, N., DeMagistris, L., Rehfeld, J. F., and Schwartz, T. W., Somatostatin cell processes as pathways for paracrine secretion. *Science* 205, 1393, 1979.
6. Hirschowitz, B., and Sachs, G., Vagal gastric secretory stimulation by 2-deoxy-D-glucose. *Am. J. Physiol.* 209, 452, 1965.
7. Bennett, N. W., Postsecretory metabolism of peptides. *Am. Rev. Respir. Dis.* 136, S27, 1987.
8. Holst, J. J., Jørgensen, P. N., Rasmussen, T. N., and Schmidt, P., Somatostatin restraint of gastrin secretion in pigs revealed by monoclonal antibody immunoneutralization. *Am. J. Physiol.* 263, G908, 1992.
9. Holst, J., Harling, H., Messell, T., and Coy, D. H., Identification of the neurotransmitter/neuromodulator functions of the neuropeptide gastrin-releasing peptide in the porcine antrum, using the antagonist (Leu[13]-ψ-CH$_2$NH-Leu[14])-bombesin. *Scand. J. Gastroenterol.* 25, 89, 1990.
10. Flemström, G., Gastric and duodenal mucosal bicarbonate secretion, in *Physiology of the Gastrointestinal Tract*, Johnson, L. R., Ed., Raven Press, New York, 1987, chap. 35.
11. Weir, G. C., and Bonner-Weir, S., Islets of Langerhans: The puzzle of intraislet interactions and their relevance to diabetes. *J. Clin. Invest.* 85, 983, 1990.
12. Kawai, K., Ipp, E., Orci, L., Perrelet, A., and Unger, R. H., Circulating somatostatin acts on the islets of Langerhans by way of a somatostatin-poor compartment. *Science* 218, 477, 1982.
13. Boyd, C. A. R., and Parsons, D. S., Effects of vascular perfusion on the accumulation, distribution and transfer of 3-O-methyl-D-Glucose within and across the small intestine. *J. Physiol. (London).* 274, 17, 1978.
14. Powell, G. M., Hughes, H. M., and Curtis, C. G., Isolated perfused liver technology for studying metabolic and toxicological problems. *Drug Metab. Drug Interact.* 7, 53, 1989.
15. Ookhtens, M. and Kaplowitz, N., The use of isolated perfused liver in studies of biological transport processes. *Methods Enzymol.* 192, 485, 1990.
16. Krzeminsksi, T., Kurcok, A., Kapustecki, J., Kowalinski, J., Slovinski, Z., and Brus, R., A new concept of the isolated perfused heart preparation with on-line computerized data evaluation. *J. Pharmacol. Methods* 25, 95, 1991.
17. Johnsson, E., and Haraldsson, B., An isolated perfused rat kidney preparation designed for assessment of glomerular permeability characteristics. *Acta Physiol. Scand.* 144, 65, 1992.
18. Rademacher, J., Klanke, B., Kastner, S., Haale, G., Schurek, H. J., Stolte, H. F., and Frolich, J. C., Effect of arginine depletion on glomerular and tubular kidney function: studies in isolated perfused rat kidneys. *Am. J. Physiol.* 261, F779, 1991.
19. Czartolomna, J., Voelkel, N. F., Chang, S. W., Permeability chracteristics of isolated perfused rat lungs. *J. Appl. Physiol.* 70, 1854, 1991.
20. Scratcherd, T., and Case, R. M., Perfusion of the pancreas. *Gut* 14, 592, 1973.
21. Karl, P. I., and Fisher, S. E., Biotin transport in microvillous membrane vesicles, cultured trophoblasts, and isolated perfused human placenta. *Am. J. Physiol.* 262, C302, 1992.
22. Lopez-Hilker, S., Martin, K. J., Sugimoto, T., and Slatopolsky, E., Biological activities of parathyroide hormone 1-34 and parathyroid hormone-related peptide 1-34 in isolated perfused rat femur. *J. Lab. Clin. Med.* 119, 738, 1992.
23. de Lange, J., van Eck, P., Elliot, G. R., de Kort, W. L., and Wolthuis, O. L., The isolated blood-perfused pig ear: an inexpensive and animal-saving model for skin penetration studies. *J. Pharmacol. Toxicol. Methods* 27, 71, 1992.
24. Eghianruwa, K. I. and Eyre, P., Isolated perfused bovine ear. A model for pharmacological study of cutaneous vasculature and anaphylaxis. *Vet. Res. Commun.* 15, 117, 1991.
25. Tseng, M. T., Liu, K. N., and Radtke, N. D., Isolated, perfused bovine eye as model for acute retinal toxicity screening. *Lens Eye Toxic. Res.* 6, 241, 1989.

26. Pawlyk, B. S., Sandberg, M. A., and Berson, E. L., Effects of IMBX on the rod ERG of the isolated perfused cat eye: antagonism with light, calcium, or L-cis-diltiazem. *Vision Res.* 31, 1093, 1991.

27. Preston, J. E., Segal, M. B., Walley, G. J., and Zlokovic, B. V., Neutral amino acid uptake by the isolated perfused sheep choroid plexus. *J. Physiol.* 408, 31, 1989.

28. Ritchie, H. D. and Hardcastle, J. D., *Isolated Organ Perfusion.* Crosby, Lockwood, and Staples, London, 1973, pp. 1-214.

29. Ross, B. D., *Perfusion Techniques in Biochemistry.* Clarendon Press, Oxford, 1972, pp. 1-479.

30. Ekblad, E., Håkanson, R., and Sundler, F., Microanatomy and chemical coding of peptide-containing neurons, in the digestive tract, in *Neuropeptide Function in the Gastrointestinal Tract*, Daniel, E. E., Ed., CRC Press, Boca Raton, 1991, pp. 131-179.

31. Jean Dodds, W., The pig model for biomedical research. *Fed. Proc.* 41, 147, 1982.

32. Miller, E. R. and Ullrey, D. E., The pig as a model for human nutrition. *Annu. Rev. Nutr.* 7, 361, 1987.

33. Balis, G. U., and Monroe, R. R., The pharmacology of chloralose. *Psychopharmacology* 6, 1, 1964.

34. Skak-Nielsen, T., Holst, J. J., and Vagn Nielsen, O., Role of gastrin-releasing peptide in the neural control of pepsinogen secretion from the pig stomach. *Gastroenterology* 95, 1216, 1988.

35. Holst, J. J., Skak-Nielsen, T., Ørskov, C., and Seier-Poulsen, S., Vagal control of the release of somatostatin, vasoactive intestinal polypeptide, gastrin releasing peptide, and HCl from porcine non-antral stomach. *Scand. J. Gastroenterol.* 27, 677, 1992.

36. Holst, J. J., Differences in the control of somatostatin release from the antrum and fundus, in *The Stomach as an Endocrine Organ.* Håkanson, R. and Sundler, F., Eds., Elsevier, Amsterdam, 1991, p. 139.

37. Lindkær Jensen, S., Kühl, C., Vagn Nielsen, O., and Holst, J. J., Isolation and perfusion of the porcine pancreas. *Scand. J. Gastroenterol.*, Suppl. 37, 57, 1976.

38. Lindkær Jensen, S., Fahrenkrug, J., Holst, J. J., Kühl, C., Vang Nielsen, O., and Schaffalitzky de Muckadell, O. B., Secretory effects of secretin on isolated perfused pancreas. *Am. J. Physiol.* 235, E381, 1978.

39. Holst, J. J., Fahrenkrug, J. F., Knuhtsen, S., Jensen, S. L., Seiere Poulsen, S., and Vagn Nielsen, O., Vasoactive intestinal polypeptide (VIP) in the pig pancreas: role of VIPergic nerves in control of fluid and bicarbonate secretion. *Regul. Pept.* 8, 245, 1984.

40. Holst, J. J., Jensen, S. L., Knuhtsen, S., and Nielsen, O. V., Automic nervous control of pancreatic somatostatin secretion. *Am. J. Physiol.* 245, E542, 1983.

41. Holst, J. J., Jensen, S. L., Knuhtsen, S., Nielsen, O. V., and Rehfeld, J. F., Effect of vagus, gastric inhibitory polypeptide, and HCl on gastrin and somatostatin release from perfused pig antrum. *Am. J. Physiol.* 244, G515, 1983.

42. Holst, J. J., Lauritsen, K., Jensen, S. L., Nielsen, O. V., and Schaffalitzky de Muckadell, O. B., Secretin release from the isolated, vascularly perfused pig duodenum. *J. Physiol.* 318, 327, 1981.

43. Messell, T., Harling H., Seier Poulsen, S., Bersani, M., and Holst, J. J., Extrinsic control of the release of galanin and VIP from intrinsic nerves of isolated, perfused, porcine ileum, *Regul. Pept.* 38, 179, 1992.

44. Schmidt, P., Rasmussen, T. N., and Holst, J. J., Nervous control of the release of substance P and neurokinin A from the isolated perefused porcine ileum. *J. Autonom. Nerv. Syst.* 38, 85, 1992.

45. Schmidt, P., Rasmussen, T. N., and Holst, J. J., Release of immunoreactive somatostatin, vasoactive intestinal polypeptide, (VIP), and galanin during propulsive complexes in isolated pig ileum. *Peptides* 14, 215, 1993.

46. Holst, J. J., Ehrhart-Bornstein, M., Messell, T., Poulsen, S. S., and Harling, H., Release of galanin from isolated perfused porcine adrenal glands: role of the splanchnic nerves. *Am. J. Physiol.* 261, E31, 1991.

47. Børglum, T., Fahrenkrug, J., and Holst, J. J., Secretion of pancreastatins from isolated, perfused, porcine adrenal glands. *Peptides,* in press.

48. Holst, J. J., Jensen, S. L., Nielsen, O. V., and Schwartz, T. W., Oxygen supply, oxygen consumption, and endocrine and exocrine secretions of the isolated, perfused, porcine pancreas. *Acta Physiol. Scand.* 109, 7, 1980.

49. Blunn, H. F. and Jandl, J. H., Control of hemoglobin function within the red cell. *N. Engl. J. Med.* 282, 1414, 1976.

50. Felker, T. E., Gantz, D., Tercyak, A. M., Oliva, C., Clark, S. B., and Small, D. M., A comparison of lipoprotein secretion, bile production and hepatic morphology in isolated livers perfused with perfluorocarbon emulsion or rat heptocytes. *Hepatology* 14, 340, 1991.

51. Windmueller, H. G., and Spaeth, A. E., Identification of ketone bodies and glutamine as the major respiratory fuels in vivo for postabsorptive rat small intestine. *J. Biol. Chem.* 253, 69, 1978.

Chapter 25

Cell Cultures as Replacements for Vertebrate Animals

Kai H.O. Pelkonen

CONTENTS

INTRODUCTION

The methodology for culturing animal cells *in vitro* has existed since the beginning of this century.[1,2] The term *in vitro* literally means "in glass". It can more broadly be interpreted to mean all research which does not involve intact higher animals, i.e., cultured animal cells, fertilized chicken eggs, frog embryo cell cultures, bacteria, etc. The terms cell culture and tissue culture somewhat overlap in common usage. The first cell culture techniques were elaborated with undisaggregated fragments of tissue, and growth was restricted to the migration of cells from the tissue fragment, with occasional mitoses in the outgrowth. The stimulus from medical research soon carried the interest in cell cultures from cold-blooded animal tissues to the use of tissues and cells from warm-blooded animals, where normal and pathological developments more closely resemble those in humans.

USE OF CELL CULTURES

The use of cell cultures is spread over various fields of research. Although cell cultures today touch every discipline of biomedical research,[3] the use of cell cultures as replacements for vertebrate animals is most clearly seen in research on toxicology and risk assessment, and areas related to it. In cooperation with the U.S. National Library of Medicine, the Institute of Laboratory Animal Resources (ILAR) publishes a supplement on alternatives to the use of live vertebrates in biomedical research and testing.[4] In the ILAR bibliography of years 1991 to 1992, of alternatives to the use of live vertebrates in biomedical research and testing, only one article of more than 200 deal with the use of cell cultures in other than research related to toxicology.[5,6] As a result of the wide range of research in which cell cultures are used, the reports are spread over a number of scientific publication series, but also specific journals are published mainly dealing with toxicology and risk assessment: e.g., *Alternatives to Laboratory Animals (ATLA), In Vitro Toxicology, Toxicology in Vitro.* Several societies and groups with a focus on *in vitro* toxicology, including the use of cells in cultures, have been formed, such as the European Research Group for Alternatives in Toxicity Testing (ERGATT), the Scandinavian Society for Cell Toxicology, the Industrial *In vitro* Toxicology Society in the U.K., the Japanese Society for Alternatives to Animal Experiments (JSAAE), and the Italian group for the application of *in vitro* toxicology, CELLTOX. Special conference series have been established to deal with *in vitro* techniques: e.g., Workshops on *In vitro* Toxicology (every two years in Europe), Practical *In vitro* Toxicology meetings (every four years in the U.K.), the

John Hopkins University Center for Alternatives to Animal Testing conferences (every 18 months in the U.S.).

A comprehensive list of research areas being conducted with cell cultures is beyond the scope of this chapter, which aims to give examples of the use of cell cultures especially as alternatives to whole sentient vertebrates, as proposed in the three Rs of Russell and Burch.[7] Because toxicological research so heavily dominates the research on substitution of insentient material for conscious living higher animals (feeling pain and distress), the discussion is mostly directed on cell culture use in toxicology, with only a few examples of other uses. The reference list at the end of this chapter should be referred to for more comprehensive and detailed information. The use of bacterial cultures and research on bacterial or viral infections in general are not discussed in this chapter.

TOXICOLOGICAL RESEARCH

Toxicology in all its aspects is a variable area of research (e.g., cardio-, cyto-, developmental-, geno-, hepato-, immuno-, nephro-, neuro-, phototoxicity, etc.). Today complete toxicological evaluation of even one chemical is complicated and may entail the sacrifice of thousands of animals and may take several years. The costs range between $ 0.5 to 1.5 million.[8] In the last decade there has been an enormous expansion of interest in *in vitro* techniques in search of alternative procedures in toxicology.

One of the most important areas of research involves the testing of toxicity or safety. This is needed for new chemicals to be used in health care, agriculture, food production and preservation, flavoring, as well as for many other synthetic materials for clothes, paints, everyday household equipment, cosmetics, etc. The introduction of animal testing in the U.S. in the 1920s was in its time a major advance in toxicity testing. In the mid-1980s the number of animals used per year for toxicity testing was estimated to be about 70 million, including 45 million mice and 15 million rats.[9] From the late 1960s there has been increasing awareness of the need to consider alternative methods to decrease the number of animals to be used in experiments. One aspect of the debate concerns the moral issue; e.g. the Fund for the Replacement of Animals in Medical Experiments (FRAME) Toxicity Committee endorses that the replacement of all animal procedures in toxicity testing is a morally desirable and scientifically defensible, long-term goal.[10] The financial side of the matter is that *in vitro* tests may frequently involve lower total costs than *in vivo* tests.

A large number of *in vitro* assays have been described for use in toxicity testing. A majority of these involve determination of cytotoxicity in different forms. Cytotoxicity can be defined as the interference of a chemical compound with structures and/or functions essential for survival and reproduction of the cell, integrity of membranes and cytoskeleton, metabolism including energy metabolism and synthesis and degradation of cellular constituents, ion regulation, and cell division.[11] A chemical is said to be generally cytotoxic if all cell types studied exhibit a similar sensitivity. It is selectively cytotoxic if there are more sensitive types of differentiated cells than others, e.g., due to specific receptors, activation by biotransformation, or specific uptake mechanisms. The toxicity of a chemical may also be due to interference with cell-specific functions that are not vitally important but may be critical for the functioning of the whole organism, like processes involved in cell-to-cell communication, synthesis, release, binding and degradation of transmitters and hormones, electrical excitability, specific biochemical pathways and specific transport processes.[11]

In cytotoxicity studies both differentiated and non-differentiated primary cells in culture and continuous cell lines are used. The number of viable cells after a certain exposure period is frequently used as the endpoint. Even though there are many possibilities to evaluate cell viability,[12] two test systems have received considerable attention: the total cellular protein assay[13] and neutral red uptake assay.[14] In both assays the cultured cells are treated with various concentrations of a test chemical (or mixture) added to the culture medium. After, e.g., 24 h of exposure, the test chemical is washed out and an analytical reagent is added. In the total cellular protein test, a reagent (kenacid blue) is added to the medium and it reacts with proteins in the cells, imparting a blue color whose density can be measured. Healthy, rapidly growing cells contain more protein than dead ones. Consequently, control dishes f will be dark blue. Dishes in which cells have been killed by the test chemical will be progressively lighter in tone. Also other methods for protein determination (e.g., the Lowry method) may be used. Cytotoxicity is expressed, e.g., as the concentration causing a 50% reduction of the final cell protein content (EC50).[15] For comparison, the effect of a test chemical can be compared with known chemical toxins in order to rank the test chemical's relative toxicity. The assay measuring neutral red uptake is essentially similar.[14]

Also other biological endpoints, such as morphology, cell adhesion, cell proliferation, membrane damage and uptake of radioactive precursors can be used.[16] In *in vitro* toxicity testing for dose-response studies it is recommended to give the dose-response curve for toxicity. If this is not possible, important details like EC50 and the slope of the curve should be included.[17] The validation and predictivity of cell culture methods are quite extensively discussed by Walum et al.[18]

With time-lapse microcinematography it is possible to obtain useful information regarding cell proliferation, mitotic and intermitotic time, morphological changes, analysis of cell motility, etc. after treatment with toxic substances.[19] The advantage of microcinematographic analysis is that reversible and irreversible changes can be detected, which is not possible by endpoint measurements. The analysis is, however, laborious and is not suitable for routine cytotoxicity tests. Recently developed computer-aided visual information image analysis gives further possibilities for this technique. Real-time effects on cell death can also be monitored in cultured cells using flow cytometry. This has been applied, e.g., in measuring chemical oxidant stress in cultured myoblast cells.[20]

Biotransformation of xenobiotics has pronounced effects on their cytotoxicity. The low capacity of most mammalian cell lines for xenobiotic metabolism is a major drawback to their use in toxicity testing as *in vitro* alternatives to animal experiments. Most cells in culture lose their enzyme systems for biotransformation quite rapidly, but to assess the role of xenobiotic metabolism *in vitro*, metabolically competent test systems are needed. The systems must have a capacity to metabolize xenobiotics and to detect corresponding alterations in cytotoxicity; e.g., mouse hepatoma cells containing a cytochrome P450 enzyme system have been used to detect toxic and monooxygenase enzyme-inducing compounds in commercially available bedding materials and diets used for laboratory rodents.[21-23] Cytotoxic and enzyme-inducing effects of the materials studied varied considerably from sample to sample, suggesting responses also in the whole animals. Use of these cultured cells as a quality control method was more sensitive as compared to the use of whole vertebrate animals.

Carcinogenicity Testing

There is a general opinion that no single *in vitro* bioassay can meet all the requirements of carcinogenicity hazard assessment. Rather, a battery of tests should be used. While negative results in a battery of *in vitro* assays may indicate low risk, a chemical that humans are commonly exposed to should still be evaluated in long-term animal bioassays.[24] A strategy based on cytochrome P450 has been used in the development of a computer program called COMPACT and of a program of enzyme induction studies as short-term tests to predict the potential toxicity and/or carcinogenicity of chemicals.[25] These programs show in a series of 100 miscellaneous chemicals excellent correlations with tumorigenicity tests from rodent assays and Ames test.

Teratogenicity Testing

Teratogenicity of chemicals has received much attention also in the public debate since the days of the thalidomide catastrophe. A number of cell systems and tissue cultures have been described as being able to screen teratogenic potential. Different important aspects connected to teratogenic mechanisms can be monitored by such systems, like cell attachment, intercellular communication, growth of human embryonal palatal mesenchyme cells, production of progesterone in the embryonic neural crest, limb bud and midbrain, and differentiation of tumor cells.[26] Effects of chemicals on Xenopus blastulae have been studied by using static-renewal assays, called FETAX (Frog Embryo Teratogenesis Assay: Xenopus).[27] The design and choice of suitable *in vitro* tests for evaluating embryotoxicity and teratogenicity has recently been reviewed, particularly with regards to potential teratogenic hazard to man.[28]

Genotoxicity Testing

Genotoxicity tests study the ability of a chemical to damage genetic material, causing gene mutation and chromosomal abnormalities. Screening of aneuploidy-inducing agents has been done, e.g., using Chinese hamster embryo cells. The method allows for the analysis of other cytogenetic endpoints such as anaphase-telophase alterations, structural chromosome aberrations and sister chromatid exchanges.[29] Cultured rat lymphocytes have been used for cytogenetic assays to assess the mutagenic potential of chemicals. Rat blood samples are easy to obtain, they can be collected under well-controlled environmental conditions, their *in vitro* growth has high reproducibility, and there is a positive response to known clastogens and a negative response to pH changes in media or hyperosmolalities.[30] The assessment of the genotoxic activity of chemical agents in rat hepatocyte DNA-repair assay *in vitro* offers the advantage that the target cells are metabolically competent, so that the patterns of metabolic activation and detoxification reflect those in the whole animal.[31]

Irritancy Tests

Among the animal test procedures, the Draize rabbit eye test is one of the most controversial, particularly when it is used to assess the ocular irritation potential of cosmetics and toiletries. In general, the best fit between *in vivo* and *in vitro* results is considered to be that between *in vitro* alternatives and the Draize test for eye irritancy.[32] Still, a mechanistic similarity between *in vivo* and *in vitro* effects would be highly valuable if *in vitro* techniques replace the *in vivo* eye irritancy tests.

Difficulties have been encountered with products which cannot be dissolved directly into the culture medium and particularly with galenic preparations. Recently a promising method has been developed, making it possible to study the cytotoxicity of non-hydrosoluble substances without adding surfactants or any other solubilization adjuvant which might contribute to the observed phenomena and bias the results.[33]

Kidney epithelial cell line A6 from a South African clawed toad (*Xenopus laevis*) is one example of a model for the corneal epithelium of the eye in order to determine ocular irritancy.[34] Toxicity is measured as transepithelial resistance and transepithelial potential difference. The authors suggest that this cell culture model could be used as one potential contributor to the replacement of the Draize eye irritancy test.

Dermal irritancy has classically been determined in rabbit, guinea pig or pig skin *in vivo*. In human reactions epidermal keratinocytes participate in dermal inflammation. In cell culture human keratinocytes have been proposed as a good model system for the assessment of dermal irritancy. The release of [³H]arachidonic acid from prelabeled cultured normal human epidermal keratinocytes (NHEK) in response to chemicals added to the tissue culture medium can be used to evaluate dermal irritancy and toxicity of the chemicals.[35] It has also been proposed that combination of results from cell cultures (as neutral red assay) and chorioallantoic membrane tests using chicken eggs can be used for comparative testing of chemicals with unknown irritant properties together with known weak and strong irritants from the same class of chemicals and standards in the test series.[36] This could be used as a preliminary screen for identifying irritants prior to performance of any *in vivo* studies, exposing the animals potentially to harmful effects of such substances.

OTHERS

The use of cell cultures as replacements for vertebrate animals is heavily dominated by research related to toxicology. Only two other areas, in which there certainly is a need for replacement, are discussed here, namely testing of pyrogens and monoclonal antibody production.

Rabbits have classically been used in pyrogenicity tests. Reactions in cultured human mononuclear cells caused by different pyrogen-containing fluids have been compared with both the sensitivity and specificity of the rabbit pyrogen test and the Limulus amoebocyte lysate, with the result that his cell culture method was considered to be suitable as an alternative *in vitro* pyrogenicity test.[37]

In 1984 the Nobel Prize was awarded to Kohler and Milstein for their work leading to production of monoclonal antibodies for use in a variety of experimental and clinical applications. The original method included injection of hybridoma cells into the peritoneal cavities of, particularly, mice and collection of ascitic fluid. A replacement for this method is recommendable, since the method evidently is painful to animals. In cell cultures monoclonal antibodies can be produced with high levels of purity. While one mouse will produce ascites for only a few days, hybridomas in cell culture can secrete antibody over 18 months. Spent culture titers from cell culture average 0.01 to 0.1 mg/ml, whereas titers from ascitic fluid average 1 to 10 mg/ml. Developments in cell culture production of monoclonal antibodies have led to substantial production capacities by using a prolonged cell culture in a bioreactor system.[38] Eventually the use of cell cultures for monoclonal antibody production will likely be replaced by production in bacterial cultures, which is presently a rapidly developing area.

COMPARISON OF CELL CULTURES AND WHOLE VERTEBRATE ANIMALS

One major topic in the evaluation of biomedical research is the dilemma between the opinions of the public and the scientists on the relevance of *in vitro* studies as "alternative methods" in biomedical research in general and in the safety evaluation of chemicals specifically. Cell cultures can certainly be used for studies of strictly cellular events. In these studies the cell cultures are not considered as replacements for animals. Types of investigations which are particularly suitable in cell culture are, e.g., studies on intracellular activities (e.g., replication and transcription of DNA, protein synthesis, energy metabolism), intracellular flux (e.g., movement of RNA, translocation of hormone receptor complexes, fluctuations in metabolite pools), "cell ecology" (e.g., nutrition, infection, virally and chemically induced transformations, drug actions), and cell-to-cell interactions (e.g., embryonic induction, cell population kinetics, cell-to-cell adhesion).[31]

Whereas whole-animal testing is difficult to standardize, the standardization of an *in vitro* test seems more straightforward. Environmental factors like temperature, gas composition, movement of the experimental container, humidity and sterility must be strictly controlled during the experiments. Even minor changes in temperature or gas composition may cause disturbances in cell growth (e.g., by synchronizing the culture).[18] When primary cultures are used, the origin of the tissue should be given in detail, including a certificate of the microbiological status of the source animals used. In addition, infections like mycoplasma should be checked. When cell lines of human origin are used, the microbial status of the cells should be most rigidly studied and documented, not only to eliminate false results, but also to protect the research personnel.

An advantage in the use of cell cultures is that usually relatively small quantities of the substance studied are needed. Thus, novel compounds available in limited amounts can easily be tested *in vitro*, and disposal problems are minimized if a compound turns out to be toxic.

Dedifferentiation of cultured cells is a clear limitation to the application of *in vitro* systems, e.g., in many areas of toxicology. As acute systemic toxicity in man can be caused by a variety of mechanisms, harmful effects or concentrations may be rather difficult to predict on the basis of only *in vitro* methods, e.g., because they may be tissue-specific or result from tissue or organ interactions. In the real exposure situation, clinical toxicity is the result of many factors. Properties of the compound, kinetics of its uptake, distribution in the body, excretion and metabolism vary in different organs. The observed *in vivo* effects are the net result of all toxic actions. It can be speculated that a combination of several *in vitro* tests could mimic the phases of absorption, distribution, metabolism and targeting of metabolites to specialized tissues.[38]

Exposure of cell cultures to chemical compounds needs special consideration. The component may be water-soluble, insoluble solid, liquid extract, insoluble compound, or volatile. In each case there may be different problems in determining the actual dose presented to the cells. In extracts the chemical composition and concentration of the individual constituents are frequently not known in detail. If insoluble compounds are used, the effects of solubilizers further complicate the situation. The cell culture medium may also modify the behavior of the compound studied in an unpredictable way. The most important undefined component in the medium is serum, which may bind the test component and lead to the masking of the toxicity. Some ions can be precipitated by components in the medium, e.g. barium is precipitated by sulfate present in most media.[17] Plastic dishes may release chemicals, or the culture flask may adsorb both test chemicals and proteins from the medium.

Primary cultures are relatively short-term experimental systems. In dividing cell cultures, after the exponential phase of growth, the confluent culture enters a stationary phase, where the cells normally remain viable for only a few days, during which their metabolism slows down and many enzymatic activities are turned off.[32] Therefore, while mammalian cells *in vitro* are suitable for studying acute and subacute toxicity, they cannot easily be used to reproduce chronic toxicity as it occurs *in vivo*, where the gradual accumulation of toxic chemicals can take place in specialized, metabolically active tissues.

In summary, studies on cell cultures are accompanied by inherent disadvantages, e.g., a reduced ability to study organism growth processes, cells, tissues, and organ systems acting in concert, integrated biochemical and metabolic pathways, behavior, recovery of damaged tissues, interaction between the organism and its environment, idiosyncratic or species-specific responses, reduced ability to distinguish between male- and female-specific phenomena and handicap to probing the unknown and phenomena not yet identified.[3]

The relevance of the results from *in vitro* cytotoxicity testing has for these reasons also been heavily debated, correlations observed being claimed to be simply fortuitous: "Why do we imagine that the death of cultured hepatocytes should be related to the mechanism of lethal poisoning involved in LD50 studies? Why should protein coagulation or damage to the vascular system of the chick's chorio-allantoic membrane be related to ocular irritation?" "If a patient dies with serum concentrations of 60 µg/ml, but a hepatocyte does not die with the concentration as high as 2000 µg/ml, we can only conclude that hepatotoxicity is not the cause of acute toxicity resulting in death."[39]

VIEW TO THE FUTURE

The development of a cell culture method as a true alternative for the use of whole vertebrates in research and testing is a multistep procedure involving several critical steps: development, validation, evaluation, and acceptance.

THE QUESTION OF VALIDATION

During the development of a method or a test all components are defined, integrated and optimized for the specific purpose. It is generally believed that validation is the key to extending the use of *in vitro* methods as supplements or alternatives to the animal testing of the systemic, target organ and local toxicities of chemicals.[40] During validation the reliability and the relevance of the new procedure are established for the purpose in question.[41] The evaluation of the new method should be made to obtain a general or official acceptance and incorporation of the new method in order to replace an animal test previously used or required by the authorities. Several hundred different *in vitro* assays of general toxicity have been proposed during the last 20 years, but only very few of them have been validated and accepted.[40]

The first step in the validation of the suitability of a cell culture for, e.g., toxicity or safety testing should be to demonstrate that the cells isolated *in vitro* have properties consonant with the cells affected by model drugs *in vivo*. Only then can one be confident enough to test unknown components; and should this confidence be sustained in use, the test procedure can become a requirement and may eventually replace some animal studies.

Recommendations for validities are proposed as follows: for screening-tests mechanistic similarity is not necessary if empirical correlation/predictivity criteria are met. For adjunct tests mechanistic related-ness is desired, but not required. For replacement tests mechanistic similarity is generally required, but exceptions could exist.[38] Recently it has been proposed that one critical rule is enough: all (*in vitro*) tests must have demonstrable mechanistic similarity to the events we wish to study *in vivo*.[39]

REGULATORY PROBLEMS

Variations in guidelines and requirements of the various regulatory agencies continue to cause great concern. Many individuals within industry and regulatory agencies find it easier to conceive non-animal methods as prescreens or as adjuncts, rather than as replacements.

If non-animal tests are to replace any of the currently accepted animal procedures, they must be no less relevant, no less reproducible, and no less useful for identifying the toxic potentials of chemicals, their toxic potencies, and the hazards they might represent under certain conditions of exposure — as a basis for risk assessment and risk limitation and/or risk management.[10] If non-animal test procedures are to meet these requirements, they must be properly developed, proceed through formal validation pro-cesses, and be independently assessed and recommended for acceptance by regulatory authorities.[10] Before being considered for screening, adjunct or replacement procedures, the new tests or test batteries should be subject to formal validation in order to establish their relevance and reliability. This validation process includes interlaboratory assessment (including blind trials), test database development, and evaluation. The results of validation studies should be published in peer-review literature. All reasonable steps should be taken to make the formal acceptance of validated non-animal procedures into regulatory practice as smooth and rapid a process as possible.[41]

DEVELOPMENT PROGRAMS AND DATABASES

A five-year program to validate *in vitro* tests for general toxicity has been organized by the Scandinavian Society for Cell Toxicology (MEIC, multicenter evaluation of *in vitro* cytotoxicity). During the project 50 test chemicals having data on acute human toxicity plus rodent oral LD50 values are investigated, aiming to be able to sort out the best combinations of *in vitro* tests predicting acute toxicity, chronic toxicity, skin irritancy, etc. and to recommend tests and batteries of tests as supplements or alternatives to animal testing of various types of general toxicity.[42] In 1991 a multicenter collaborative research project ECITTS, the ERGATT/CFN integrated toxicity testing scheme started. Its aim is to employ non-animal methods to assess the toxicological properties of chemicals, and to improve this assessment through the use of knowledge about mechanisms of toxic action.[32]

As a special effort the CTFA (Cosmetic, Toiletry and Fragrance Association) Evaluation of Alternatives Program, Animal Welfare Task Force has recently organized a program designed to evaluate the effectiveness and limitation(s) of *in vitro* tests in predicting the ocular irritation potential of generic/cosmetic personal care product formulations. It is designed as a correlation analysis of the relationship between Draize primary eye irritation test data and comparative data from a selection of *in vitro* tests.[43]

Acute toxicity and irritancy are areas of research and testing causing great concern due to the apparent discomfort and suffering inherent in the scope of the test. The second report of the FRAME Toxicity Committee states, e.g., that "...concerted effort should be concentrated on the validation of non-animal tests and test batteries, the use in both acute toxicity and irritancy studies".[44] Alternative protocols have been adopted recently by regulatory agencies such as the U.S. Food and Drug Administration (FDA) and Environmental Protection Agency (EPA) and the Japanese Ministry of Health and Welfare, and the EEC has recently accepted a fixed dose procedure as an alternative to the oral LD50 test.[45] Procedures for the notification, consideration, consensus agreement and adoption of new test methods are available also by the EEC and the OECD.[10]

At present no specific strategies at the international level have been developed to obtain special information from biomedical databases with reference to the "Three Rs", but in Germany in 1989 the Centre for Documentation and Evaluation of Alternative Methods to Animal Experiments (ZEBET) at the German Federal Health Office started a data bank to meet requirements of the German Animal Protection Act. The data bank comprises two types of evaluation: whether a specific method contributes to the Three Rs concept and whether the method meets the criteria of validation of toxicity test procedures. The language of ZEBET is German, but it contains English summaries, key words and updated list of references.[46]

In the U.K., FRAME has an active research program, which involves collaboration with industrial companies and research scientists in Europe and the U.S. INVITTOX, a data bank aimed at providing state-of-the-art technical information on the use of alternative methods in toxicology and toxicity testing is presently run in collaboration with FRAME and the European Research Group for Alternatives in Toxicity testing (ERGATT) with the financial support of the Commission of the European Communities (CEC). The ERGATT/FRAME *In vitro* Toxicology data bank in the U.K. concentrates on up-to-date methodological protocols and includes literature references.[47] The *In vitro* Toxicity Testing (IVT) database in the U.S. gives access to current *in vitro* toxicity testing data from all participants and presently mainly concentrates on alternatives to replace ocular irritation testing.[48] A database on the references of alternatives to animal testing is under development in Japan (ALTDBASE), and the Italian database (DATABASE)[46] is planned to provide a comprehensive list of the methods on alternative methods to animal testing. The Yellow List (Gelbe Liste) in Germany[49] covers three fields of interest: pharmacological, medical and biological research.

CONCLUSIONS

There are still several obvious advantages in the use of whole animals in testing. The whole animal provides an integrated biological system that can be used to assess the outcome of exposure by different routes and over long periods. Whole animal tests can also predict whether or not particular effects are reversible. To have even nearly the same information, possibly one *in vitro* test for every potential target-cell type in the body is needed. The problem of how immunological processes may be involved in the effects must also be solved. Simulation of different routes of exposure, e.g., inhalation, ingestion, skin contact, may be extremely difficult in cell culture systems.

In vitro cytotoxicity and target organ toxicity tests, used intelligently in combination with predictive computer modeling, may play a major role in improving the quality and scientific basis of hazard prediction.[38] In the present situation it can be accepted/proposed generally that in risk assessment one *in vitro* test is insufficient to obtain the information needed, and thus batteries of *in vitro* tests should be used. The ultimate goal would be to make the risk assessment without laboratory animals. If appropriate, for human use it would be most advantageous to use human cells. An obvious advantage of this is reduction of risks in extrapolation from animals to man. The availability of different types of human cells is not presently very good, but this will improve in the future. More resources should be devoted especially to human cell studies for the development of biomonitoring methods for detecting genetic damage in somatic cells. Even if cells from animals are used, the *in vitro* results obtained still can reduce the number of animals needed for conclusive results.

The obstacles of *in vitro* testing and experiments in general must be weighed against the disadvantages of whole animal use: animal discomfort, pain and death, species-extrapolation problems, and excessive time and expense needed in animal experiments. Before the use of vertebrate animals can be replaced by alternatives, including cell cultures, also the critical steps of method development, validation, evaluation and acceptance must be completed.

Finally, for *in vitro* tests or cell cultures to be useful they do not need to replace whole animal use totally. They can contribute to chemical evaluation and be used in sophisticated experimental designs with highly specified target questions. They can be incorporated into the early stages of risk assessment, or used to identify the mechanism by which a new chemical affects. In this way they can reduce the number of animals needed, and thereby reduce the suffering of animals. Their use may also save money and time.

REFERENCES

1. Harrison, R.G.: Observations on the living developing nerve fiber. *Proc. Soc. Exp. Biol. Med.,* 4, 104, 1907.
2. Carrel, A. On the permanent life of tissues outside the organism. *J. Exp. Med.,* 15, 516, 1912.
3. Office of Technology Assessment of the U.S. Congress: *Alternatives to Animal Use in Research, Testing and Education.* Marcel Dekker, New York, 1988.
4. ILAR: Alternatives to the use of live vertebrates in biomedical research and testing: an annotated bibliography. *ILAR News,* 31(1), A1, 1989.
5. Cosmides, G.J., Stafford, R.S., Lu, P.-Y.: Alternatives to the use of live vertebrates in biomedical research and testing: An annotated bibliography, *ILAR News,* 33(3), S1, 1991.
6. Cosmides, G.J., Stafford, R.S., Lu, P.-Y.: Alternatives to the use of live vertebrates in biomedical research and testing: An annotated bibliography, *ILAR News,* 34(3), S1, 1992.
7. Russell, W.M.S., Burch, R.L.: Principles of Humane Experimental Technique. Charles C Thomas, Springfield, IL, 1959.
8. Goldberg, A.M., Frazier, J.M.: Alternatives to animals in toxicity testing. *Sci. Am.,* 261, 16, 1989.
9. Rowan, A.N.: *Of mice, models & men: A critical evaluation of animal research.* State University of New York Press, Albany, NY, 1984.
10. FRAME: Animals and alternatives in toxicology: Present status and future prospects (The second report of the FRAME Toxicity Committee). *ATLA,* 19, 116, 1991.
11. Seibert, H., Gülden, M., Kolossa, M., Schepers, G.: Evaluation of the relevance of selected *in vitro* toxicity test systems for acute systemic toxicity. *ATLA,* 20, 240, 1992.
12. Cook, J.A., Mitchell, J.B.: Viability measurements in mammalian cell systems. *Anal. Biochem.,* 179, 1, 1989.
13. Knox, P., Uphill, P.F., Fry, J.R., Benford, D., Balls, M.: The FRAME multicentre project on *in vitro* toxicology. *Food Chem. Toxicol.,* 28, 457, 1986.
14. Borenfreund, E., Puerner, J.A.: A simple quantitative procedure using monolayer cultures for cytotoxicity assays (HTD/NR90). *J. Tissue Cult. Meth.,* 9, 7, 1984.
15. Shopsis, C., Eng, B.: Rapid cytotoxicity testing using a semi-automated protein determination on cultured cells. *Toxicol. Lett.,* 26, 1, 1985.
16. Balls, M., Fentem, J.H.: The use of basal cytotoxicity and target organ toxicity tests in hazard identification and risk assesment. *ATLA,* 20, 368, 1992.
17. Syversen, T.: Factors important to the quality of cell culture toxicology. *ATLA,* 19, 234, 1991.
18. Walum, E., Stenberg, K., Jenssen, D.: *Understanding Cell Toxicology.* Ellis Horwood, Chichester, U.K., 1990.
19. Cervinka, M.: Time-lapse phase-contrast microphotography of cell populations as a basis for improvement of *in vitro* toxicity assessment. *ATLA,* 20, 302,1992.
20. Sen, C.K., Agrawal, Y., Hänninen, O.: Manuscript submitted, 1993.
21. Pelkonen, K., Kärenlampi, S., Haasio, K., Törrönen, R.: *In vivo* and *in vitro* effects of substances in rodent beddings. *Scand. J. Lab. Anim. Sci.,* 16, Suppl. 1, 117, 1989.

22. Törrönen, R., Pelkonen, K., Kärenlampi, S.: Enzyme inducing effects of wood-based materials used as bedding for laboratory animals. Comparison by a cell culture study. *Life Sci.,* 45, 559, 1989.

23. Törrönen, R., Kärenlampi, S., Pelkonen, K.: Cytotoxic and aryl hydrocarbon hydroxylase-inducing effects of laboratory rodent diets. A cell culture study. *Life Sci.,* 48, 1945, 1991.

24. Santella, R.M.: *In vitro* testing of carcinogens and mutagens. In: Brandt-Rauf, P.W. (ed) *Occupational Cancer and Carcinogenesis.* Vol 2 No 1, Occupational Medicine, 39, Hanley and Belfus, Philadelphia, 1987.

25. Parke, D.V., Ioannides, C., Lewis, D.F.V.: Computer modelling and *in vitro* tests in the safety evaluation of chemicals — strategic applications. *Toxicol. in Vitro,* 4, 680, 1990.

26. Welsh, J.J.: Teratological research using *in vitro* systems. IV. Cells in culture. *Environ. Health Perspect.,* 72, 225, 1987.

27. Bantle, J.A., Fort, D.J., Rayburn, J.R., DeYoung, D.J., Bush, S.J.: Further validation of FETAX: Evaluation of the developmental toxicity of five known mammalian teratogens and non-teratogens. *Drug Chem. Toxicol.,* 13, 267, 1990.

28. Peters, P.W.J., Piersma, A.H.: *In vitro* embryotoxicity and teratogenicity studies. *Toxicol. in Vitro,* 4, 570, 1990.

29. Dulout, F.N., Natarajan, A.T.: A simple and reliable *in vitro* test system for the analysis of induced aneuploidy as well as other cytogenetic endpoints using Chinese hamster cells. *Mutagenesis,* 2, 212, 1987.

30. Sinha, A.K., Gollapudi, B.B., Linscombe, V.A., McClintock, M.L.: Utilization of rat lymphocytes for the *in vitro* chromosomal aberration assay. *Mutagenesis,* 4, 147, 1989.

31. Freshney, R.I.: *Culture of Animal Cells.* Alan R. Liss, New York, 1987.

32. Walum, E., Balls, M., Bianchi, V., Blaauboer, B., Bolcsfoldi, G., Guillouzo, A., Moore, G.A., Odland, L., Reinhardt, C., Spielmann, H.: ECITTS: An integrated approach to the application of *in vitro* test systems to the hazard assessment of chemicals. *ATLA,* 20, 406, 1992.

33. Boue-Gabot, M., Halaviat, B., Pinon, J.F.: A simple method for cytotoxicity studies of non-hydrosoluble substances. Possible application as an alternative to the Draize test for cosmetics and toiletries. *ATLA,* 20, 307, 1992.

34. Bjerregaard, H.F.: Electrophysiological measurements of toad renal epithelial cell line (A6) assay for predicting ocular eye irritancy. *ATLA,* 20, 218, 1992.

35. Segal, L., Riedel, D., Ritter, L.: Evaluation of normal human epidermal keratinocyte cultures as a test system for the assessment of the dermal irritancy of pesticides. *Toxicol. in Vitro,* 4, 277, 1990.

36. Sterzal, W., Bartnik, F.G., Matthies, W., Kästner, W., Künstler, K.: Comparison of two *in vitro* and two *in vivo* methods for the measurement of irritancy. *Toxicol. in Vitro,* 4, 698, 1990.

37. Hansen, E.W., Christensen, J.D.: Comparison of cultured human mononuclear cells, Limulus Amoebocyte lysate, and rabbits in the detection of pyrogens. *J. Clin. Pharmacol.,* 15, 425, 1990.

38. Evans, T.L., Miller, R.A.: Large scale production of murine monoclonal antibodies using hollow fiber bioreactors. *Biotechnology,* 6, 734, 1988.

39. Flint, O.P.: *In vitro* test validation: A house built on sand. Editorial. *ATLA,* 20, 196, 1992.

40. Ekwall, B., Bondesson, I., Hellberg, S., Högberg, J., Romert, L., Stenberg, K., Walum, E.: Validation of *in vitro* cytotoxicity tests — past and present strategies. *ATLA,* 19, 226, 1991.

41. Balls, M., Blaauboer, B., Brusick, D., Frazier, J., Lamb, D., Pemberton, M., Reinhardt, C., Robefroid, M., Rosenkranz, H., Schmid, B., Spielmann, H., Stammati, A.L., Walum, E.: Report and recommendations of the CAAT/ERGATT Workshop on the Validation of Toxicity Test Procedures. *ATLA,* 18, 313, 1990.

42. Ekwall, B.: Features and prospects of the MEIC cytotoxicity evaluation project. Lecture at the *5th Annual Meeting of the Japanese Society for Alternatives to Animal Experiments,* 1991.

43. Gettings, S.D., Bagley, D.M., Chudkowski, M., Demetrulias, J.L., DiPasquale, L.C., Galli, C.L., Gay, R., Hintze, K.L., Janus, J., Marenus, K.D., Muscatiello, M.J., Pape, W.J.W., Renskens, K.J., Roddy, M.T., Schnetzinger, R.: Development of potential alternatives to the Draize Eye Test: The CTFA Evaluation of Alternatives Program. Phase II: Review of materials and methods. *ATLA,* 20, 164, 1992.

44. FRAME: Second report of the FRAME Toxicity Committee. In: *Animals and Alternatives in Toxicology: Present Status and Future Prospects.* Balls, M., Bridges, J.W., Southee, J.A. (eds), 345, MacMillan, VHC Publishers, London, 1991.

45. Van den Heuvel, M.J., Clarke, D.G., Fielder, R.J., Koundakijan, P.P., Oliver, G.J., Pelling, D., Tomlinson, N.J., Walker, A.P.: The international validation of a fixed-dose procedure as an alternative to the classical LD50 test. *Food Chem. Toxicol.,* 28, 469, 1990.

46. Spielmann, H., Grune-Wolff, B., Ewe, S., Skolik, S., Liebsch, M., Traue, D., Heuer, J.: ZEBET's data bank and information service on alternatives to the use of experimental animals in Germany. *ATLA,* 20, 362, 1992.

47. Warren, M., Atkinson, K., Steer, S.: Introducing INVITTOX: the ERGATT/FRAME *in vitro* toxicology data bank. *ATLA,* 16, 332, 1989.

48. Green, M.R.: IVT Data bank. *Alternat. Rep.,* 3, 42, 1991.

49. *Akademie für Tierschutz des Deutschen Tierschutzbundes* e.V.: Gelbe Liste, 1-3. Bonn, Köllen Druck, 1987.

Chapter 26

Computers as Alternatives to Animals in Biomedical Science

Richard T. Fosse

CONTENTS

INTRODUCTION

A leading theme in laboratory animal science is that of the Three Rs of Russel and Burch: Replacement, Refinement, and Reduction. Each of these serves to contribute to a more humane use of animals in biomedical research. Many scientific methods have elements of the Three Rs inherently included in their mode of action. One of the methods that is almost universally found in most areas of biomedical investigation is the use of computer technology, which has come to play a ubiquitous role in almost all phases of research. Computers are used for control of instruments, statistical analysis, simulation modeling, image analysis, to mention but a few.

Access to advanced computers has meant that researchers can extend the depth of information analysis needed to derive relevant and significant results from experimentation. Implicit in this process is the idea that more research has been made possible using fewer resources. Statistical analysis of results has allowed researchers to draw conclusions at an early phase of an experiment and potentially, obviates the need for unnecessary repeated experiments. This has implications for experiments that make use of animals as a part of the model or protocol. With the Three Rs as a driving ideology, there are clear spin-off effects from any process that would tend to reduce animal usage.

Computer technology has direct benefits to experimentation involving animals. Table 1 shows some of the areas in which computers play a direct role in fulfilling the Three Rs. There are several extensive reviews and databases that list computer software in education.[1,2]

When discussing the role played by computers in biomedical research, it is essential that one distinguishes between the use of computer technology in education and in research.

THE USE OF COMPUTERS IN RESEARCH AND EDUCATION

The advent of computer technology has brought about a revolution in the way information can be used in biomedical research and education. Computers enable us to manipulate the vast quantities of information that are produced in the course of research and rapidly make this available for teachers when instructing students. This chapter will deal with those aspects of computer technology that have led to simulations, emulations, courseware, interactive video, computer-controlled mannequins and virtual reality. There are several other important areas in which computer technology plays important roles. These include the field of molecular modeling and its related disciplines of computer-aided drug design (CADD), and Quantitative Structure-Activity Relationships (QSAR).[3-5] It is beyond the scope of this chapter to cover all these areas and will therefore focus primarily on uses in education. Computers in

Table 1. Examples of computer systems that play a role in experimentation with animals and lead to reduction and refinement, and in some cases replacement.

System	Benefit	R?
Statistics	Rapid result analysis	Refinement
	Correct numbers of animals for experiment	Reduction
Data logging	Real time analysis of results during the course of an experiment	Refinement
Control and monitoring instruments	Rapid response to subtle parameter changes that may not be noticed by human operators	Refinement
Calibration and standardisation of instruments	Increased accuracy when measuring resulting in fewer errors	Refinement
Quantitative Structural Activity Relationships (QSAR)	Computer generated molecule models with estimation of toxicological or pharmacologic effects	Replace & Refinement
Computer aided drug design (CADD)	Computer generated cell membrane structures matched with software-generated biologically active compounds	Replacement
Simulation of biomedical processes	Teaching physiology, pharmacology to students of biomedicine	Replace & Refinement
Virtual reality	Simulated real-time experience in surgery training	Replace

education serve as a good example of an area in which computer technology is actively in use and in which there are good replacements for animals that otherwise would have been used for student courses. It is important that one differentiates between the use of computer technology as a research tool and as an educational method. By definition, research involves the clarification and uncovering of knowledge that is previously unknown. Education involves the transfer of previously known, proven knowledge from a source (teacher, book) to a recipient (student). At the same time, the student will often benefit by having the impression that he or she is discovering the information for the first time. The prime goal for the teacher is to place a mental image of the system in the minds of the student in such a way that the problem and its solution takes on the form of a *de novo* investigation comprising a hypothesis and solution. In other words, biomedical education is often based on students performing "experiments". Computers can take the place of the experimental animal in this process.

SIMULATION

Many of the processes involved in biomedical research can be defined and expressed in terms of mathematical models. Biomedical research has, as one of its goals, the expression of experimentally derived data as statistically expressible results. Increasing in-depth investigation has given rise to information regarding biological phenomena that can be described mathematically. There is a historical development that has refined the depth of information from fairly simple global physiological data —

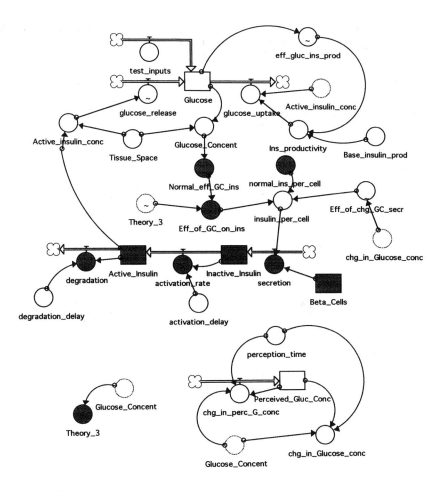

Figure 1. The Stella® simulation system used to describe the interrelationship between glucose and insulin in diabetes dynamics.[10]

cutting the vagus brings about a speeding up of the heart, to complex interrelated feedback models that involve hormonal, neurochemical and electric data. As a system is investigated the level of information that becomes available increases, and sets of complex interrelationships will often develop. Simulation theory allows each element that plays a role in description of a biological model to be expressed as mathematical models, each of which describes a biomedical subsystem. The global system can in turn be expressed as an algorithm that allows the model to be manipulated and displayed graphically.[6,8] Computers enable us to describe and visualize complex biological phenomena.

Computerized description can either consist of static graphs or as real-time displays of parameters. Such phenomena can consist of many subsystems that ordinarily would be difficult to integrate and display. Simulation theory is used as a research tool in its own right, in that systems with high degrees of complexity can be analyzed. Changes in single phenomena sets can be predictively studied in terms of the whole system. There are many simulations that have been written for biomedical education,[2] and simulation models have been described for many of the processes encountered when teaching biomedical subject matter.[9] The STELLA® simulation of the effect of insulin on blood glucose is a good example of computer simulation that encompasses multiple subsystems (Figure 1, Table 2).[10] This particular simulation can be used both as an educational and a research tool. Knowledge about the regulation of the blood level of glucose was initiated by the discovery of the effect of the pancreatic hormone insulin and its effects. The first system that was described was the dose/concentration relationship between insulin and circulating blood glucose. It soon became apparent that this was not sufficient and that several other unknown factors must play a role. As research progressed, many other factors were investigated and clarified. As each of these was defined the original model had to be modified. Figure 1 shows the interrelated subsystems that are used to build a simulation model for the regulation of blood glucose.

Table 2. Examples of some of the equations used in the diabetes model shown in Figure 1. The equations apply to cells marked grey in Figure 1.

The concentration of active insulin

Active Insulin = Active Insulin + dt * (activation rate - degradation) INIT(Active Insulin) = 300

The concentration of inactive insulin

Inactive Insulin = Inactive Insulin + dt * (-activation rate + secretion) INIT(Inactive Insulin) = normal ins per cell*Beta Cells*activation delay

The effect of glucose concentration on insulin concentration

Eff of GC on ins = IF TIME > 200 THEN Theory 3 ELSE Normal eff GC ins
{Implements Theory 3 — reduced responsiveness of insulin secretion to Glucose Concentration}

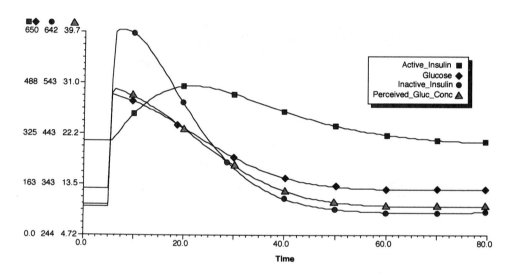

Figure 2. Graphic output showing the concentration/time interrelationship between active insulin, glucose, inactive insulin and perceived glucose concentrations in the serum.

Figure 2 shows a computer-generated integrated simulation curve for the interrelationship between blood glucose and active insulin concentration.

By modifying input into each element, the global effects of a subsystem can be studied in relation to its effect. Each equation element can be modified so as to exert an influence on the total model. This is the strength of the use of computers as simulation tools. Equally important is that the strength of the simulation model is only as strong as its weakest link. The computer model shown here is based entirely on knowledge that has been derived from previous research on animals. The above table gives some idea of the current state of the art of the field of hormonal regulation of glucose. As research progresses, several of the equation subsystems will inevitably be changed. This will be reflected in a modified simulation model and potentially could result in a change in the graphic output.

EMULATION

In the previous section, the use of of the computer was described in the simulation of the biological system that regulates blood glucose and insulin. The model that is used is based on a series of mathematical equations and the output result is numerically "correct", i.e., it reflects a true biological situation. It is, in other words, quantitatively representative.

It is also possible to present computer presentations of biological systems that mimic the system in a qualitative non-numerical fashion. This type of program is commonly seen in biomedical education. Here the student wishes to study the principles of a system and is interested in cause/relationship manipulation,

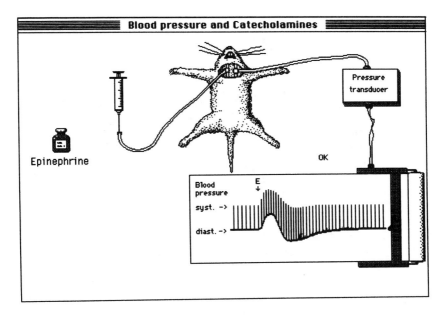

Figure 3. An experiment from the PharmaTutor emulation.[11] The experimental setup shows a rat with a catheter placed in the jugular for drug administration, and a pressure transducer catheter in the carotid artery. Blood pressure and heart rate are displayed following the administration of epinephrine.

rather than true numerical value/relationship expression. An example of this type of program is the FFVFF PharmaTutor® program.[11] In this program several "experiments" are available. Figure 3 shows one of the experiments: the effects of catecholamines on heart rate and blood pressure in the rat. Adrenalin (epinephrine) has been given via the jugular catheter and changes in blood pressure and heart rate are shown. Several factors are apparent when working with this program: The heart rate and blood pressure (systolic and diastolic) presented are not true for the rat. There is no possibility of modifying the parameters that are used. The results are always the same (no variability). These factors should be compared to the diabetes dynamics models presented in the section on simulations.

COURSEWARE

Traditional teaching methods have made use of paper-based materials: books, manuals. These have been supplemented by other methods: slides, tape cassettes, film, video presentations. Computer technology has brought about a new generation of teaching methods based on software and the production of teaching materials on disk. Computer simulations and emulations are a part of the concept of courseware and are often an integral part of courseware. Courseware is an extended concept and encompasses the integration of several forms. The main element in the production of courseware is the presentation of text on the computer monitor. Text can then be linked to relevant simulations or emulations, while simultaneously providing access to video materials or other picture elements that may be needed for study or presentation of a subject. *Anesthesia and Analgesia of Laboratory Animals,*[12] is a typical example of courseware that is used to teach researchers and other users anesthesia techniques. This program has a fourfold purpose: (1) to formally teach the subject of anesthesia and analgesia in small laboratory rodents; (2) to allow users to acquaint themselves with principles before using animals; (3) to provide a tool for laboratory use in the form of dose calculations, volume calculations and source of physiological data; (4) to provide animated emulations of reflex responses that can be used as alternatives to animals when studying the theory of anesthesia.

This courseware program is representative of "one way" teaching systems in which the student receives information from the computer and has a limited degree of interaction.

Graphic presentation of information can be linked to specific textual information or to relevant animations that provide additional information. This can be in the form of active zones (buttons) on the screen that can be clicked on (Figure 4) or via key word searches though dialogue boxes.

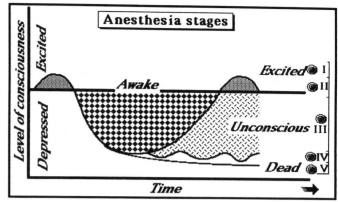

Figure 4. The classic dose-response curve for the intravenous administration of pentobarbital in the rabbit. Active zones in the form of buttons on the curve allow the user to examine the curve in detail. The curve is a part of the Anesthesia and Analgesia courseware program.[12]

Courseware of this type commonly makes use of a programming language known as HyperText. HyperText-based systems are combinations of text and image in which areas on visual images can be linked with text and visa versa. Text can also be linked to other text files or statements. The implication of this is that a particular subject can be programmed and placed on a disk or other computer medium. Through programming, text or image in the courseware file can be linked to other subjects on other computers and at foreign locations. This can be compared to cross referencing in encyclopedias. The implications of this somewhat abstract concept can be made more apparent if one considers a courseware program that concerns, e.g., kidney physiology. The program can be used in its own right and without modification. Within the program there may be a visual representation of an interstitial cell fluid model that has relevance to courseware on gas exchange in the lung. A HyperText link can then be created that will access and retrieve the information from the relevant section and present it to a student involved with lung physiology. The student will not be aware of the link's existence and will appear to be reading material as if it were an integral part of the subject. The link could be performed between files on the same computer or via networks on computers on different continents. The immediate importance of this is that there is a vast increase in the amount of information that can be accessed and retrieved by students in the course of study.

INTERACTIVE VIDEO

Conventional video film is recorded linearly on tape. This makes access to sequences difficult and slow. It is possible to record video (still pictures and film sequences) on laser discs which can be played back on television. Laser discs contain large numbers of picture sequences and computers can be used to control them. Furthermore, in contrast to conventional taped video-recording, video material can be recorded onto laser discs in any sequence and order. The material on the disc is registered on a directory and the directory is used to access the desired sequences. Software is available that allows control of a laser disc as part of courseware. This software can be written as part of courseware or as separate control programs that can be used in conjunction with manuals or books that are printed with bar codes embedded in the text.[13] The user then uses a bar code reader or pen to read the codes and the computer-controlled disk will play the desired sequence.

The laser disc produced by the Department of Laboratory Animal Science, Utrecht University,[14] is typical of a system that uses software to control the disc and displays the video on the computer monitor. The disc consists of several hundred sequences. It is controlled by a courseware program that is used to teach anesthesia. The video sequences can be shown on television or as a "window" on the monitor of the computer. In contrast to recording the sequences on video tape, the laser disc allows rapid access to material irrespective of placement on the disc or order of recording. Furthermore, software based semi-expert systems allow the disc to be used in conjunction with strategic questions. The Utrecht disc runs in conjunction with training software. Administration of anesthetic to a rat will elicit a pain response that is appropriate to the dose given. If the student then decides to proceed with surgery, the computer will respond with a question that asks the student to evaluate reflexes again and the disc will display the relevant response. The computer will also inform the student as to the appropriateness of his/her actions.

The advantage of this type of system is that it allows access to real picture sequences instead of animations or graphic presentations. The disadvantage is that there is a need for special equipment in the

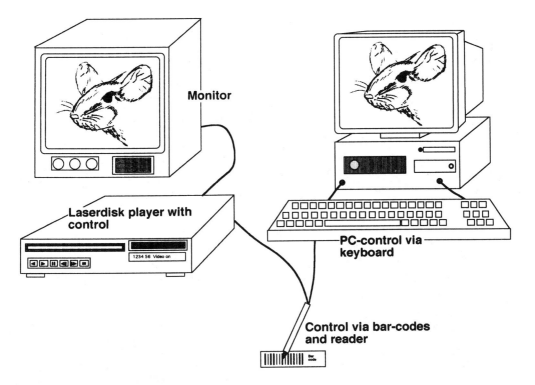

Figure 5. Interactive video by means of laser disc. Video images and sequences on the disc can be played directly on a television monitor, controlled by computers and integrated within courseware or controlled by bar codes embedded in text.

form of a laser disc player. From an alternatives viewpoint, there is a need for filming of real procedures with animals. This must be weighed up against the fact that once a procedure has been successfully filmed, it can be used for many different teaching purposes. There are no limitations as to the type of courseware that can make use of a laser disc. Unlike a video tape which is limited to the format of the edited copy, laser discs can be used independently of their format.

Courseware software can be used in one- or two-way teaching systems. In a one-way system, the student uses the computer as a source of information and has little interaction with the teaching material. In the two-way system, the student interacts with the software and receives as well as gives information in conjunction with the computer. The interactive multimedia teaching programs on muscle physiology are good examples of this type of courseware.[15]

Figure 5 shows a typical setup with a laser disc player linked to and controlled by a computer or bar code reader, with a display on the computer monitor and adjacent television monitor. There are several difficulties in using interactive laser disc-driven software teaching packages: (1) the system is dependent on expensive and complex hardware, (2) there are a limited number of laser discs currently available, (3) it is expensive and complicated to make new laser discs, and (4) people with special programming competence are needed in order to produce software. There are also several advantages in using laser disc teaching: (1) new developments in software make it easy for students with little or no computer skills to use the programmes, (2) students can study individually and at their leisure, without having to have a teacher at their sides, (3) depending on the software design, the teaching value of the systems is high, (4) students can repeat the "experiment" as often as they desire without having to use new animals every time, and (5) errors are possible and do not involve wasting animals every time the student makes such an error.

COMPUTER-CONTROLLED MANNEQUINS

Medical education has a long history of using models when illustrating anatomical structures. These models were often made of wax or wood and were designed to copy idealized structures. Modern materials have made it possible to produce sophisticated mannequins that both look and feel like organs and that have simulated physiological functions that are controlled by computer software. Such mannequins are no longer static reproductions of organs or organ systems but are able to realistically reproduce many physiological and pathological conditions as well as giving realistic tissue responses. This type of model has been developed for anesthesia training. The best known model is that of the human respiratory anaesthetic model. In this model, a computer is used to control the respiratory and cardiovascular responses in a model of a human torso. The model is used to simulate several conditions including hemorrhage, pulmonary collapse, thoracic hernia, to mention a few. Drugs can be given to the patient and cardiovascular response studied.[16]

A field in which computer-driven models have been used with considerable success is that of the use of models in car crash research.[17] The General Motors Corporation BIOSID model was developed using data derived from animal-based testing. The BIOSID model and a similar General Motors computer-driven model, HYBRID III, have to a large extent replaced the use of dogs and pigs in crash testing.[17]

VIRTUAL REALITY

Virtual reality is a relatively new form of presenting visual and sound imagery to an observer. The topic has been extensively described by several authors.[18,19] In essence, all human sensory and motor response is based on input of sensory information in the form of sound, sight, and smell, together with the ability to spatially associate the sensory input with a location within space and time. Sound and images have been available in forms that readily allow computerization. Examples of this are discussed in the section on laser disc technology. The idea behind virtual reality is based on an integration of these elements in forms that give the user an impression of participation within the sound/picture synthesis. This can best be described by looking at the way pictures are presented on computers. In a conventional display system, this is done by means of a screen that displays a television-like image to the viewer. Similarly, sound is presented via loudspeakers and may be stereo or monaural. New technology has brought about totally different concepts in image presentation. The aerospace industry has long since had so-called head up displays in which instruments are displayed on semitransparent glass screens that allow aircraft pilots to read instruments without looking down and keeping the surrounding field of view in place. This has led to specially designed helmets being made that allow a viewer to see the computer image within a floating field of vision. This gives the impression of being inside the image. At the same time, sound is presented through a stereo headset. The illusion is developed further by wearing gloves with sensors that analyze the posting of the hands and fingers and translate this into spatial information that can be analyzed and used in controlling the image in the helmet. Images are recorded on laser discs capable of storing the vast number of sequences needed and computer software controls the integration of imagery with sound and spatial information derived from gloves or other body-mounted sensors.[18,19]

Several models have been proposed for virtual reality imagery. The most likely of these is the development of surgery or radiotherapy training systems in which three-dimensional anatomy images are controlled by the computer. The user holds surgical instruments and "operates" on the computer image. The spatial sensory information that comes from the gloves is used to relate the position of the instrument to the computerized image. This would allow the surgeon to cut though blood vessels which would bleed or through other structures which would then respond accordingly.[20,21]

The technology is still at a very early stage of development but will probably develop rapidly as computing power increases and image storage improves. There is considerable promise for this type of technology as a replacement for animals used for surgery training or anatomical dissection.

CONCLUSION

There are several other areas in which computer technology plays a role in either refining or replacing animal experimentation (Table 1). It is beyond the scope of this chapter to describe them all in detail. However, it is increasingly apparent that this type of technology will contribute to the replacement of animals in experimentation, refinement of models that make use of animals, and thereby bring about reductions in the numbers of animals used in biomedical research.

ACKNOWLEDGMENTS

The diabetes simulation model (graphic representation, system equations and concentration curve) using the Stella® Simulation software system has been reproduced with the kind permission of High Performance Systems, Inc.© 1986-92. The model was created by Barry Richmond.

REFERENCES

1. Engler, K. and Larson, J., Alternatives to animals in biomedical education, U.S. Dept. of Agriculture, Animal Welfare Center, 1989.
2. Smith, A., Smith, I. and Fosse, R. T., Database on audiovisual and computer based training methods, Norwegian College of Veterinary Medicine, Oslo, 1993.
3. Weiner, S. J., Kollman, P. A., Nguyen, D. T. and Case, D. A., An all atomic force field for simulations of proteins and nucleic acids, *J. Comput. Chem.,* 7, 230, 1986.
4. Ferrin, T. E., Huang, C. C., Jarvis, L. E. and Langridge, R., The MIDAS display system, *J. Mol. Graphics,* 6, 13, 1988.
5. Dahl, S. G., Edvardsen, O. and Sylte, I., Molecular modeling of antipsychotic drugs and G protein coupled receptors, *Therapie,* 46, 453, 1991.
6. Hughes, I., Computer with mouse; a new experimental animal?, in *UFAW Directory of Audio Visual Alternatives,* Universities Federation for Animal Welfare, London, 1988.
7. Hughes, I. E., Computer simulation of cardiovascular responses from in-vivo preparations, *Alt. Lab. Anim.* II, 204, 1987.
8. Blackman, J. G., Microcomputer simulation of pharmacokinetic behaviour of drugs for teaching and learning, *Br. J. Pharmacol.,* 80, 589, 1983.
9. Brown, G. J. and Dewhurst, D. G., Interactive teaching programmes in physiology and pharmacology for the BBC microcomputer, *Br. J. Pharmacol.,* 92, 790, 1987.
10. Richmond, B., Diabetes dynamics using STELLA?, High Performance Systems, Hannover, NH, 1990.
11. Keller, D., PharmaTutor, *FFVFF,* Zürich, 1991.
12. Fosse, R. T. and Hem, A., Anesthesia and analgesia of laboratory animals, NIF Software (*Norwegian Resource Group for Laboratory Animal Science),* Oslo, 1992.
13. Smith, A., Department of Laboratory Animal Science, Norwegian College of Veterinary Medicine, Personal communication, 1992.
14. Nab, J., *Anesthesia in the rat,* Department of Laboratory Animal Science, Utrecht University, Utrecht, 1990.
15. Meijer, N. W., *Teaching animal physiology interactively,* Alternatives to Animals in Toxicology, Zürich, 1992.
16. Anon., Resusci Torso, Lærdal Medical, Stavanger, 1992.
17. Smiler, K., General Motors Corporation, Biomedical Science Department, Personal communication, 1992.
18. Woolley, B., *Virtual Worlds,* Blackwell Publishers, Oxford, 1992.
19. Pimentel, K. and Texeira, K., *Virtual Reality — Through the New Looking Glass,* Intel/Windcrest/ McGraw Hill, New York, 1993.
20. Sherhouse, G. W., Bourland, J. D., Reynolds, K., McMurry, H. L., Mitchell, T. P. and Chaney, E.L., Virtual simulation in the clinical setting: some practical considerations., *Int. J. Radiat. Oncol. Biol. Phys.,* 19, 1059, 1990.
21. Sherhouse, G. W. and Chaney, E. L., The portable virtual simulator, *Int. J. Radiat. Oncol. Biol. Phys.,* 21, 475, 1991.

INDEX